Introductory
Clinical
Pharmacology

Introductory
Clinical
Pharmacology

Fifth Edition

Jeanne C. Scherer, RN, BSN, MS

Former Assistant Director and Medical-Surgical Coordinator
Sisters School of Nursing
Buffalo, New York

Sally S. Roach, RN, BSN, MSN, CNS

Assistant Professor
University of Texas at Brownsville and Texas Southmost College
Brownsville, Texas

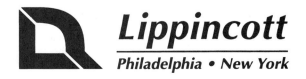

Lippincott
Philadelphia • New York

Acquiring Editor: Margaret Belcher
Coordinating Editorial Assistant: Emily Cotlier
Project Editor: Erika Kors
Indexer: David Amundson
Senior Design Coordinator: Kathy Kelley-Luedtke
Cover Designer: Lou Fuiano
Production Manager: Helen Ewan
Production Coordinator: Patricia McCloskey

5th Edition

Library of Congress Cataloging-in-Publications Data

Scherer, Jeanne C.
    Introductory clinical pharmacology / Jeanne C. Scherer,
Sally S. Roach. — 5th ed.
        p.   cm.
    Includes index.
    ISBN 0-397-55247-5 (alk. paper)
    1. Clinical pharmacology. 2. Nursing. I. Roach, Sally S.
II. Title.
    [DNLM: 1. Pharmacology, Clinical—nurses' instruction.
2. Drug Therapy—nurses' instruction.   QV 38 S326i   1996]
RM301.28.S34   1992
615.5'8—dc20
DNLM/DLC
for Library of Congress   95-4484
                                                                CIP

The material contained in this volume was submitted as previously
unpublished material, except in the instances in which credit has
been given to the source from which some of the illustrative material
was derived.

Any procedure or practice described in this book should be applied by
the health-care practitioner under appropriate supervision in
accordance with professional standards of care used with regard to
the unique circumstances that apply in each practice situation. Care
has been taken to confirm the accuracy of information presented and
to describe generally accepted practices. However, the authors,
editors, and publisher cannot accept any responsibility for errors or
omissions or for any consequences from application of the
information in this book and make no warranty, express or implied,
with respect to the contents of the book.

The authors and publisher have exerted every effort to ensure that
drug selection and dosage set forth in this text are in accordance with
current recommendations and practice at the time of publication.
However, in view of ongoing research, changes in government
regulations, and the constant flow of information relating to drug
therapy and drug reactions, the reader is urged to check the package
insert for each drug for any change in indications and dosage and for
added warnings and precautions. This is particularly important when
the recommended agent is a new or infrequently employed drug.

Materials appearing in this book prepared by individuals as part of
their official duties as U.S. Government employees are not covered
by the above-mentioned copyright.

9 8 7 6 5 4 3 2 1

Preface

The fifth edition of *Introductory Clinical Pharmacology* reflects the ever-changing science of pharmacology and the nurse's responsibilities in administering pharmacologic agents. The information contained in this textbook has been revised and updated according to the latest available information.

Purpose

This text is designed for those wishing a clear, concise introduction to pharmacology. The basic explanations presented in this text are not intended to suggest that pharmacology is an easy subject. Drug therapy is one of the most important and complicated treatment modalities in modern healthcare. Because of its importance and complexity, and the frequent additions and changes in the field of pharmacology, it is imperative that healthcare professionals constantly review and update their knowledge.

New Features

The fifth edition has incorporated several new features which the authors hope will clarify the contents of each chapter.

- *Chapter Outlines* — contain the major headings of the chapter
- *Key Terms* — list the new words appearing in the chapter
- *Nursing Management Sections* — discuss nursing actions applicable to a type or class of drugs
- *Nursing Alerts* — identify urgent nursing considerations to be implemented in the management of the patient receiving each type of drug
- *Critical Thinking Exercises* — help the student create realistic patient care situations from the application of the material contained in the chapter

Organization

This text has been reorganized and is presented in fifty-one chapters, which are divided into nine units. Reorganization of the text in this manner allows the reader to move about the text when these general areas are covered in the curriculum. While pharmacological agents are presented in specific units, a disease entity may be treated with more than one type of drug, which may require consulting one or more units.

UNIT I presents a foundation for the study of pharmacology and covers general principles of pharmacology, the administration of medications, a review of arithmetic and calculation of drug dosages, a discussion of the nursing process as applicable to pharmacology, and an overview of the general areas to be considered when doing patient and family teaching.

UNIT II contains nine chapters that present the antiinfective drugs, grouped according to classification. These shorter chapters allow for more inclusive coverage of the types of antiinfectives and the appropriate nursing management for each class of drug.

UNIT III includes two chapters that present agents used in the management of pain: the narcotic and nonnarcotic analgesics and the narcotic antagonists.

UNIT IV consists of eleven chapters that discuss drugs that affect the nervous system. These chapters include coverage of adrenergic and adrenergic blocking drugs; cholinergic and cholinergic blocking drugs; sedatives and hypnotics; central nervous system stimulants; anticonvulsant drugs; antiparkinsonism drugs; psychotherapeutic drugs; antiemetic and antivertigo drugs; and anesthetic agents.

UNIT V includes two chapters on drugs that affect the respiratory system. One chapter discusses antihistamines, bronchodilators, and decongestants and the other presents antitussives, mucolytics, and expectorants.

UNIT VI covers drugs that affect the cardiovascular system. It is divided into five chapters: cardiotonics; antiarrhythmic drugs; anticoagulant and thrombolytic drugs; antianginal, peripheral vasodilating, and antihyperlipidemic drugs; and antihypertensive drugs.

UNIT VII consists of two chapters on drugs that affect the urinary system: diuretics; urinary anti-infectives; and miscellaneous agents.

UNIT VIII discusses drugs that affect the endocrine system and consists of five chapters: insulin and oral hypoglycemic agents; pituitary and adrenocortical hormones; thyroid and antithyroid drugs; male and female hormones; and drugs acting on the uterus.

UNIT IX consists of ten chapters that discuss types of drugs that are not members of a particular class or group. This unit contains chapters on drugs that affect other body systems such as the gastrointestinal, immune, and musculoskeletal systems, as well as drugs that affect the skin, eyes, and ears. Also included in this unit are chapters that discuss antineoplastic drugs, fluids and electrolytes, vitamins, and heavy metal antagonists. The last chapter presents a general discussion of substance abuse, including two newer substances subject to abuse.

Chapter Content

Each chapter opens with chapter learning objectives, an outline of the major headings of the chapter, and a list of key terms used and defined in the chapter. Less commonly used medical terms are also defined within the chapter.

The body of each chapter contains the actions, uses, and adverse reactions of the class or type of drug being discussed, followed by specific nursing management considerations and a section devoted to the nursing process. To promote easy retrieval of information, each of these areas is identified by a heading in large type.

- *Drug Actions* — a basic explanation of how the drug accomplishes its intended activity
- *Drug Uses* — the more common uses of the drug class or type are provided. No unlabelled or experimental uses of drugs are given in the text because these uses are not approved by the FDA. Students should be reminded that under certain circumstances some physicians may prescribe drugs for a condition not labelled or may prescribe an experimental drug.

When discussing the uses of antibiotics, this text does not list specific microorganisms. Microorganisms can become resistant to antibiotic drugs very rapidly. Because of this, the authors feel that listing specific microorganisms or types of infections for an antibiotic may be misleading to the text user. Instead, when antibiotics are needed, the authors recommend consulting culture and sensitivity studies to indicate which antibiotic has the most potential for controlling the infection.

- *Adverse Drug Reactions* — the most common adverse drug reactions are listed under this heading
- *Nursing Management* — specific points of nursing management are discussed, with important nursing actions highlighted by nursing alerts
- *Nursing Process* — with a few exceptions, the nursing process is used in most chapters of the text and geared specifically to the administration of pharmacologic agents
- *Chapter Summary* — chapters end with a bulleted summary of the material covered in the chapter
- *Critical Thinking Exercises* — each chapter includes critical thinking exercises that provide the user with the challenge of applying chapter content to specific clinical situations
- *Summary Drug Tables* — the extensively revised Summary Drug Tables contain commonly used drugs representative of the class of drugs discussed in the chapter. Important drug information is provided, including generic and trade names, adverse reactions, and dose ranges. In these tables, generic drug names are followed by trade names; when a drug is available under several trade names, a sample of the available trade names is given.

The more common or more serious adverse reactions associated with the drug are also listed. It should be noted that some patients may exhibit adverse reactions not listed in this text. Because of this, the nurse, when administering any drug, should consider any sign or symptom as a **possible** adverse reaction until the cause of the problem is decided by the physician.

The adverse reactions are followed by the dose ranges for the drug. In most cases, the adult dose **ranges** are given in these tables because space does not permit the inclusion of all possible dosages for various types of disorders. Space limitations do not permit an **accurate** presentation of pediatric dose ranges due to the complexity of determining the pediatric dose of many pharmacologic agents; many drugs given to children are determined on the basis of weight or body surface area and have a variety of dosage schedules. When drugs are given to the pediatric patient, the practitioner is encouraged to consult references that give **complete** and **extensive** pediatric dosages.

The student and practitioner should remember that information about drugs, such as dosage and new forms, is constantly changing. Likewise, there may be new drugs on the market that were not FDA-approved at the time of publication of the text. The reader may find that certain drugs or drug dosages, available when this textbook was published, may no longer be available. For the most current drug information and dosages, the practitioner is advised to consult references such as the *Physician's Desk Reference* or *Facts and Comparisons*, and the package inserts that accompany most drugs. If reliable references are not available, the hospital pharmacist or physician should be contacted for information concerning a specific drug, including dosage, adverse reactions, or administration.

Pedagogic Aids

As in previous editions, learning objectives appear at the beginning of each chapter. The fifth edition also includes a chapter outline and a list of key terms. Nursing management is presented as a separate entity to allow the user to identify directly nursing activities associated with a specific type or class of drug. The nursing process is used throughout the text. As mentioned before, a Chapter Summary provides a review of the important material discussed in the chapter. Critical Thinking Exercises are presented at the end of the chapter and are based on the material presented in the chapter.

Critical Thinking

Critical thinking encourages the user to look at a problem and state the nursing actions that may be necessary to solve it. Critical thinking gives practice in analyzing and utilizing information critical to the practicing nurse and provides an opportunity to use problem-solving techniques.

Teaching/Learning Package

The *Student Study Guide to Accompany Introductory Clinical Pharmacology*, Fifth Edition, correlates with the textbook chapter by chapter. The *Study Guide* contains true or false questions, multiple choice questions, and critical thinking exercises. Multiple choice questions have been written using the same format as currently used in the CAT-PN examinations. Each multiple choice question is followed by the identification of the specific patient need and the specific part of the nursing process pertaining to each question.

The *Instructional Testing Program to Accompany Introductory Clinical Pharmacology*, Fifth Edition, contains additional true or false questions, multiple choice questions, and critical thinking exercises derived from the textbook.

Acknowledgments

The authors wish to thank those involved in the fifth edition of this textbook. The guidelines offered by Margaret Belcher, Senior Acquisitions Editor, provided the framework for the changes in the format of this edition and gave us support during the preparation of this manuscript. Emily Cotlier, Editorial Assistant, promptly took care of any problems that arose during preparation of the manuscript. Helen Ewan, Production Manager, Erika Kors, Project Editor, Kathy Luedtke, Senior Designer, and Patricia McCloskey, Production Coordinator, were responsible for the design and production of this text.

Special recognition must go to Melva Martinez who helped with the many little problems that arose and always seemed to be there when we needed help. The authors would also like to thank our families and friends for the support given during the preparation of this manuscript.

Jeanne C. Scherer, RN, BSN, MS
Sally S. Roach, RN, BSN, MSN, CNS

Contents

Foundations
of Clinical
Pharmacology

I

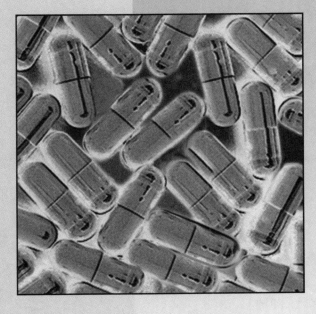

1

General Principles of Pharmacology

Key Terms

Additive drug reaction
Adverse drug reaction
Agonist
Allergic Reaction
Anaphylactic Shock
Angioedema
Antagonist
Antibodies
Antigen
Cumulative drug effect
Drug idiosyncrasy
Drug tolerance
Hypersensitivity
Macromolecule
Pharmacodynamics
Pharmacology
Polypharmacy
Receptor
Sensitized
Synergistic
Toxic

Chapter Outline

Chapter Objectives

On completion of this chapter the student will:

- *Define pharmacology*
- *Identify the different names of drugs*
- *Identify factors that influence drug action*
- *Discuss the types of drug interactions that may be seen with drug administration*
- *Discuss the various types of adverse drug reactions*
- *Define drug tolerance, cumulative drug effect, and drug idiosyncrasy*
- *Identify factors that may influence drug response.*
- *Discuss the nursing implications associated with drug actions, interactions, and effects*
- *Discuss the laws governing the manufacture, distribution, and sale of drugs*

*P*harmacology is the study of drugs and their action on living organisms. A sound knowledge of drug effects, interactions, and reactions is essential if the nurse is to safely monitor patients receiving drug therapy. This chapter gives an overview of the general principles used by the nurse to administer drugs safely and assess patients receiving those drugs.

DRUG NAMES

Drugs may have several names assigned to them: a chemical name, a generic name (nonproprietary name), a trade name (proprietary name), and an official name. This is confusing unless the nurse has a clear understanding of the different names used. Table 1-1 identifies the different names and provides an explanation of each.

DRUG ACTION

Drug action occurs at the cellular level at the target site(s) of action. There are two main mechanisms of action: (1) alteration in cellular environment and (2) alteration in cellular function.

Alteration in Cellular Environment

The first way drugs act on the body is by changing the cellular environment, either physically or chemically. Physical changes in the cellular environment

that cause drug action include changes in osmotic pressure, lubrication, and absorption, or changes in the conditions on the surface of the cell membrane. For example, Mannitol produces a change in the osmotic pressure in brain cells, causing a reduction in cerebral edema. An example of a drug action caused by altering absorption is the administration of activated charcoal orally to absorb a toxic chemical ingested into the gastrointestinal tract.

Chemical changes in the cellular environment include inactivation of cellular functions or the alteration of the chemical components of body fluid, such as a change in the pH. For example, antacids are given to patients with peptic ulcers to neutralize gastric acidity.

Alteration in Cellular Function

The second way that drugs act on the body is by altering cellular function. A drug cannot completely change the function of a cell but it can alter its function. The function of a cell can be altered when a drug interacts with a *receptor* cell. A *receptor* is a specialized *macromolecule* (a large group of molecules linked together) that attaches (binds) to the drug molecule. This alters the function of the cell and produces the therapeutic response of the drug.

For a drug-receptor reaction to occur, a drug must be attracted to a particular receptor. Drugs bind to a receptor much like a piece of a puzzle. The closer the shape, the better the fit, and the better the therapeutic response. *Agonists* are drugs that bind with a receptor to produce a therapeutic response. Drugs that bind only partially to the receptor will most probably have some, although slight, therapeutic response. Figure 1-1 identifies the different drug-receptor interactions.

Antagonists join with a receptor to prevent the action of an agonist. Drugs that act as *antagonists* produce no pharmacologic effect. An example of an antagonist is Narcan, a narcotic antagonist that completely blocks the effects of morphine, including the respiratory depression. It is useful in reversing opioid (narcotic) overdosage effects.

DRUG EFFECT

All drugs produce more than one effect in the body. The primary effect of a drug is the desired or therapeutic effect. Secondary effects are all other effects produced by the drug whether desirable or undesirable.

Table 1-1. Drug Names

Drug Name	Explanation
Chemical name	Gives the exact chemical make-up of the drug and placing of the atoms or molecular structure
Generic name (nonproprietary)	Name given to a drug before it becomes official; may be used in all countries, by all manufacturers; it is not capitalized
Official name (proprietary)	Name listed in *The United States Pharmacopoeia-National Formulary*; may be the same as the generic name
Trade name (brand name)	Name that is registered by the manufacturer and is followed by the trademark symbol; the name can only be used by the manufacturer; a drug may have several trade names, depending on the number of manufacturers; the first letter of the name is capitalized

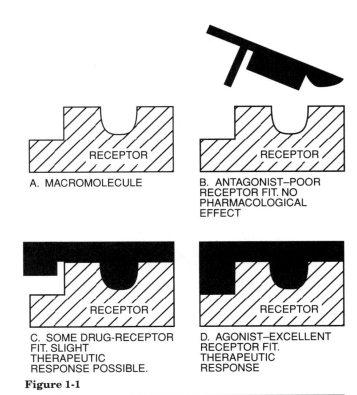

A. MACROMOLECULE

B. ANTAGONIST–POOR RECEPTOR FIT. NO PHARMACOLOGICAL EFFECT

C. SOME DRUG-RECEPTOR FIT. SLIGHT THERAPEUTIC RESPONSE POSSIBLE.

D. AGONIST–EXCELLENT RECEPTOR FIT. THERAPEUTIC RESPONSE

Figure 1-1

Drug-receptor interactions. (Adapted from Reiss & Evans, *Pharmacological Aspects of Nursing Care,* 3rd ed.)

The effects of a drug are influenced by the number of receptor sites available for it to interact with. If only a few receptor sites are occupied even though many sites are available, the response will be small. If the drug dose is increased then more receptor sites can be used and the response will increase. If only a few receptor sites are available, however, the response will *not* be increased if more of the drug is administered.

DRUG INTERACTIONS

Drug-Drug Interactions

A drug-drug interaction occurs when one drug interacts with or interferes with the action of another drug. An example of one drug interfering with the action of another is the effect of taking certain types of antacids at the same time the antibiotic tetracycline is taken orally. The antacid may chemically interact with the tetracycline and impair its absorption into the bloodstream, thus reducing the effectiveness of the tetracycline. Drugs known to cause interactions include oral anticoagulants, oral hypoglycemics, antiinfectives, antiarrhythmics, cardiac glycosides, and alcohol.

Drug-drug interactions can produce effects that are additive, synergistic, or antagonistic. An *additive drug reaction* occurs when the combined effect of two drugs is equal to the sum of each drug given alone. For example, taking the drug heparin with alcohol will increase bleeding. The equation $1 + 1 = 2$ is sometimes used to illustrate the additive effect of drugs.

Drug interactions can also be *synergistic*. Drug synergism may occur when drugs interact with each other and produce an effect that is *greater than* the sum of their separate actions.

An example of drug synergism is seen in the person taking more than the prescribed dose of a hypnotic (a drug that induces sleep). If alcohol is also taken at the same time or shortly before or after the hypnotic is taken, the action of the hypnotic is increased. The individual is likely to experience a drug effect that is greater than if either of these two agents were taken alone. On occasion, the occurrence of a synergistic drug effect can be serious and even fatal.

An *antagonist* drug reaction occurs when one drug interferes with the action of another, causing a neutralization or a decrease in the effect of one of the drugs. For example, protamine sulfate is a heparin antagonist. This means that the administration of protamine sulfate completely neutralizes the effects of heparin in the body.

Drug-Food Interactions

Depending on the oral drug given, food may impair or enhance its absorption. Eating certain foods at the same time a specific drug is taken may also influence the action of some drugs. When a drug is taken on an empty stomach, it is absorbed into the bloodstream at a faster rate than when taken with food in the stomach. Some drugs, especially those capable of irritating the stomach, result in nausea or vomiting and epigastric distress and are best given with food or meals.

Some drugs *must* be taken on an empty stomach to achieve an optimal effect. Other drugs should be taken with food. When it is necessary to take a drug on an empty stomach or with food, manufacturers give these directions in the package inserts. Approved drug references also give this information. When the drug is dispensed by a pharmacist, this same information is placed on the prescription label. In the hospital, this information may or may not be on the drug label. If it is not provided, the nurse must check approved references for information regarding the administration of a specific oral drug.

DRUG REACTIONS

Adverse Drug Reactions

Patients may experience one or more *adverse reactions* (side effects) when they are given a drug. *Adverse reactions* are undesired drug effects. Adverse reactions may be common or may occur infrequently. They may be mild, severe, or life-threatening. They may occur after the first dose, after several doses, or even after many doses. An adverse reaction often is unpredictable, although some drugs are known to cause certain adverse reactions in a large number of patients. For example, drugs used in the treatment of cancer are very toxic and are known to produce adverse reactions in most of the patients receiving them. Other types of drugs, although capable of producing adverse reactions, do so in a smaller number of patients. Some adverse reactions are fairly predictable, but many adverse drug reactions occur without warning.

Allergic Reactions

An allergic reaction is also called a *hypersensitivity reaction*. Allergy to a drug usually begins to occur after more than one dose of the drug is given. On occasion, the nurse may observe an allergic reaction the first time a drug is given because the patient has received or taken the drug in the past. A drug allergy occurs because the individual has become *sensitized* to the drug, that is, the drug has become an *antigen*, which stimulates the body to produce *antibodies*. If the patient takes the drug after the antigen/antibody response has occurred, an *allergic reaction* results. This can be compared to an allergy produced by ragweed pollen (hay fever). The ragweed pollen is the antigen and the response of the individual to exposure to ragweed is an allergic reaction, which often consists of itching and watering of the eyes, increased nasal discharge, swollen nasal membranes, and sneezing.

Allergic reactions to drugs can range from very mild to extremely serious and even life-threatening. Even a mild reaction can become serious if it goes unnoticed and the drug is given again. This is why even the most mild allergic reactions must be detected early and reported to the physician before the next dose of the drug is given. Serious allergic reactions require contacting the physician immediately because emergency treatment may be necessary.

Some allergic reactions occur within minutes (even seconds) after the drug is given; others may be delayed for hours or days. Allergic reactions that occur immediately often are the most serious.

Allergic reactions may be manifested by a variety of signs and symptoms that are observed by the nurse or reported by the patient. Examples of some allergic symptoms include itching, various types of skin rashes, hives (urticaria), difficulty breathing, wheezing, cyanosis, a sudden loss of consciousness, and swelling of the eyes, lips, or tongue.

Anaphylactic shock is an extremely serious allergic drug reaction that usually occurs shortly after the administration of a drug to which the individual is sensitive. This type of allergic reaction requires immediate medical attention. Symptoms of anaphylactic shock are listed in Table 1-2.

All or only some of these symptoms may be present. Anaphylactic shock can be fatal if the symptoms are not observed and treatment obtained immediately. Treatment is aimed at raising the blood pressure, improving breathing, restoring cardiac function, and treating other symptoms as they occur.

Angioedema (angioneurotic edema) is another type of allergic drug reaction. It is manifested by the collection of fluid in subcutaneous tissues. The areas that may be affected are the eyelids, lips, mouth, throat, hands, and feet, although other areas may also be affected. Angioedema can be dangerous when the mouth is affected because the swelling may block the airway and asphyxia may occur. Any patient with swelling of any area of the body occurring after a drug is given is closely observed for difficulty in breathing. The physician is contacted immediately if *any* signs of angioedema occur.

Table 1-2. Symptoms of Anaphylactic Shock	
Respiratory	Bronchospasm
	Dyspena (difficult breathing)
	Feeling of fullness in the throat
	Cough
	Wheezing
Cardiovascular	Extremely low blood pressure
	Tachycardia (heart rate over 100)
	Palpations
	Syncope (fainting)
	Cardiac arrest
Integumentary	Urticaria
	Angioedema
	Pruritus (itching)
	Sweating
Gastrointestinal	Nausea
	Vomiting
	Abdominal pain

Drug Idiosyncrasy

Drug idiosyncrasy is a term used to describe any unusual or abnormal reaction to a drug. It is any reaction that is different from the one normally expected of a specific drug and dose. For example, a patient may be given a drug to help him or her sleep (eg, a hypnotic). Instead of falling asleep, the patient remains wide awake and shows signs of nervousness or excitement. This response is different from what is expected from this type of drug. Another patient may receive the same drug and dose, fall asleep, and after 8 hours find it difficult to awaken. This, too, is abnormal and can be described as an over-response to the drug.

The cause of drug idiosyncrasy is not clear. It is believed to be due to a genetic deficiency that makes the patient unable to tolerate certain chemicals, including drugs.

Drug Tolerance

Drug tolerance is a term used to describe a *decreased* response to the dose of a drug, usually requiring an *increase* in dosage to give the desired effect. Drug tolerance may develop when certain drugs, for example, narcotics and tranquilizers, are taken for a long time. The individual taking these drugs at home may have a tendency to increase the dose when the expected drug effect does not occur. The development of drug tolerance is one of the signs of drug addiction (see Chap. 51). Drug tolerance may also occur in the hospitalized patient. Drug tolerance (and possibly drug addiction) is *suspected* when the patient receiving a narcotic for more than 10 to 14 days begins to ask for the drug at more frequent intervals.

Cumulative Drug Effect

A *cumulative drug effect* may be seen in those with liver or kidney disease because these organs are the major sites for the breakdown and excretion of most drugs. This drug effect occurs when the body is unable to metabolize and excrete one (normal) dose of a drug before the next dose is given. Thus, if a second dose of this same drug is given, some of the drug from the first dose remains in the body. A cumulative drug effect can be serious because too much of the drug can accumulate in the body and lead to toxicity.

Patients with liver or kidney disease are usually given drugs with caution because a cumulative effect may occur. In some instances, the physician lowers the dose of the drug to prevent a toxic drug reaction due to failure to excrete the drug at a normal rate and the accumulation of the drug in the body.

Toxic Reactions

Most drugs are capable of producing *toxic* or poisonous reactions if administered in large dosages or when blood concentration levels exceed the therapeutic level. When a drug is administered in dosages that exceed the normal level or if the kidneys are not functioning properly and cannot excrete the drug, toxic levels can build up causing a severe reaction. Some toxic effects are immediately visible; others may not be evident for weeks or months.

Drug toxicity can be reversible or irreversible, depending on the organs involved. Damage to the liver may be reversible because liver cells can regenerate. However, with the administration of the anti-infective, streptomycin, hearing loss due to damage to the eighth cranial nerve may be permanent. Nurses must carefully monitor patient's blood levels of drugs to assure that they remain within the therapeutic range. Any deviation should be reported to the physician.

FACTORS INFLUENCING DRUG RESPONSE

Certain factors may influence drug response and must be taken into account when the physician prescribes and the nurse administers a drug.

Age

The age of the patient may influence the effects of a drug. Infants and children almost always require smaller doses of a drug than adults do. Immature organ function, particularly liver and kidney, can affect the ability of infants and young children to metabolize drugs. An infant's immature kidneys impair the elimination of drugs in the urine. Liver function is poorly developed in infants and young children. Drugs metabolized by the liver may produce more intense effects for longer periods of time. Parents must be taught the potential problems associated with administering drugs to their children. For example, a safe dose of a nonprescription drug for a 4-year-old child may be dangerous for a 6-month-old infant.

Elderly patients may also require smaller doses, although this may depend on the type of drug administered. For example, the elderly patient may be given the same dose of an antibiotic as a younger adult, but may require a smaller dose of a drug that depresses the central nervous system, such as a narcotic or a drug to induce sleep (a hypnotic).

Changes that occur with aging may affect the *pharmacodynamics* of a drug. *Pharmacodynamics* refers to the absorption, distribution, metabolism, and excretion of drugs. Any of these may be altered due to the physiological changes that occur with aging. Table 1-3 summarizes the changes that occur with aging and the effect on pharmacodynamics.

Additionally, the practice of *polypharmacy* (the taking of large numbers of drugs) in the elderly can lead to an increase in the number of adverse reactions experienced by the patient. While multiple drug therapy is necessary to treat certain disease states, it always increases the possibility of adverse reactions. Close observation of the patient and good assessment skills for the nurse are necessary to detect any problems when monitoring the geriatric patient's response to drug therapy.

Weight

In general, dosages are based on a weight of approximately 150 pounds, which is calculated to be the "average" weight of men and women. A drug dose may sometimes be increased or decreased because the patient's weight is significantly higher or lower than the average. In the case of narcotics, for example, higher or lower than average dosages may be necessary to produce relief of pain in the patient who weighs significantly more than or less than average.

Sex

The sex of an individual may influence the action of some drugs. Women may require a smaller dose of some drugs than men. This is based on the fact that many women are smaller than men and have a different ratio of body fat and water than men do.

Disease

The presence of disease may influence the action of some drugs, and, in some instances, may be an indication for not prescribing a drug or for reducing the dose of a certain drug. In liver disease, for example, the ability to metabolize or detoxify a specific type of drug may be impaired. If the average or normal dose of the drug is given, the liver may be unable to metabolize the drug at a normal rate. Consequently, the drug may be excreted from the body at a much slower rate than normal. The physician may then decide to prescribe a lower dose and lengthen the time between doses because liver function is abnormal.

Patients with kidney disease may exhibit drug toxicity and a longer duration of drug action. The dosage of drugs may be reduced to prevent the accumulation of toxic levels in the blood or further injury to the kidney.

Route of Administration

Intravenous administration of a drug produces the most rapid drug action. Next in order of time of action is the intramuscular route, followed by the subcutaneous route. Giving a drug orally usually produces the slowest drug action. Some drugs can be given only by one route, for example, antacids are only given orally. Other drugs are available in oral and parenteral forms. The physician selects the

Table 1-3. Factors Altering Drug Response in the Elderly	
Pharmacodynamic Effect	**Age-Related Change**
Absorption decreased	Decrease in gastric acidity, gastric emptying and in intestinal blood flow
Distribution of drug is less	Alteration in body fluid composition, decline in body water and decreased cardiac output
Metabolism is decreased	Decrease in the number of receptors, decreased ability of the liver to detoxify drugs
Excretion of drug is decreased	Decrease kidney function causes increase in blood levels of the drug

route of administration based on many factors including the desired rate of action. For example, the patient with a severe cardiac problem may require intravenous administration of a drug that affects the heart, whereas another patient with a mild cardiac problem will respond well to oral administration of the same drug.

NURSING IMPLICATIONS

Many factors can influence drug action. Appropriate references or the hospital pharmacist should be consulted if there is any question about the dosage of a drug; about whether other drugs the patient is receiving will interfere with the drug being given; or about whether the oral drug should or should not be given with food.

Drug reactions are potentially serious. All patients should be observed for adverse drug reactions, drug idiosyncrasy, and evidence of drug tolerance (when applicable). All drug reactions or any unusual drug effect should be reported to the physician. The nurse must use judgment as to when *adverse drug reactions* (unusual drug effects) are reported to the physician. Accurate observation and evaluation of the circumstances are essential; all observations are recorded in the patient's record. If there is any question regarding the events that are occurring, the drug can usually be withheld but the physician must be contacted immediately.

DRUG LEGISLATION

The *Pure Food and Drug Act,* passed in 1906, was the first attempt by the government to regulate and control the manufacture, distribution, and sale of drugs. Before 1906, any substance could be called a drug, and no testing or research was required before placing the drug on the market. Before this time, drug potency and the purity of many drugs were questionable and some were even dangerous for human use.

The *Harrison Narcotic Act* of 1914 regulated the sale of narcotic drugs. Before the passage of this act, any narcotic could be purchased without a prescription.

In 1938, Congress passed the *Pure Food, Drug, and Cosmetic Act,* which gave the Food and Drug Administration control over the manufacture and sale of drugs, as well as food and cosmetics. Before the passage of this act, some drugs, as well as foods and cosmetics, contained chemicals that were often harmful to humans. This law requires that these substances are safe for human use. It also requires pharmaceutical companies to perform toxicology tests before a new drug is submitted to the Food and Drug Administration for approval. Following Food and Drug Administration review of the tests performed on animals, as well as other research data, approval may be given to market the drug.

The *Comprehensive Drug Abuse Prevention and Control Act* was passed by Congress in 1970. This act was written because of the growing problem of drug abuse. It regulates the manufacture, distribution, and dispensation of drugs that have the potential for abuse. Title II of this law, the *Controlled Substances Act,* deals with control and enforcement. The Drug Enforcement Agency within the U.S. Department of Justice is the leading federal agency responsible for the enforcement of this act.

Drugs under jurisdiction of the Controlled Substances Act are divided into five schedules based on their potential for abuse and physical and psychological dependence. These schedules are as follows:

Schedule I (C-I)—high abuse potential and no accepted medical use (heroin, marijuana, LSD)
Schedule II (C-II)—high abuse potential with severe dependence liability (narcotics, amphetamines, barbiturates)
Schedule III (C-III)—less abuse potential than schedule II drugs and moderate dependence liability (nonbarbiturate sedatives, nonamphetamine stimulants, limited amounts of certain narcotics)
Schedule IV (C-IV)—less abuse potential than schedule III drugs and limited dependence liability (some sedatives and antianxiety agents, nonnarcotic analgesics)
Schedule V (C-V)—limited abuse potential; primarily small amounts of narcotics (codeine) used as antitussives or antidiarrheals

Prescriptions for controlled substances must include the name and address of the patient and the Drug Enforcement Agency number of the physician. Prescriptions for these drugs cannot be filled more than 6 months after the prescription was written or be filled more than five times. Under federal law, limited quantities of certain C-V drugs may be purchased without a prescription, with the purchase recorded by the dispensing pharmacist.

PREGNANCY CATEGORIES

The use of any medication, prescription or nonprescription, carries a risk of causing birth defects in the developing fetus. The Food and Drug Administration has established five categories indicating the potential of a drug for causing birth defects. Information regarding the pregnancy category of a specific drug is found in reliable drug literature, such as the inserts accompanying drugs and approved drug references.

Pregnancy category A—Studies have not demonstrated a risk to the fetus in the first trimester of pregnancy and there is no evidence of risk in the second and third trimesters.

Pregnancy category B—This category includes two distinctions. One is that animal studies have not demonstrated a risk to the fetus but there are no adequate studies in pregnant women. The other is that animal studies have demonstrated an adverse effect but adequate studies on pregnant women have not demonstrated a risk to the human fetus during the first, second, or third trimester of pregnancy.

Pregnancy category C—This category includes two distinctions. One is that animal studies have shown an adverse effect on the fetus but there are no adequate studies in humans. The other is that there are no animal reproduction studies and no adequate studies performed in humans.

Pregnancy category D—Evidence indicates a risk to the human fetus. However, the potential benefit from the use of the drug may outweigh the risk to the fetus.

Pregnancy category X—Studies in animals and humans demonstrate fetal abnormalities or reports indicate evidence of fetal risk. The risk of using these drugs outweigh any possible benefit.

During pregnancy, no woman should consider taking *any* drug, legal or illegal, prescription or nonprescription, unless the use of the drug is prescribed or recommended by the physician. Smoking or drinking any type of alcoholic beverage also carries risks, such as low birth weight, premature birth, and fetal alcohol syndrome. Children born of mothers using addictive drugs such as cocaine or heroin are often born with an addiction to the drug abused by the mother.

Chapter Summary

- Nurses are responsible for safely and accurately administering drugs in a number of different settings. Without a thorough understanding of the basic principles of pharmacology this is impossible to accomplish. Drugs can cause serious and even lethal consequences if the nurse fails to administer them accurately and correctly or if the nurse fails to monitor and report adverse reactions in a timely manner.

Critical Thinking Exercises

1. Judy Martin, a student nurse, has just administered an antibiotic to Mr. Green. When she returns to the room about one half hour later she finds Mr. Green flushed, complaining of a lump in his throat, and experiencing difficulty breathing. What actions should the student nurse take?

2. Ms. James, an 80-year-old woman, is receiving Demerol, a narcotic analgesic, postoperatively for pain. Her daughter questions the dosage, stating that she received a larger dose after her surgery and is afraid that her mother's pain will not be adequately relieved. What rationale can the nurse give Ms. James's daughter that would ease her mind?

2

The Administration of Medication

Key Terms

Buccal
Extravasation
Infiltration
Inhalation
Intradermal
Intramuscular
Intravenous
Parenteral
Subcutaneous
Sublingual
Transdermal
Unit dose
Universal precautions
Z-track

Chapter Outline

Chapter Objectives

On completion of this chapter the student will:

- *Name the six rights of drug administration*
- *List the various routes by which a drug may be given*
- *Discuss the administration of oral and parenteral medications*
- *Discuss the administration of medications through the skin and mucous membranes*
- *Discuss nursing responsibilities before, during, and after a drug is administered*

The administration of medication is a fundamental responsibility of the nurse. An understanding of the basic concepts of administering medication is critical if the nurse is to perform this task safely and accurately. In addition to administering the medication, the nurse monitors the therapeutic response and reports adverse reactions. In the home setting, the nurse is responsible for teaching the patient and family members the necessary information to administer medication safely in an outpatient setting.

THE SIX RIGHTS OF DRUG ADMINISTRATION

The nurse preparing and administering a drug to a patient assumes responsibility for this procedure. Responsibility entails preparing and administering the prescribed drug. There are six "rights" in the administration of drugs:

Right patient
Right drug
Right dose
Right route
Right time
Right documentation

Medication errors occur because one or more of these has not been followed. Each time a drug is prepared and administered, the six rights *must* be a part of the procedure.

After the administration of any drug, the process must be recorded immediately. Immediate documentation is particularly important when medications are given on an as needed basis (prn medications). For example, most analgesics require 20 to 30 minutes before the medication begins to relieve pain. A patient may forget that he or she received a medication for pain; may not have been told that the administered medication was for pain; or may not know that pain relief is not immediate and may ask another nurse for medication. If the administration of the analgesic were not recorded, the patient might receive a second dose of the analgesic shortly after the first dose. This kind of situation can be extremely serious, especially when narcotics or other central nervous system depressants are administered. Immediate documentation prevents accidental administration of a drug by another individual. Proper documentation is essential to the process of administering medications correctly.

Medication errors must be reported immediately so that any necessary steps to counteract the action of the drug or any observation can be made as soon as possible. In most institutions, an incident report must be completed and the physician notified.

In addition to the six rights just discussed, the nurse must have factual knowledge of *each* drug given; the reasons for use of the drug; the drug's general action; the more common adverse reactions associated with the drug; special precautions in administration (if any); and the normal dose ranges.

Some drugs may be given frequently; the nurse becomes familiar with pharmacologic information about a specific drug. Other drugs may be given less frequently, or a new drug may be introduced, requiring the nurse to obtain information from reliable sources such as the drug package insert or the hospital department of pharmacy. *It is of utmost importance to check current and approved references for all drug information.*

GENERAL PRINCIPLES OF DRUG ADMINISTRATION

Before giving any medication for the first time ask the patient about any known allergies and any family history of allergies. This not only includes allergies to medications but to food, pollen, animals, and so on. Patients with a personal or family history of allergies are more likely to develop additional allergies and must be monitored closely.

Immediately before administering any drug to a patient, verify the patient's identity. This usually is done by checking the identification band attached to the patient's wrist. On occasion, identification bands become illegible or have been removed. If the medication must be given immediately, ask an alert patient his or her name; the response can confirm the patient's identity. Replace the patient's identification band as soon as possible.

If the patient makes any statement about the medication or if there is any change in the patient, these must be carefully considered *before* the medication is given. Examples of situations that require consideration before a drug is given include the following:

1. Problems that may be associated with the drug, such as nausea, dizziness, ringing in the ears, and difficulty walking. Any comments made by the patient *may* indicate the occurrence of an adverse reaction. The drug should be withheld until references are consulted and the physician is contacted. The decision to withhold the drug must have a sound rationale and must be based on a knowledge of pharmacology.

2. Comments stating that the medication looks different from the one previously received, that the medication was just given by another nurse, or that the patient thought the physician discontinued the medication.

3. A change in the patient's condition, a change in one or more vital signs, or the appearance of new symptoms. Depending on the drug being administered and the patient's diagnosis, these changes *may* indicate that the drug should be withheld and the physician contacted.

Preparing a Drug for Administration

When preparing a drug for administration, observe the following guidelines:

1. *Obtain a physician's written order for the administration of all drugs.* The physician's order must include the patient's name, the drug name, the dosage form and route, the dosage to be administered, and the frequency of administration. The physician's signature must follow the drug order. In an emergency, the nurse may administer a drug with a verbal order from the physician. However, the physician must write and sign the order as soon as the emergency is over.

2. *Question any order that is unclear.* This includes unclear directions for the administration of the drug, illegible handwriting on the physician's order sheet, or a drug dose that is higher or lower than the dosages given in approved references.

3. *Always check the physician's written orders.*

4. *Prepare medications for administration in a quiet, well-lit area.*

5. *Check the label of the drug three times:* (1) when the drug is taken from its storage area, (2) immediately before removing the drug from the container, and (3) before returning the drug to its storage area.

6. *Never remove a drug from an unlabeled container or from a container whose label is illegible.*

7. *Wash the hands* immediately before preparing a drug for administration.

8. *Do not let the hands touch capsules or tablets.* To remove an oral drug from the container, the correct number of tablets or capsules is shaken into the cap of the container and from there into the medicine cup.

9. *Observe aseptic technique when handling syringes and needles.*

10. *Be alert for drugs with similar names.* Some drugs have names that sound alike but are very different. To give one drug when another is ordered could cause serious consequences. For example, digoxin and digitoxin sound alike but are different drugs.

11. *Replace the caps of drug containers immediately after the drug is removed.*

12. *Return those drugs requiring special storage to the storage area immediately after they are prepared for administration.* This rule applies mainly to the refrigeration of drugs but may also apply to those drugs that must be protected from exposure to light or heat.

13. *Never crush tablets or open capsules without first checking with the pharmacist.* Some tablets can be crushed or capsules can be opened and the contents added to water or a tube feeding when the patient cannot swallow a whole tablet or capsule. Some tablets have a special coating that delays the absorption of the drug. Crushing the tablet may destroy this drug property and result in problems such as improper absorption of the drug or gastric irritation. Capsules are gelatin and dissolve on contact with a liquid. The contents of some capsules do not mix well with water and therefore are best left in the capsule. If the patient cannot take an oral tablet or capsule, consult the physician because the drug may be available in liquid form.

14. *Never give a drug that someone else has prepared.* The individual preparing the drug **must** administer the drug.

15. *When using a unit-dose system, do not remove the wrappings of the unit dose until the drug reaches the bedside of the patient who is to receive it.* The method of administering drugs by the *unit dose* system is widely used. Many drugs are packaged by their manufacturers in *unit doses.* That is, each package is labeled by the manufacturer and contains one tablet or capsule, a premeasured amount of a liquid medication, a prefilled syringe, or one suppository. Hospital pharmacists may also prepare *unit doses.* The *unit dose* system uses portable carts with a drawer for each patient containing a 24-hour supply of medications. The pharmacist restocks the cart each day with the medications needed for the next 24-hour period. The nurse takes the drug cart into each patient's room. After administering the drug, the nurse charts immediately on the *unit dose* drug form (Fig. 2-1). Some hospitals are using a bar-code scanner in the adminis-

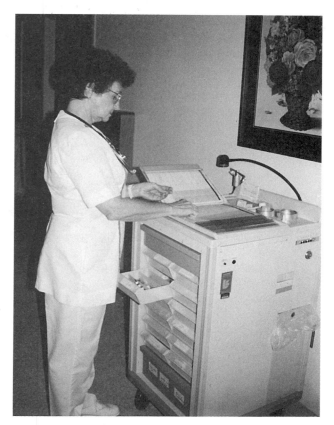

Figure 2-1

The mobile cart and the Kardex or Medication Administration Record (MAR) are taken to the patient's room when medications are given. Each patient's medications are stored in a separate drawer numbered according to the patient's room. Note that the nurse carefully checks the medication she will give with the MAR. Between uses, the cart is stored near the nurses' station. The cart is kept locked when not in use.

tration of unit dose medications. To utilize this system a bar code is placed on the patient's hospital identification band when the patient is admitted to the hospital. These bar codes, along with bar codes on the medication unit dose packages, are used to identify the patient, as well as to record and charge routine and prn medications. The scanner also keeps an ongoing inventory of controlled substances which eliminates the need for narcotic counts at the end of each shift.

ADMINISTRATION OF DRUGS BY THE ORAL ROUTE

The oral route is the most frequent route of drug administration and rarely causes physical discomfort. Oral drug forms include tablets, capsules, and liq-

uids. Some capsules and tablets contain sustained release drugs, which dissolve over an extended period of time. Administration is relatively easy for patients who are alert and can swallow.

Nursing Responsibilities

Observe the following points when giving an oral drug:

1. See that the patient is placed in an upright position. It is difficult, as well as dangerous, to swallow a solid or liquid when lying down.
2. Make sure that a full glass of water is readily available.
3. Assess the patient's need for assistance in removing the tablet or capsule from the container, holding the container, holding a medicine cup, or holding a glass of water. Some patients with physical disabilities cannot handle or hold these objects and may require assistance.
4. Advise the patient to take a few sips of water before placing a tablet or capsule in the mouth.
5. Instruct the patient to place the pill or capsule on the back of the tongue and tilt the head back to swallow a tablet or slightly forward to swallow a capsule. Encourage the patient first to take a few sips of water to move the drug down the esophagus and into the stomach, and then to finish the whole glass.
6. Give the patient any special instructions, such as drinking extra fluids or remaining in bed, that are pertinent to the drug being administered.
7. *Never* leave a medication at the patient's bedside to be taken later unless there is a specific order by the physician to do so. There are a few drugs (eg, antacids and nitroglycerin tablets) that may be ordered to be left at the bedside.
8. Patients with a nasogastric feeding tube may be given their oral medications through the tube. Liquid medications are diluted and flushed through the tube. Tablets, however, must be crushed and dissolved in water. Prior to administration, check the tube for placement. It is important that the tube be flushed with water after the drugs are placed in the tube to completely clear the tubing.
9. *Buccal* medications are placed against the mucous membranes of the cheek in either the upper or the lower jaw. These medications are given for a local rather than systemic effect. They are absorbed slowly from the mucous membranes of the mouth. Examples of drugs given buccally are lozenges and troches.

10. Certain drugs are also given *sublingually* (eg, placed under the tongue.) These drugs must not be swallowed or chewed and must be dissolved completely before the patient eats or drinks. Nitroglycerin is commonly given sublingually.

ADMINISTRATION OF DRUGS BY THE PARENTERAL ROUTE

Parenteral drug administration means the giving of a drug by the *subcutaneous* (SC), *intramuscular* (IM), *intravenous* (IV), or *intradermal* route (Fig. 2-2). Other routes of *parenteral* administration that may be used by the physician are intralesional (into a lesion), intraarterial (into an artery), intracardiac (into the heart), and intraarticular (into a joint). In some instances, intraarterial drugs are administered by a nurse. However, administration is not by direct arterial injection but by means of a catheter that has been placed in an artery.

Nursing Responsibilities

Observe the following points when giving a drug by the parenteral route:

1. After selecting the site for injection, cleanse the skin. Most hospitals have a policy regarding the type of skin antiseptic used for cleansing the skin before parenteral drug administration. Cleanse the skin with a circular motion, starting at an inner point and moving outward.

2. After inserting the needle for SC and IM administration, pull back the syringe barrel to aspirate the drug. If blood appears in the syringe, remove the needle so the drug is not injected. Discard the medication, needle, and syringe and prepare another injection. If no blood appears in the syringe, the medication may be injected. Aspiration is not necessary when giving an intradermal injection.

3. After inserting a needle into a vein for IV drug administration, pull back the syringe barrel. Blood should flow back into the syringe. After a back flow of blood is obtained, the medication can safely be injected.

4. After removing the needle from an IM, SC, or IV injection site, place pressure on the area. Patients with bleeding tendencies often require prolonged pressure on the area.

5. Syringes are *not* recapped and are disposed of according to agency policy. Needles and syringes are discarded into clearly marked, appropriate containers. Most agencies have a "sharps" container located in each room for immediate disposal of needles and syringes after use.

6. Gloves may be worn for protection from the potential of a blood spill when giving parenteral medications if desired or if this is a policy of the healthcare agency. The risk of exposure to infected blood is increasing for all healthcare workers. The Centers for Disease Control recommend that gloves be worn when touching blood and/or body fluids, mucous membranes, or any broken skin area. This recommendation

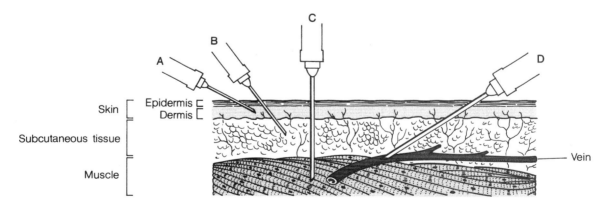

Figure 2-2

Needle insertion for parenteral medication: (**A**) Intradermal injection: a 26-gauge, 3/8-inch long needle is inserted at a 10° to 15° angle. (**B**) Subcutaneous injection: a 25-gauge, 1/2-inch long needle is inserted at an angle that depends on the size of the patient. (**C**) Intramuscular injection: a 20-gauge to 23-gauge, 1-inch to 3-inch long needle is inserted into the relaxed muscle at a 90° angle with a dart-throwing type of hand movement. (**D**) Intravenous injection: the diameter and length of the needle used depend on the substance to be injected and on the site of injection.

is referred to as *Standard Precautions*, which combine *Universal Precautions for Blood and Body Fluids* with *Body Substance Isolation*.

7. A new type of needle is available that is designed to prevent sticks. This needle has a plastic guard that slips over the needle as it is withdrawn from the injection site. The guard locks in place and eliminates the need to recap.

Administration of Drugs by the Subcutaneous Route

An SC injection places the drug into the tissues between the skin and the muscle (Fig. 2-2B). Drugs administered in this manner are absorbed more slowly than intramuscular injections. Heparin and insulin are two of the drugs most commonly given subcutaneously.

Nursing Responsibilities

Observe the following points when giving a drug by the subcutaneous route:

1. A volume of 0.5 to 1 mL is used for SC injection. Larger volumes (eg, more than 1 mL) are best given as IM injections. If a larger volume is ordered by the SC route, the injection is given in two sites with separate needles and syringes.
2. The sites for SC injection are the upper arms, the upper abdomen, and the upper back (Fig. 2-3). Injection sites must be rotated to assure proper absorption and minimize tissue damage.
3. When giving a drug by the SC route, the needle is most often inserted at a 45-degree angle. However, to place the medication in the subcutaneous tissue, select the needle length and angle of insertion based on the patient's body weight. Obese patients have excess subcutaneous tissue, and the injection may need to be given at a 90-degree angle. If the patient is thin or cachectic, there usually is less SC tissue. For these patients, the upper abdomen is the best site for injection. Generally, a syringe with a 23- to 25-gauge needle that is 1/2″ to 5/8″ in length is most suitable for an SC injection.

Administration of Drugs by the Intramuscular Route

An IM injection is the administration of a drug into a muscle (Fig. 2-2C). Drugs given by this route are absorbed more rapidly than drugs given by the SC

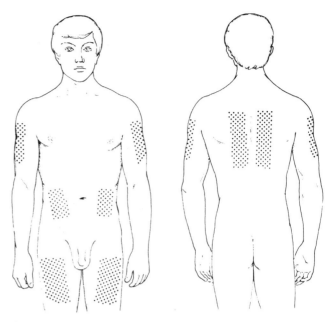

Figure 2-3

Sites on the body at which subcutaneous injections can be given.

route because of the rich blood supply in the muscle. Drugs that are irritating to subcutaneous tissue can be given IM. In addition, a larger volume (1–3 mL) can be given at one site. Volumes larger than 3 mL will not be absorbed properly.

Z-Track Technique

The *Z-track* method of IM injection is used when a drug is highly irritating to SC tissues or has the ability to permanently stain the skin. The procedure below is followed when using the Z-track technique (Fig. 2-4):

1. Draw the drug up into the syringe.
2. Discard the needle and place a new needle on the syringe. This prevents any solution that may remain in the needle (that was used to draw the drug into the syringe) from contacting tissues as the needle is put into the muscle.
3. Pull the plunger down to draw approximately 0.1 to 0.2 mL of air into the syringe. The air bubble in the syringe follows the drug into the tissues and seals off the area where the drug was injected, thereby preventing oozing of the drug up through the extremely small pathway created by the needle.
4. See that the patient is placed in the correct position (see below) for administration of an intramuscular injection.
5. Cleanse the skin.

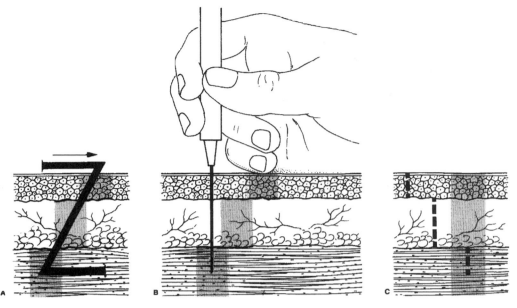

Figure 2-4

Z-track injection: (**A**) The tissue is tensed laterally at the injection site before the needle is inserted. This pulls the skin, subcutaneous tissue, and fat planes into a Z formation. (**B**) After the tissue has been displaced, the needle is thrust straight into the muscular tissue. (**C**) After injection, tissues are released while the needle is withdrawn. As each tissue plane slides by the other, the track is sealed.

6. Pull the skin, subcutaneous tissues, and fat (that are over the injection site) laterally, displacing the tissue to the side.
7. While holding the tissues in the lateral position, insert the needle and inject the drug. After the drug is injected, release the tissues and withdraw the needle. This technique prevents the back flow of medication into the subcutaneous tissue.

Nursing Responsibilities

Observe the following points when giving a drug by the IM route:

1. If an injection is more than 3 mL, it should be divided and given as two separate injections. A 22-gauge needle that is 1 1/2 inches in length is most often used for IM injections.
2. The sites for IM administration are the deltoid muscle (upper arm), the ventrogluteal or dorsogluteal sites (hip), and the vastus lateralis (thigh; Fig. 2-5). The vastus lateralis site is frequently used for infants and small children because it is often more developed than the gluteal or deltoid sites. This site may also be used for adults.
3. When giving a drug by the IM route, insert the needle at a 90-degree angle. When injecting a

drug into the ventrogluteal or dorsogluteal muscles, place the patient in a comfortable position, preferably in a prone position with the toes pointing inward. When injecting the drug into the deltoid, a sitting or lying down position may be used. Place the patient in a recumbent position for injection of a drug into the vastus lateralis.

Administration of Drugs by the Intravenous Route

A drug administered by the IV route is given directly into the blood by a needle inserted into a vein. Drug action occurs almost immediately.

Drugs administered IV may be given:

- Slowly, over 1 or more minutes
- Rapidly (IV push)
- By piggy-back infusions (medications are mixed with 50 to 100 mL of compatible IV fluid and administered over 30 to 60 minutes piggy-backed onto the primary IV)
- Into an existing IV line (the IV port)
- Into an intermittent venous access device called a heparin lock (a small IV catheter in the patient's vein connected to a small fluid reservoir with a

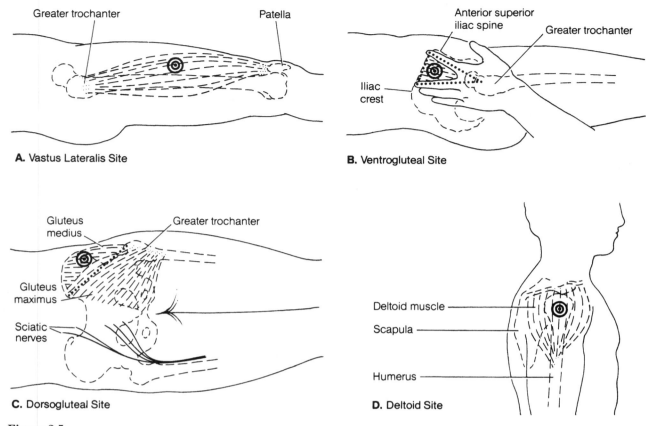

Greater trochanter   Patella

A. Vastus Lateralis Site

Anterior superior
iliac spine   Greater trochanter

Iliac
crest

B. Ventrogluteal Site

Gluteus
medius   Greater trochanter

Gluteus
maximus

Sciatic
nerves

C. Dorsogluteal Site

Deltoid muscle

Scapula

Humerus

D. Deltoid Site

Figure 2-5

(**A**) Vastus Lateralis Site: the patient is supine or sitting. (**B**) Ventrogluteal Site: the nurse's palm is placed on the greater trochanter and the index finger is placed on the anterior superior iliac spine: the injection is made into the middle of the triangle formed by the nurse's fingers and the iliac crest. (**C**) Dorsogluteal site: to avoid the sciatic nerve and accompanying blood vessels, an injection site is chosen above and lateral to a line drawn from the greater trochanter to the posterior superior iliac spine. (**D**) Deltoid Site: the mid-deltoid area is located by forming a rectangle, the top of which is at the level of the lower edge of the acromion, and the bottom of which is at the level of the axilla; the sides are one third and two thirds of the way around the outer aspect of the patients arm.

rubber cap through which the needle is inserted to administer the medication)

• By being added to an IV solution and allowed to infuse into the vein over a longer period.

When administering a drug into a vein by a venipuncture, place a tourniquet *above* the selected vein. Tighten the tourniquet so that venous blood flow is blocked but there is arterial blood flow. Allow the veins to fill (distend). Then, pull the skin taut (to anchor the vein and the skin) and insert the needle into the vein, bevel up, and at a short angle to the skin (Fig. 2-6). Blood should immediately flow into the syringe if the needle is properly inserted into the vein.

Performing a venipuncture requires practice. Some veins are difficult to enter, and a suitable vein for venipuncture may be hard to find. At no time should the nurse repeatedly and unsuccessfully at-

tempt a venipuncture. Depending on clinical judgment, three unsuccessful attempts on the same patient warrant having a more skilled individual attempt the procedure.

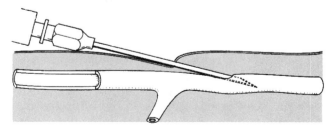

Figure 2-6

Needle bevel position for venipuncture. (From N.M. Metheny and W.D. Snively, Jr., 1983. *Nurses Handbook of Fluid Balance*, 4th ed., Philadelphia: J.B. Lippincott.

Some drugs are added to an IV solution such as 1000 mL of dextrose 5% and water. The drug is usually added to the IV fluid container immediately before adding the fluid to the IV line. Whenever a drug is added to an IV fluid, the bottle *must* have a label attached indicating the drug and drug dose added to the IV fluid. In some hospitals, a pharmacist is responsible for adding specific drugs to IV fluids.

Intravenous Infusion Controllers and Pumps

Electronic infusion devices are classified as either infusion controllers or infusion pumps (Fig. 2-7). The primary difference between the two is that an infusion pump adds pressure to the infusion, while a controller does not. An infusion pump may be used to deliver the desired number of drops per minute. An alarm is set to sound if the IV is more than or less than the preset rate.

Controllers and pumps have detectors and alarms that alert the nurse to various problems, such as air in the line, an occlusion, low battery, completion of an infusion, or an inability to deliver the preset rate. When any problem is detected by the device, an alarm is activated to alert the nurse. Potential complications in *intravenous* therapy are the same as those with peripheral lines.

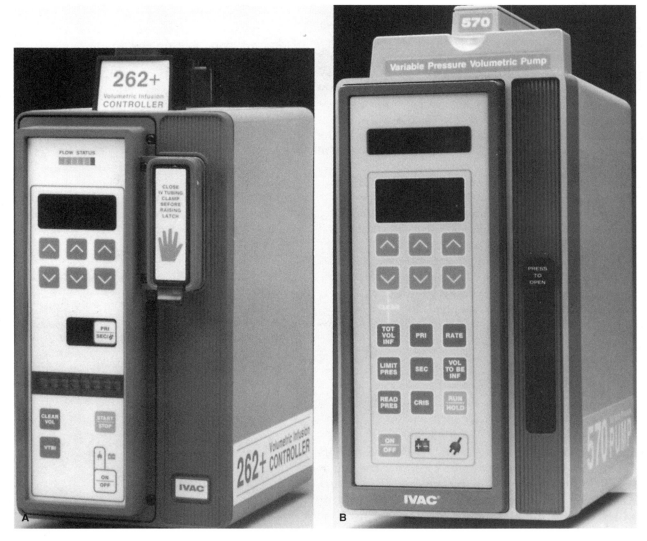

Figure 2-7

Two types of infusion control devices (ICDs) are pictured: an infusion controller (**A**) and infusion pump (**B**). Hospitals use these types of devices to provide safer intravenous therapy for patients. Since a number of manufacturers are producing ICDs, nurses must inquire about the type used and follow specific instructions for each particular device.

Nursing Alert

Use of an infusion pump or controller still requires nursing supervision and frequent monitoring of the IV infusion. Infiltration can progress rapidly because the increased pressure will not slow the infusion until considerable edema has occurred. Monitor frequently for signs of infiltration such as edema or redness at the site. Careful monitoring of the pump or controller is also necessary to make sure the flow rate is correct.

Nursing Responsibilities

After the start of an IV infusion, record the type of IV fluid and, when applicable, the drug added to the IV solution on the patient's chart. Check the infusion rate every 15 to 30 minutes. At this time, also inspect the needle site for signs of redness, swelling, or other problems. Swelling around the needle may indicate that the needle is no longer in the vein and the IV fluid is being deposited in SC tissue. One of two events may have occurred: extravasation or infiltration. *Extravasation* refers to the escape of fluid from a blood vessel into surrounding tissues while the needle or catheter is in the vein. *Infiltration* is the collection of fluid into tissues (usually SC tissue) when the needle or catheter is out of the vein. Both events necessitate discontinuation of the infusion and insertion of an IV line in another vein. Some drugs are capable of causing severe tissue damage if extravasation or infiltration occurs.

If extravasation or infiltration should occur, the IV must be stopped and restarted in another vein. The physician should be contacted if a drug, for example, norepinephrine (Levophed), capable of causing tissue damage has escaped into the tissues surrounding the needle insertion site.

Administration of Drugs by the Intradermal Route

Drugs given by the *intradermal* route are usually agents for sensitivity tests, for example, the tuberculin test or allergy skin testing (see Fig. 2-2A). Absorption is slow and allows for good results when testing for allergies or administering local anesthetics.

Nursing Responsibilities

Observe the following points when administering drugs by the intradermal route:

1. The inner part of the forearm and the upper back may be used for intradermal injections. The area should be hairless; areas near moles, scars, or pigmented skin areas should be avoided. Cleanse the area in the same manner as for SC and IM injections.
2. A 1-mL syringe with a 25- to 27-gauge needle that is 1/4″ to 5/8″ long is best suited for intradermal injections. Small volumes (usually less than 0.1 mL) are used for intradermal injections and administered with the bevel up.
3. Insert the needle at a 15-degree angle between the upper layers of the skin. Do not aspirate the syringe or massage the area. Injection produces a small wheal (raised area) on the outer surface of the skin. If a wheal does not appear on the outer surface of the skin, there is a good possibility that the medication entered the subcutaneous tissue and any test results would be inaccurate.

Other Parenteral Routes of Drug Administration

The physician may administer a drug by the intracardial, intralesional, intraarterial, or intraarticular routes. The nurse may be responsible for preparing the drug for administration. The physician should be asked what special materials will be required for administration.

Venous access ports are totally implanted ports with a self-sealing septum that is attached to a catheter leading to a large vessel, usually the vena cava. These devices are most commonly used for chemotherapy or other long-term therapy. Drugs are administered through injections made into the portal through the skin. These medications are administered by the physician or registered nurse. These devices require surgical insertion and removal.

ADMINISTRATION OF DRUGS THROUGH THE SKIN AND MUCOUS MEMBRANES

Drugs may be applied to the skin and mucous membranes using several routes. Drugs may be applied on the outer layers of the skin or topically. Certain drugs may be applied, transdermally, through a patch on which the medication has been implanted. Drugs may also be inhaled through the membranes of the upper respiratory tract.

Administration of Drugs by the Topical Route

Most topical drugs are not absorbed through the skin, and their action is to the skin, not the structures lying below the skin surface. Topical drugs may be in the form of ointments, lotions, liquids, solids, or creams. When applied to the skin for their local effect, they are used to soften, disinfect, or lubricate the skin. A few topical drugs are enzymes that have the ability to remove superficial debris, such as the dead skin and purulent matter present in skin ulcerations. Other topical agents are used to treat minor, superficial skin infections.

The various forms of topical applications include the following:

- Creams, lotions, or ointments applied to the skin with a tongue blade, gloved fingers, or gauze
- Sprays applied to the skin or into the nose or oral cavity
- Liquids inserted into body cavities such as fistulas
- Liquids inserted into the bladder or urethra
- Solids (eg, suppositories) or jellies inserted into the urethra
- Liquids dropped into the eyes, ears, or nose
- Ophthalmic ointments applied to the eyelids or dropped into the lower conjunctival sac
- Solids (eg, suppositories, tablets), foams, liquids, and creams inserted into the vagina
- Continuous or intermittent wet dressings applied to skin surfaces
- Solids (eg, tablets, lozenges) dissolved in the mouth
- Sprays or mists inhaled into the lungs
- Liquids, creams, or ointments applied to the scalp
- Solids (eg, suppositories), liquids, or foams inserted into the rectum

Nursing Responsibilities

Consider the following points when administering drugs by the topical route:

1. The physician may write special instructions for the application of a topical drug, for example, to apply the drug in a thin, even layer or to cover the area following application of the drug to the skin.
2. Other drugs may have special instructions provided by the manufacturer, such as to apply the drug to a clean, hairless area or to let the drug dissolve slowly in the mouth. All of these instructions are important because drug action may depend on correct administration of the agent.

Administration of Drugs by the Transdermal Route

Drugs administered by the *transdermal* route are readily absorbed from the skin to provide systemic effects. This type of administration is called transdermal drug delivery system. The drug dosages are implanted in a small patch-type bandage. The backing is removed and the patch is applied to the skin where the drug is gradually absorbed into the systemic circulation. This type of drug system maintains a relatively constant blood concentration and reduces the possibility of toxicity. The use of drugs transdermally causes fewer adverse reactions and administration is less frequent than when the drugs are given by another route. Nitroglycerin (used to treat cardiac problems) and scopolamine (used to treat dizziness and nausea) are two drugs given frequently by the transdermal route.

Nursing Responsibilities

Observe the following points when administering drugs by the transdermal route:

1. Apply transdermal patches to clean, dry, nonhairy areas of intact skin.
2. Remove the patch when the next dose is applied and a new site is used. Sites for transdermal patches are rotated to prevent skin irritation. The chest, flank, or upper arm are the most commonly used sites. Do not shave the area to apply the patch; shaving may cause skin irritation.
3. Ointments are sometimes used and come with a special paper marked in inches. Measure the correct length (onto the paper). Place the paper with the drug ointment side down on the skin and secure with tape. Prior to the next dose, remove the paper and tape and cleanse the skin. Rotate sites to prevent irritation to the skin.

ADMINISTRATION OF DRUGS THROUGH INHALATION

Drug droplets, vapor, or gas are administered through the mucous membranes of the respiratory tract with the use of a face mask, a nebulizer, or positive-pressure breathing machine. Bronchodilators, mucolytics, and some anti-inflammatory drugs can be administered with positive-pressure breathing machines or nebulizers (inhalers) to produce primarily a local effect in the lungs. Drugs administered in this way are delivered through *inhalation*.

Nursing Responsibilities

The primary nursing responsibility is to provide the patient with the proper instructions for administering the drug. For example, many patients with asthma use a metered-dose inhaler to dilate the bronchi and make breathing easier. Without proper instruction on how to use the inhaler, much of the medication can be deposited on the tongue rather that in the respiratory tract. This decreases the therapeutic effect of the drug. Instructions may vary with each inhaler. To be certain that the inhaler is used correctly, the patient is referred to the instructions accompanying each device. Figure 2-8. illustrates the proper use of one type of inhaler.

Nursing Responsibilities After Drug Administration

After the administration of any type of drug, the nurse is responsible for the following:

1. *Recording the administration of the drug.* This task is completed as soon as possible. This is particularly important when prn medications (especially narcotics) are given.
2. *Recording (when necessary) any information concerning the administration of the drug.* This includes information such as the IV flow rate, the site used for *parenteral* administration, problems with administration (if any), and vital signs taken immediately before administration.
3. *Evaluating and recording the patient's response to the drug* (when applicable). Evaluation may include such facts as relief of pain, decrease in body temperature, relief of itching, decrease in the number of stools passed, and so on.
4. *Observing the adverse reactions.* The frequency of these observations will depend on the drug administered. All suspected adverse reactions are recorded, as well as reported, to the physician. Serious adverse reactions are reported to the physician immediately.

Chapter Summary

- The administration of medication is an important responsibility for the nurse. The well-being of the patient depends on the nurse's knowledge of this important task and her application of the principles of drug administration in a timely and accurate manner.
- Preparation of medication must be done methodically and accurately. Observation of the "six rights" provides guidelines to ensure safe administration of medication.
- The nurses' responsibility does not end with proper administration of the drug. The nurse is also responsible for monitoring the therapeutic response, as well as observing and reporting any adverse reaction the patient experiences.

Critical Thinking Exercises

1. Ms. Benson, a nurse on your clinical unit, tells you that the head nurse is upset with her because she has not been recording the administration of narcotics immediately after they are given. What rationales could you give to Ms. Benson to stress the importance of recording the administration of narcotics immediately after they are given.
2. A nurse is to give a subcutaneous injection of heparin to a patient. What information would the nurse need to know about the patient before preparing the injection? How would this information affect the preparation of the injection and the technique used to give the subcutaneous injection?

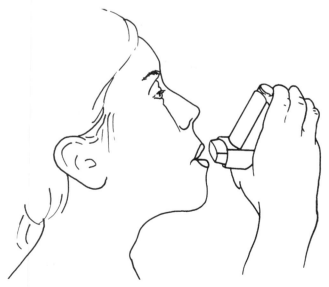

Figure 2-8

A respiratory inhalant is used to deliver medication directly into the lungs. To deliver a dose of the drug, the patient takes a slow, deep breath while depressing the top of the canister.

3

Review of Arithmetic and Calculation of Drug Dosages

Chapter Outline

Chapter Objectives

On completion of this chapter the student will:

- *Accurately perform mathematical calculations when they are necessary to compute drug dosages*

Review of Arithmetic

FRACTIONS

The two parts of a fraction are the numerator and the denominator.

$$\frac{2}{3} \begin{array}{l}\leftarrow\text{numerator} \\ \leftarrow\text{denominator}\end{array}$$

A **proper fraction** may be defined as a part of a whole or any number less than a whole number. An **improper fraction** is a fraction having a numerator the same as or larger than the denominator.

$$\text{Proper Fraction} \quad \frac{1}{2}$$

$$\text{Improper Fraction} \quad \frac{7}{3}$$

The numerator and the denominator *must be of like entities or terms,* that is:

Correct (like terms)	Incorrect (unlike terms)
$\frac{2\text{ acres}}{3\text{ acres}}$	$\frac{2\text{ acres}}{3\text{ miles}}$
$\frac{2\text{ grams}}{3\text{ grams}}$	$\frac{2\text{ grams}}{5\text{ milliliters}}$

Mixed Numbers and Improper Fractions

A **mixed number** is a whole number and a proper fraction. A whole number is a number that stands alone. 3, 25, and 117 are examples of whole numbers. A proper fraction is a fraction whose numerator is *smaller than* the denominator. 1/8, 2/5, and 3/7 are examples of proper fractions.

These are mixed numbers

2⅔ 2 is the whole number and ⅔ is the proper fraction

3¼ 3 is the whole number and ¼ is the proper fraction

When doing certain calculations, it is sometimes necessary to change a mixed number to an improper fraction or change an improper fraction to a mixed number. An improper fraction is a fraction whose numerator is *larger than* the denominator. 5/2, 16/3, and 123/2 are examples of improper fractions.

To change a **mixed number to an improper fraction**, multiply the denominator of the fraction by the whole number, add the numerator, and place the sum over the denominator.

EXAMPLE mixed number 3⅗

1. Multiply the denominator of the fraction (5) by the whole number (3) or 5 X 3 = 15:

$$3 \times\nwarrow \frac{3}{5}$$

2. Add the result of multiplying the denominator of the fraction (15) to the numerator (3) or 15 + 3 = 18:

$$3 \begin{array}{c}\nearrow \\ \times\nwarrow\end{array} \frac{3}{5}$$

3. Then place the sum (18) over the denominator of the fraction:

$$\frac{18}{5}$$

To change an **improper fraction to a mixed number**, divide the denominator into the numerator. The quotient (the result of the division of these two numbers) is the whole number. Then place the remainder over the denominator of the improper fraction.

EXAMPLE improper fraction 15/4

$$\frac{15}{4} \begin{array}{l}\leftarrow\text{numerator} \\ \leftarrow\text{denominator}\end{array}$$

1. Divide the denominator (4) into the numerator (15) or 15 divided by 4 (15 ÷ 4)

$$\begin{array}{r} 3 \quad \leftarrow\textbf{quotient} \\ 4\overline{)15} \\ \underline{12} \\ 3 \quad \leftarrow\textbf{remainder} \end{array}$$

2. The **quotient** (3) becomes the whole number

$$3\frac{3}{4}$$

3. The **remainder** (3) now becomes the numerator of the fraction of the mixed number

$$3\frac{3}{}$$

4. And the denominator of the improper fraction (4) now becomes the denominator of the fraction of the mixed number

$$3\frac{3}{4}$$

Adding Fractions with Like Denominators

When the denominators are the *same*, fractions can be added by adding the numerators and placing the sum of the numerators over the denominator.

EXAMPLES

$$2/7 + 3/7 = 5/7$$

$$1/10 + 3/10 = 4/10$$

$$2/9 + 1/9 + 4/9 = 7/9$$

$$1/12 + 5/12 + 3/12 = 9/12$$

$$2/13 + 1/13 + 3/13 + 5/13 = 11/13$$

When giving a final answer, fractions are *always* reduced to the lowest possible terms. In the examples above, the answers of 5/7, 7/9, and 11/13 cannot be reduced. The answers of 4/10 and 9/12 can be reduced to 2/5 and 3/4.

To reduce a fraction to the lowest possible terms, determine if any number, which always must be the same, can be divided into both the numerator and the denominator.

4/10   the numerator **and** the denominator can be divided by 2

9/12   the numerator **and** the denominator can be divided by 3

$$\text{For example: } \frac{4}{10} \div \frac{2}{2} = \frac{2}{5}$$

If when adding fractions the answer is an improper fraction, it may then be changed to a mixed number.

$$2/5 + 4/5 = 6/5 \text{ (improper fraction)}$$

6/5 changed to a mixed number is 1 1/5

Adding Fractions with Unlike Denominators

Fractions with *unlike denominators* cannot be added until the denominators are changed to like numbers or numbers that are the same. The first step is to find the *lowest common denominator,* which is the lowest number divisible by (or that can be divided by) all the denominators.

EXAMPLE add 2/3 and 1/4

$$\frac{2}{3} \quad \frac{1}{4}$$

The lowest number that can be divided by these two denominators is 12; therefore, 12 is the lowest common denominator

1. Divide the lowest common denominator (which in this example is 12) by each of the denominators in the fractions (in this example 3 and 4)

$$\frac{2}{3} = \frac{}{12} \quad (12 \div 3 = 4)$$

$$\frac{1}{4} = \frac{}{12} \quad (12 \div 4 = 3)$$

2. Multiply the results of the divisions by the numerator of the fractions (12 ÷ 3 = 4 X the numerator 2 = 8 and 12 ÷ 4 = 3 X the numerator 1 = 3) and place the results in the numerator

$$\frac{2}{3} = \frac{}{12} \quad \frac{\mathbf{8}}{12}$$

$$\frac{1}{4} = \frac{}{12} \quad \frac{\mathbf{3}}{12}$$

3. Add the numerators (8 + 3) and place the result over the denominator (12)

$$\frac{8}{12}$$
$$\frac{3}{12}$$
$$\overline{\quad}$$
$$\frac{11}{12}$$

Adding Mixed Numbers or Fractions with Mixed Numbers

When adding two or more mixed numbers or adding fractions and mixed numbers, the mixed number is first changed to an improper fraction.

EXAMPLE Add 3 3/4 and 3 3/4

$$3\frac{3}{4} \text{ changed to an improper fraction} \rightarrow \frac{15}{4}$$

$$3\frac{3}{4} \text{ changed to an improper fraction} \rightarrow \frac{15}{4}$$

$$\text{The numerators are added} \rightarrow \frac{30}{4} = 7\,2/4 = 7\,1/2$$

The improper fraction (30/4) is changed to a mixed number (7 2/4) and the fraction of the mixed number (2/4) changed to the lowest possible terms (1/2).

EXAMPLE Add 2 1/2 and 3 1/4

$$2\frac{1}{2} \text{ changed to an improper fraction} \quad \frac{5}{2}$$

$$3\frac{1}{4} \text{ changed to an improper fraction} \quad \frac{13}{4}$$

In the example above, 5/2 and 13/4 cannot be added because the denominators are not the same. It will be necessary to find the lowest common denominator first.

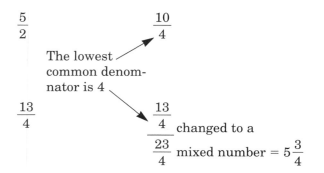

$$\frac{13}{4}$$ changed to a $$\frac{23}{4}$$ mixed number $= 5\frac{3}{4}$

Comparing Fractions

When fractions with *like* denominators are compared, the fraction with the *largest numerator* is the *largest* fraction.

EXAMPLES

Compare 5/8 and 3/8 Answer: **5/8** is larger than **3/8**

Compare 1/4 and 3/4 Answer: **3/4** is larger than **1/4**

When the denominators are *not* the same, for example, comparing 2/3 and 1/10, the lowest common denominator must first be determined. The same procedure is followed when adding fractions with unlike denominators (see above).

EXAMPLE Compare 2/3 and 1/10 (fractions with unlike denominators)

$$\frac{2}{3} = \frac{20}{30}$$
lowest common denominator
$$\frac{1}{10} = \frac{3}{30}$$

The largest numerator in these two fractions is 20; therefore, 2/3 is larger than 1/10.

Multiplying Fractions

When fractions are multiplied, the numerators are multiplied *and* the denominators are multiplied.

EXAMPLES

$$\frac{1}{8} \times \frac{1}{4} = \frac{1}{32} \quad \frac{1}{2} \times \frac{2}{3} = \frac{2}{6} = \frac{1}{3}$$

In the above examples, it was necessary to reduce one of the answers to its lowest possible terms.

Multiplying Whole Numbers and Fractions

When whole numbers are multiplied with fractions, the numerator is multiplied by the whole number and the product is placed over the denominator. When necessary, the fraction is reduced to its lowest possible terms. If the answer is an improper fraction, it may be changed to a mixed number.

EXAMPLES

$$2 \times \frac{1}{2} = \frac{2}{2} = 1 \text{ (answer reduced to lowest possible terms)}$$

$$2 \times \frac{3}{8} = \frac{6}{8} = \frac{3}{4} \text{ (answer reduced to lowest possible terms)}$$

$$4 \times \frac{2}{3} = \frac{8}{3} = 2\frac{2}{3} \text{ (improper fraction changed to a mixed number)}$$

Multiplying Mixed Numbers

To multiply mixed numbers, the mixed numbers are changed to *improper fractions* and then multiplied.

EXAMPLES

$$2\frac{1}{2} \times 3\frac{1}{4} = \frac{5}{2} \times \frac{13}{4} = \frac{65}{8} = 8\frac{1}{8}$$

$$3\frac{1}{3} \times 4\frac{1}{2} = \frac{10}{3} \times \frac{9}{2} = \frac{90}{6} = 15$$

Multiplying a Whole Number and a Mixed Number

To multiply a whole number and a mixed number, *both* numbers must be changed to improper fractions.

EXAMPLES

$$3 \times 2\frac{1}{2} = \frac{3}{1} \times \frac{5}{2} = \frac{15}{2} = 7\frac{1}{2}$$

$$2 \times 4\frac{1}{2} = \frac{2}{1} \times \frac{9}{2} = \frac{18}{2} = 9$$

A whole number is converted to an improper fraction by placing the whole number over 1. In the above examples, 3 becomes 3/1 and 2 becomes 2/1.

Dividing Fractions

When fractions are divided, the *second* fraction (the divisor) is inverted (turned upside down) and then the fractions are multiplied.

EXAMPLES

$$\frac{1}{3} \div \frac{3}{7} = \frac{1}{3} \times \frac{7}{3} = \frac{7}{9}$$

$$\frac{1}{8} \div \frac{1}{4} = \frac{1}{8} \times \frac{4}{1} = \frac{4}{8} = \frac{1}{2}$$

$$\frac{3}{4} \div \frac{1}{2} = \frac{3}{4} \times \frac{2}{1} = \frac{6}{4} = 1\frac{1}{2}$$

In the above examples, the second answer was reduced to its lowest possible terms and the third answer, which was an improper fraction, was changed to a mixed number.

Dividing Fractions and Mixed Numbers

Some problems of division may be expressed as (1) fractions and mixed numbers, (2) two mixed numbers, (3) whole numbers and fractions, or (4) whole numbers and mixed numbers.

Mixed Numbers and Fractions

When a mixed number is divided by a fraction, the whole number is first changed to a fraction.

EXAMPLES

$$2\frac{1}{3} \div \frac{1}{4} = \frac{7}{3} \div \frac{1}{4} = \frac{7}{3} \times \frac{4}{1} = \frac{28}{3} = 9\frac{1}{3}$$

$$2\frac{1}{2} \div \frac{1}{2} = \frac{5}{2} \div \frac{1}{2} = \frac{5}{2} \times \frac{2}{1} = \frac{10}{2} = 5$$

Mixed Numbers

When two mixed numbers are divided, they are both changed to improper fractions.

EXAMPLE

$$3\frac{3}{4} \div 1\frac{1}{2} = \frac{15}{4} \div \frac{3}{2} = \frac{15}{4} \times \frac{2}{3} = \frac{30}{12}$$

$$= 2\frac{6}{12} = 2\frac{1}{2}$$

Whole Numbers and Fractions

When a whole number is divided by a fraction, the whole number is changed to an improper fraction by placing the whole number over 1.

EXAMPLE

$$2 \div \frac{2}{3} = \frac{2}{1} \div \frac{2}{3} = \frac{2}{1} \times \frac{3}{2} = \frac{6}{2} = 3$$

Whole Numbers and Mixed Numbers

When whole numbers and mixed numbers are divided, the whole number is changed to an improper fraction and the mixed number is changed to an improper fraction.

EXAMPLE

$$4 \div 2\frac{2}{3} = \frac{4}{1} \div \frac{8}{3} = \frac{4}{1} \times \frac{3}{8} = \frac{12}{8} = 1\frac{4}{8} = 1\frac{1}{2}$$

RATIOS

A ratio is a way of expressing *a part of a whole* or *the relation of one number to another*. For example, a ratio written as 1:10 means 1 in 10 parts, or 1 to 10. A ratio may also be written as a fraction; thus 1:10 can also be expressed as 1/10.

EXAMPLES

1:1000 is 1 part in 1000 parts, or 1 to 1000, or 1/1000

1:250 is 1 part in 250 parts, or 1 to 250, or 1/250

Some drug solutions are expressed in ratios, for example 1:100 or 1:500. These ratios mean that there is 1 part of a drug in 100 parts of solution or 1 part of the drug in 500 parts of solution.

PERCENTAGES

The term *percentage or percent (%)* means *parts per hundred*.

EXAMPLES

25% is 25 parts per hundred

50% is 50 parts per hundred

A percentage may also be expressed as a fraction.

EXAMPLES

>   25% is 25 parts per hundred or 25/100
>
>   50% is 50 parts per hundred or 50/100
>
>   30% is 30 parts per hundred or 30/100

The above fractions may also be reduced to their lowest possible terms:

>   25/100 = 1/4, 50/100 = 1/2, 30/100 = 3/10.

Changing a Fraction to a Percentage

To change a fraction to a percentage, divide the denominator by the numerator and multiply the results (quotient) by 100 and then add a percent sign (%).

EXAMPLES

Change 4/5 to a percentage

$$4 \div 5 = 0.8$$

$$0.8 \times 100 = 80\%$$

Change 2/3 to a percentage

$$2 \div 3 = 0.666$$

$$0.666 \times 100 = 66.6\%$$

Changing a Ratio to a Percentage

To change a ratio to a percentage, the ratio is first expressed as a fraction with the first number or term of the ratio becoming the numerator and the second number or term becoming the denominator. For example, the ratio 1:500 when changed to a fraction becomes 1/500. This fraction is then changed to a percentage by the same method shown in the preceding section.

EXAMPLE

Change 1:125 to a percentage
1:125 written as a fraction is 1/125

$$1 \div 125 = 0.008$$

$$0.008 \times 100 = 0.8$$

adding the percent sign = 0.8%

Changing a Percentage to a Ratio

To change a percentage to a ratio, the percentage becomes the numerator and is placed over a denominator of 100.

EXAMPLES

Changing 5% and 10% to ratios

$$5\% \text{ is } \frac{5}{100} = \frac{1}{20} \text{ or } 1{:}20$$

$$10\% \text{ is } \frac{10}{100} = \frac{1}{10} \text{ or } 1{:}10$$

PROPORTIONS

A proportion is a method of expressing equality between two ratios. An example of two ratios expressed as a proportion is
3 is to 4 as 9 is to 12
This may also be written as

>   3:4 as 9:12

or

>   3:4::9:12

or

$$\frac{3}{4} = \frac{9}{12}$$

Proportions may be used to find an unknown quantity. The unknown quantity is assigned a letter, usually X. An example of a proportion with an unknown quantity is 5:10::15:X.

The first and last terms of the proportion are called the *extremes*. In the above expression 5 and X are the extremes. The second and third terms of the proportion are called the *means*. In the above proportion, 10 and 15 are the means.

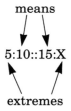

$$\underset{\text{mean}}{\overset{\text{extreme}}{}} \frac{5}{10} = \frac{15}{X} \underset{\text{extreme}}{\overset{\text{mean}}{}}$$

To solve for X:

1. Multiply the extremes and place the product (result) to the *left* of the equal sign.

>   5:10::15:X
>
>   5X =

2. Multiply the means and place the product to the *right* of the equal sign.

$$5:10::15:X$$
$$5X = 150$$

3. Solve for X by dividing the number to the right of the equal sign by the number to the left of the equal sign ($150 \div 5$).

$$5X = 150$$
$$X = 30$$

4. To prove the answer is correct, substitute the answer (30) for X in the equation.

$$5:10::15:X$$
$$5:10::15:30$$

Then multiply the means and place the product to the left of the equal sign. Then multiply the extremes and place the product to the right of the equal sign.

$$5:10::15:30$$
$$150 = 150$$

If the numbers are the same on both sides of the equal sign, the equation has been solved correctly.

If the proportion has been set up as a fraction, cross multiply and solve for X.

$$\frac{5}{10} = \frac{15}{X}$$

5 times X = 5X and 10 times 15 = 150

$$5\,X = 150$$
$$X = 30$$

To set up a proportion, remember that a *sequence must be followed*. If a sequence is not followed, the proportion will be stated incorrectly.

EXAMPLES

If a man can walk 6 **miles** in 2 **hours**, how many **miles** can he walk in 3 **hours**?

MILES is to HOURS as MILES is to HOURS

or

MILES:HOURS::MILES:HOURS

or

$$\frac{\text{MILES}}{\text{HOURS}} = \frac{\text{MILES}}{\text{HOURS}}$$

The unknown fact is the number of miles walked in 3 hours

6 miles:2 hours::X miles:3 hours

$$2X = 18$$

X = 9 miles (he can walk 9 miles in 3 hours)

If there are 15 **grains** in 1 **gram**, 30 **grains** equals how many **grams**?

15 grains:1 gram::30 grains:X grams

$$15\,X = 30$$

X = 2 grams (30 grains equals 2 grams)

DECIMALS

Decimals are used in the metric system. A **decimal** is a fraction in which the denominator is 10 or some power of 10. For example, 2/10 (read as two tenths) is a fraction with a denominator of 10; 1/100 (one one-hundredth) is an example of a fraction with a denominator that is a power of ten (ie, 100).

A power (or multiple) of 10 is the *number 1 followed by one or more zeros*. Therefore, 100, 1000, 10,000 and so on are powers of 10 because the number 1 is followed by two, three, and four zeros, respectively. Fractions whose denominators are 10 or a power of 10 are often expressed in decimal form.

Parts of a Decimal

There are three parts to a decimal:

$$1 \cdot 25$$

number(s)	d	number(s)
to the	e	to the
left of	c	right of
the	i	the
decimal	m	decimal
	a	
	l	

Types of Decimals

A decimal may consist only of numbers to the right of the decimal point. This is called a **decimal fraction.** Examples of decimal fractions are 0.05, 0.6, and 0.002.

A decimal may also have numbers to the *left* and *right* of the decimal point. This is called a **mixed decimal fraction.** Examples of mixed decimal fractions are 1.25, 2.5, and 7.5.

Both decimal fractions and mixed decimal fractions are commonly referred to as decimals. When there is no number to the left of the decimal, a zero may be written, for example, 0.25. Although in general mathematics the zero may not be required, it should be used in the writing of drug doses in the metric system. *Use of the zero lessens the chance of medication errors,* especially when the dose of a drug is hurriedly written and the decimal point is indistinct. For example, a drug order for dexamethasone is written as dexamethasone .25 mg by one physician and written as dexamethasone 0.25 by another. If the decimal point in the first written order is indistinct, the order might be interpreted as 25 mg, which is 100 times the prescribed dose!

Reading Decimals

To read a decimal, the position of the number to the left or right of the decimal point indicates how the decimal is to be expressed.

Adding Decimals

When adding decimals, place the numbers in a column so that the whole numbers are aligned to the left of the decimal and the decimal fractions are aligned to the right of the decimal.

EXAMPLE

20.45 + 2.56 is written as: 2 + 0.25 is written as:
20.45   2.00
 2.56   0.25
------   ------
23.01   2.25

Subtracting Decimals

When subtracting decimals, the numbers are aligned to the left and right of the decimal in the same manner as for the addition of decimals.

EXAMPLE

20.45 − 2.56 is written as: 9.74 − 0.45 is written as:
20.45   9.74
 2.56   0.45
------   ------
17.89   9.29

Multiplying a Whole Number by a Decimal

To multiply a whole number by a decimal, move the decimal point of the product (answer) as many places to the left as there are places to the right of the decimal point.

EXAMPLE

500   there are two places to the right
.05   ←of the decimal

2500.   the decimal point is moved two places
           to the left

After moving the decimal point, the answer reads 25.

250   there are two places to the right
.3   ←of the decimal
------
750.   the decimal point is moved two places
           to the left

After moving the decimal point, the answer reads 75.

Multiplying a Decimal by a Decimal

To multiply a decimal by a decimal, move the decimal point of the product (answer) as many places to the left as there are places to the right in *both* decimals.

EXAMPLE

          there are two places to the right
2.75 ←of the decimal
0.5   ←plus one place to the right of the decimal

1375.   move the decimal point three places
          to the left

After moving the decimal point, the answer reads 1.375

Dividing Decimals

The **divisor** is a number that is divided into the dividend.

EXAMPLE

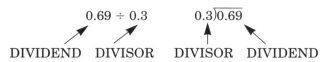

DIVIDEND   DIVISOR   DIVISOR   DIVIDEND

This may be written or spoken as 0.69 divided by 0.3. To divide decimals:

1. The *divisor* is changed to a whole number. In this example, the decimal point is moved one place to the right so that 0.3 now becomes 3, which is a whole number.

$$0.3\,)\overline{0.69}$$

2. The decimal point in the *dividend* is now moved the *same number of places* to the right. In this example, the decimal point is moved one place to the right, the same number of places the decimal point in the divisor was moved.

$$3\,)\overline{0.69}$$

3. The numbers are now divided.

$$3\,)\overline{6.9}^{\,2.3}$$

When only the dividend is a decimal, the decimal point is carried to the quotient (answer) in the same position.

EXAMPLES

$$2\,)\overline{0.750}^{\,.375} \qquad 2\,)\overline{3.472}^{\,1.736}$$

To divide when only the divisor is a decimal, for example,

$$.3\,)\overline{66}$$

1. The divisor is changed to a whole number. In this example the decimal point is moved one place to the right.

$$.3\,)\overline{66}$$

2. The decimal point in the dividend must also be moved one place to the right.

$$.3\,)\overline{66.0}$$

3. The numbers are now divided.

$$3\,)\overline{660}^{\,220}$$

Whenever the decimal point is moved in the dividend *it must also be moved* in the divisor, and whenever the decimal point in the divisor is moved *it must be moved* in the dividend.

Changing a Fraction to a Decimal

To change a fraction to a decimal, divide the numerator by the denominator.

EXAMPLE

$$\frac{1}{5} = 5\,)\overline{1.0}^{\,.2} \qquad \frac{3}{4} = 4\,)\overline{3.00}^{\,.75} \qquad \frac{1}{6} = 6\,)\overline{1.000}^{\,.166}$$

Changing a Decimal to a Fraction

To change a decimal to a fraction:

1. Remove the decimal point and make the resulting whole number the numerator: 0.2 = 2

2. The denominator is stated as 10 or a power of 10. In this example, 0.2 is read as two *tenths,* and therefore the denominator is 10.

$$0.2 = \frac{2}{10}$$ reduced to the lowest possible number is $$\frac{1}{5}$$

ADDITIONAL EXAMPLES

$$0.75 = \frac{75}{100} = \frac{3}{4} \qquad 0.025 = \frac{25}{1000} = \frac{1}{40}$$

Calculation Of Drug Dosages

Although most hospital pharmacies dispense drugs as single doses or in a unit dose system, there are occasions when the nurse must compute a drug dosage since it differs from the dose of the drug that is available. This is particularly true of small hospitals, nursing homes, physician's offices, and outpatient clinics that may not have a complete range of all available doses for a particular drug. Because certain situations may require computing the desired amount of drug to be given, nurses must be familiar with the calculation of all forms of drug dosages.

SYSTEMS OF MEASUREMENT

There are three systems of measurement of drug dosages: the **metric system, the apothecaries' system,** and **household measurements.** The metric system is the most commonly used system of measurement in medicine. A physician may prescribe a drug dosage in the apothecaries' system, but for the most part this ancient system of measurements is only occasionally used. The household system is rarely used in a hospital setting, but may be used to measure drug dosages in the home.

The Metric System

The metric system uses decimals (or the decimal system). In the metric system, the **gram** is the unit of weight, the **liter** the unit of volume, and the **meter** the unit of length.

Table 3-1 lists the measurements used in the metric system. The abbreviations for the measurements are given in parenthesis.

The Apothecaries' System

The apothecaries' system uses whole numbers and fractions. Decimals are *not* used in this system. The whole numbers are written as lower case Roman numerals, for example x instead of 10, or v instead of 5.

The units of weight in the apothecaries' system are **grains, drams,** and **ounces.** The units of volume are **minims, fluid drams,** and **fluid ounces.** The units of measurement in this system are not based on exact measurements.

Table 3-2 lists the measurements used in the apothecaries' system. The abbreviations (or symbols) for the measurements are given in parenthesis.

Table 3-1. Metric Measurements

WEIGHT

The unit of weight is the gram
1 kilogram (kg) = 1000 grams (g)
1 milligram (mg) = 0.001 gram (g)
1 microgram (mcg) = 0.000001 gram (g)
1 nanogram (ng) = 0.000000001 gram (g)

VOLUME

The unit of volume is the liter
1 decaliter (dL) = 10 liters (L)
1 liter (L) = 1000 milliliters (mL)
1 milliliter (mL) = 0.001 liter (L)

LENGTH

The unit of length is the meter
1 meter (m) = 100 centimeters (cm)
1 centimeter (cm) = 0.01 meter (m)
1 millimeter (mm) = 0.001 meter (m)

Table 3-2. Apothecaries' Measurements

WEIGHT

The units of weight are grains, drams, and ounces
60 grains (gr) = 1 dram (ʒ)
1 ounce (ʒ) = 480 grains (gr)

VOLUME

The units of volume are minims, fluid drams, and fluid ounces
1 fluid dram (fl ʒ) = 60 minims (ℳ)
1 fluid ounce = (fl ʒ) = 8 fluid drams

Household Measurements

When used, household measurements are for volume only. In the hospital, household measurements are rarely used because they are inaccurate when used to measure drug dosages. On occasion, the nurse may use the pint, quart, or gallon when ordering, irrigating, or sterilizing solutions or stock solutions. For ease in taking a medication at home the physician may order a drug dosage in household measurements.

Table 3-3 lists the more common household measurements.

Conversion Between Systems

To convert between systems, it is necessary to know the equivalents, or what is equal to what in each system. Table 3-4 lists the more common equivalents. These equivalents are only *approximate* because the three systems are different and are not truly equal to each other.

Several methods may be used to convert from one system to another using an equivalent, but most conversions can be done by using proportion.

EXAMPLES Convert 120 mg (metric) to grains (apothecaries')

Using proportion and the known equivalent 60 mg = gr i (1 grain)

$$1 \text{ gr}:60 \text{ mg}::X \text{ gr}:120 \text{ mg}$$
$$60 X = 120$$
$$X = 2 \text{ gr (grains or gr ii)}$$

Table 3-3. Household Measurements

3 teaspoons (tsp) = 1 tablespoon (tbsp)
2 tablespoons (tbsp) = 1 ounce (oz)
2 pints (pt) = 1 quart (qt)
4 quarts (qt) = 1 gallon

Table 3-4. Approximate Equivalents		
Metric	**Apothecaries'**	**Household**
WEIGHT		
0.1 mg	gr $\frac{1}{600}$	
0.15 mg	gr $\frac{1}{400}$	
0.2 mg	gr $\frac{1}{300}$	
0.3 mg	gr $\frac{1}{200}$	
0.4 mg	gr $\frac{1}{150}$	
0.6 mg	gr $\frac{1}{100}$	
1 mg	gr $\frac{1}{60}$	
2 mg	gr $\frac{1}{30}$	
4 mg	gr $\frac{1}{15}$	
6 mg	gr $\frac{1}{10}$	
8 mg	gr $\frac{1}{8}$	
10 mg	gr $\frac{1}{6}$	
15 mg	gr $\frac{1}{4}$	
20 mg	gr $\frac{1}{3}$	
30 mg	gr ss ($\frac{1}{2}$)	
60 mg	gr 1	
100 mg	gr i ss (1$\frac{1}{2}$)	
120 mg	gr ii	
1 g (1000 mg)	gr xv	
VOLUME		
0.06 mL	min (ɱ) i	
1 mL	min (ɱ) xv or xvi	
4 mL	fluidram (fl ʒ) i	1 teaspoon (tsp)
15 mL	fluidrams (fl ʒ) iv	$\frac{1}{2}$ ounce (oz)
30 mL	fluid ounce (fl ʒ) i	1 ounce (oz)
500 mL	1 pint (pt)	1 pint (pt)
1000 mL (1 liter)	1 quart (qt)	1 quart (qt)

Note the use of the abbreviations gr and mg when setting up the proportion. This shows that the proportion was stated correctly and helps in identifying the answer as 2 *grains*.

Convert gr 1/100 (apothecaries') to mg (metric)

Using proportion and the known equivalent 60 mg = 1 gr:

If there are 60 milligrams in 1 grain, there are X milligrams in 1/100 gr

$$60 \text{ mg:1 gr::X mg:1/100 gr}$$

$$X = 60 \times \frac{1}{100} = \frac{60}{100} = \frac{3}{5}$$

$$X = \frac{3}{5} \text{ mg}$$

or

$$\frac{60 \text{ mg}}{1 \text{ gr}} = \frac{X \text{ mg}}{1/100} \text{ gr}$$

$$X = 60 \text{ X} \frac{1}{100} = \frac{60}{100} = \frac{3}{5}$$

$$X = \frac{3}{5} \text{ mg}$$

Fractions are *not* used in the metric system, therefore the fraction must be converted to a decimal by dividing the denominator into the numerator, or 3 ÷ 5 = 0.6 or

$$5 \overline{)3.0}^{.6}$$

Therefore, gr 1/100 is equal to 0.6 mg.

When setting up the proportion, the apothecaries' system was written in Arabic numbers instead of Roman numerals, and their order was reversed (1 gr instead of gr i) so that all numbers and abbreviations are uniform in presentation.

Convert 0.3 milligrams (mg) [metric] to grains (gr) [apothecaries'].

Using proportion and the known equivalent 1 mg = gr 1/60

$$1/60 \text{ gr:1 mg::X gr:0.3 mg}$$

$$X = \frac{1}{60} \times 0.3 = \frac{0.3}{60} = \frac{3}{600} = \frac{1}{200}$$

$$X = \frac{1}{200} \text{ grain}$$

or

$$\frac{1/60}{1 \text{ mg}} = \frac{X \text{ gr}}{0.3 \text{ mg}}$$

$$X = \frac{1}{60} \times 0.3 = \frac{0.3}{60} = \frac{3}{600} = \frac{1}{200}$$

$$X = \frac{1}{200 \text{ gr}}$$

Therefore, 0.3 mg equals gr 1/200

There is no rule stating which equivalent must be used. In the above problem, another equivalent (60 mg = 1 grain) also could have been used. If 60 mg = 1 gr is used, the proportion would be

$$60 \text{ mg:1 gr::0.3 mg:X gr}$$

$$60 \text{ X} = 0.3$$

$$X = 0.005$$

or

$$\frac{60 \text{ mg}}{1 \text{ gr}} = \frac{0.3 \text{ mg}}{X \text{ gr}}$$

$$60 \text{ X} = 0.3$$

$$X = 0.005$$

Therefore 0.3 mg equals 0.005 grains.

Because decimals are not used in the apothecaries' system, this decimal answer must be converted to a fraction. 0.005 is 5/1000, which, when reduced to its lowest terms, is 1/200. The final answer is now 0.3 mg equals gr 1/200.

Converting Within a System

Sometimes it is necessary to convert within the same system, for example, changing grams (g) to milligrams (mg) or milligrams to grams. Proportion and a known equivalent also may be used for this type of conversion.

EXAMPLE

Convert 0.1 gram (g) to milligrams (mg)
Using proportion and the known equivalent 1000 mg = 1 g

$$1000 \text{ mg}:1 \text{ g}::X \text{ mg}: 0.1 \text{ g}$$
$$X = 1000 \times 0.1$$
$$X = 100 \text{ mg}$$

or

$$\frac{1000 \text{ mg}}{1 \text{ g}} = \frac{X \text{ mg}}{0.1 \text{ g}}$$
$$X = 1000 \times 0.1$$
$$X = 100 \text{ mg}$$

Therefore 0.1 gram (g) equals 100 milligrams (mg)

ORAL DOSAGES OF DRUGS

Under certain circumstances, it may be necessary to compute an oral drug dosage, because the dosage ordered by the physician may not be available, or the dosage may have been written in the apothecaries' system and the drug or container label is in metric.

Tablets and Capsules

To find the correct dosage of a solid oral preparation, the following formula may be used:

$$\frac{\text{dose desired}}{\text{dose on hand}} = \text{dose administered (the unknown or X)}$$

This formula may be abbreviated as

$$\frac{D}{H} = X$$

When the dose ordered by the physician (dose desired) is written in the *same system* as the dose on the drug container (dose on hand), these two figures may be inserted into the formula.

EXAMPLE

The physician orders ascorbic acid 100 mg (metric)
The drug is available as ascorbic acid 50 mg (metric)

$$\frac{D}{H} = X$$

$$\frac{100 \text{ mg}}{50 \text{ mg}} \begin{array}{l}\text{(dose desired)}\\\text{(dose on hand)}\end{array} = 2 \text{ tablets of 50 mg ascorbic acid}$$

If the physician had ordered ascorbic acid 0.5 g and the drug container was labeled ascorbic acid 250 mg, a *conversion of grams to milligrams* (because the drug container is labeled in milligrams) would be necessary before this formula can be used. If the 0.5 g were *not* converted to milligrams, the fraction of the formula would look like this:

$$\frac{0.5 \text{ grams}}{250 \text{ milligrams}}$$

A fraction **must** be stated in *like terms*; therefore proportion may be used to convert grams to milligrams.

$$1000 \text{ mg}: 1 \text{ g}::X \text{ mg}:0.5 \text{ g}$$
$$X = 1000 \times 0.5$$
$$X = 500 \text{ mg}$$
$$\frac{D}{H} = X$$
$$\frac{500 \text{ mg}}{250 \text{ mg}} = 2 \text{ tablets of 250 mg ascorbic acid}$$

As with all fractions, the numerator and the denominator must be of like terms, for example, milligrams over milligrams or grams over grams. Errors in using this and other drug formulas, as well as proportions, will be reduced if the entire dose is written rather than just the numbers.

$$\frac{100 \text{ mg}}{50 \text{ mg}} \text{ rather than } \frac{100}{50}$$

This will eliminate the possibility of using *unlike* terms in the fraction.

Even if the physician's order was written in the apothecaries' system, the drug container will most likely be labeled in the metric system. A conversion of *apothecaries' to metric* will now be necessary because the drug label is written in the metric system.

EXAMPLE

The physician's order reads: codeine sulfate gr 1/4 (apothecarie's)

The drug container is labeled: codeine sulfate 15 mg (metric)

Grains must be converted to milligrams OR milligrams converted to grains.

Grains to milligrams

$$60 \text{ mg:}1 \text{ gr::X mg:}1/4 \text{ gr}$$

$$X = 60 \times \frac{1}{4}$$

$$X = 15 \text{ mg}$$

or

$$\frac{60 \text{ mg}}{1 \text{ gr}} = \frac{X \text{ mg}}{1/4 \text{ gr}}$$

$$X = 60 \times \frac{1}{4}$$

$$X = 15 \text{ mg}$$

Therefore, 1/4 grain is approximately equivalent to 15 mg

Milligrams to grains

$$60 \text{ mg:}1 \text{ gr::}15 \text{ mg:X gr}$$

$$60 \text{ X} = 15$$

$$X = 1\backslash4 \text{ gr}$$

or

$$\frac{60 \text{ mg}}{1 \text{ gr}} = \frac{15 \text{ mg}}{X \text{ gr}}$$

$$60 \text{ X} = 15$$

$$X = \frac{1}{4} \text{ grain}$$

Therefore, 15 mg is approximately equivalent to 1/4 grain

The formula $\dfrac{D}{H} = X$ can now be used

$$\frac{D}{H} = X$$

$$\frac{15 \text{ mg}}{15 \text{ mg}} = 1 \text{ tablet}$$

or

$$\frac{1/4 \text{ gr}}{1/4 \text{ gr}} = 1 \text{ tablet}$$

Liquids

In liquid drugs, there is a specific amount of drug in a given volume of solution. For example, if a container is labeled as 10 mg per 5 mL (or 10 mg/5 mL),

this means that for every 5 mL of solution there is 10 mg of drug.

As with tablets and capsules, the prescribed dose of the drug may not be the same as what is on hand (or available). For example, the physician may order 20 mg of an oral liquid preparation and the bottle is labeled as 10 mg/5 mL.

The formula for computing the dosage of oral liquids is

$$\frac{\text{dose desired}}{\text{dose on hand}} \times \text{quantity} = \text{volume administered}$$

This may be abbreviated as

$$\frac{D}{H} \times Q = X$$

The quantity (or **Q**) in this formula is the amount of liquid in which the available drug is contained. For example, if the label states that there is 15 mg/5 mL, 5 mL is the *quantity* (or volume) in which there is 15 mg of this drug.

EXAMPLE

The physician orders oxacillin sodium 125 mg PO oral suspension. The drug is labeled as 250 mg/5 mL. The 5 mL is the amount (quantity or **Q**) that contains 250 mg of the drug.

$$\frac{D}{H} \times Q = X \text{ (the liquid amount to be given)}$$

$$\frac{125 \text{ mg}}{250 \text{ mg}} \times 5 = X$$

$$\frac{1}{2} \times 5 = 2.5 \text{ mL}$$

Therefore, 2.5 mL contains the desired dose of 125 mg of oxacillin oral suspension.

Liquid drugs may also be ordered in drops (gtt) or minims. With the former, a medicine dropper is usually supplied with the drug and is always used to measure the ordered dosage. Eye droppers are not standardized, and therefore the size of a drop from one eye dropper may be different than one from another eye dropper.

To measure an oral liquid drug in minims, a measuring glass *calibrated in minims* must be used.

PARENTERAL DOSAGES OF DRUGS

Drugs for parenteral use must be in liquid form before they are administered. Parenteral drugs may be available in the following forms:

1. As liquids in disposable cartridges or disposable syringes that contain a specific amount of

a drug in a specific volume, for example, meperidine 50 mg/mL. After administration, the cartridge or syringe is discarded.

2. In ampules or vials that contain a specific amount of the liquid form of the drug in a specific volume. The vials may be single-dose vials or multidose vials. A multidose vial contains more than one dose of the drug.
3. In ampules or vials that contain powder or crystals, to which a liquid (called a **diluent**) must be added before the drug can be removed from the vial and administered. Vials may be single dose or multidose vials.

Parenteral Drugs in Disposable Syringes or Cartridges

There may be instances when a specific dosage strength is not available and it will be necessary to administer less than the amount contained in the syringe.

EXAMPLE

The physician orders diazepam 5 mg IM. The drug is available as a 2 mL disposable syringe labeled 5 mg/mL.

$$\frac{D}{H} \times Q = X$$

$$\frac{5\ mg}{10\ mg} \times 2\ mL = X$$

$$X = \frac{1}{2} \times 2 = 1\ mL$$

Note that since the syringe contained 2 mL of the drug and that *each* mL contains 5 mg of the drug, there is a total of 10 mg of the drug in the syringe. Because there is 10 mg of the drug in the syringe, half of the liquid in the syringe (1 mL) is discarded and the remaining half (1 mL) is administered to give the prescribed dose of 5 mg.

Parenteral Drugs in Ampules and Vials

If the drug is in liquid form in the ampule or vial, the desired amount is withdrawn from the ampule or vial. In some instances, the entire amount is used; in others, only part of the total amount is withdrawn from the ampule or vial and administered.

Whenever the dose to be administered is different from the label, the volume to be administered must be calculated. To determine the volume to be administered, the formula for liquid preparations is used. The calculations are the same as for parenteral drugs in disposable syringes or cartridges given in the preceding section.

EXAMPLES

The physician orders chlorpromazine 12.5 mg IM. The drug is available as chlorpromazine 25 mg/mL in a 1 mL ampule

$$\frac{D}{H} \times Q = X$$

$$\frac{12.5\ mg}{25\ mg} \times 1\ mL = X$$

$$\frac{1}{2} \times 1\ mL = \frac{1}{2}\ mL\ (or\ 0.5\ mL)\ volume\ to\ be\ administered.$$

The physician orders hydroxyzine 12.5 mg
The drug is available as hydroxyzine 25 mg/mL in 10 mL vials.

$$\frac{D}{H} \times Q = X$$

$$\frac{12.5\ mg}{25\ mg} \times 1\ mL = \frac{1}{2}\ mL\ (or\ 0.5\ mL)$$

Therefore 0.5 mL is withdrawn from the 10 mL multidose vial and administered. In this example, the amount in this or any multidose vial is *not* entered into the equation. What is entered into the equation as quantity (Q) is the amount of the available drug that is contained in a specific volume.

When the dose is less than 1 mL, it may be necessary, in some instances, to convert the answer to minims. A conversion factor of 15 or 16 minims/mL may be used.

EXAMPLES

The physician orders chlorpromazine 10 mg IM
The drug is available as chlorpromazine 25 mg/mL

$$\frac{10\ mg}{25\ mg} \times 1\ mL = X$$

$$\frac{2}{5} \times 1\ mL = \frac{2}{5}\ mL$$

$$\frac{2}{5} \times 15\ minims = 6\ minims$$

In this example 15 minims = 1 mL is used because 15 can be divided by 5.

The physician's order reads methadone 2.5 mg IM
The drug is available as methadone 10 mg/mL

$$\frac{2.5\ mg}{10\ mg} \times 1\ mL = X$$

$$\frac{1}{4} \times 1\ mL = X$$

$$\frac{1}{4} \times 16\ minims = 4\ minims$$

Because 16 (and not 15) minims can be divided by 4, the conversion factor of 16 is used.

WARNING: ALWAYS CHECK DRUG LABELS CAREFULLY. Some may be labeled in a manner different from others.

EXAMPLE

a **2**-mL ampule labeled: **2** mL = 0.25 mg

a **2**-mL ampule labeled: **1** mL = 5 mg

In these two examples, one manufacturer states the entire dose contained in the ampule: 2 mL = 0.25 mg. The other manufacturer gives the dose per milliliter: 1 mL = 5 mg. In this 2-mL ampule, there is a total of 10 mg.

Parenteral Drugs in Dry Form

Some parenteral drugs are available as a crystal or a powder. Because these drugs have a short life in liquid form, they are available in ampules or vials in dry form and must be made a liquid (reconstituted) before they are removed and administered. Some of these products have directions for reconstitution on the label or on the enclosed package insert. The manufacturer may give either of the following information for reconstitution: (1) the name of the diluent(s) that must be used with the drug, or (2) the amount of diluent that must be added to the drug.

In some instances, the manufacturer supplies a diluent with the drug. If a diluent is supplied, no other stock diluent should be used. Before a drug is reconstituted, the label is carefully checked for instructions.

EXAMPLES

Methicillin sodium: To reconstitute 1 g vial add 1.5 mL of Sterile Water for Injection or Sodium Chloride for Injection. Each reconstituted mL contains approximately 500 mg of methicillin.

Mechlorethamine: Reconstitute with 10 mL of Sterile Water for Injection or Sodium Chloride Injection. The solution now contains 1 mg/mL of mechlorethamine.

If there is any doubt about the reconstitution of the dry form of a drug and there are no manufacturer's directions, the hospital pharmacist should be consulted.

Once a diluent is added, the volume to be administered is determined. In some cases, the entire amount is given; in others, a part (or fraction) of the total amount contained in the vial or ampule is given.

Following reconstitution of any multidose vial, the following information *must* be added to the label:

- amount of diluent added
- dose of drug in mL (500 mg/mL, 10 mg/2 mL, etc.)
- the date of reconstitution
- the expiration date (the date after which any unused solution is discarded)

Calculating IV Flow Rates

When the physician orders a drug added to an IV fluid, the amount of fluid to be administered over a specified period, such as 125 mL/h or 1000 mL over 8 hours must be included in the written order. If no infusion rate had been ordered, 1 L (1000 mL) of IV fluid should infuse over 6 to 8 hours.

To allow the IV fluid to infuse over a specified period, the IV flow rate must be determined. Before using one of the methods below, the drop factor must be known. Drip chambers on the various types of IV fluid administration sets vary. Some deliver 15 drops/mL and others deliver more or less than this number. This is called the *drop factor*. The drop factor (number of drops/mL) is given on the package containing the drip chamber and IV tubing. Three methods for determining the IV infusion rate follow. Methods 1 and 2 can be used when the known factors are the total amount of solution, the drop factor, and the number of hours over which the solution is to be infused are known.

METHOD 1

Step 1. Total amount of solution ÷ number of hours = number of mL/hour

Step 2. mL/hour ÷ 60 minutes/hr = number of mL/minute

Step 3. mL/minute X drop factor = number of drops/minute

EXAMPLE

1000 mL of an IV solution is to infuse over a period of 8 hours. The drop factor is 14.

Step 1. 1000 mL ÷ 8 hours = 125 mL/hour

Step 2. 125 ÷ 60 minutes = 2.08 mL/minute

Step 3. 2.08 × 14 = 29 drops/minute

METHOD 2

Step 1. Total amount of solution ÷ number of hours = number of mL/h

Step 2. mL/h × drop factor ÷ 60 = number of drops per minute

EXAMPLE

1000 mL of an IV solution is to infuse over a period of 6 hours. The drop factor is 12

Step 1. 1000 mL ÷ 6 = 166.6 mL/hour

Step 2. 166.6 × 12 ÷ 60 = 33.33 (33 to 34) drops/minute

METHOD 3

This method may be used when the desired amount of solution to be infused in 1 hour is known or written as a physician's order.

$$\frac{\text{drops/mL of given set (drop factor)}}{60 \text{ (minutes in an hour)}} \times \text{total hourly volume} = \text{drops/minute}$$

EXAMPLE

If a set delivers 15 drops/minute and 240 mL is to be infused in 1 hour:

$$\frac{15}{60} \times 240 = \frac{1}{4} \times 240 = 60 \text{ drops/minute}$$

Oral or Parenteral Drug Dosages Based on Weight

The dosage of an oral or parenteral drug may be based on the patient's weight. In many instances, references give the dosage based on the weight in kilograms (kg) rather than pounds (lb). There are 2.2 pounds in 1 kilogram.

When the dosage of a drug is based on weight the physician, in most all instances, computes and orders the dosage to be given. However, errors can occur for any number of reasons. The nurse should be able to calculate a drug dosage based on weight to detect any type of error that may have been made in the prescribing or dispensing of a drug whose dosage is based on weight.

To convert a known weight in kilograms to pounds, multiply the known weight by 2.2.

EXAMPLES

Patient's weight in kilograms is 54

$54 \times 2.2 = 118.8$ (or 119) pounds

Patient's weight in kilograms is 61.5

$61.5 \times 2.2 = 135.3$ (or 135) pounds

To convert a known weight in pounds to kilograms divide the known weight by 2.2

EXAMPLES

Patient's weight in pounds is 142

$142 \div 2.2 = 64.5$ kilograms

Child's weight in pounds is 43

$43 \div 2.2 = 19.5$ kilograms

Once the weight is converted to pounds or kilograms, this information is used to determine drug dosage.

EXAMPLES

A drug dose is 5 mg/kg/day.

The patient weighs 135 lb which is converted to 61.2 kg

61.2 kg X 5 mg = 306.8 mg

Proportion also can be used:

5 mg:1 kg::X mg:61.2 kg

X = 306.8 mg

A drug dose is 60 mg/kg/day IV in three equally divided doses.

The patient weighs 143 lb which is converted to 65 kg

65 kg X 60 mg = 3900 mg/day

3900 mg ÷ 3(doses per day) = 1300 mg each dose

If the drug dose is based on body surface area (m^2) the same method of calculation may be used.

EXAMPLE

A drug dose is 60 to 75 mg/m^2 as a single IV injection.

The body surface area of a patient is determined by means of a nomogram for estimating body surface area (see appendix) and is found to be 1.8 m^2. The physician orders 60 mg/m^2.

60 mg $\times$ 1.8 m^2 = 108 mg

Proportion also can be used:

60 mg:1 m^2:: X mg: 1.8 m^2

X = 108 mg

TEMPERATURES

Two scales used in the measuring of temperatures are **Fahrenheit (F)** and **Celsius (C)** (also known as **centigrade**). On the Fahrenheit scale, the freezing point of water is 32° F and the boiling point of water is 212° F. On the Celsius scale, 0° C is the freezing point of water and 100° C is the boiling point of water.

To convert from Celsius to Fahrenheit the following formula may be used:

F = 9/5 C + 32 [9/5 times the temperature in Celsius then add 32]

EXAMPLE

Convert 38° C to Fahrenheit

$$F = \frac{9}{5} \times 38° + 32$$

$$F = 68.4 + 32$$

$$F = 100.4°$$

To convert from Fahrenheit to Celsius the following formula may be used:

C = 5/9 (°F − 32) [5/9 times the temperature in Fahrenheit minus 32]

EXAMPLE

Convert 100° F to Celsius

$$C = \frac{5}{9} \times (100 - 32)$$

$$C = \frac{5}{9} \times 68$$

$$C = 37.77 \text{ or } 37.8°$$

Instead of remembering two formulas, a single formula may be used to convert to either scale.

$$\frac{9}{5} C = F - 32$$

To convert 101.4° F to C

$$\frac{9}{5} C = 101.4 - 32$$

$$\frac{9}{5} C = 69.4$$

$$C \frac{5}{9} = 69.4 \times —$$

$$C = 38.55°$$

To convert 38.2° C to F

$$\frac{9}{5} C = F - 32$$

$$\frac{9}{5} \times 38.2 = F - 32$$

$$68.76 = F - 32$$

$$F = 68.76 + 32$$

$$F = 100.76° \text{ (or } 100.8°)$$

A single proportion also may be used to convert Celsius to Fahrenheit or Fahrenheit to Celsius. When proportion is used only one formula need be remembered.

C:F−32::5:9

EXAMPLES

Convert 30° Celsius to Fahrenheit	*Convert 50° Fahrenheit to Celsius*
C:F − 32::5:9	C:F − 32::5:9
30:F − 32::5:9	C:50 − 32::5:9
270 = 5 F − 160	9 C = 5(50 − 32)
5 F = 270 + 160	9 C = 5 × 18
5 F = 430	9 C = 90
F = 86°	C = 10°

PEDIATRIC DOSAGES

The dosages of drugs given to children are usually less than those given to adults. The dosage may be based on age, weight, or body surface area (BSA).

Body Surface Area

Charts are used to determine the BSA in square meters according to the child's height and weight. Once the BSA is determined, the following formula is used:

$$\frac{\text{surface area of the child in square meters}}{\text{surface area of an adult in square meters*}} \times \text{usual adult dose} = \text{pediatric dose}$$

Weight

Pediatric as well as adult dosages may also be based on the patient's weight in pounds or kilograms. The method of converting pounds to kilograms or kilograms to pounds is explained in a previous section.

EXAMPLE

5 mg/kg

0.5 mg/lb

Today, most pediatric dosages are clearly given by the manufacturer, thus eliminating the need for formulas except for determining the dose of some drugs based on the child's weight or BSA.

SOLUTIONS

A **solute** is a substance dissolved in a **solvent.** A solvent may be water or some other liquid. Usually water is used for preparing a solution unless another liquid is specified. Solutions are prepared by using a solid (powder, tablet) and a liquid, or a liquid and a liquid. Today, most solutions are prepared by a pharmacist and not by the nurse.

Examples of how solutions may be labeled include:

10 mg/mL—10 mg of the drug in each milliliter
1:1000—a solution denoting strength or 1 part of the drug per 1000 parts
5 mg/teaspoon—5 mg of the drug in each teaspoon (home use)

The figure for the average BSA of an adult in square meters is 1.7.

4

The Nursing Process

Key Terms

Assessment
Evaluation
Implementation
Independent nursing
actions
Nursing diagnosis
Nursing process
Objective data
Planning
Subjective data

Chapter Outline

Chapter Objectives

On completion of this chapter the student will:

- *List the five parts of the nursing process*
- *Discuss assessment, nursing diagnosis, planning, implementation, and evaluation as they apply to the administration of pharmacologic agents*
- *Differentiate between objective and subjective data*
- *Discuss and demonstrate how the nursing process may be used in daily life, as well as when administering pharmacologic agents*

Scherer JC, Roach S: INTRODUCTORY CLINICAL PHARMACOLOGY,
FIFTH EDITION © 1996 Lippincott-Raven Publishers

The *nursing process* is a framework for nursing action consisting of problem-solving steps that help members of the healthcare team provide effective patient care.

The nursing process is a specific and orderly plan that is used to identify patient problems, develop and implement a plan of action, and then evaluate the results of nursing activities, including the administration of drugs.

The five parts of this process are used not only in nursing but in our daily lives. For example, when buying a television, we may first think about whether we need it and then price it in different stores (assessment). We may have to decide how to pay for the television (planning) and then buy it (implementation). After purchase and use, we evaluate the television set (evaluation).

Using the nursing process requires practice, experience, and a constant updating of knowledge. The nursing process is used in this text only as it applies to drug administration. It is not within the scope of this textbook to list *all* of the assessments, plans, implementations, and evaluations for the medical diagnosis that require the administration of a specific pharmacologic agent.

THE FIVE PARTS OF THE NURSING PROCESS

Although there are various ways of describing the nursing process, it generally consists of five parts: *assessment, nursing diagnosis, planning, implementation,* and *evaluation.* Each part is applicable, with modification, to the administration of drugs.

Assessment

Assessment involves collecting *objective* and *subjective* data. *Objective data* are facts obtained by means of a physical assessment or physical examination. *Subjective data* are facts supplied by the patient or the patient's family.

Assessments are both initial and ongoing. An *initial* assessment is made based on objective and subjective data collected when the patient is first seen in a hospital, outpatient clinic, physician's office, or other type of healthcare facility. The initial assessment usually is more thorough and provides a data base from which decisions can be made. The initial assessment also provides information that is analyzed to identify problems that can be resolved or alleviated by nursing actions.

Objective data are obtained during an initial assessment through activities such as examining the skin, obtaining vital signs, palpating a lesion, and auscultating the lungs. A review of any recent laboratory tests and diagnostic studies also are part of the initial physical assessment. Subjective data are acquired during an initial assessment by obtaining information from the patient, such as a family history of disease, allergy history, occupational history, a description (in the patient's words) of the current illness or chief complaint, a medical history, and a drug history.

An *ongoing* assessment is one that is made at the time of each patient contact and may include the collection of objective data, subjective data, or both. The scope of an ongoing assessment depends on many factors, such as the patient's diagnosis, the severity of illness, the response to treatment, and the prescribed medical or surgical treatment.

The assessment phase of the nursing process can be applied to the administration of drugs with objective and subjective data collected before and after administration of a drug. Examples of objective data include blood pressure, pulse, respiratory rate, temperature, weight, examination of the skin, examination of an intravenous infusion site, and auscultation of the lungs. Subjective data include any statement made by the patient about relief or nonrelief of pain or other symptoms after administration of a drug.

The extent of the assessment and collection of objective and subjective data before and after a drug is administered will depend on the type of drug and the reason for administering the drug.

Nursing Diagnosis

After the data collected during assessment are analyzed, the patient's needs (problems) are identified and one or more nursing diagnoses are formulated. A nursing diagnosis is not a medical diagnosis, but a description of the patient's problems and their probable or actual related causes, based on the subjective and objective data in the data base. A nursing diagnosis identifies those problems that can be solved or prevented by *independent nursing actions*. Independent nursing actions are actions that do not require a physician's order and may be legally performed by a nurse.

The North American Nursing Diagnosis Association (NANDA) has approved a list of diagnostic categories to be used in formulating a nursing diagnosis. This list of diagnostic categories is periodically revised and updated. Some of the nursing diagnoses developed by NANDA may be used to identify patient's problems associated with drug therapy. In some instances, nursing diagnoses may apply to a specific group or type of drug, for example, fluid volume deficit related to diuresis secondary to administration of a diuretic.

Planning

After data are collected, they are sorted and analyzed, and a plan of action or patient care plan is developed. For example, during the initial assessment interview to collect subjective data, the patient may report an allergy to penicillin. This information is important, and the nurse must now plan the best method of informing all members of the health team of the patient's allergy to penicillin.

Planning also involves the setting of goals, which are patient-oriented. For example, a patient may need to apply a skin ointment after discharge from the hospital. The planned goal for this patient is stated as "will be able to demonstrate the technique of ointment application."

The planning phase also lays the groundwork or plans the steps for carrying out nursing activities that are specific and that will meet the stated goals. This phase also anticipates the implementation phase, or the carrying out of nursing actions that are specific for the drug being administered. If, for example, the patient is to receive a medication by the intravenous route, the nurse must plan the materials needed and the patient instruction for administration of the drug by this route. In this instance, the planning phase occurs immediately before the implementation phase and is necessary to carry out the technique of intravenous administration correctly. Failing to plan effectively may result in forgetting to obtain all of the materials necessary for drug administration.

Setting goals that are patient-oriented and planning for nursing actions that are specific for the drug to be administered can result in greater accuracy in drug administration, patient understanding of the drug regimen, and improved patient compliance with the prescribed drug therapy after discharge from the hospital.

Implementation

Implementation is the carrying out of a plan of action, and is a natural outgrowth of the assessment and planning phases of the nursing process. When related to the administration of pharmacologic agents, implementation refers to the preparation and administration of one or more drugs to a specific patient. Before administering a drug, the nurse reviews the subjective and objective data obtained on admission and considers any additional data, such as blood pressure, pulse, or a statement made by the patient. The decision of whether to administer the drug is based on an analysis of all information. For example, a patient is hypertensive and is supposed to receive a medication to lower his blood pressure. Objective data obtained at the time of admission included a blood pressure of 188/110. Additional objective data obtained immediately before the administration of the drug included a blood pressure of 182/110. A decision was made by the nurse to administer the drug because there was minimal change in his blood pressure. If, however, the patient's blood pressure was 132/88 and this was only the second dose of medication, the nurse could decide to withhold the medication and contact the physician. Giving or withholding a medication or contacting the patient's physician are nursing activities related to the implementation phase of the nursing process.

Evaluation

Evaluation is a decision-making process and determines the effectiveness of nursing management. When related to the administration of pharmacologic agents, this part of the nursing process can be used to evaluate the patient's response to drug therapy. Evaluation also may be used to determine if the patient or family member has understood the medication regimen.

To evaluate the patient's response to therapy, and depending on the drug administered, the nurse may check the patient's blood pressure in an hour, inquire whether pain has been relieved, or monitor the pulse every 15 minutes. After evaluation, certain other decisions may need to be made and plans of action implemented, for example, notifying the physician of a marked change in a patient's pulse and respiratory rate after a drug was administered or changing the bed linen because sweating occurred after administration of a drug to lower the patient's elevated temperature.

The nurse can evaluate the patient or family's understanding of the medication regimen by noting if one or both appear to understand the material that has been presented. Facial expressions may indicate that one or both do or do not understand what has been explained. The nurse also may ask questions about the information that has been given.

Chapter Summary

- The nursing process is a framework for nursing action consisting of problem-solving steps that help members of the healthcare team provide effective patient care.
- The five parts of the nursing process are: assessment, nursing diagnosis, planning, implementation, and evaluation.
- Assessment involves the collection of *objective* and *subjective* data.
- A nursing diagnosis is a description of the patient's problems and their probable or actual related causes based on the subjective and objective data in the data base.
- Planning involves setting patient-oriented goals.
- Implementation is carrying out a plan of action, and is a natural outgrowth of the assessment and planning phases of the nursing process.
- Evaluation is a decision-making process; it determines the effectiveness of nursing management.

Critical Thinking Exercise

Ms. Taylor is receiving three drugs for the treatment of difficulty breathing and swelling of her legs. When giving these drugs for the first time, what questions would you ask Ms. Taylor to obtain subjective data?

5

Patient and Family Teaching

Key Terms

Assessment
Evaluation
Implementation
Learning
Motivation
Nursing process
Planning
Teaching

Chapter Outline

Chapter Objectives

On completion of this chapter the student will:

- *Define teaching and learning*
- *Explain how the nursing process can be used to develop a teaching plan*
- *Identify important aspects of the teaching/learning process*
- *Identify nursing considerations included in a patient and family teaching plan*

*Scherer JC, Roach S: INTRODUCTORY CLINICAL PHARMACOLOGY,
FIFTH EDITION © 1996 Lippincott-Raven Publishers*

Patient teaching is an integral part of nursing. When a drug is prescribed, the patient and the family must be made aware of all information concerning the drug. The nurse is responsible for supplying the patient with accurate and up-to-date information about the drugs that are prescribed. The teaching/learning process is the means through which the patient is made aware of the medication regimen.

THE TEACHING/LEARNING PROCESS

Teaching is defined as an interactive process that promotes learning. Both the patient and the nurse must be actively involved if teaching is to be effective. *Learning* is acquiring new knowledge or skills. For learning to occur, a patient must be motivated (have the desire or see the need) to learn and have the ability to learn. The nurse is responsible for evaluating the patient's ability to learn.

Teaching strategies must reflect individual learning needs and ability. For example, a patient who speaks and reads only Spanish will not benefit from discharge instructions given in English or from instructions written in English. Other strategies must be implemented such as providing instructions written in Spanish or communicating the necessary information to the patient through another nurse who is fluent in the Spanish language.

Motivation depends on the patient's perception of the need to learn. Education concerning the disease process may be necessary for the patient to become motivated to learn. Encouraging patient participation in planning realistic and attainable goals promotes motivation as well.

Creating an accepting and positive atmosphere enhances learning. Physical discomfort affects the patient's ability to learn. A patient in pain is not able to concentrate and learning may be limited or impossible.

THE NURSING PROCESS AS A FRAMEWORK FOR PATIENT TEACHING

The *nursing process* is a systematic method of identifying patient health needs, devising a plan of care to meet the identified needs, initiating the plan, and evaluating its effectiveness. The nursing process provides the necessary framework to develop an effective teaching plan. The teaching plan differs from the nursing process, however, in that the nursing process encompasses all of the patient's healthcare needs while the teaching plan focuses primarily on the patient's learning needs. Nurses must be actively involved in teaching if they are to educate their patients about the proper way to take their medication, the possibility of adverse reactions, and the signs and symptoms of toxicity (if applicable).

Assessment

Assessment is the data-gathering phase of the nursing process. To develop an effective teaching plan, the nurse must first determine the patient's needs. Needs stem from two areas: (1) information the patient or family needs to know about a particular drug and (2) the patient or family member's ability to learn, accept, and use information.

Some drugs require relatively little information or teaching. For example, applying a nonprescription ointment to the skin requires only minimal teaching. Other drugs, such as insulin, require detailed information that may need to be given over several days.

At times, assessing an individual's ability to learn may be difficult. Most people readily understand what is being taught, but some cannot. For example, a visually impaired patient may be unable to read a label or printed directions supplied by the physician, pharmacist, or nurse. A printed card with directions for taking the medication is of little value in such a case. Another means of learning will have to be found.

Language and literacy skills must be evaluated. Some patients may not have the ability to read well. The nurse must carefully assess the patient's ability to communicate. Without accurate communication learning will not occur. If the patient has a learning impairment, perhaps a family member or friend can be included in the teaching process.

The nurse, through the assessment, determines what barriers or obstacles (if any) may prevent the patient or family member from fully understanding the material being presented. The assessment assists the nurse in choosing the best teaching methods and individualizing the teaching plan.

Nursing Diagnoses

The nursing diagnosis is formulated after analyzing the information obtained during the assessment phase. Most often nursing diagnoses related to the administration of drugs are associated with a risk for ineffective management, knowledge deficit, or noncompliance. Examples of nursing diagnoses related to the administration of drugs include the following:

Risk for Ineffective Management of Therapeutic Regimen related to lack of knowledge, indifference, other factors

Noncompliance with medication regimen related to indifference, lack of knowledge, other factors

Nursing diagnoses related to specific drug classifications are found in subsequent chapters.

Planning and Implementation

Planning is the actual development of strategies to be used in the teaching plan and the selection of information to be taught. The nurse develops a teaching plan based on the assessment. *Implementation* is the actual performance of the interventions identified in the teaching plan.

The teaching plan should include the following information: (1) therapeutic response expected from the drug; (2) adverse reactions to expect when taking the drug; (3) adverse reactions to report to the nurse and/or physician; (4) dosage and route; and (5) any special considerations of the particular drug prescribed.

Additional education may be necessary for special considerations of certain drugs, such as techniques of giving injections, applying topical patches, and instilling eye drops. Any special precautions for a particular drug are also included.

Teaching is individualized and done at an appropriate time for each patient. For example, patient teaching should *not* be done when there are visitors (unless they are to be involved in the administration of the patient's medications) immediately before discharge from the hospital, or if the patient has been sedated or is in pain.

Teaching is begun a day or more before discharge, at a time when the patient is alone and alert, and continued each day until dismissal. The nurse should gear teaching to the patient's level of understanding and, when necessary, provide written, as well as oral, instruction. If much information is given, it is often best to present the material in two or more sessions.

Evaluation

To determine the effectiveness of patient teaching, the nurse must evaluate the patient's knowledge of the material presented. *Evaluation* can be done in

several ways depending on the nature of the information. For example, if the patient is being taught to administer insulin, several demonstrations can be scheduled, followed by a demonstration by the patient with the nurse observing to evaluate the patient's technique effectively.

Questions such as "Do you understand?" or "Is there anything you don't understand?" are usually avoided because the patient may feel uncomfortable admitting a lack of understanding. When factual material is being evaluated, the nurse periodically asks the patient to list or repeat some of the information that was presented.

NURSING CONSIDERATIONS WHEN DEVELOPING A TEACHING PLAN

Teaching plans must be individualized because patients do not have identical needs and may lack knowledge about their prescribed medications. Areas covered in an individualized teaching plan vary depending on the drug prescribed, the physician's preference for including or excluding specific facts about the drug, and what the patient needs to know to take the drug correctly.

In teaching patients and their families, the nurse must select information relevant to a specific drug. Patient and family teaching is adapted to the individual's level of understanding. Medical terminology is avoided unless terms are explained or defined.

Drugs, Drug Containers, and Drug Storage

The following are important facts about drugs, drug containers, and the storage of drugs that must be considered when developing a teaching plan:

1. The term *drug* applies to both nonprescription and prescription drugs.
2. A drug must be kept in the container in which it was dispensed or purchased. Some drugs require special containers, such as light-resistant (brown) bottles to prevent deterioration that may occur on exposure to light.
3. If any drug changes color or develops a new odor, a pharmacist must be consulted immediately about continued use of the drug.
4. The original label on the drug container must not be removed while it is used to hold the drug.

5. Two or more different drugs must never be mixed in one container, even for a brief time, because one drug may chemically affect another. Mixing drugs can also lead to mistaking one drug for another, especially when the size and color are similar.

6. The lid or cap of the container must be replaced immediately after removing the drug from the container. The lid or cap must be firmly snapped or screwed in place. Exposure to air or moisture shortens the life of most drugs.

7. Drugs requiring refrigeration are so labeled. The container must be returned to the refrigerator immediately after removing the medication.

8. *All* drugs must be kept out of the reach of children.

9. Unless otherwise directed, drugs must be stored in a cool, dry place.

10. Do not expose a drug to excessive sunlight, heat, cold, or moisture because deterioration may occur.

11. The *entire* label of the prescription or nonprescription drug container must be read, including the recommended dosage and warnings.

12. All directions printed on the label (eg, "shake well before using," "keep refrigerated," "take before meals") must be followed to ensure drug effectiveness.

13. In some instances, especially when an ointment or liquid drug is prescribed, some medication may remain after it is used or taken for the prescribed time. Some drugs have a short life (a few weeks to a few months) and may deteriorate or change chemically after a time. A prescription must *never* be saved for later use unless the physician so advises.

The Dosage Regimen

The dosage regimen is an important aspect of the teaching plan. The following general points must be taken into consideration when teaching about the dosage regimen:

1. Capsules or tablets should be taken with water unless the physician or pharmacist directs otherwise (eg, take with food, milk, or an antacid). Some liquids such as coffee, tea, fruit juice, and carbonated beverages may interfere with the action of some drugs.

2. A full glass of water is used when taking an oral drug. In some instances, it may be necessary to drink extra fluids during the day while taking certain medications.

3. Capsules are not to be chewed before swallowing; they must be swallowed whole. Tablets are not chewed unless labeled as "chewable." Some tablets have special coatings that are required for purposes such as proper absorption of the drug or prevention of irritation of the lining of the stomach.

4. The dose of a drug or the time interval between doses is *never* increased or decreased unless directed by a physician. A prescription drug or a physician-recommended nonprescription drug is not stopped or omitted except on the advice of a physician.

5. A prescribed or recommended drug is *not* discontinued unless advised by a physician.

6. If the symptoms for which a drug was prescribed do not improve, or become worse, the physician must be contacted as soon as possible because a change in dosage or a different drug may be necessary.

7. If a dose of a drug is omitted or forgotten, the next dose must *not* be doubled or the drug taken at more frequent intervals unless advised by a physician.

8. Other physicians, dentists, nurses, and health personnel must *always* be informed of all drugs (prescription and nonprescription) currently being taken on a regular or occasional basis.

9. The exact names of all prescription and nonprescription drugs currently being taken should be kept in a wallet or purse for instant reference when seeing a physician or dentist.

10. Check prescriptions carefully when obtaining refills from the pharmacy and report *any* changes in the prescription (eg, changes in color, size, shape) to the pharmacist or physician before taking the drug since an error may have occurred.

11. Wear a Medic-Alert bracelet or other type of identification when taking a drug for a long time, especially drugs such as anticoagulants, steroids, oral hypoglycemic agents, insulin, or digitalis. In case of an emergency, the bracelet ensures that medical personnel are aware of health problems and current drug therapy.

Adverse Drug Effects

Teaching the patient about adverse drug effects of the prescribed drug is essential when developing a teaching plan. The patient is taught the following general points about adverse drug effects:

1. All drugs cause adverse reactions (side effects). Examples of some of the more common adverse reactions are nausea, vomiting, diarrhea, constipation, skin rash, dizziness, drowsiness, and dry mouth. Some may be mild and disappear with time or when the physician adjusts the dosage. In some instances, mild reactions such as dry mouth may have to be tolerated. Some adverse reactions are potentially serious and even life-threatening.
2. Adverse effects are *always reported* to the physician as soon as possible.
3. Medical personnel must be informed of all drug allergies *before* any treatment or drug is given.

Family Members

The following points concerning family members are considered when developing a teaching plan:

1. A drug prescribed for one family member is *never* given to another family member, relative, or friend unless directed to do so by a physician.
2. Family members or relatives should be made aware of all drugs, prescription and nonprescription, that are currently being taken.

Chapter Summary

- Patient teaching is an important aspect of nursing care. Patients must be knowledgeable about the drugs prescribed if they are to follow the proper drug regimen to obtain a therapeutic response and monitor for adverse reactions.

- The teaching/learning process is the method by which patients learn about their drug regimen. Teaching is an interactive process that promotes learning. Learning is a process in which new information or skills are obtained. To be effective, the teaching plan must be individualized to meet the patient's learning needs.
- The nursing process provides the framework to develop a teaching plan. After assessing the patient's knowledge of the medication and learning needs, the nurse plans, implements, and evaluates the teaching program. The teaching plan includes: (1) the therapeutic response expected from the drug; (2) side effects to expect when taking the drug; (3) side effects to report; (4) the dosage and route; and (5) any special considerations for the particular drug(s) prescribed.

Critical Thinking Exercises

1. Locate the clinical educator in any healthcare agency in your community whose job it is to do patient education. Ask that person to share with you their thoughts and feelings on patient education, as well as any problems or pitfalls he or she has identified.
2. Interview friends or relatives about their knowledge of the medication(s) prescribed by their physician. Discuss with them the teaching they received prior to taking the drugs by nurses or other healthcare providers. What areas could have been included that were not discussed? How was the teaching/learning process evaluated? Can you identify any areas that could be improved?

The
Antiinfectives

II

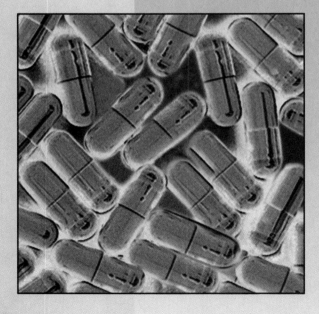

6

The Penicillins

Key Terms

Anaphylactic shock
Angioedema
Bacterial resistance
Bactericidal
Bacteriostatic
Cross-allergenicity
Cross-sensitivity
Culture and sensitivity tests
Hypersensitivity
Nonpathogenic
Pathogenic
Penicillinase
Prophylaxis
Pseudomembranous colitis
Superinfection

Chapter Outline

Chapter Objectives

On completion of this chapter the student will:

- *List the actions and uses of the penicillins*
- *List the adverse reactions associated with the administration of the penicillins*
- *Discuss the nursing implications associated with the administration of the penicillins*
- *Use the nursing process when administering a penicillin*

After the introduction of the sulfonamides, newer and more effective drugs were developed for the treatment of infections. The antibacterial properties of penicillin were recognized in 1928 by Sir Arthur Fleming while doing research on influenza. Ten years later British scientists studied the effects of penicillin on disease-causing microorganisms. It was not until 1941 that penicillin was used clinically in the treatment of infections. After the introduction of penicillin, more antibiotics were introduced.

With the increased early use of the penicillins, drug-resistant strains of microorganisms developed, making the penicillins less effective in treating infections.

The Penicillins

There are two types of penicillin: natural penicillin and the semisynthetic derivatives of penicillin (Summary Drug Table 6-1). The natural penicillins include penicillin G and penicillin V. The semisynthetic penicillins include: penicillin-resistant penicillins, such as cloxacillin and methicillin; aminopenicillins such as amoxicillin and ampicillin; and the extended-spectrum penicillins such as carbenicillin and piperacillin.

One problem seen with the natural penicillins is the increased incidence of *bacterial resistance*. Bacterial resistance is the ability of bacteria to produce the enzyme *penicillinase*, which inactivates the penicillin. The natural penicillins also have a narrow spectrum of activity, which means that they are effective against only a few strains of bacteria.

The semisynthetic penicillins partially solved the problems associated with the natural penicillins. The semisynthetic penicillins are a result of chemical treatment of a biological precursor to penicillin. Because of their chemical modifications, they are more slowly excreted by the kidneys and have a somewhat wider spectrum of antibacterial activity.

ACTIONS OF THE PENICILLINS

Both the natural and semisynthetic penicillins basically have the same type of action against bacteria. Penicillin prevents bacteria from using a substance (muramic acid peptide) that is necessary for the maintenance of their outer cell wall. Unable to use this substance for cell wall maintenance, the bacteria swell, rupture, assume unusual shapes, and are finally destroyed.

The penicillins may be *bactericidal* (destroy bacteria) or *bacteriostatic* (slow or retard the multiplication of bacteria). They are bactericidal against sensitive microorganisms (eg, those microorganisms that will be affected by penicillin) provided there is an adequate concentration of penicillin in the body. An adequate concentration of any drug in the body is referred to as the blood level. An inadequate concentration (or inadequate blood level) of penicillin may produce bacteriostatic activity, which may or may not control the infection.

To determine if a specific type of bacteria is sensitive to penicillin, *culture and sensitivity tests* are performed. A culture is the placing of the infectious material obtained from areas such as the skin, respiratory tract, and blood on a special growing medium of a culture plate, which is "food" for the bacteria. After a specified time, the bacteria are examined under a microscope and identified. The sensitivity test involves placing the infectious material on a separate culture plate and then placing small disks, which are impregnated with various antibiotics, over the area. After a specified time, the culture plate is examined. If there is little or no growth around a disk, then the bacteria are considered *sensitive* to the antibiotic that was impregnated in the disk and the infection will be controlled by this particular antibiotic. If there is considerable growth around the disk, then the bacteria are considered *resistant* to the antibiotic impregnated in the disk and that the infection will *not* be controlled by this particular antibiotic. After receiving a culture and sensitivity report, the strain of microorganisms causing the infection is known and the antibiotic to which these microorganisms are sensitive and resistant are identified. The physician then selects the antibiotic to which the microorganism is sensitive.

USES OF THE PENICILLINS

The natural and semisynthetic penicillins are used in the treatment of infections due to susceptible microorganisms. Examples of the infectious microorganisms that may respond to penicillin therapy include gonococci, staphylococci, streptococci, and pneumococci. Culture and sensitivity tests are performed whenever possible to determine which penicillin will best control an infection caused by a specific strain of bacteria. Penicillin is of no value in the treatment of viral or fungal infections.

Penicillin may be prescribed for the treatment of a *potential* infection in certain high-risk individuals, such as those with a history of rheumatic fever. This is called *prophylaxis* (prevention). Penicillin is taken

Summary Drug Table 6-1. The Penicillins

Generic Name	Trade Name*	Uses	Adverse Reactions	Dose Ranges
NATURAL PENICILLINS				
penicillin G (aqueous), parenteral	Pfizerpen, *generic*	Treatment of infections due to susceptible microorganisms	Hypersensitivity reactions, superinfection, hemato-poietic changes	Up to 24 million U/d IV; up 2 million U IM; dosage may also be based on weight
penicillin G benzathine, parenteral	Bicillin L-A, Permapen	Same as pencillin G (aqueous), parenteral	Same as penicillin G (aqueous), parenteral	Up to 2.4 million U per dose IM
pencillin G benzathine and procaine combined	Bicillin C-R, Bicillin C-R 900/300	Same as pencillin G (aqueous), parenteral	Same as penicillin G (aqueous), parenteral	Up to 2.4 million U per dose IM
pencillin G potassium oral	Pentids '400', Pentids '800', *generic*	Same as pencillin G (aqueous), parenteral	Same as penicillin G (aqueous), parenteral	200,000–500,000 U PO q6–8h or 400,000–800,000 U PO q6–8–12h
penicillin G pro-caine, aqueous (APPG)	Wycillin, Crysti-cillin 300 and 600 A.S., Pfizerpen-AS	Same as pencillin G (aqueous), parenteral	Same as penicillin G (aqueous), parenteral	Up to 4.8 million U/day IM
penicillin V potassium	Betapen-VK, V-Cillin K *generic*	Same as pencillin G (aqueous), parenteral	Same as pencillin G (aqueous), parenteral	125–500 mg PO bid-qid
SEMISYNTHETIC PENICILLINS				
Penicillinase-Resistant Penicillins				
cloxacillin sodium	Tegopen, *generic*	Same as penicillin G (aqueous), parenteral	Same as pencillin G (aqueous), parenteral	250–500 mg PO q6h
dicloxacillin sodium	Dynapen, Dycill, *generic*	Same as penicillin G (aqueous), parenteral	Same as pencillin G (aqueous), parenteral	125–250 mg PO q6h
methicillin sodium	Staphcillin	Same as penicillin G (aqueous), parenteral	Same as pencillin G (aqueous), parenteral	4–12 g/d q4–6h IM, IV
nafcillin sodium	Unipen, Nafcil, Nallpen, *generic*	Same as penicillin G (aqueous), parenteral	Same as pencillin G (aqueous), parenteral	250 mg to 1 g PO, IM q4–6h; 3–6 g/d IV
oxacillin sodium	Prostaphilin, Bactocill, *generic*	Same as penicillin G (aqueous), parenteral	Same as pencillin G (aqueous), parenteral	500 mg to 1 g PO q4–6h; 250 mg to 1 g q4–6h IM, IV
Aminopenicillins				
ampicillin, oral	Polycillin, Omni-pen, *generic*	Same as penicillin G (aqueous), parenteral	Same as pencillin G (aqueous), parenteral	250 mg PO q6h
ampicillin sodium, parenteral	Polycillin-N, Omnipen-N *generic*	Same as penicillin G (aqueous), parenteral	Same as pencillin G (aqueous), parenteral	1–12 g/d IM, IV in divided doses q4–6h
ampicillin sodium and sulbactam sodium	Unasyn	Same as pencillin G (aqueous), parenteral	Same as pencillin G (aqueous), parenteral	1.5–3 g IM, IV q6h
amoxicillin	Amoxil, Polymox, *generic*	Same as pencillin G (aqueous), parenteral	Same as pencillin G (aqueous), parenteral	250–500 mg PO q8h
amoxicillin and clavulanate potassium	Augmentin	Same as pencillin G (aqueous), parenteral	Same as pencillin G (aqueous), parenteral	One '250' or '500' tablet q8h
bacampicillin	Spectrobid	Same as pencillin G (aqueous), parenteral	Same as pencillin G (aqueous), parenteral	400–800 mg PO q12h
Extended Spectrum Penicillins				
carbenicillin indanyl sodium	Geocillin	Same as pencillin G (aqueous), parenteral	Same as pencillin G (aqueous), parenteral	382–764 mg PO qid
mezlocillin sodium	Mezlin	Same as pencillin G (aqueous), parenteral	Same as pencillin G (aqueous), parenteral	1.5–2g IM q6–8h; 1.5–3 g IV q6–8h; 4 g IV pre-operative prophylaxis

(continued)

Summary Drug Table 6-1 (Continued)

Generic Name	Trade Name*	Uses	Adverse Reactions	Dose Ranges
piperacillin sodium	Pipracil	Same as pencillin G (aqueous), parenteral	Same as pencillin G (aqueous), parenteral	12–24 g/d IV in divided doses; 2 g IM
piperacillin sodium and tazobactam sodium	Zosyn	Same as pencillin G (aqueous), parenteral	Same as pencillin G (aqueous), parenteral	12 g piperacillin and 1.5 g tazobactam/d IV in divided doses
ticarcillin disodium	Ticar	Same as pencillin G (aqueous), parenteral	Same as pencillin G (aqueous), parenteral	150–300 mg/kg/d IV in divided doses q3,4 or 6h; 1 g IM
ticarcillin and clavulanate potassium	Timentin	Same as pencillin G (aqueous), parenteral	Same as pencillin G (aqueous), parenteral	3.1 g IV q4–6h or 200– 300 mg/kg/d IV in divided doses q4–6h

*The term *generic* indicates that the drug is available in generic form.

several hours or, in some instances days, before and after an operative procedure, such as dental, oral or upper respiratory tract procedures, which can result in bacteria entering the bloodstream. Normally, this does not present a problem in healthy persons. Taking penicillin before and after the procedure will usually prevent a bacterial infection in these high risk patients.

Penicillin also may be given prophylactically and on a continuing basis to those with rheumatic fever and chronic ear infections.

ADVERSE REACTIONS ASSOCIATED WITH THE ADMINISTRATION OF PENICILLIN

A *hypersensitivity* (allergic) reaction may occur with the use of any drug. A *superinfection* is an adverse reaction that may be seen with penicillin, as well as mostly all antibiotics.

Hypersensitivity Reactions

A hypersensitivity (or allergy) reaction to a drug occurs in some individuals, especially those with a history of allergy to many substances. Signs and symptoms may include any one or more of the following: skin rash; urticaria (hives); sneezing; wheezing; pruritus (itching); bronchospasm (spasm of the bronchi); laryngospasm (spasm of the larynx); *angioedema* (also called angioneurotic edema), characterized by swelling of the skin and mucous membranes espe-

cially around and in the mouth and throat; hypotension, which can progress to shock; and signs and symptoms resembling serum sickness (chills, fever, edema, joint and muscle pain, and malaise). *Anaphylactic shock*, which is a severe form of hypersensitivity reaction, can also occur (see Chap. 1). Signs of anaphylactic shock include severe hypotension, loss of consciousness, and acute respiratory distress. Anaphylactic shock, if not immediately treated, can be fatal.

Once an individual is allergic to one penicillin, he or she is most likely allergic to all of the penicillins. Those allergic to penicillin also have a higher incidence of allergy to the cephalosporins (see Chap. 7). Allergy to drugs in the same or related groups is called *cross-sensitivity* or *cross-allergenicity*.

Superinfections

A superinfection is an overgrowth of bacterial or fungal microorganisms not affected by the antibiotic being administered and may occur with the use of any antibiotic, especially when these drugs are given for a long time or when repeated courses of therapy are necessary. When a superinfection occurs, the antibiotic being given not only was bactericidal against *pathogenic* (disease-causing) microorganisms but also affected *nonpathogenic* (not disease-causing) microorganisms that normally exist in the body. This allows other pathogenic microorganisms (bacteria or fungi), which are often resistant to usual antibiotic therapy, to cause a secondary infection, which can be potentially serious and even life-threatening.

Diarrhea may be an indication of *pseudomembranous colitis*, which is one type of a bacterial superinfection. This potentially life-threatening problem develops because of an overgrowth of the microorganism *Clostridia difficile*, which produces a toxin that affects the lining of the colon. Signs and symptoms include fever, abdominal cramps and severe diarrhea with visible blood and mucus. This adverse reaction usually requires immediate discontinuation of the antibiotic. Severe cases may require treatment with intravenous fluids and electrolytes, protein supplementation, and the antibiotics vancomycin (Vancocin) or metronidazole (Flagyl).

Another type of superinfection may occur because of an overgrowth of the yeastlike fungi that usually exist in small numbers in the vagina. The multiplication rate of these microorganisms is normally slowed and kept under control because of the presence of a strain of bacteria (*Döderlein's bacillus*) in the vagina. If penicillin therapy destroys the normal microorganisms of the vagina, for example, *Döderlein's bacillus,* the fungi are now uncontrolled, multiply at a rapid rate, and cause symptoms of a fungal infection called candidiasis (or moniliasis).

A fungal superinfection often occurs in the mouth, vagina, and around the anal and genital areas. Signs and symptoms include anal or vaginal itching, vaginal discharge, and lesions in the mouth. Bacterial superinfections may vary in location but are often seen in the bowel with diarrhea being the most prominent symptom.

Other Adverse Reactions

Other adverse reactions associated with penicillin are hematopoietic changes such as anemia, thrombocytopenia (low platelet count), leukopenia (low white blood cell count), and bone marrow depression. When given orally, glossitis (inflammation of the tongue), stomatitis (inflammation of the mouth), dry mouth, gastritis, nausea, vomiting, and abdominal pain may be seen. When penicillin is given intramuscularly (IM), there may be pain at the injection site. Irritation of the vein and phlebitis (inflammation of a vein) may be seen with intravenous (IV) administration.

NURSING MANAGEMENT

Penicillin may be ordered in units or milligrams. Each unit is approximately equivalent to 0.0006 gram. The exact equivalency usually is stated on the container or package insert.

When preparing a parenteral form of penicillin, shake the vial thoroughly before withdrawing the drug to ensure even distribution of the drug in the solution. Some forms of penicillin are in powder or crystalline form and must be made into a liquid (reconstituted) before being withdrawn from the vial. The manufacturer's directions regarding reconstitution are printed on the label or package insert. If no directions for reconstitution are given, the amount of water or saline used depends on the vial size and the dosage to be given. An example of using judgment to determine the amount of fluid (diluent) to be added to the vial that has no manufacturer's recommendation for reconstitution is as follows:

1. Dose in the vial is 1 g.
2. The dose ordered is 0.5 g.
3. The vial will hold up to 4 mL of fluid.
4. 2 mL of sterile water or normal saline may be added to the 1 g of powder, mixed thoroughly, and then half of the amount in the vial withdrawn to give the dose of 0.5 g.

The manufacturer may indicate the type of diluent to be used when reconstituting a specific drug. Some powdered or crystalline drugs, when reconstituted with a given amount of diluent, may yield slightly more or less than the amount of the diluent added to the vial. If there is any question regarding the reconstitution of this or any drug, a pharmacist is consulted.

To be effective, adequate blood levels of the drug must be maintained. Accidental omission or delay of a dose results in decreased blood levels, which then reduce the effectiveness of the antibiotic. Oral penicillins are best given on an empty stomach, 1 hour before or 2 hours after a meal. Bacampicillin (Spectrobid), penicillin V (Pen-Vee K), and amoxicillin (Amoxil) may be given without regard to meals.

Nursing Process
The Patient Receiving Penicillin

■ *Assessment*
Before the administration of the first dose of penicillin, obtain or review the patient's general health history. The health history includes an allergy history, a history of all medical and surgical treatments, a drug history, and the present symptoms of the infection. If the patient has a history of allergy, particularly a drug allergy, this area must be explored to ensure the patient is not allergic to penicillin or a cephalosporin.

Take and record vital signs. When appropriate, obtain a description of the signs and symptoms of the infection from the patient or family. Assess the infected area (when possible) and record findings on the patient's chart. It is important to describe accurately any signs and symptoms related to the patient's infection, such as color and type of drainage from a wound, pain, redness and inflammation, color of sputum, or presence of an odor. Note the patient's general appearance. A culture and sensitivity test is almost always ordered and must be obtained *before* the first dose of penicillin is given.

The results of a culture and sensitivity test take several days because time must be allowed for the bacteria to grow on the culture media. However, infections are treated as soon as possible. In a few instances, the physician may determine that a penicillin is the choice of treatment until the results of the culture and sensitivity tests are known. In many instances, the physician selects a broad-spectrum antibiotic, for example, an antibiotic that is effective against many types or strains of bacteria, for initial treatment because of the many penicillin-resistant strains of microorganisms.

■ Nursing Diagnoses

Depending on the drug, dose, and reason for administration, one or more of the following may apply to a person receiving penicillin:

- **Risk for Altered Body Temperature: Hyperthermia related to infection**
- **Anxiety** related to diagnosis, route of drug administration (IM, IV), discomfort of injection, other factors (specify)
- **Diarrhea** related to superinfection secondary to penicillin therapy
- **Noncompliance** related to indifference, lack of knowledge, other factors
- **Ineffective Management of Therapeutic Regimen** due to insufficient knowledge of medication regimen

■ Planning and Implementation

The major goals of the patient may include a reduction in anxiety and an understanding of and compliance to the prescribed treatment regimen. To make these goals measurable, more specific criteria must be added.

Warn the patient that at the time the drug is injected into the muscle, there may be a stinging or burning sensation. Discomfort at the time of injection occurs because the drug is irritating to the tissues. Inspect previous areas used for injection for

---

Nursing Alert

Question the patient about allergy to penicillin or the cephalosporins before administering the first dose, even when an accurate drug history has been taken. Tell patients that the drug they are receiving is penicillin because information regarding a drug allergy may have been forgotten at the time the initial drug history was obtained. If a patient states he or she is allergic to penicillin or a cephalosporin, withhold the drug and contact the physician.

---

continued redness, soreness, or other problems. Inform the physician if previously used areas for injection appear red or the patient complains of pain in the area.

Evaluate the patient daily for a response to therapy, such as a decrease in temperature, the relief of symptoms caused by the infection (such as pain or discomfort), an increase in appetite, and a change in the appearance or amount of drainage (when originally present). Once an infection is controlled, patients often look better and even state that they feel better. Record these evaluations on the patient's chart. Notify the physician if signs and symptoms of the infection appear to worsen.

Additional culture and sensitivity tests may be performed during therapy because microorganisms causing the infection may become resistant to penicillin or a superinfection may have occurred. A urinalysis, complete blood count, and renal and hepatic function tests also may be performed at intervals during therapy.

Fever. Take vital signs every 4 hours or as ordered by the physician. Report any increase in temperature to the physician because additional treatment measures, such as administration of an antipyretic drug or change in the drug or dosage, may be necessary. An increase in body temperature several days after the start of therapy may indicate a secondary bacterial infection or failure of the drug to control the original infection.

Adverse Drug Reactions

Nursing Alert

Observe the patient closely for a hypersensitivity reaction, which may occur any time during therapy with the penicillins. If it should occur, contact the physician immediately and withhold the drug until the patient is seen by a physician.

Treatment of minor hypersensitivity reactions may include administration of an antihistamine (for a rash or itching). Major hypersensitivity reactions, such as bronchospasm, laryngospasm, hypotension, and angioneurotic edema require immediate treatment with drugs such as epinephrine, cortisone, or an IV antihistamine. When respiratory difficulty occurs, a tracheostomy may need to be performed.

The administration of oral penicillin may result in a superinfection in the oral cavity. To detect this problem early, inspect the patient's mouth daily for evidence of glossitis, sore tongue, ulceration, or a black, furry tongue. Closely observe the patient for a bacterial or fungal superinfection. Signs and symptoms of a fungal superinfection include itching around the anal area, and vaginal itching or discharge. Diarrhea, chills, fever, sore mouth, and sore throat may indicate a bacterial superinfection. Report any signs and symptoms of a superinfection to the physician before the next dose of the drug is administered. When these are severe, additional treatment measures may be necessary, such as administration of an antipyretic agent for fever or an antifungal agent.

Diarrhea. Diarrhea may be an indication of a superinfection of the gastrointestinal tract or pseudomembranous colitis. Inspect all stools and notify the physician if diarrhea occurs because it may be necessary to stop the drug. If diarrhea does occur and there appears to be blood and mucus in the stool, save a sample of the stool and test for occult blood using a test such as Hemoccult. If the stool tests positive for blood, the sample is saved for possible further laboratory analysis.

Anxiety. Patients may have varying degrees of anxiety related to their diagnosis or the fact that the IM injections are uncomfortable or painful. Reassure the patient that the discomfort or pain is due to the drug but will decrease in a short time. Rotate IM injection sites to reduce discomfort when these drugs are given for a long time.

Noncompliance. When a penicillin is to be taken for a long time for prophylaxis the patient may feel well despite the need for long-term antibiotic therapy. There may be a tendency to omit one or more doses or even neglect to take the medication for an extended time. Stress the importance of uninterrupted therapy to help the patient and family understand the reason for and the importance of therapy.

■ *Patient and Family Teaching*

Carefully review the dose regimen with the patient and family. Develop a teaching plan to include one or more of the following:

- Prophylaxis—Take the drug as prescribed until the physician discontinues therapy.
- Infection—Complete the *full* course of therapy. Do not stop the drug even if the symptoms have disappeared unless directed to do so by the physician.
- Take the drug at the prescribed times of day because it is important to keep an adequate amount of drug in the body throughout the entire 24 hours of each day.
- Penicillin (oral)—Take the drug on an empty stomach either 1 hour before or 2 hours after meals (*exception*—bacampicillin, penicillin V, amoxicillin).
- Take each dose with a full glass of water.
- Notify the physician immediately if any one or more of the following should occur: skin rash, hives (urticaria), severe diarrhea, vaginal or anal itching, sore mouth, black furry tongue, sores in the mouth, swelling around the mouth or eyes, breathing difficulty or gastrointestinal disturbances such as nausea, vomiting, and diarrhea. Do not take the next dose of the drug until the problem is discussed with the physician.
- Oral suspensions—Keep the container refrigerated (if so labeled); shake the drug well before pouring (if so labeled); return the drug to the refrigerator immediately after pouring the dose. Drugs that are kept refrigerated lose their potency when kept at room temperature. A small amount of the drug may be left after the last dose is taken and should be discarded because the drug (in suspension form) begins to lose its potency after a few weeks.
- Never give this drug to another individual even though the symptoms appear to be the same.
- Notify the physician if the symptoms of the infection do not improve or if the condition becomes worse.

■ *Expected Outcomes for Evaluation*

- Anxiety is reduced
- Adverse reactions are identified and reported to the physician
- Patient complies to the prescribed drug regimen
- Patient and family demonstrate understanding of drug regimen
- Patient verbalizes importance of complying with the prescribed therapeutic regimen

Chapter Summary

- There are two types of penicillin: natural penicillin and the semisynthetic derivatives of penicillin; both are used in the treatment of infections due to susceptible microorganisms.

- Both the natural and semisynthetic penicillins basically have the same type of action against bacteria and may be bactericidal or bacteriostatic.
- Penicillin prevents bacteria from using a substance (muramic acid peptide) that is necessary for the maintenance of their outer cell wall. Unable to use this substance for cell wall maintenance, the bacteria swell, rupture, assume unusual shapes, and are finally destroyed.
- Culture and sensitivity tests may be used to determine if a specific type of bacteria is sensitive to penicillin.
- Adverse reactions associated with penicillin administration include hypersensitivity reactions, superinfections, hematopoietic changes such as anemia, thrombocytopenia, leukopenia, and bone marrow depression. When given orally, glossitis, stomatitis, dry mouth, gastritis, nausea, vomiting, and abdominal pain may be seen. When penicillin is given IM, there may be pain at the injection site.

Irritation of the vein and phlebitis may be seen with IV administration.

Critical Thinking Exercises

1. Ms. Barker had a bowel resection 4 days ago. Following a culture and sensitivity test of her draining surgical wound, the physician orders penicillin G aqueous IV as a continuous drip. What questions would you ask Ms. Barker before the penicillin was added to the intravenous solution?
2. Ms. Evans took 5-year-old Tommy to the pediatrician because he had a cold. The pediatrician suggested acetaminophen (Tylenol) for his fever, forced fluids, and bed rest. Ms. Evans tells you that she is upset because the physician did not order penicillin for Tommy's cold. What explanation would you give Mrs. Evans?

7

The Cephalosporins

Key Terms

Aplastic anemia
Bactericidal
Epidermal necrolysis
Nephrotoxicity
Stevens-Johnson syndrome

Chapter Outline

Chapter Objectives

On completion of this chapter the student will:

- *List the actions and uses of the cephalosporins*
- *List the adverse reactions associated with the administration of the cephalosporins*
- *Use the nursing process when administering a cephalosporin*
- *Discuss the nursing implications associated with the administration of the cephalosporins*

The effectiveness of penicillin in the treatment of infections prompted research directed toward finding additional antibiotics with a wider range of antibacterial activity. Although not the first group of drugs arising from continued research, the cephalosporins are a valuable group of drugs that are effective in the treatment of almost all of the strains of bacteria affected by the penicillins, as well as some strains of bacteria that have become resistant to penicillin.

The cephalosporins (Summary Drug Table 7-1) are structurally and chemically related to penicillin. Cefoxitin (Mefoxin), loracarbef (Lorabid) and cefotetan (Cefotan) are drugs similar to the cephalosporins. They have basically the same pharmacologic action and are included with the cephalosporins in many references.

The Cephalosporins

The cephalosporins are divided into three groups: first, second, and third-generation agents. Particular cephalosporins may also be differentiated within each group according to the microorganisms that are sensitive to them. Generally, progression from the first to the second, and then to the third generation shows an increase in the sensitivity of gram-negative microorganisms and a decrease in the sensitivity of gram-positive microorganisms. For example, a first-generation cephalosporin would have more use against gram-positive microorganisms than would a third-generation cephalosporin.

The following are examples of first, second, and third-generation cephalosporins:

First generation—cephalexin (Keflex), cefazolin (Ancef)
Second generation—cefaclor (Ceclor), cefoxitin (Mefoxin)
Third generation—cefixime (Suprax), cefoperazone (Cefobid)

ACTIONS OF THE CEPHALOSPORINS

Cephalosporins affect the bacterial cell wall, making it defective and unstable. This action is similar to the action of penicillin. The cephalosporins are usually *bactericidal* (capable of destroying bacteria).

USES OF THE CEPHALOSPORINS

The cephalosporins are used in the treatment of infections due to susceptible microorganisms. Examples of microorganisms that may be susceptible to the cephalosporins include streptococci, staphylococci, citrobacter, gonococci, shigella, and clostridium. Culture and sensitivity tests (see Chap. 6) are performed whenever possible to determine which antibiotic, including a cephalosporin, will best control an infection caused by a specific strain of bacteria.

The cephalosporins also may be used perioperatively, that is during the preoperative, intraoperative, and postoperative periods, to prevent infection in those having surgery on a contaminated or potentially contaminated area, such as the gastrointestinal tract or vagina. In some instances, a specific drug may be recommended for postoperative prophylactic use only.

ADVERSE REACTIONS ASSOCIATED WITH THE ADMINISTRATION OF THE CEPHALOSPORINS

The most common adverse reactions seen with administration of the cephalosporins are gastrointestinal disturbances such as nausea, vomiting, and diarrhea.

Hypersensitivity (allergic) reactions may occur with administration of the cephalosporins and range from mild to life-threatening. Mild hypersensitivity reactions include pruritus, urticaria, and skin rashes. More serious hypersensitivity reactions include *Stevens-Johnson syndrome* (fever, cough, muscular aches and pains, headache, and the appearance of lesions on the skin, mucous membranes, and eyes), hepatic and renal dysfunction, *aplastic anemia* (anemia due to deficient red blood cell production), and *epidermal necrolysis* (death of the epidermal layer of the skin).

Because of the close relation of the cephalosporins to penicillin, a patient allergic to penicillin may also be allergic to the cephalosporins.

Other adverse reactions that may be seen with administration of the cephalosporins are headache, dizziness, *nephrotoxicity* (damage to the kidneys by a toxic substance), malaise, heartburn, and fever. Intramuscular administration often results in pain, tenderness, and inflammation at the injection site. Intravenous administration has resulted in thrombophlebitis and phlebitis.

Therapy with antibiotics may result in a superinfection. Diarrhea may be an indication of pseudomembranous colitis, which is one type of bacterial

Summary Drug Table 7-1. The Cephalosporins

Generic Name	Trade Name*	Uses	Adverse Reactions	Dose Ranges
cefaclor	Ceclor	Treatment of infections due to susceptible microorganisms	Nausea, vomiting, diarrhea, hypersensitivity reactions, superinfection, hematologic changes, nephrotoxicity, headache	250 mg PO q8h
cefamandole nafate	Mandol	Same as cefaclor	Same as cefaclor	500 mg to 1 g IM, IV q4–8h
cefazolin sodium	Kefzol, Ancef, *generic*	Same as cefaclor	Same as cefaclor plus perioperative prophylaxis	250 mg to 1 g IM, IV 6–12h; perioperative: 0.5 to 1g IM, IV
cefixime	Suprax	Same as cefaclor	Same as cefaclor	400 mg/d PO or 200 mg PO q12h
cefoperazone sodium	Cefobid	Same as cefaclor	Same as cefaclor	2–4 g/d IM, IV in equally divided doses
cefotaxime sodium	Claforan	Same as cefaclor	Same as cefaclor plus perioperative prophylaxis	1–2 g IM, IV q4–12h; perioperative: 1 g IM, IV
cefotetan disodium	Cefotan	Same as cefaclor	Same as cefaclor plus perioperative prophylaxis	1–6 g IM, IV in equally divided doses; perioperative: 1–2 g IV
cefoxitin sodium	Mefoxin	Same as cefaclor	Same as cefaclor plus - perioperative prophylaxis	1–2 g IM q6–8h; 1–12 g/d IV in equally divided doses; perioperative: 1–2 g IV
cefpodoxime proxetil	Vantin	Same as cefaclor	Same as cefaclor	200–800 mg/d PO in equally divided doses
cefprozil	Cefzil	Same as cefaclor	Same as cefaclor	500 mg/d PO in single or divided doses; up to 1 g/d PO in divided doses
ceftazidime	Fortaz, Tazidime, Ceptaz	Same as cefaclor	Same as cefaclor	250 mg to 2 g IM, IV q8–12h
ceftizoxime sodium	Cefizox	Same as cefaclor	Same as cefaclor	2–12 g/d IV in divided doses; 1–6 g/d IM in divided doses
ceftriaxone sodium	Rocephin	Same as cefaclor	Same as cefaclor plus preoperative prophylaxis	1–2 g/d IM, IV as a single or divided dose; preoperative: 1 g IM, IV'; gonorrhea—250 mg IM as a single dose
cefuroxime	Ceftin, Kefurox, Zinacef	Same as cefaclor	Same as cefaclor plus preoperative prophylaxis	250 mg PO bid; 750 mg to 1.5 g IM, IV q8h; preoperative: 1.5 g IV
cephalaxin monohydrate	Keflex, *generic*	Same as cefaclor	Same as cefaclor	1–4 g/d PO in divided doses
cephalothin sodium	Keflin Neutral, *generic*	Same as cefaclor	Same as cefaclor plus preoperative prophylaxis	500 mg to 1 g IM, IV q4–6h; perioperative: 1–2 g IV
loracarbef	Lorabid	Same as cefaclor	Same as cefaclor	200–400 mg PO q12h or 200 mg/d PO

*The term, *generic,* indicates that the drug is available in generic form.

superinfection. See Chapter 6 for a discussion of these two adverse reactions.

NURSING MANAGEMENT

Some cephalosporins are available as powder for a suspension and are reconstituted by a pharmacist. This form of the drug must be kept refrigerated until used.

Give oral preparations with food or milk. Cefpodoxime (Vantin) and cefuroxime (Kefurox) are given with food to increase gastrointestinal absorption of the drug.

Some cephalosporins are given intravenously by direct intravenous (IV), intermittent infusion, or continuous IV infusion. When the direct IV method is used, the dose is given directly into a vein. Intermittent IV infusion is given by means of Y-tubing while another solution is being given on a continuous basis. When this method is used, the intravenous fluid given on a continuous basis is clamped off while the drug is allowed to infuse. Continuous IV infusion requires adding the drug to a specified amount of an intravenous solution at a drip rate or volume per hour prescribed by the physician.

Nursing Alert

Read the manufacturer's package insert for each drug for instructions regarding reconstitution of powder for injection, storage of unused portions, life of the drug following reconstitution, methods of IV administration, and precautions to be taken when the drug is administered.

When a cephalosporin in given intramuscularly (IM), inject the drug into a large muscle mass such as the gluteus muscle or lateral aspect of the thigh.

Nursing Process
The Patient Receiving a Cephalosporin

■ *Assessment*

Before the administration of the first dose of a cephalosporin, obtain a general health history. The health history includes an allergy history, a history of all medical and surgical treatments, a drug history, and the present symptoms of the infection. If the patient has a history of allergy, particularly a drug allergy, this area must be explored to ensure the patient is not allergic to a cephalosporin. Pa-

tients with a history of an allergy to penicillin, may also be allergic to a cephalosporin (see Chap. 6) even though they have never received one of these drugs. If an allergy to either of these drug groups is suspected, the physician is informed of this before the first dose of the drug is given.

■ *Nursing Diagnoses*
- **Risk for Altered Body Temperature: Hyperthermia** related to infection
- **Anxiety** related to diagnosis, route of drug administration (IM, IV), discomfort of injection, other factors (specify)
- **Diarrhea** related to superinfection secondary to cephalosporin therapy
- **Risk for Ineffective Management of Therapeutic Regimen** due to insufficient knowledge of medication regimen

■ *Planning and Implementation*

The major goals of the patient may include a reduction in anxiety, an absence of adverse drug effects, and an understanding of and compliance to the prescribed treatment regimen. To make these goals measurable, more specific criteria must be added.

Question the patient about allergy to penicillin or the cephalosporins before administering the first dose, even when an accurate drug history has been taken. Tell patients that the drugs they are receiving are related to the penicillins because information regarding a drug allergy may have been forgotten at the time the initial drug history was obtained. If a patient gives a history of possible penicillin or cephalosporin allergy, withhold the drug and contact the physician.

Nursing Alert

Warn the patient that at the time the drug is injected into the muscle, there may be a stinging or burning sensation and the area may be sore for a short period of time. Inform the physician if previously used areas for injection appear red or the patient complains of continued pain in the area.

When the drug is given IV inspect the needle insertion site for signs of extravasation or infiltration (see Chapter 2). In addition, inspect the needle insertion site and the area above the site several times a day for signs of redness, which may indicate thrombophlebitis (inflammation of a vein with formation of a clot within the vein) or phlebitis (inflammation of a vein). If this problem occurs, the physician is contacted and the IV must be discontinued and restarted in another vein, preferably in another extremity.

Evaluate the patient daily for a response to therapy, such as a decrease in temperature, the relief of symptoms caused by the infection (such as pain or discomfort), an increase in appetite, and a change in the appearance or amount of drainage (when originally present). Notify the physician if symptoms of the infection appear to worsen.

Fever. Take vital signs every 4 hours or as ordered by the physician. Report any increase in temperature to the physician because additional treatment measures, such as administration of an antipyretic drug or change in the drug or dosage, may be necessary.

Adverse Drug Reactions. Observe the patient closely for any adverse drug reactions, particularly signs and symptoms of a hypersensitivity reaction. If a hypersensitivity reaction should occur, contact the physician immediately and withhold the drug until the patient is seen by a physician.

Nursing Alert

The Stevens-Johnson syndrome is manifested by fever, cough, muscular aches and pains, headache, and the appearance of lesions on the skin, mucous membranes, and eyes. The lesions appear as red wheals or blisters, often starting on the face, in the mouth or on the lips, neck, and extremities. This syndrome, which also may occur with the administration of other types of drugs, can be fatal.

Closely observe the patient for signs and symptoms of a bacterial or fungal superinfection, such as itching around the anal area, vaginal itching or discharge (fungal superinfection) or diarrhea, chills, fever, sore mouth, and sore throat (bacterial superinfection). If any one or more of these should occur, contact the physician before the next dose of the drug is due.

Nephrotoxicity may occur with the administration of these drugs. Early signs of this adverse reaction may become apparent by a decrease in the urine output. Measure and record the intake and output and notify the physician if the output is less than 500 mL/day. Any changes in the intake and output ratio or in the appearance of the urine may indicate nephrotoxicity and are reported to the physician promptly.

Anxiety. Patients may have varying degrees of anxiety related to their diagnosis, to the fact that the IM injections are uncomfortable or painful, or that prolonged IV administration of the drug is necessary.

Reassure the patient that the discomfort or pain at the injection site is due to the drug but will decrease in a short time. Rotate IM injection sites to help reduce discomfort.

Diarrhea. Frequent liquid stools may be an indication of a superinfection or pseudomembranous colitis. If pseudomembranous colitis does occur, it is usually seen 4 to 10 days after treatment was started.

Inspect each bowel movement and immediately report the occurrence of diarrhea or loose stools containing blood and mucus to the physician because it may be necessary to discontinue the drug and institute treatment for diarrhea, a superinfection, or pseudomembranous colitis.

If there appears to be blood and mucus in the stool, save a sample of the stool and test for occult blood using a test such as Hemoccult. If the stool tests positive for blood, the sample is saved for possible laboratory testing for blood.

■ *Patient and Family Teaching*

Carefully review the dose regimen with the patient and family. Develop a teaching plan to include one or more of the following:

- Complete the *full* course of therapy. Do not stop the drug even if the symptoms have disappeared unless directed to do so by the physician.
- Take the drug at the prescribed times of day because it is important to keep an adequate amount of drug in the body throughout the entire 24 hours of each day.
- Take each dose with food or milk unless directed otherwise by the physician or pharmacist.
- Notify the physician immediately if any one or more of the following should occur: vomiting, skin rash, hives (urticaria), severe diarrhea, vaginal or anal itching, sores in the mouth, swelling around the mouth or eyes, breathing difficulty or gastrointestinal disturbances, such as nausea, vomiting, and diarrhea. Do not take the next dose of the drug until the problem is discussed with the physician.
- Oral suspensions—Keep the container refrigerated (if so labeled); shake the drug well before pouring (if so labeled); return the drug to the refrigerator immediately after pouring the dose. Drugs that are kept refrigerated lose their potency when kept at room temperature. A small amount of the drug may be left after the last dose is taken and should be discarded because the drug (in suspension form) begins to lose potency after a few weeks.
- Never give this drug to another individual even though the symptoms appear to be the same.

- Notify the physician if the symptoms of the infection do not improve or if the condition becomes worse.

■ *Expected Outcomes for Evaluation*
- Anxiety is reduced
- Adverse reactions are identified and reported to the physician
- Patient and family demonstrate understanding of drug regimen
- Patient verbalizes importance of complying with the prescribed therapeutic regimen

Chapter Summary

- The cephalosporins are structurally and chemically related to penicillin. Cefoxitin (Mefoxin), loracarbef (Lorabid) and cefotetan (Cefotan) are drugs similar to the cephalosporins, have basically the same pharmacologic action, and are included with the cephalosporins in many references.
- The cephalosporins are divided into three groups: first, second, and third-generation agents. Particular cephalosporins may also be differentiated within each group according to the microorganisms that are sensitive to them. Generally, progression from the first to the second, and then to the third generation shows an increase in the sensitivity of gram-negative microorganisms and a decrease in the sensitivity of gram-positive microorganisms.
- Cephalosporins, which are usually bactericidal, affect the bacterial cell wall, making it defective and unstable. This group of antibiotics is used in the treatment of infections due to susceptible microorganisms.
- The most common adverse reactions seen with administration of the cephalosporins are gastrointestinal disturbances such as nausea, vomiting, and mild to severe diarrhea. Additional adverse reactions include hypersensitivity reactions, superinfection, pseudomembranous colitis, Stevens-Johnson syndrome, hepatic and renal dysfunction, aplastic anemia, superinfection, epidermal necrolysis, hematologic changes, headaches, dizziness, nephrotoxicity, malaise, heartburn, glossitis, and fever. Intramuscular administration often results in pain, tenderness, and inflammation at the injection site. Intravenous administration has resulted in thrombophlebitis and phlebitis.
- Because of the close relation of the cephalosporins to penicillin, a patient allergic to penicillin may also be allergic to the cephalosporins.

Critical Thinking Exercises

1. Mr. Jonas is receiving a cephalosporin IM. He tells you that he has had to get out of bed several times this morning because he has diarrhea. What questions would you ask Mr. Jonas? What steps would you take to resolve this problem?
2. A patient who is a recent immigrant to the United States is seen in the outpatient clinic for a severe upper respiratory infection. The physician prescribed a cephalosporin and asks you to given the patient instructions for taking the drug. You note that the patient appears to understand little English. How would you solve this problem?

8

The Tetracyclines, Macrolides, and Lincosamides

Key Terms

Bactericidal

Bacteriostatic

Photosensitivity reaction

Chapter Outline

Chapter Objectives

On completion of this chapter the student will:

- *Discuss the actions and uses of the tetracyclines, macrolides, and lincosamides*
- *List some of the adverse reactions associated with the administration of the tetracyclines, macrolides, or lincosamides*
- *Discuss the nursing management of the patient receiving a tetracycline, macrolide, or lincosamide*
- *Use the nursing process when administering a tetracycline, macrolide, or lincosamide*

After penicillin was introduced, it was widely used for almost every infection. In some patients, penicillin was either partially or totally ineffective; in others, the infection was controlled. Continued use, as well as overuse, of penicillin began to produce penicillin-resistant strains of bacteria, thus making penicillin ineffective for many types of infections. Continued research developed the cephalosporins (see Chap. 7) and a variety of broad-spectrum antibiotics. Although the penicillins still remain important antibiotics, the physician now has a wide variety of drugs to treat an infection.

The Tetracyclines, Macrolides, and Lincosamides

This chapter discusses three groups of broad-spectrum antibiotics: the tetracyclines, the macrolides, and the lincosamides.

Examples of the tetracyclines include doxycycline (Vibramycin), methacycline (Rondomycin), minocycline (Minocin), and tetracycline (Sumycin). Examples of the macrolides include azithromycin (Zithromax), clarithromycin (Biaxin), and erythromycin (E-Mycin). The lincosamides include clindamycin (Cleocin) and lincomycin (Lincocin). Summary Drug Table 8-1 lists the types of broad-spectrum antibiotics discussed in this chapter.

ACTIONS OF THE TETRACYCLINES, MACROLIDES, AND LINCOSAMIDES

The tetracyclines, macrolides, and lincosamides exert their effect by inhibiting bacterial protein synthesis, which is a process that is necessary for reproduction of the microorganism. The ultimate effect of this action is that the bacteria are either destroyed or their multiplication rate is slowed. The tetracyclines are bacteriostatic (capable of slowing or retarding the multiplication of bacteria) whereas the macrolides and lincosamides may be bacteriostatic or bactericidal (capable of destroying bacteria).

USES OF THE TETRACYCLINES, MACROLIDES, AND LINCOSAMIDES

These antibiotics are effective in the treatment of infections caused by a wide range of gram-negative and gram-positive microorganisms. Culture and sensitivity tests (see Chap. 6) are performed to determine which antibiotic will best control the infection. These drugs are of no value in the treatment of infections caused by a virus or fungus. There may be times when a secondary bacterial infection has occurred or potentially will occur when the patient has a fungal or viral infection. The physician may then order one of the broad-spectrum antibiotics, but its purpose is for the prevention (prophylaxis) or treatment of a secondary bacterial infection that could potentially develop following the primary fungal or viral infection.

ADVERSE REACTIONS ASSOCIATED WITH THE ADMINISTRATION OF THE TETRACYCLINES, MACROLIDES, AND LINCOSAMIDES

Superinfections, pseudomembranous colitis, and hypersensitivity reactions (see Chap. 6) may occur with the use of these drugs.

The Tetracyclines

Gastrointestinal reactions that may occur during tetracycline administration include nausea, vomiting, diarrhea, epigastric distress, stomatitis, and sore throat. Skin rashes may also be seen. A photosensitivity (phototoxic) reaction may be seen with this group of drugs, manifested by an exaggerated sunburn reaction when the skin is exposed to sunlight even for brief periods. Demeclocycline has been known to cause the most serious photosensitivity reaction. Minocycline is least likely to cause this type of reaction.

The tetracyclines are not given to children under 8 years of age unless their use is absolutely necessary because these drugs may cause permanent yellow-gray-brown discoloration of the teeth.

The Macrolides

Most of the adverse reactions seen with the administration of azithromycin and clarithromycin are related to the gastrointestinal tract and include nausea, vomiting, diarrhea, and abdominal pain.

Abdominal cramping, nausea, vomiting, diarrhea, and allergic reactions have been reported with the administration of the erythromycins. There appears to be a low incidence of adverse reactions with oral use with normal doses of the erythromycins.

Summary Drug Table 8-1. The Tetracyclines, Macrolides, and Lincosamides

Generic Name	Trade Name*	Uses	Adverse Reactions	Dose Ranges
THE TETRACYCLINES				
demeclocycline	Declomycin	Treatment of infections due to susceptible microorganisms	Nausea, vomiting, diarrhea, hypersensitivity reactions, photosensitivity reactions, pseudomembranous colitis, hematologic changes	150 mg PO qid or 300 mg PO bid; gonorrhea: 600 mg PO initially then 300 mg PO q12h for 4 d
doxycycline	Vibramycin, *generic*	Same as demeclocycline	Same as demeclocycline	100 mg PO q12h first day then 100 mg/d PO; gonorrhea: 200 mg PO immediately and 100 mg PO hs then 100 mg PO bid for 3 d; 200 mg IV first day then 100–200 mg/d IV
methacycline	Rondomycin	Same as demeclocycline	Same as demeclocycline	600 mg/d PO in 2–4 divided doses
minocycline	Minocin, Minocin IV	Same as demeclocycline	Same as demeclocycline	200 mg PO, IV initially then 100 mg q12h
tetracycline	Panmycin, generic	Same as demeclocycline	Same as demeclocycline	1–2 g/d PO in 2–4 divided doses; 250 mg once a day IM or 150 mg q8–12h IM; 250–500 mg IV q12h
THE MACROLIDES				
azithromycin	Zithromax	Same as demeclocycline	Nausea, vomiting, diarrhea, abdominal pain, hypersensitivity reactions, pseudomembranous colitis	500 mg PO first day then 250 mg PO daily for 4 d
clarithromycin	Biaxin	Same as demeclocycline	Same as azithromycin	500 mg PO bid
erythromycin base	E-Mycin, Eryc, *generic*	Same as demeclocycline	Same as azithromycin	250 mg PO q6h
erythromycin ethylsuccinate	EryPed, E.E.S. 400	Same as demeclocycline	Same as azithromycin	400 mg PO q6h
erythromycin estolate	Ilosone, *generic*	Same as demeclocycline	Same as azithromycin	250 mg PO q6h
erythromycin I.V.	*generic*	Same as demeclocycline	Same as azithromycin	Up to 4 g/d by continuous or intermittent IV infusion
THE LINCOSAMIDES				
clindamycin	Cleocin, *generic*	Same as demeclocycline	Abdominal pain, esophagitis, nausea, vomiting, diarrhea, skin rash, blood dyscrasias, pseudomembranous colitis, hypersensitivity reactions	150–450 mg PO q6h; 600–1200 mg/d IM in 2–4 equal doses; up to 4.8 g/d IV
lincomycin	Lincocin, Lincorex	Same as demeclocycline	Same as clindamycin	500 mg PO q6h; 600 mg IM q12–24h; up to 8 g/d IV

*The term, generic, indicates the drug is available in generic form.

The Lincosamides

Abdominal pain, esophagitis, nausea, vomiting, diarrhea, skin rash, and blood dyscrasias may be seen with the use of these drugs. These drugs can also cause pseudomembranous colitis, which may range from mild to very severe. Discontinuing the drug may relieve the mild symptoms.

NURSING MANAGEMENT

When given orally, erythromycin, azithromycin, and lincomycin are given on an empty stomach, that is, 1 hour before or 2 hours after a meal and with a full glass of water. The tetracyclines also are given on an empty stomach and are not to be taken with dairy products (milk or cheese). The exceptions are doxycycline (Vibramycin) and minocycline (Minocin), which may be taken with dairy products or food.

Nursing Alert

The tetracyclines are not given along with antacids, laxatives, or products containing iron. When these drugs are prescribed, they are given 2 hours before or after the administration of a tetracycline.

Clindamycin is given with food or a full glass of water. Troleandomycin and clarithromycin can be given without regard to meals.

When these drugs are given intramuscularly, inspect previous injection sites for signs of pain or tenderness, redness, and swelling. Some antibiotics may cause temporary local reactions but persistence of a localized reaction should be reported to the physician. Rotate injection sites, and record the site used for injection in the patient's chart.

When these drugs are given intravenously (IV), inspect the needle site and area around the needle for signs of extravasation of the intravenous fluid or signs of tenderness, pain, and redness (which may indicate phlebitis or thrombophlebitis). If these symptoms are apparent, restart the IV in another vein and bring the problem to the attention of the physician.

Nursing Process
The Patient Receiving a Tetracycline, Macrolide, or Lincosamide

■ *Assessment*

Before the administration of any antibiotic, identify and record the signs and symptoms of the infection. Signs and symptoms may vary and often depend on the organ or system involved and whether the infection is external or internal. Examples of some of the signs and symptoms of an infection in various areas of the body are pain, drainage, redness, changes in the appearance of sputum, general malaise, chills and fever, cough, and swelling.

Obtain a thorough allergy history, especially a history of drug allergies. Some antibiotics have a higher incidence of hypersensitivity reactions in those with a history of allergy to drugs or other substances. If the patient has a history of allergies and has not told the physician, do not administer the first dose of the drug until this problem is discussed with the physician.

It is also important to take and record vital signs before the first dose of the antibiotic is given. The physician may order culture and sensitivity tests, and these should also be performed before the first dose of the drug is given. Other laboratory tests such as renal and hepatic function tests, complete blood count, and urinalysis may also be ordered by the physician.

■ *Nursing Diagnoses*

One or more of the following nursing diagnoses may apply to a person receiving one of these drugs. Additional nursing diagnoses, based on the patient's symptoms, may be required.
- **Risk for Altered Body Temperature: Hyperthermia** related to infectious process
- **Anxiety** related to infection, seriousness of illness, route of administration, other factors (specify)
- **Diarrhea** related to superinfection secondary to antibiotic therapy, adverse drug reaction
- **Noncompliance** related to indifference, lack of knowledge, other factors
- **Risk for Ineffective Management of Therapeutic Regimen** due to insufficient knowledge of medication regimen

■ *Planning and Implementation*

The major goals of the patient may include a reduction in anxiety, an absence of adverse drug effects, and an understanding of and compliance to the prescribed treatment regimen. To make these goals measurable more specific criteria must be added.

Vital Signs. Take vital signs every 4 hours or as ordered by the physician. Notify the physician if there are changes in the vital signs, such as a significant drop in blood pressure, an increase in the pulse or respiratory rate, or a sudden increase in temperature. Closely monitor the temperature of those with a body temperature over 101°F (38.3°C).

Response to Therapy. Each day compare the present signs and symptoms of the infection against the initial signs and symptoms and record specific findings in the patient's chart. When an antibiotic is ordered for the prevention of a secondary infection (prophylaxis), observe the patient for those signs and symptoms that may indicate the beginning of an infection despite the prophylactic use of the antibiotic. If signs and symptoms of an infection should occur, report this to the physician.

Adverse Drug Reactions. Review the adverse reactions associated with the administration of a specific antibiotic before therapy is started. A review of these reactions often determines the assessments and nursing tasks that will be necessary for identification of some of these adverse reactions.

Observe the patient at frequent intervals, especially during the first 48 hours of therapy. Report the occurrence of any adverse reaction to the physician before the next dose of the drug is due. Report serious adverse reactions, such as a severe hypersensitivity reaction, respiratory difficulty, severe diarrhea, or a decided drop in blood pressure, to the physician immediately because a serious adverse reaction may require emergency intervention.

Observe the patient for the signs and symptoms of a bacterial or fungal superinfection, such as vaginal or anal itching, sore throat, sores in the mouth, diarrhea, fever, chills, and sore throat. Any new signs and symptoms occurring during antibiotic therapy are reported to the physician, who must then decide if these problems are part of the original infection or if a superinfection has occurred.

Diarrhea. Diarrhea may be an indication of a superinfection or pseudomembranous colitis, both of which can be serious. Inspect all stools for the presence of blood or mucus. If diarrhea does occur and there appears to be blood and mucus in the stool, save a sample of the stool and test for occult blood using a test such as Hemoccult. If the stool tests positive for blood, save the sample for possible further laboratory analysis.

Anxiety. Patients may exhibit varying degrees of anxiety related to their illness and infection and the necessary drug therapy. When these drugs are given by the parenteral route, anxiety may be experienced because of the discomfort or pain that accompanies an intramuscular injection or intravenous administration of fluids. Assure the patient that every effort will be made to reduce pain and discomfort but there are times when this may not be possible. Warn the patient at the time the first intramuscular injection is given that some pain or discomfort may be experienced at the time the drug is injected and for a short time after.

Noncompliance. It is most important that the patient and family understand the prescribed therapeutic regimen. It is not uncommon for patients to stop taking a prescribed drug because they feel better. Develop a detailed plan of teaching to reduce the incidence of this problem.

■ *Patient and Family Teaching*

Explain in easy to understand terms the adverse reactions associated with the specific prescribed antibiotic. Advise the patient to contact the physician if any of these should occur. Potentially serious adverse reactions such as hypersensitivity reactions, moderate to severe diarrhea, sudden onset of chills and fever, sore throat, or sores in the mouth are explained, along with the necessity of contacting the physician immediately should these occur. Caution the patient to avoid the use of alcoholic beverages during therapy unless use has been approved by the physician.

When tetracycline has been prescribed, warn the patient to avoid exposure to the sun or any type of tanning lamp or bed. When exposure to direct sunlight is unavoidable, advise the patient to completely cover the arms and legs and wear a wide-brimmed hat to protect the face and neck. Advise the patient that application of a sunscreen may or may not be effective and to consult the physician before using a sunscreen to prevent a photosensitivity reaction.

Develop a teaching plan to include one or more of the following:
- Take the drug at the prescribed time intervals. These time intervals are important because a certain amount of the drug must be in the body at all times for the infection to be controlled.
- Do not increase or omit the dose unless advised to do so by the physician.
- Complete the entire course of treatment. Do not stop the drug, except on the advice of a physician, before the course of treatment is completed even though symptoms improve or have disappeared. Failure to complete the prescribed course of treatment may result in a return of the infection.
- Take each dose with a full glass of water. Follow the directions given by the pharmacist regarding taking the drug on an empty stomach or with food.
- Notify the physician if symptoms of the infection become worse or there is no improvement in the original symptoms after about 5 days.

■ *Expected Outcomes for Evaluation*
- Anxiety is reduced
- Adverse reactions are identified and reported to the physician

- Patient and family demonstrate understanding of drug regimen
- Patient verbalizes importance of complying with the prescribed therapeutic regimen

Chapter Summary

- This chapter discusses three groups of broad-spectrum antibiotics: the tetracyclines, the macrolides, and the lincosamides.
- The tetracyclines, macrolides, and lincosamides exert their effect by inhibiting protein synthesis of microorganisms. The ultimate effect of this action is that the bacteria are either destroyed or their multiplication rate is slowed.
- The tetracyclines, macrolides, and lincosamides are effective in the treatment of infections caused by a wide range of gram-negative and gram-positive microorganisms. Culture and sensitivity tests (see Chap. 6) are performed to determine which antibiotic will best control the infection.
- Adverse reactions that may be seen with the administration of any antibiotic include superinfection and hypersensitivity reactions. Adverse reactions of the tetracyclines are primarily related to the gastrointestinal tract. Photosensitivity reactions also may be seen.
- Most of the adverse reactions seen with the administration of azithromycin and clarithromycin are related to the gastrointestinal tract and include nausea, vomiting, diarrhea, and abdominal pain. Abdominal cramping, nausea, vomiting, diarrhea, and allergic reactions have been reported with the administration of the erythromycins.
- Abdominal pain, esophagitis, nausea, vomiting, diarrhea, skin rash, and blood dyscrasias may be seen with the use of the administration of the lincosamides.

Critical Thinking Exercises

1. Ms. Jonas has been prescribed minocycline. To decrease the possibility of noncompliance to the treatment regimen, how would you stress the importance of taking the medication as prescribed by the physician?
2. Mr. Park, a patient in a nursing home, has been receiving clarithromycin for an upper respiratory infection for 8 days. The nurse assistant reports that he has been incontinent of feces for the past 2 days. Should this matter be investigated? Why?

9

The Fluoroquinolones and Aminoglycosides

Key Terms

Bactericidal

Nephrotoxicity

Neuromuscular blockade

Neurotoxicity

Ototoxicity

Photosensitivity reaction

Chapter Outline

Chapter Objectives

On completion of this chapter the student will:

- *Discuss the uses of the fluoroquinolones and aminoglycosides*
- *List some of the adverse reactions associated with the administration of the fluoroquinolones and aminoglycosides*
- *Discuss the nursing management of the patient receiving a fluoroquinolone or aminoglycoside*
- *Use the nursing process when administering a fluoroquinolone or aminoglycoside*

The fluoroquinolones and aminoglycosides are two groups of broad-spectrum antibiotics that resulted from research into different types of drugs that would be effective in treating infections due to microorganisms that were becoming resistant to antibiotics in current use.

The Fluoroquinolones and Aminoglycosides

The fluoroquinolones include ciprofloxacin (Cipro), enoxacin (Penetrax), lomefloxacin (Maxaquin), ofloxacin (Floxin). The aminoglycosides include amikacin (Amikin), gentamicin (Garamycin), kanamycin (Kantrex), neomycin (Mycifradin), netilmicin (Netromycin), paromomycin (Humatin), streptomycin, and tobramycin (Nebcin). Summary Drug Table 9-1 lists the fluoroquinolones and aminoglycosides discussed in this chapter.

ACTIONS OF THE FLUOROQUINOLONES AND AMINOGLYCOSIDES

The fluoroquinolones exert their *bactericidal* (bacteria-destroying) effect by interfering with an enzyme (DNA gyrase) needed by bacteria for the synthesis of DNA. The aminoglycosides exert their bactericidal effect by blocking a step in protein synthesis necessary for bacterial multiplication.

USES OF THE FLUOROQUINOLONES AND AMINOGLYCOSIDES

The fluoroquinolones and aminoglycosides are used in the treatment of infections caused by susceptible microorganisms. The fluoroquinolones are effective in the treatment of infections caused by gram-positive and gram-negative microorganisms. The aminoglycosides are used primarily in the treatment of infections caused by gram-negative microorganisms. Culture and sensitivity tests (see Chap. 6) are performed to determine which antibiotic will best control the infection. As with other antibiotics, these drugs are of no value in the treatment of viral or fungal infections.

The oral aminoglycosides kanamycin (Kantrex) and neomycin (Mycifradin) are used preoperatively to reduce the number of bacteria normally present in the intestine ("bowel prep"). A reduction in intestinal bacteria is thought to lessen the possibility of abdominal infection that may occur after surgery on the bowel. These two drugs and paromomycin are also used orally in the management of hepatic coma. In this disorder, liver failure results in an elevation of blood ammonia levels. By reducing the number of ammonia-forming bacteria in the intestines, blood ammonia levels may be lowered, thereby temporarily reducing some of the symptoms associated with this disorder.

ADVERSE REACTIONS ASSOCIATED WITH THE ADMINISTRATION OF THE FLUOROQUINOLONES AND AMINOGLYCOSIDES

Bacterial or fungal superinfections and pseudomembranous colitis (see Chap. 6 for a discussion of these adverse reactions) may be seen. The administration of any drug may result in a hypersensitivity reaction, which can range from mild to severe and, in some cases, be life-threatening. Mild hypersensitivity reactions may only require discontinuing the drug, whereas the more serious reactions require immediate treatment. See Chapters 1 and 6 for a discussion of hypersensitivity reactions.

The Fluoroquinolones

The more common adverse effects seen with the administration of these agents include nausea, diarrhea, headache, abdominal pain or discomfort, and headache. A serious adverse reaction seen with the administration of the fluoroquinolones, especially lomefloxacin, is a *photosensitivity reaction*; this is manifested by an exaggerated sunburn reaction when the skin is exposed to the ultraviolet rays of sunlight or sunlamps.

The Aminoglycosides

The aminoglycosides are capable of causing *nephrotoxicity* (damage to the kidneys by a toxic substance) and *ototoxicity* (damage to the organs of hearing by a toxic substance). Signs and symptoms of nephrotoxicity may include protein in the urine (proteinuria), hematuria, increase in the blood urea nitrogen, decrease in urine output, and an increase in the serum creatinine. Signs and symptoms of ototoxicity in-

Summary Drug Table 9-1. The Fluoroquinolones and Aminoglycosides

Generic Name	Trade Name*	Uses	Adverse Reactions	Dose Ranges
THE FLUOROQUINOLONES				
ciprofloxacin	Cipro, Cipro I.V.	Treatment of infections due to susceptible microorganisms	Nausea, diarrhea, headache, abdominal pain or discomfort, photosensitivity reaction, superinfection, hypersensitivity reactions, pseudomembranous colitis	250–750 mg PO q12h; 200–400 mg IV q12h
enoxacin	Penetrex	Same as ciprofloxacin	Same as ciprofloxacin	200–400 mg PO q12h
lomefloxacin hydrochloride	Maxaquin	Same as ciprofloxacin	Same as ciprofloxacin	400 mg PO once daily
norfloxacin	Noroxin Minocin IV	Urinary tract infections, uncomplicated gonorrhea	Same as ciprofloxacin	400 mg PO q12h; 800 mg PO as single dose for gonorrhea
ofloxacin	Floxin,	Same as ciprofloxacin	Same as ciprofloxaci	200–400 mg PO, IV q12h
THE AMINOGLYCOSIDES				
amikacin	Amikin, *generic*	Same as ciprofloxacin	Nephrotoxicity, ototoxicity, neurotoxicity, nausea, vomiting, anorexia, hypersensitivity reaction, superinfection, pseudomembranous colitis	15 mg/kg/d IM, IV in 2–3 equal doses
gentamicin	Garamycin, *generic*	Same as ciprofloxacin	Same as amikacin	3 mg/kg/d IM, IV in 3 equally divided doses 8qh (higher doses may be used in some cases)
kanamycin sulfate	Kantrex, *generic*	IM, IV use same as ciprofloxacin; oral use suppression of intestinal bacteria, hepatic coma	Same as amikacin	15 mg/kg/d IM, IV in 2 divided doses q6, 8, or 12h; suppression of intestinal bacteria: 1 g PO qh ×4 then 1 g PO q6h for 36–72 h; hepatic coma 8–12 g/d PO in divided doses
neomycin sulfate	Mycifradin, *generic*	Suppression of intestinal bacteria, hepatic coma	Same as amikacin	Suppression of intestinal bacteria (day 1 before surgery): 1 g PO at 1 PM, 2 PM, 11 PM; hepatic coma: 4–12 g/d PO in divided doses
netilmicin sulfate	Netromycin	Same as ciprofloxacin	Same as amikacin	Up to 6.5 mg/kg/d IM, IV in divided doses
paromomycin	Humatin	Hepatic coma	Same as amikacin	4 g/d PO in divided doses
streptomycin sulfate	*generic*	Tuberculosis, infections caused by susceptible microorganisms	Same as amikacin	Tuberculosis: up to 1 g/d IM or 25–30 mg/kg IM 2–3 times a week
tobramycin sulfate	Nebcin, *generic*	Same as ciprofloxacin	Same as amikacin	3–5 mg/kg/d IM, IV in 3 equal doses q8h

*The term, *generic*, indicates the drug is available in generic form.

clude tinnitus, dizziness, roaring in the ears, vertigo, and a mild to severe loss of hearing. If hearing loss occurs, it is most often permanent. Ototoxicity may occur during drug therapy but may also not occur until after the drug is discontinued. Nephrotoxicity is usually reversible once the drug is discontinued.

The short-term administration of kanamycin and neomycin as a preparation for bowel surgery rarely causes these two adverse reactions.

Neurotoxicity (damage to the nervous system by a toxic substance) may also be seen with the administration of the aminoglycosides. Signs and symptoms of neurotoxicity include numbness, skin tingling, circumoral (around the mouth) paresthesia, peripheral paresthesia, tremors, muscle twitching, convulsions, muscle weakness, and *neuromuscular blockade* (acute muscular paralysis and apnea).

Additional adverse reactions may include nausea, vomiting, anorexia, rash, and urticaria. When these agents are given, individual drug references, such as the package insert, should be consulted for more specific adverse reactions.

NURSING MANAGEMENT

Encourage patients receiving the fluoroquinolones to increase their fluid intake. Norfloxacin and enoxacin are given on an empty stomach (eg, 1 hour before or 2 hours after meals). Ciprofloxacin and lomefloxacin can be given without regard to meals, however, the manufacturer recommends that the preferred dosing time is 2 hours after a meal. The oral aminoglycosides may be given without regard to meals. If there is any doubt about administration of these drugs with or without food, consult the hospital pharmacist.

When kanamycin or neomycin are given for suppression of intestinal bacteria prior to surgery, the physician's orders regarding the timing of the administration of the drug are extremely important. Omission of a dosage or failure to give the drug at the specified time may result in inadequate suppression of intestinal bacteria. When neomycin is given, enteric coated erythromycin (see Chap. 8) may be given at the same time as part of the bowel preparation.

When kanamycin or neomycin are given orally as treatment for hepatic coma, exercise care when giving the drug. During the early stages of this disorder, various changes in the level of consciousness may be seen. At times, the patient may appear lethargic and respond poorly to commands. Because of these changes in the level of consciousness, there may be difficulty swallowing and a danger of aspiration. If the patient appears to have difficulty taking an oral medication, withhold the drug and contact the physician.

Nursing Process
The Patient Receiving a Fluoroquinolone or Aminoglycoside

■ *Assessment*
Before the administration of these drugs, identify and record the signs and symptoms of the infection. It is particularly important to obtain a thorough al-

lergy history, especially a history of drug allergies. Take and record vital signs as well.

The physician may order culture and sensitivity tests, and the culture is obtained before the first dose of the drug is given. When an aminoglycoside is to be given, laboratory tests such as renal and hepatic function tests, complete blood count, and urinalysis may also be ordered.

When kanamycin or neomycin is given for hepatic coma, the patient's level of consciousness and ability to swallow must be evaluated.

■ *Nursing Diagnoses*
One or more of the following nursing diagnoses may apply to a person receiving an antibiotic. Additional nursing diagnoses, based on the patient's symptoms, may be required.

- **Risk for Altered Body Temperature: Hyperthermia** related to infectious process
- **Anxiety** related to infection, seriousness of illness, route of administration, other factors (specify)
- **Diarrhea** related to superinfection secondary to antibiotic therapy, adverse drug reaction
- **Noncompliance** related to indifference, lack of knowledge, other factors
- **Risk for Ineffective Management of Therapeutic Regimen** due to insufficient knowledge of medication regimen

■ *Planning and Implementation*
The major goals of the patient may include a reduction in anxiety, an absence of adverse drug effects, and an understanding of and compliance to the prescribed treatment regimen. To make these goals measurable, more specific criteria must be added.

Each day compare the initial signs and symptoms of the infection, which were recorded during the initial assessment, to the present signs and symptoms and record these findings in the patient's chart. When kanamycin or neomycin are given for hepatic coma, evaluate and record the patient's general condition daily.

Vital Signs. Monitor vital signs every 4 hours or as ordered by the physician. Notify the physician if there are changes in the vital signs, such as a significant drop in blood pressure, an increase in the pulse or respiratory rate, or a sudden increase in temperature.

When an aminoglycoside is being administered, monitor the patient's respiratory rate because neuromuscular blockade has been reported with the administration of these drugs. Report any changes in the respiratory rate or rhythm to the physician because immediate treatment may be necessary.

Adverse Drug Reactions. A variety of adverse reactions can be seen with the administration of the fluoroquinolones or aminoglycosides. Review the reactions associated with a specific drug to determine which assessments and nursing tasks will be necessary to identify the adverse reactions that may occur during therapy with that drug. Observe the patient, especially during the first 48 hours of therapy. Report the occurrence of any adverse reaction to the physician before the next dose of the drug is due. Contact the physician immediately if a serious adverse reaction, such as a hypersensitivity reaction, respiratory difficulty, severe diarrhea, or a decided drop in blood pressure, occurs.

Always listen, evaluate, and report any complaints the patient may have; certain complaints may be an early sign of an adverse drug reaction. All changes in the patient's condition and any new problems that occur, for example, nausea or diarrhea, should be brought to the attention of the physician as soon as possible. It is then up to the physician to decide if these changes or problems are a part of the patient's infectious process or due to an adverse drug reaction.

> ### Nursing Alert
>
> The aminoglycosides are potentially nephrotoxic, ototoxic, and neurotoxic and cause permanent damage to these organs and structures. Notify the physician immediately when one or more signs and symptoms of these adverse reactions is suspected.

Measure and record the intake and output and notify the physician if the output is less than 500 mL/day. Any changes in the intake and output ratio or in the appearance of the urine may indicate nephrotoxicity and are reported to the physician promptly. To detect ototoxicity, carefully evaluate the patient's complaints or comments related to hearing, such as a ringing or buzzing in the ears or difficulty hearing. If hearing problems do occur, report this problem to the physician immediately.

INTRAMUSCULAR ADMINISTRATION. With the exception of paromomycin, all of the aminoglycosides can be given intramuscularly. None of the fluoroquinolones are given by this route of administration. Inspect previous injection sites for signs of pain or tenderness, redness, and swelling. Inform the physician of any persistence in a localized reaction of pain,

redness, or extreme tenderness. Rotate injection sites and record the site used on the patient's chart.

INTRAVENOUS ADMINISTRATION. With the exception of paromomycin and streptomycin, all of the aminoglycosides can be given intravenously (IV). Ciprofloxacin and ofloxacin are the only fluoroquinolones given by this route. Inspect the needle site and area around the needle every hour for signs of extravasation of the IV fluid. Perform these assessments more frequently if the patient is restless or uncooperative. Check the rate of infusion every 15 minutes and adjust as needed. Inspect the vein used for the IV infusion every 4 hours for signs of tenderness, pain, and redness (which may indicate phlebitis or thrombophlebitis). If these are apparent, restart the IV in another vein and bring the problem to the attention of the physician. Measure the intake and output.

SUPERINFECTION AND PSEUDOMEMBRANOUS COLITIS. A superinfection can occur during therapy with any antibiotic. Signs and symptoms of a fungal superinfection include sores in the mouth, itching around the anogenital area, and vaginal itching and discharge. Signs and symptoms of a bacterial superinfection include diarrhea, fever, chills, and sore throat.

Check the patient's stools and report any incidence of diarrhea immediately as this event may be an indication of a superinfection or pseudomembranous colitis. If diarrhea does occur and there appears to be blood and mucus in the stool, save a sample of the stool and test for occult blood using a test such as Hemoccult. If the stool tests positive for blood, the sample is saved for possible additional laboratory tests.

Anxiety. Some patients may show varying degrees of anxiety due to their illness and infection and the prescribed treatment modality. Parenteral administration of the drug may result in pain or discomfort. Make an effort to relieve discomfort by nursing measures, such as supporting the extremity used for IV administration or turning the patient to relieve pressure on an injection site. Reassure the patient that every effort will be made to reduce pain and discomfort but there may be times when this may not be possible.

■ *Patient and Family Teaching*

Explain all adverse reactions associated with the specific prescribed antibiotic to the patient. Alert the patient to the signs and symptoms of potentially serious adverse reactions, such as hypersensitivity reactions, which include moderate to severe diarrhea, sudden onset of chills and fever, sore throat, sores in the mouth, or extreme fatigue. Reinforce the necessity of contacting the physician immediately if such symptoms should occur. Caution patients against the use of alcoholic beverages during therapy unless approved by the physician.

To reduce the incidence of noncompliance to the treatment regimen, develop a teaching plan to include one or more of the following:

* Take the drug at the prescribed time intervals. These time intervals are important because a certain amount of the drug must be in the body at all times for the infection to be controlled.
* Drink six to eight large glasses of fluids while taking these drugs and take each dose with a full glass of water.
* Do not increase or omit the dose unless advised to do so by the physician.
* Complete the entire course of treatment. Do not stop the drug, except on the advice of a physician, before the course of treatment is completed even if symptoms improve or have disappeared. Failure to complete the prescribed course of treatment may result in a return of the infection.
* Follow the directions supplied with the prescription regarding taking the drugs with meals or on an empty stomach. For drugs that must be taken on an empty stomach: take 1 hour before or 2 hours after a meal.
* Notify the physician if symptoms of the infection become worse or there is no improvement in the original symptoms after 5 to 7 days of drug therapy.

Specific instructions for the fluoroquinolones:
* Avoid any exposure to sunlight or ultraviolet light (tanning beds, sunlamps) while taking these drugs and for several weeks after completing the course of therapy.

Specific instructions for a preoperative preparation of the bowel:
* Take the prescribed drug at the exact times indicated on the prescription container.

■ Expected Outcomes for Evaluation
* Adverse reactions are identified and reported to the physician
* Anxiety is reduced
* Patient and family demonstrate understanding of drug regimen
* Patient verbalizes importance of complying with the prescribed therapeutic regimen

Chapter Summary

* The fluoroquinolones and aminoglycosides are two groups of broad-spectrum antibiotics.
* The fluoroquinolones exert their bactericidal effect by interfering with an enzyme (DNA gyrase) needed by bacteria for the synthesis of DNA. The aminoglycosides exert their bactericidal effect by blocking a step in protein synthesis necessary for bacterial multiplication.
* The fluoroquinolones and aminoglycosides are used in the treatment of infections caused by susceptible microorganisms. The fluoroquinolones are effective in the treatment of infections caused by gram-positive and gram-negative microorganisms. The aminoglycosides are used primarily in the treatment of infections caused by gram-negative microorganisms. Kanamycin and neomycin are also used in preparing the bowel for surgery. These two drugs and paromomycin are also used orally in the management of hepatic coma.
* Superinfections, pseudomembranous colitis and hypersensitivity reactions may occur with the use of any antibiotic.
* The more common adverse effects seen with the administration of the fluoroquinolones include nausea, diarrhea, headache, abdominal pain or discomfort, and headache. A photosensitivity reaction also may be seen.
* The aminoglycosides are potentially nephrotoxic, ototoxic, and neurotoxic and cause permanent damage to these organs and structures.

Critical Thinking Exercises

1. Mr. Baker is receiving amikacin (Amikin) IV as treatment for a bacterial septicemia. When checking a drug reference you note that this drug is an aminoglycoside. There are two major and serious toxic effects associated with this group of drugs. What daily assessments would you perform to detect early signs and symptoms of these adverse drug effects?
2. Mr. Carson is seen in the outpatient clinic for a severe respiratory infection and is prescribed ciprofloxacin. What would you include in the teaching plan for this patient?

10

Miscellaneous Antiinfectives

Key Terms

Aerobic
Anaerobic
Bactericidal
Bacteriostatic
Nephrotoxicity
Neurotoxicity
Ototoxicity
Paresthesias

Chapter Outline

Chapter Objectives

On completion of this chapter the student will:

- *Discuss the uses of the drugs presented in this chapter*
- *List and describe any three serious adverse reactions that may be seen with the administration of the drugs presented in this chapter*

(continued)

Chapter Objectives *(continued)*

- *Give one or more nursing assessments that are performed when a drug is potentially neurotoxic, nephrotoxic, or ototoxic*
- *Discuss the nursing implications to be considered when administering the drugs presented in this chapter*
- *Use the nursing process when administering the drugs presented in this chapter*

The antiinfectives discussed in this chapter (see Summary Drug Table 10-1) are singular drugs, that is, they are not related to each other and do not belong to any one of the drug groups discussed in Chapters 6 through 9. Some of these drugs are only used for the treatment of one type of infection whereas other ones may be limited to the treatment of serious infections not treatable by other antiinfectives.

Atovaquone

ACTIONS AND USES OF ATOVAQUONE

Atovaquone (Mepron) is used in the treatment of mild to moderate *Pneumocystis carinii* pneumonia, which is seen in persons with inadequate function of their immune system, primarily those with acquired immunodeficiency syndrome. The mechanism of action against the microorganism *P. carinii* is not known.

ADVERSE REACTIONS ASSOCIATED WITH THE ADMINISTRATION OF ATOVAQUONE

Some of the adverse reactions associated with this drug include fever, rash, nausea, diarrhea, vomiting, insomnia, and headache.

NURSING MANAGEMENT

The drug is taken three times a day for 21 days. The importance of completing the full course of therapy is emphasized. Some of the adverse reactions associated with atovaquone may be difficult to distinguish from those that may be caused by acquired immun-

odeficiency syndrome. Any problem or complaint that the patient may have is reported to the physician, who must then determine the probable cause.

> **Nursing Alert**
>
> This drug is given orally and *must* be given with meals because food increases the absorption of the drug and thereby increases the concentration of the drug in the blood.

Aztreonam

ACTION AND USES OF AZTREONAM

Aztreonam (Azactam) is a synthetic antiinfective, which exerts its *bactericidal* (bacteria-destroying) activity by inhibiting the synthesis of the bacterial cell wall. This antiinfective is chemically related to, but not in the same class as, the penicillins and cephalosporins.

Aztreonam is used in the treatment of disorders such as urinary tract infections, lower respiratory infections, septicemia, surgical wound infections, and gynecologic infections caused by gram-negative *aerobic* (requiring oxygen to live and grow) bacteria.

ADVERSE REACTIONS ASSOCIATED WITH THE ADMINISTRATION OF AZTREONAM

The adverse effects associated with the administration of aztreonam include bacterial or fungal superinfection (see Chap. 6) and hypersensitivity reactions (see Chap. 1 and 6). Other adverse reactions include skin rash, diarrhea, nausea, and vomiting. Localized thrombophlebitis or phlebitis may be seen after intravenous (IV) administration.

NURSING MANAGEMENT

Patients allergic to penicillin and the cephalosporins may be allergic to aztreonam. A careful drug history, particularly a history of drug allergy is essential. Discomfort at the site of intramuscular (IM) injection may occur. Prior to giving each injection, warn the patient that some discomfort may be felt as the drug is injected, as well as for a brief time afterwards.

Summary Drug Table 10-1. Miscellaneous Antiinfectives

Generic Name	Trade Name*	Uses	Adverse Reactions	Dose Ranges
atovaquone	Mepron	Treatment of mild to moderate *Pneumocystis carinii* pneumonia	Fever, rash, nausea, diarrhea, vomiting, insomnia, headache	750 mg PO tid with food for 21 d
aztreonam	Azactam	Treatment of susceptible gram-negative infections	Superinfection, rash, diarrhea, nausea, vomiting, phlebitis or thrombophlebitis with IV administration	500 mg to 1 g IM q8 or 12h; 500 mg to 2 g IV q6, 8, or 12h
chloramphenicol	Chloromycetin, *generic*	Treatment of serious, susceptible infections in which other less potentially dangerous drugs are ineffective or contraindicated	Serious to fatal blood dyscrasias, super infection, hypersensitivity reactions, nausea, vomiting, headache	50–100 mg/kg/d PO, IV in divided doses q8h
furazolidone	Furoxone	Bacterial or protozoal diarrhea	Hypersensitivity reactions, headache, malaise, nausea, vomiting, disulfiram-like reaction with alcohol ingestion	100 mg PO qid
imipenem-cilastatin	Primaxin I.M., Primaxin I.V.	Treatment of serious, susceptible gram-positive and gram-negative infections	Hypersensitivity reactions, superinfection, pseudomembranous colitis, thrombophlebitis and phlebitis (IV use), pain at the injection site (IM use), nausea, diarrhea, vomiting, fever, chest discomfort, rash	250 mg to 1 g IV q6–8h; 500–750 mg IM q12h
metronidazole	Flagyl, Protostat, *generic*	Infections caused by susceptible anaerobic microorganisms	Nausea, anorexia, vomiting, diarrhea, seizures, numbness, hypersensitivity reactions, disulfiram-like reaction with alcohol ingestion	7.5–15 mg/kg IV q6h; 7.5 mg/kg PO q6h
novobiocin	Albamycin	Treatment of serious, susceptible infections caused by *S. aureus*	Superinfection, hypersensitivity reactions, blood dyscrasias, jaundice, nausea, vomiting, diarrhea	250 mg PO q6h or 500 mg PO q12h
pentamidine isethionate	Pentam 300, NebuPent	Treatment of *Pneumocystis carinii* pneumonia (IM, IV); prevention of *Pneumocystis carinii* (inhalation)	Leukopenia, severe hypotension, hypoglycemia, thrombocytopenia	4 mg/kg IM, IV once a day; 300 mg once every 4 w aerosol
polymyxin-B sulfate	Aerosporin, *generic*	Treatment of gram-negative infections especially susceptible strains of *Pseudomonas aeruginosa*	Nephrotoxicity, neurotoxicity, fever, rash, pain at IM injection site, thrombophlebitis (IV use)	15,000–25,000 units/kg/d IV; 25,000–30,000 units/kg/d IM in divided doses q4–6h
spectinomycin	Trobicin	Gonorrhea	Urticaria, dizziness, rash, chills, fever, hypersensitivity reactions, soreness at injection site	2 g IM as single dose; disseminated gonococcal infections: 2 g IM q12h
vancomycin	Vancocin, Lyphocin, *generic*	Treatment of serious, susceptible gram-positive infections not responding to treatment with other antibiotics	Nephrotoxicity, ototoxicity, nausea, chills, fever, urticaria, rash, sudden fall in blood pressure (IV use)	500 mg to 2 g/d PO in 3–4 divided doses; 500 mg IV q6h or 1 g IV q12h

*The term, *generic*, indicates the drug is available in generic form.

Chloramphenicol

ACTIONS AND USES OF CHLORAMPHENICOL

Chloramphenicol (Chloromycetin) interferes with or inhibits protein synthesis, a process necessary for the growth and multiplication of microorganisms. Serious and sometimes fatal blood dyscrasias are the chief adverse reaction seen with the administration of chloramphenicol and therefore limit its usefulness except in serious infections when less potentially dangerous drugs are ineffective or contraindicated.

ADVERSE REACTIONS ASSOCIATED WITH THE ADMINISTRATION OF CHLORAMPHENICOL

In addition to blood dyscrasias, superinfection, hypersensitivity reactions, nausea, vomiting, and headache, may also be seen. It is recommended that patients receiving oral chloramphenicol be hospitalized so that patient observation and frequent blood studies can be performed during treatment with this drug.

NURSING MANAGEMENT

When given orally, the drug is given on an empty stomach. If gastrointestinal distress occurs, the drug may be given with food. Chloramphenicol is also given IV.

Nursing Alert

The blood dyscrasias may occur with the administration of chloramphenicol during either short- or long-term therapy. Observe patients closely for signs and symptoms that may indicate a blood dyscrasia, namely fever, sore throat, sores in the mouth, easy bruising, and extreme fatigue.

Furazolidone

ACTIONS AND USES OF FURAZOLIDONE

Furazolidone (Furoxone) exerts its bactericidal activity by interfering with several bacterial enzyme systems, thus decreasing the chance of development of resistant strains of bacteria. This drug is used specifically for treatment of diarrhea due to bacteria or protozoa.

ADVERSE REACTIONS ASSOCIATED WITH THE ADMINISTRATION OF FURAZOLIDONE

Although used in treatment of a GI disorder, this drug does not alter the normal bowel flora and administration does not result in a fungal superinfection of the bowel. Adverse effects that may be seen include hypersensitivity reactions, headache, malaise, nausea, and vomiting. If the patient drinks an alcoholic beverage while taking this drug, a disulfiram-like reaction (see Chap. 51) may be seen. This reaction is characterized by fever, flushing, lightheadedness, dyspnea, and nausea and vomiting.

NURSING MANAGEMENT

Furazolidone is given orally. Inform the patient that the drug may turn the urine brown and that this is normal. When this drug is given on an outpatient basis, instruct the patient to avoid drinking any type of alcoholic beverage during and for 4 days after therapy is completed. Also instruct the patient to avoid all over-the-counter medications (especially those used for hay fever, nasal congestion, appetite suppression, and colds) unless use has been approved by the physician. If the drug is taken for more than 5 days, instruct the patient to avoid foods high in tyramine because marked hypertension or a hemorrhagic stroke may occur during or after therapy with this drug. The length of time the patient must avoid these foods is decided by the physician. Examples of tyramine-containing foods are sharp or aged cheeses, sour cream, yogurt, bananas, chicken liver, beer, sherry wine, and coffee. A complete list of foods containing tyramine can be obtained from the dietitian and given to the patient.

Imipenem-Cilastatin

ACTIONS AND USES OF IMIPENEM-CILASTATIN

Imipenem-cilastatin (Primaxin I.V., Primaxin I.M.) exerts its bactericidal activity by inhibiting synthesis of the bacterial cell wall. This drug is used to treat serious infections, such as lower respiratory tract, urinary tract, and intraabdominal infections caused by susceptible aerobic gram-positive and gram-negative microorganisms.

ADVERSE REACTIONS ASSOCIATED WITH THE ADMINISTRATION OF IMIPENEM-CILASTATIN

Hypersensitivity reactions, superinfection, pseudomembranous colitis, and localized thrombophlebitis and phlebitis can occur when this drug is given IV. Pain is possible at the injection site when given IM. Nausea, diarrhea, vomiting, fever, chest discomfort, and rash may be seen with the administration of imipenem-cilastatin.

NURSING MANAGEMENT

Reconstitute the drug with the appropriate diluents as directed on the container and package insert. If the drug was prepared for administration (eg, reconstituted) by the pharmacist, follow the pharmacist's or package insert directions regarding storage and use. When given IM, reconstitute the drug with a 1% lidocaine (*without* epinephrine) solution as directed in the package insert. Lidocaine, a local anesthetic, reduces discomfort following intramuscular injection. Inject the drug is injected into a large muscle mass, such as the gluteus muscle.

> **Nursing Alert**
>
> Patients allergic to penicillin may experience a hypersensitivity reaction to imipenem-cilastatin. A careful drug allergy history is essential.

Metronidazole

ACTIONS AND USES OF METRONIDAZOLE

The mode of action of metronidazole (Flagyl) is not well understood. This drug may be used in the treatment of serious infections, such as intraabdominal, bone, soft tissue, lower respiratory, and central nervous system (CNS) infections caused by susceptible *anaerobic* (able to live without oxygen) microorganisms.

ADVERSE REACTIONS ASSOCIATED WITH THE ADMINISTRATION OF METRONIDAZOLE

The most common adverse reactions to this drug are related to the gastrointestinal tract and may include nausea, anorexia, and occasionally vomiting and diarrhea. The most serious adverse reaction is related to the CNS with seizures and numbness of the extremities. Hypersensitivity reactions may also be seen. Thrombophlebitis may occur withIV use.

NURSING MANAGEMENT

When prepared by the nurse, the package insert should be consulted for reconstitution of the powder form because the directions for the order of preparation for IV administration *must* be followed. When given orally, the drug is given with meals to avoid gastrointestinal upset. Inform the patient that an unpleasant metallic taste may be noted during therapy. When given on an outpatient basis, advise the patient to avoid drinking alcoholic beverages because a disulfiram-like reaction may occur.

Novobiocin

ACTIONS AND USES OF NOVOBIOCIN

Novobiocin (Albamycin) exerts its *bacteriostatic* (slow or retard the multiplication of bacteria) effect by interfering with bacterial cell wall synthesis. Novobiocin is used in the treatment of serious infections due to a *Staphylococcus aureus* infection when other antiinfectives are ineffective.

ADVERSE REACTIONS ASSOCIATED WITH THE ADMINISTRATION OF NOVOBIOCIN

Superinfection and hypersensitivity reactions may be seen with the administration of this drug. Additional adverse reactions include blood dyscrasias, jaundice, nausea, vomiting, and diarrhea.

NURSING MANAGEMENT

> **Nursing Alert**
>
> Novobiocin, which is given orally, has a high rate of hypersensitivity reactions. Closely observe the patient for skin rash and urticaria, two of the most common indications of a hypersensitivity reaction with the administration of this drug.

Pentamidine Isethionate

ACTIONS AND USES OF PENTAMIDINE ISETHIONATE

Pentamidine isethionate (Pentam 300, the parenteral form; NebuPent, the aerosol form) is used in the treatment (parenteral form) or prevention (aerosol form) of *Pneumocystis carinii* pneumonia, a pneumonia seen in those with acquired immunodeficiency syndrome. The mode of action of this drug is not fully understood.

ADVERSE REACTIONS ASSOCIATED WITH THE ADMINISTRATION OF PENTAMIDINE ISETHIONATE

More than half of the patients receiving this drug by the parenteral route experience some adverse reaction. Severe and sometimes life-threatening reactions include leukopenia (low white blood cell count), hypoglycemia (low blood sugar), thrombocytopenia (low platelet count), and hypotension. Moderate or less severe reactions include changes in some laboratory tests, such as the serum creatinine and liver function tests. Nausea and anorexia may also be seen. Aerosol administration may result in fatigue, a metallic taste in the mouth, shortness of breath, and anorexia.

NURSING MANAGEMENT

When given IM or IV, prepare the drug according to the manufacturer's directions. When given by the IV route, infuse the drug over 1 hour. When given by aerosol, use a special nebulizer (Respirgard II) and deliver the drug until the chamber is empty. Explain or demonstrate the use of the nebulizer to the patient.

Polymyxin B

ACTIONS AND USES OF POLYMYXIN B

Polymyxin B (Aerosporin) exerts its bactericidal effect against susceptible gram-negative bacilli, especially severe infections caused by *Pseudomonas aeruginosa*. It acts by increasing the permeability of bacterial cell wall membranes, which, in turn, results in death of the cell.

ADVERSE REACTIONS ASSOCIATED WITH THE ADMINISTRATION OF POLYMYXIN B

The most serious adverse reactions to this drug are *nephrotoxicity* (damage to the kidneys by a toxic substance) and *neurotoxicity* (damage to the nervous system by a toxic substance). A superinfection also may occur with the use of this drug. Additional adverse reactions include rash, fever, pain at the IM injection site, and thrombophlebitis at the IV injection site.

The signs and symptoms of neurotoxicity include facial flushing, dizziness, *paresthesias* (numbness) of the extremities or around the mouth (circumoral paresthesia), and drowsiness. Signs and symptoms of nephrotoxicity are related to laboratory abnormalities, such as albumin in the urine (albuminuria) and rise in the blood urea nitrogen.

NURSING MANAGEMENT

The manufacturer recommends reconstituting the drug with 2 mL of 1% procaine when the IM route is used to reduce the discomfort associated with this route of administration. When given IV by continuous infusion, inspect the needle site for signs of thrombophlebitis, namely redness and pain along the path of the vein used for administration. Observe the patient for signs of neurotoxicity and any decrease in the urinary output, which may indicate nephrotoxicity.

Spectinomycin

ACTIONS AND USES OF SPECTINOMYCIN

Spectinomycin (Trobicin) is chemically related to but different from the aminoglycosides (see Chap. 9). This drug exerts its action by interfering with bacterial protein synthesis. Spectinomycin is used for treatment of gonorrhea.

ADVERSE REACTIONS ASSOCIATED WITH THE ADMINISTRATION OF SPECTINOMYCIN

Soreness at the injection site, urticaria, dizziness, rash, chills, fever, and hypersensitivity reactions may be seen with the administration of this drug.

NURSING MANAGEMENT

Spectinomycin may be given as a single dose but multiple doses may be prescribed for complicated, widespread gonorrhea. The patient is warned that the IM injection may be uncomfortable and that soreness at the injection site may be noted for a brief time. Emphasis is placed on the importance of following the physician's recommendations regarding a follow-up examination to determine if the infection has been eliminated.

Vancomycin

ACTIONS AND USES OF VANCOMYCIN

Vancomycin (Vancocin) acts against susceptible gram-positive bacteria by inhibiting bacterial cell wall synthesis and increasing cell wall permeability. This drug is used in the treatment of serious gram-positive infections not responding to treatment with other antiinfectives. It also may be used in treating antiinfective-associated pseudomembranous colitis caused by *Clostridium difficile.*

ADVERSE REACTIONS ASSOCIATED WITH THE ADMINISTRATION OF VANCOMYCIN

Nephrotoxicity and *ototoxicity* (damage to the organs of hearing by a toxic substance) may be seen with the administration of this drug. Additional adverse reactions include nausea, chills, fever, urticaria, sudden fall in blood pressure with parenteral administration, and skin rashes.

NURSING MANAGEMENT

Vancomycin may be given orally or by intermittent IV infusion. Unused portions of reconstituted oral suspensions and parenteral solutions are stable for 14 days when refrigerated after reconstitution.

Nursing Alert

Administer each IV dose of the drug over 60 minutes. Too rapid an infusion may result in a sudden and profound fall in blood pressure and shock. When giving the drug IV, the infusion rate must be closely monitored.

Report patient complaints of difficulty hearing or tinnitus (ringing in the ears) to the physician before the next dose is due. Monitor the intake and output and bring any decrease in the urinary output to the attention of the physician.

Nursing Process
The Patient Receiving a Miscellaneous Antiinfective

■ *Assessment*

Before administering these drugs, take and record the patient's vital signs, and identify and record the symptoms of the infection. A thorough allergy history, especially a history of drug allergies, is most important. Aztreonam and imipenem-cilastatin have a higher incidence of hypersensitivity reactions in those with a history of allergy to penicillin or the cephalosporins.

■ *Nursing Diagnoses*

One or more of the following nursing diagnoses may apply to a person receiving an antiinfective. Additional nursing diagnoses, based on the patient's symptoms, may be required.

- **Anxiety** related to infection, seriousness of illness, route of administration, other factors (specify)
- **Diarrhea** related to adverse drug reaction, superinfection
- **Pain** related to intramuscular injection
- **Risk for Ineffective Management of Therapeutic Regimen** related to insufficient knowledge of medication regimen

■ *Planning and Implementation*

The major goals of the patient may include a reduction in anxiety, an absence of adverse drug effects, and an understanding of and compliance to the prescribed treatment regimen. To make these goals measurable, more specific criteria must be added.

When culture and sensitivity tests are ordered, these procedures must be performed before the first dose of the drug is given. Other laboratory tests such as renal and hepatic function tests, complete blood count, and urinalysis may also be ordered before and during drug therapy for early detection of toxic reactions.

Vital Signs. Monitor vital signs every 4 hours or as ordered by the physician. Notify the physician if there are changes in the vital signs, such as a significant drop in blood pressure, an increase in the pulse or respiratory rate, or a sudden increase in temperature.

Adverse Drug Reactions. Observe the patient at frequent intervals, especially during the first 48 hours of therapy. Report the occurrence of any adverse reaction to the physician before the next dose of the drug is due. Immediately report serious adverse reactions, such as signs and symptoms of a hypersensitivity reaction or superinfection, respiratory difficulty, or a marked drop in blood pressure.

Polymyxin-B and Vancomycin are potentially nephrotoxic drugs; some patients may experience a change in kidney function. Measure and record intake and output during the time the patient is receiving either of these drugs. Report any changes in the intake and output ratio or in the appearance of the urine because these may indicate nephrotoxicity.

Polymyxin-B is potentially neurotoxic. Observe the patient for signs and symptoms of this adverse reaction. Vancomycin is potentially ototoxic. Evaluate and report the patient's complaints related to hearing, particularly comments about a ringing or buzzing in the ears or an inability to hear.

IM Administration. When giving these drugs IM, inspect previous injection sites for signs of pain or tenderness, redness, and swelling. Report any persistent local reaction to the physician. Develop a plan for rotation of injection sites and record the site used for each injection.

IV Administration. When giving these drugs IV, inspect the needle site and area around the needle at frequent intervals for signs of extravasation of the IV fluid. Perform more frequent assessments if the patient is restless or uncooperative.

Check the rate of infusion every 15 minutes and adjust as needed. This is especially important when administering vancomycin because rapid infusion of the drug can result in severe hypotension and shock. Inspect the vein used for the IV infusion every 4 to 8 hours for signs of tenderness, pain, and redness (which may indicate phlebitis or thrombophlebitis). If these symptoms are apparent, restart the IV in another vein and bring the problem to the attention of the physician.

Diarrhea. Diarrhea may be a sign of a superinfection or pseudomembranous colitis, both of which are problems that may be seen with the administration of any antiinfective. Check each stool and report any changes in color or consistency. When vancomycin is given as part of the treatment for pseudomembranous colitis, record the color and consistency of each stool to determine the effectiveness of therapy.

Pain. Pain at the injection site may occur when these drugs are given IM. Warn the patient that discomfort may be felt when it is injected and that additional discomfort may be experienced for a brief time afterwards.

Anxiety. Patients may exhibit varying degrees of anxiety related to their illness and infection and the necessary drug therapy. When these drugs are given by the parenteral route, patients may experience anxiety because of the discomfort or pain that accompanies an IM injection or IV administration. Reassure the patient that every effort will be made to reduce pain and discomfort, although complete pain relief but may not always be possible.

■ *Patient and Family Teaching*

Atovaquone, chloramphenicol, furazolidine, metronidazole, novobiocin, and vancomycin can be given orally and prescribed for outpatient use. Patients requiring oral chloramphenicol are usually hospitalized so that blood studies can be done during treatment.

When pentamidine is prescribed for aerosol use at home, review the use of the special nebulizer, as well as directions for cleaning and maintaining the nebulizer equipment.

When furazolidone or metronidazole is prescribed, warn the patient to avoid the use of alcoholic beverages because a severe reaction may occur.

It is most important that the patient and family understand the prescribed treatment regimen. To decrease the chance of noncompliance, the following points are emphasized:

- Take the drug at the prescribed time intervals. These time intervals are important because a certain amount of the drug must be in the body at all times for the infection to be controlled.
- Take the drug with food or on an empty stomach as directed on the prescription container.
- Do not increase or omit the dose unless advised to do so by the physician.
- Complete the entire course of treatment. Do not stop the drug, except on the advice of a physician, before the course of treatment is completed even if symptoms have improved or have disappeared. Failure to complete the prescribed course of treatment may result in a return of the infection.
- Notify the physician if symptoms of the infection become worse or there is no improvement in the original symptoms after about 5 to 7 days.
- Contact the physician as soon as possible if a rash, fever, sore throat, diarrhea, chills, extreme fatigue, easy bruising, or other problems occur.
- Avoid drinking alcoholic beverages unless use has been approved by the physician.

■ *Expected Outcomes for Evaluation*
- Pain or discomfort following IM or IV administration is relieved or eliminated
- Anxiety is reduced
- Adverse reactions are identified and reported to the physician
- Patient and family demonstrate understanding of drug regimen

Chapter Summary

- The antiinfectives discussed in this chapter are singular drugs. They are not related to each other and do not belong to any one of the drug groups discussed in Chapters 6 through 9. Some of these drugs are only used for the treatment of one type of infection, whereas the use of other drugs may be limited to the treatment of serious infections not treatable by other antiinfectives.
- Some of these drugs have the potential to cause serious adverse reactions, such as blood dyscrasias, neurotoxicity, nephrotoxicity, and ototoxicity.
- In many instances, the nursing management during administration of these drugs requires close observation of the patient for serious adverse reactions.

Critical Thinking Exercises

1. The charge nurse asks you to discuss the drug metronidazole (Flagyl) at a team conference. What specific points regarding administration and patient and family teaching would you discuss at the conference?
2. Mr. Stone is receiving vancomycin. One adverse reaction that may be seen with the administration of this drug is ototoxicity. Rather than ask Mr. Stone directly whether he is having any problem with his hearing, how might you determine if ototoxicity might be occurring?
3. Mr. Reeves, who is receiving polymyxin-B, complains of numbness around his mouth and numbness in the tips of his fingers. Why is this complaint significant?

11

The Sulfonamides

Key Terms

Agranulocytosis

Anorexia

Antibacterial

Antiinfective

Aplastic anemia

Bacteriostatic

Leukopenia

Pruritus

Stevens-Johnson
syndrome

Stomatitis

Thrombocytopenia

Urticaria

Chapter Outline

Chapter Objectives

On completion of this chapter the student will:

- *Describe the actions of the sulfonamides*
- *List the adverse reactions associated with the administration of the sulfonamides*
- *Describe the signs and symptoms associated with Stevens-Johnson syndrome*
- *Discuss the nursing implications associated with the administration of the sulfonamides*
- *Use the nursing process when administering a sulfonamide*

Scherer JC, Roach S: INTRODUCTORY CLINICAL PHARMACOLOGY,
FIFTH EDITION © 1996 Lippincott-Raven Publishers

The sulfonamides ("sulfa") drugs were the first effective agents used in the treatment of infections. The use of sulfonamides began to decline following the introduction of more effective antiinfectives, such as the penicillins and other antibiotics. These drugs still remain important antiinfectives in the treatment of certain types of infections.

The Sulfonamides

Sulfonamides are *antibacterial* agents, that is, they are active against (anti) bacteria. Another term that may be used to describe the general action of these drugs is *antiinfective* because they are used to treat infections caused by certain bacteria. Sulfadiazine, sulfisoxazole (Gantrisin), and sulfamethizole (Thiosulfil Forte) are examples of sulfonamide preparations.

ACTIONS OF THE SULFONAMIDES

The sulfonamides are primarily *bacteriostatic*, which means they slow or retard the multiplication of bacteria.

The sulfonamides have bacteriostatic activity because of their antagonism to para-aminobenzoic acid, a substance that some, but not all, bacteria need to multiply. Once the rate of bacterial multiplication is slowed, the body's own defense mechanisms (white blood cells) are able to rid the body of the invading microorganisms and therefore control the infection.

USES OF THE SULFONAMIDES

The sulfonamides are often used to control urinary tract infections caused by certain bacteria such as *Escherichia coli, Staphylococcus aureus,* and *Klebsiella-Enterobacter*. Additional uses of the sulfonamides are given in Summary Drug Table 11-1.

Sulfasalazine (Azulfidine) is used for the management of ulcerative colitis but also has shown effectiveness in the treatment of other disorders such as Crohn's disease and colitis. Mafenide (Sulfamylon) and silver sulfadiazine (Silvadene) are topical sulfonamides used in the treatment of second-degree and third-degree burns. Silver sulfadiazine is also discussed in Chapter 48.

The combination of sulfamethoxazole and the antiinfective trimethoprim (Septra) is used in the treatment of urinary tract infections, acute otitis media, and traveler's diarrhea.

ADVERSE REACTIONS ASSOCIATED WITH THE ADMINISTRATION OF THE SULFONAMIDES

The sulfonamides are capable of causing a variety of adverse reactions. Some of these are serious or potentially serious; others are mild. The hematologic changes that may occur during therapy are an example of a serious adverse reaction. Hematologic changes include *agranulocytosis*, a decrease in or lack of granulocytes, which are a type of white blood cell; *thrombocytopenia*, a decrease in the number of platelets; *aplastic anemia*, anemia due to deficient red blood cell production in the bone marrow; and *leukopenia*, a decrease in the number of white blood cells, any of which may require discontinuation of sulfonamide therapy. A marked decrease in the white blood cell count may result in signs and symptoms of an infection, such as fever, sore throat, and cough. A marked decrease in the number of platelets may result in easy bruising and unusual bleeding following trauma to the skin or mucous membranes. *Anorexia* (loss of appetite) is an example of a mild adverse reaction. Unless it becomes severe and pronounced weight loss occurs, it may not be necessary to discontinue sulfonamide therapy.

Various types of hypersensitivity (allergic) reactions may be seen during sulfonamide therapy and include *Stevens-Johnson syndrome, urticaria* (hives), *pruritus* (itching), and generalized skin eruptions. Stevens-Johnson syndrome is manifested by fever, cough, muscular aches and pains, and headache, all of which are signs and symptoms of many other disorders. The appearance of lesions on the skin, mucous membranes, eyes, and other organs are diagnostically significant and may be the first conclusive signs of this syndrome. The lesions appear as red wheals or blisters, often starting on the face, in the mouth or on the lips, neck, and extremities. This syndrome, which also may occur with the administration of other types of drugs, can be fatal.

Other adverse reactions that may occur during therapy are nausea, vomiting, diarrhea, abdominal pain, chills, fever, and *stomatitis* (inflammation of the mouth). In some instances, these may be mild, whereas at other times they may cause serious problems requiring discontinuation of the drug. Sulfasalazine may cause the urine and skin to be an orange-yellow color; this is not abnormal.

Crystalluria (crystals in the urine) may occur during administration of a sulfonamide, although this problem occurs less frequently with some of the newer sulfonamide preparations. Crystalluria is potentially a serious problem that often can be prevented by increasing fluid intake during sulfonamide therapy.

Summary Drug Table 11-1. The Sulfonamides

Generic Name	Trade Name*	Uses	Adverse Reactions	Dose Ranges
SINGLE AGENTS				
sulfadiazine	*generic*	Urinary tract infections due to susceptible microorganisms, chancroid, acute otitis media, *Haemophilus influenzae* and meningococcal meningitis, rheumatic fever	Hematologic changes, Stevens-Johnson syndrome, nausea, vomiting, headache, diarrhea, chills, fever	Loading dose: 2–4 g PO; maintenance dose: 4–8 g/d PO in 4–6 divided doses
sulfamethizole	Thiosulfil Forte	Urinary tract infections due to susceptible microorganisms	Same as sulfadiazine	0.5–1 g PO tid, qid
sulfamethoxazole	Gantanol, *generic*	Urinary tract infections due to susceptible microorganisms, meningococcal meningitis, acute otitis media	Same as sulfadiazine	Initial dose: 2 g PO; maintenance dose: 1 g PO bid, tid
sulfasalazine	Azulfidine, Azulfidine Entabs, *generic*	Ulcerative colitis	Same as sulfadiazine	Initial therapy: 1–4 g/d PO in divided doses; maintenance dose: 500 mg PO qid
sulfisoxazole	Gantrisin, *generic*	Same as sulfadiazine	Same as sulfadiazine	Loading doses: 2–4 g PO; maintenance dose: 4–8 g/d PO in 4–6 divided doses
MULTIPLE PREPARATIONS				
trimethoprim (TMP) and sulfamethoxazole (SMZ)	Bactrim, Bactrim DS, Septra, Septra DS, *generic*	Urinary tract infections due to susceptible microorganisms, acute otitis media, traveler's diarrhea due to *E. coli*	GI disturbances, allergic skin reactions, hematologic changes, Stevens-Johnson syndrome, headache	160 mg TMP/ 800 mg SMZ PO q12h; 8–10 mg/kg/d (based on TMP) IV in 2–4 divided doses
MISCELLANEOUS SULFONAMIDE PREPARATIONS				
mafenide	Sulfamylon	Second and third degree burns	Pain or burning sensation, rash, itching, facial edema	Apply to burned area 1–2 times/d
silver sulfadiazine	Silvadene, Thermazene	Same as mafenide	Leukopenia, skin necrosis, skin discoloration, burning sensation	Same as mafenide

*The term, *generic*, indicates that the drug is available in generic form.

The most frequent adverse reaction seen with the application of mafenide is a burning sensation or pain when the drug is applied to the skin. Other possible allergic reactions include rash, itching, edema, and urticaria. Burning, rash, and itching may also be seen with the use of silver sulfadiazine. It may be difficult to distinguish between an adverse reaction due to the use of mafenide or silver sulfadiazine and reactions that may occur from the severe burn injury or from other agents used at the same time for the management of the burns.

NURSING MANAGEMENT

The patient receiving a sulfonamide drug almost always has an active infection. However, some patients may be receiving one of these drugs to prevent an infection (prophylaxis) or as part of the management of a disease such as ulcerative colitis.

Unless the physician orders otherwise, sulfonamides are given on an empty stomach, that is, 1 hour before or 2 hours after meals. Sulfasalazine may be given with food or immediately after meals if gastrointestinal irritation occurs. Instruct the patient to drink a full glass of water when taking an oral sulfonamide and to drink at least eight large glasses of water each day until therapy is finished.

When mafenide or silver sulfadiazine is used in the treatment of burns, the treatment regimen is outlined by the physician or the burn treatment unit. There are various burn treatment regimens, such as whirlpool baths, special dressings, and cleansing of the burned area. The use of a specific treatment regimen often depends on the extent of the burned area, the degree of the burns, and the physical condition and age of the patient. Other concurrent problems, such as lung damage due to smoke or heat or physical injuries that occurred at the time of the burn injury, may also influence the treatment regimen.

When instructed to do so, clean and remove debris present on the surface of the skin before each application of mafenide or silver sulfadiazine and apply these drugs with a sterile gloved hand. Warn the patient that stinging or burning may be felt during and for a short time after mafenide is applied. Some burning may also be noted with the application of silver sulfadiazine.

It is most important to inspect the burned areas every 1 to 2 hours because some treatment regimens require keeping the affected areas covered with the mafenide or silver sulfadiazine ointment at all times. Note any adverse reactions that have occurred and report this to the physician immediately.

Nursing Process
The Patient Receiving a Sulfonamide

■ *Assessment*
Before the initial administration of the drug, assess the patient's general appearance and take and record the vital signs. Obtain information regarding the symptoms experienced by the patient, and the length of time these symptoms have been present. Depending on the type and location of the infection or disease, review the results of tests such as a urine culture, urinalysis, complete blood count, intravenous pyelogram, renal function tests, and examination of the stool.

■ *Nursing Diagnoses*
Depending on the drug, dose, and reason for administration, one or more of the following nursing diagnoses may apply to a person receiving a sulfonamide:
- **Anxiety** related to diagnosis, symptoms of infection, other factors

- **Noncompliance** related to indifference, lack of knowledge, other factors
- **Risk for Ineffective Management of Therapeutic Regimen** due to insufficient knowledge of medication regimen

■ *Planning and Implementation*
The major goals of the patient may include a reduction in anxiety, absence of adverse drug reactions, and an understanding of and compliance to the prescribed treatment regimen. To make these goals measurable, more specific criteria must be added.

Evaluate the patient at periodic intervals for response to the drug, that is, a relief of symptoms and a decrease in temperature (if it was elevated before therapy started), as well as the occurrence of any adverse reactions. Closely observe patients receiving sulfasalazine for ulcerative colitis for evidence of the relief or intensification of the symptoms of the disease. Inspect all stool samples and record their number and appearance.

Anxiety. The symptoms of infection, for example frequent urination or burning on urination in those with a bladder infection, may result in anxiety. Reassure the patient that symptoms will most likely diminish after a few days of drug therapy.

Mafenide and sometimes silver sulfadiazine causes a stinging or burning sensation, resulting in anxiety before, during, and after application of the drug. While it may not be possible to completely prevent this problem, use a gentle touch in applying the drug to reduce some of the discomfort associated with the application of a drug to a burned area.

Adverse Drug Reactions. Observe the patient for adverse reactions, especially an allergic reaction. If one or more adverse reactions should occur, withhold the next dose of the drug and notify the physician.

Nursing Alert
Stevens-Johnson syndrome is a serious and sometimes fatal hypersensitivity reaction. Be alert for lesions on the skin and mucous membranes, a diagnostically important symptom of this syndrome. In addition to notifying the physician and withholding the next dose of the drug, exercise care to prevent injury to the involved areas.

Vital Signs. Monitor the temperature, pulse, respiratory rate, and blood pressure every 4 hours or as ordered by the physician. If fever is present and the patient's temperature suddenly increases or if the temperature was normal and suddenly increases, contact the physician immediately.

Fluids. Encourage patients to increase their fluid intake to 2000 mL or more a day to prevent crystalluria and stone formation in the genitourinary tract, as well as to aid in the removal of microorganisms from the urinary tract. Measure and record the intake and output every 8 hours and notify the physician if the urinary output decreases or the patient fails to increase his or her oral intake.

Patients With Diabetes Mellitus. Sulfonamides may inhibit the (hepatic) metabolism of the oral hypoglycemic drugs tolbutamide (Orinase) and chlorpropamide (Diabinese) and thereby increase the possibility of a hypoglycemic reaction.

Nursing Alert

Patients who are diabetic and receiving the oral hypoglycemic agents tolbutamide or chlorpropamide should be observed closely for episodes of hypoglycemia (see Chap 37).

Noncompliance. When a sulfonamide is prescribed for an infection, some outpatients have a tendency to discontinue the drug once symptoms have been relieved. Emphasize the importance of completing the prescribed course of therapy to be sure all microorganisms causing the infection have been eradicated. Failure to complete a course of therapy may result in a recurrence of the infection.

■ *Patient and Family Teaching*

Develop a teaching plan to include the following:
- Take the medication as prescribed.
- Take the drug on an empty stomach either 1 hour before or 2 hours after a meal (exception: sulfasalazine which may be taken with food or immediately after a meal if gastrointestinal upset occurs).
- Take the medication with a full glass of water. Do not increase or decrease the time between doses unless directed to do so by the physician.
- Complete the full course of therapy. Do not discontinue this medication (unless advised to do so by the physician) even though the symptoms of the infection have disappeared.
- Drink *at least* 8 to 10 eight-ounce glasses of fluid every day.
- Prolonged exposure to sunlight may result in skin reactions similar to a severe sunburn (photosensitivity reactions). When going outside, cover exposed areas of the skin or apply a protective sun screen to exposed areas.
- Notify the physician immediately if the following should occur: fever, skin rash or other skin problems, nausea, vomiting, unusual bleeding or bruising, sore throat, or extreme fatigue.
- Keep all follow-up appointments to ensure the infection is controlled.
- When taking sulfasalazine, the skin or urine may turn an orange-yellow color; this is not abnormal. Take this drug with food if stomach irritation occurs. If wearing soft contact lenses, a permanent yellow stain of the lenses may occur. Seek the advice of an ophthalmologist regarding corrective lenses while taking this drug.

■ *Expected Outcomes for Evaluation*
- Anxiety is reduced
- No evidence of adverse reactions
- Patient verbalizes importance of complying with the prescribed treatment regimen
- Patient and family demonstrate understanding of drug regimen
- Patient verbalizes an understanding of treatment modalities and importance of continued follow-up care

Chapter Summary

- Sulfonamides are antibacterial agents that are primarily bacteriostatic but also may be bactericidal.
- The bacteriostatic activity of these drugs is caused by their antagonism to para-aminobenzoic acid. Once the rate of bacterial multiplication is slowed, the body's own defense mechanisms are able to rid the body of the invading microorganisms and therefore control the infection.
- Some of the adverse reactions associated with sulfonamide therapy include hematologic changes, such as agranulocytosis, thrombocytopenia, aplastic anemia, and leukopenia, anorexia, nausea, vomiting, diarrhea, abdominal pain, chills, fever, crystalluria, and stomatitis.
- Hypersensitivity reactions include Stevens-Johnson syndrome, urticaria (hives), pruritus (itching), and generalized skin eruptions.
- Stevens-Johnson syndrome, also called erythema multiforme, is manifested by fever, cough, muscular aches and pains, headache, and the appearance of lesions on the skin, mucous membranes, eyes, and other organs.

- The most frequent adverse reaction seen with the application of mafenide is a burning sensation or pain when the drug is applied to the skin. Burning, rash, and itching may also be seen with the use of silver sulfadiazine.

Critical Thinking Exercises

1. Ms. Bartlett, age 77, has been prescribed a sulfonamide for a urinary tract infection and is to take the medication for 10 days. You note that Ms. Bartlett seems forgetful and at times confused. What problems might be associated with Ms. Bartlett's mental state and her possible noncompliance to her prescribed treatment regimen?

2. Mr. Adams is receiving sulfisoxazole for a recurrent bladder infection. When keeping an outpatient clinic appointment he tells you that he developed a fever and sore throat yesterday. What steps would you take to investigate his recent problem? Give a reason for your answers.

12

Antitubercular and Leprostatic Agents

Key Terms

Antitubercular agents
Bacteriostatic
Extrapulmonary
Leprosy
Mycobacterium leprae
Mycobacterium tuberculosis
Nephrotoxicity
Ototoxicity
Peripheral neuropathy
Prophylactic
Tuberculosis

Chapter Outline

Chapter Objectives

On completion of this chapter the student will:

- ***Discuss the drugs used in the treatment of tuberculosis***
- ***Discuss the adverse reactions associated with the administration of drugs used in the treatment of tuberculosis***
- ***Use the nursing process when administering an antitubercular agent***
- ***Discuss aspects of nursing management to be considered when administering an antitubercular agent***
- ***Discuss the drugs used in the treatment of leprosy***
- ***Discuss the adverse reactions associated with the administration of drugs used in the treatment of leprosy***
- ***Use the nursing process when administering a leprostatic agent***
- ***Discuss aspects of nursing management to be considered when administering a leprostatic agent***

Scherer JC, Roach S: INTRODUCTORY CLINICAL PHARMACOLOGY,
FIFTH EDITION © 1996 Lippincott-Raven Publishers

The antitubercular and the leprostatic agents are used in the treatment of tuberculosis and leprosy. *Tuberculosis* is an acute or chronic infection spread by inhalation of droplet nuclei when infected persons cough or sneeze. The disorder primarily affects the lungs but can spread through the lymphatic system to other areas of the body. Tuberculosis responds well to long-term treatment with a combination of two or more antitubercular drugs.

Leprosy is a chronic, communicable disease spread by prolonged, intimate contact with an infected person. Peripheral nerves are affected and skin involvement is present. Lesions may be confined to a few isolated areas or may be fairly widespread over the entire body. Treatment with the leprostatic agents provides a good prospect for controlling the disease and preventing complications.

Antitubercular Agents

Tuberculosis is an infectious disease caused by the *Mycobacterium tuberculosis* bacillus. Although tuberculosis primarily affects the lungs, other organs are also affected. People with acquired immunodeficiency syndrome (AIDS) are prone to develop *extrapulmonary* (outside of the lungs) tuberculosis. *Antitubercular agents* are used to treat active cases of tuberculosis and as a *prophylactic* to prevent the spread of tuberculosis.

Antitubercular drugs are classified as primary and secondary agents. Primary agents provide the foundation for treatment. Secondary agents are less effective and more toxic than primary agents. The most effective treatment of active tuberculosis is the combination of three primary drugs (isoniazid, rifampin, and pyrazinamide) for 2 months followed by isoniazid and rifampin for 4 months. For patients who cannot take pyrazinamide, the physician may order a 9-month treatment program consisting of the administration of isoniazid and rifampin. If laboratory studies reveal that the patient is resistant to isoniazid, the physician may order a combination of rifampin and ethambutol for a minimum of 12 months. Various other combinations may be used based on the results of laboratory tests indicating to which drugs the organism is sensitive.

Secondary agents are used to treat extrapulmonary tuberculosis or drug-resistant organisms. The drugs used in the treatment of tuberculosis do not "cure" the disease but they render the patient noninfectious to others.

The primary and secondary drugs used in the treatment of tuberculosis are listed in Summary Drug Table 12-1.

ACTIONS OF THE ANTITUBERCULAR AGENTS

The antitubercular drugs are *bacteriostatic* (slow or retard the growth of bacteria) against the *M. tuberculosis* bacillus. These drugs usually act to inhibit bacterial cell wall synthesis, which slows the multiplication rate of the bacteria.

USES OF THE ANTITUBERCULAR AGENTS

Antitubercular drugs are used in the treatment of active tuberculosis. Isoniazid (INH) is the only antitubercular agent used alone. In addition to its use in combination with other drugs for the treatment of primary tuberculosis, INH is used in preventive therapy (prophylaxis) for the following:

- Household members and other close associates of those recently diagnosed as having tuberculosis
- Those whose tuberculin skin test has become positive in the last 2 years
- Those with positive skin tests whose radiographic findings indicate nonprogressive, healed, or quiescent (causing no symptoms) tubercular lesions
- Those at risk of developing tuberculosis (eg, those with Hodgkin's disease, severe diabetes mellitus, leukemia, and other serious illnesses and those receiving corticosteroids or drug therapy for a malignancy)
- All patients under age 35 (primarily children up to age 7) who have a positive skin test.
- Persons with AIDS, or those who are positive for the human immunodeficiency virus and have a positive tuberculosis skin test or a negative tuberculosis skin test but a history of a prior significant reaction to purified protein derivative (a skin test for tuberculosis).

Bacterial resistance develops, sometimes rapidly, with the use of antitubercular drugs. To slow the development of bacterial resistance, the physician may use two or more drugs with initial therapy, as well as in retreatment. Using a combination of drugs appears to slow the development of bacterial resistance.

Summary Drug Table 12-1. Antitubercular and Leprostatic Agents

Generic Name	Trade Name*	Uses	Adverse Reactions	Dose Ranges
ANTITUBERCULAR DRUGS				
Primary Agents				
isoniazid (INH)	Laniazid, *generic*	Tuberculosis: preventive therapy for specific situations	Peripheral neuropathy, fever, skin eruptions, agranulocytosis anemia, jaundice, nausea, vomiting, hypersensitivity reactions	Treatment of tuberculosis: up to 300 mg/d PO; preventive treatment: 300 mg/d PO
rifampin	Rifadin, Rimactane	Tuberculosis	Heartburn, epigastric distress, anorexia, nausea, vomiting, hypersensitivity reactions	600 mg/d PO, IV
ethambutol hydrochloride	Myambutol	Tuberculosis	Decrease in visual acuity, dermatitis, anaphylactoid reactions, pruritus	15–25 mg/kg/d PO
streptomycin sulfate	*generic*	Tuberculosis, nontuberculous infections due to susceptible microorganisms	Nephrotoxicity, ototoxicity, numbness, tingling, tinnitus, nausea, vomiting, circumoral or peripheral paresthesia, dizziness, vertigo	1 g/d IM
pyrazinamide	*generic*	Tuberculosis	Hepatotoxicity, nausea, vomiting, diarrhea, fever	15–30 mg/kg/d PO once daily
Secondary Agents				
aminosalicylate	Teebacin, *generic*	Tuberculosis	Nausea, vomiting, diarrhea, abdominal pain	14–16 g/d PO in 2–3 divided sodium (PAS) doses
capreomycin sulfate	Capastat	Tuberculosis	Nephrotoxicity, ototoxicity, leukocytosis, leukopenia	1 g/d IM
cycloserine	Seromycin	Tuberculosis	Convulsions, drowsiness, skin rash, headache	500 mg to 1 g/d PO in divided doses
LEPROSTATIC AGENTS				
clofazimine	Lamprene	Leprosy	Skin pigmentation, abdominal pain, diarrhea, nausea, vomiting	100–200 mg/d PO
dapsone	*generic*	Leprosy, dermatitis herpetiformis	Blood cell hemolysis, nausea, vomiting, anorexia, blurred vision	Leprosy: 50–100 mg/d PO; dermatitis herpetiformis: 50–300 mg/d PO

*The term, *generic*, indicates that the drug is availabe in a generic form.

ADVERSE REACTIONS ASSOCIATED WITH THE ADMINISTRATION OF ANTITUBERCULAR AGENTS

The following adverse reactions may be seen during administration of antitubercular drugs.

Isoniazid. Incidence of adverse reactions appears to be higher when larger doses of isoniazid are prescribed. Adverse reactions include hypersensitivity reactions, hematologic changes, jaundice, fever, skin eruptions, nausea, vomiting, and epigastric distress. Severe, and sometimes fatal, hepatitis has been associated with isoniazid therapy and may appear after many months of treatment. *Peripheral neuropathy* (numbness and tingling of the extremities) is the most common symptom of toxicity.

Rifampin (Rifadin). Nausea, vomiting, epigastric distress, heartburn, and diarrhea may be seen with administration of rifampin.

Ethambutol (Myambutol). A decrease in visual acuity, which appears to be related to the dose given and the duration of treatment, has occurred in some patients receiving ethambutol. Usually, this adverse reaction disappears when the drug is discontinued. Other adverse reactions are dermatitis, pruritus, anaphylactoid reactions, joint pain, anorexia, nausea, and vomiting.

Streptomycin. *Nephrotoxicity* (damaging to the kidneys), *ototoxicity* (damaging to the organs of hearing by a toxic substance), numbness, tingling, tinnitus, nausea, vomiting, dizziness, vertigo, and circumoral (around the mouth) paresthesia may be noted with the administration of streptomycin. Soreness at the injection site may also be noted, especially when the drug is given for a long time.

Pyrazinamide. Hepatotoxicity is the principal adverse reaction seen with pyrazinamide use. Symptoms of hepatotoxicity may range from none (except for slightly abnormal hepatic function tests) to a more severe reaction such as jaundice. Nausea, vomiting, and diarrhea may also be seen.

Aminosalicylate (PAS). The most common adverse reactions associated with aminosalicylate are related to the gastrointestinal (GI) tract and include nausea, vomiting, diarrhea, and abdominal pain. Hypersensitivity reactions have also been reported.

Capreomycin (Capastat). The two major adverse reactions associated with capreomycin are ototoxicity and nephrotoxicity. Leukocytosis and leukopenia have also occurred. The physician may order a complete blood count and renal function tests at periodic intervals. Hearing testing may also be done periodically.

Cycloserine (Seromycin). The major adverse reactions are emotional and behavioral disturbances, including psychosis. Doses of cycloserine larger than 500 mg/day have been reported to cause headache, drowsiness, and convulsions in some patients. A skin rash, which is not related to the size of the dosage, may also occur.

Ethionamide (Trecator S.C.). GI intolerance, peripheral neuritis, and psychic disturbances may be seen with the administration of ethionamide. Patients with diabetes mellitus who are taking this drug may require adjustments of their insulin or oral hypoglycemic dosages.

NURSING MANAGEMENT

If the antitubercular drug is given by the parenteral route, rotate injection sites. At the time of each injection, inspect previous injection sites for signs of swelling, redness, and tenderness. If a localized reaction persists or if the area appears to be infected, notify the physician.

Give antitubercular medications by the oral route and on an empty stomach unless gastric upset occurs. If gastric upset occurs, notify the physician before the next dose is given.

Since the antitubercular drugs must be taken for prolonged periods of time, compliance to the treatment regimen becomes a problem and increases the risk of the development of resistant strains of tuberculosis. To help prevent the problem of noncompliance use Direct Observation Therapy (DOT) to administer these drugs. When using DOT, the patient makes periodic visits to the doctor's office or the health clinic where the medication is taken in the presence of the nurse. In some cases, the nurse uses the DOT method to administer the antitubercular drug in the patient's home, place of employment, or school.

Observe patients daily for the appearance of adverse drug reactions. These observations are especially important when a drug is known to be nephrotoxic or ototoxic. Report any adverse drug reactions to the physician. Monitor vital signs daily or as frequently as every 4 hours when the patient is hospitalized.

Include the following interventions in the nursing management of patients receiving antitubercular agents.

Isoniazid. Give on an empty stomach, at least 1 hour before or 2 hours after meals. If GI upset occurs, this drug can be taken with food. Alcohol consumption is minimized because of increased risk of hepatitis. To prevent pyridoxine (vitamin B_6) deficiency, 6 to 50 mg of pyridoxine may be given daily to prevent occurrence of deficiency.

Nursing Alert

Severe and sometimes fatal hepatitis may occur with isoniazid therapy. All patients must be carefully monitored at least monthly for any evidence of liver dysfunction. Instruct patients to report any of the follow symptoms: anorexia, nausea, vomiting, fatigue, weakness, yellowing of the skin or eyes, darkening of the urine, or numbness in the hands and feet.

Rifampin. Administer once daily on an empty stomach at least 1 hour before or 2 hours after meals. Urine, feces, saliva, sputum, sweat, and tears may be colored red-orange.

Ethambutol. Administer once every 24 hours at the same time each day. Give with food to prevent gastric upset. If a dose is missed, do *not* double the dose the next day. Monitor for any changes in visual acuity and report to the physician promptly. Vision changes are usually reversible if the drug is discontinued as soon as symptoms appear. Urine, feces, saliva, sputum, sweat, and tears may be colored brown-orange. Psychic disturbances may occur. If the patient appears depressed, withdrawn, noncommunicative, or has other personality changes, report the problem to the physician.

Aminosalicylate. Administer with food or meals to prevent gastric upset. Use sugarless gum, juice, or mouthwash if an aftertaste occurs. Aminosalicylate is rendered ineffective if exposed to direct sunlight, excessive heat or becomes wet.

Streptomycin and Capreomycin. These drugs may cause ototoxicity resulting in hearing loss. Monitor for any signs of hearing loss, including tinnitus (ringing in the ears) and vertigo (dizziness).

Drug Resistance

Of increasing concern is the development of mutant strains of tuberculosis resistant to many of the drugs currently in use. Tuberculosis caused by drug-resistant organisms should be considered in patients who are not responding to therapy and in patients who have been treated in the past. Treatment is individualized and based on laboratory studies identifying the drugs to which the organism is susceptible. The physician may order the administration of at least 3 drugs to which the organism is susceptible for 1 to 2 years.

Nursing Process
The Patient Receiving an Antitubercular Agent

■ *Assessment*
Once the diagnosis of tuberculosis is confirmed, the physician selects the drug that will best control the spread of the disease and make the patient noninfectious to others. Many laboratory and diagnostic tests may be necessary before starting drug therapy, for example, radiographic studies, culture and sensitivity tests, and various types of laboratory tests such as CBC.

Assessment may also include a family history and a history of contacts if the patient has active tuberculosis.

Depending on the severity of the disease, patients may be treated initially in the hospital and then discharged to their home for supervised follow-up care, or they may have all treatment instituted on an outpatient basis.

■ *Nursing Diagnoses*
Depending on the individual and the methods of treatment, one or more of the following nursing diagnoses may apply to the patient receiving an antitubercular drug:
* **Anxiety** related to diagnosis, long-term therapeutic regimen, other factors (specify)
* **Noncompliance** related to indifference, lack of knowledge, other factors
* **Risk of Ineffective Management of Therapeutic Regimen** related to indifference, lack of knowledge, other factors

■ *Planning and Implementation*
The patient's major goals may include a reduction in anxiety and an understanding of and compliance to the prescribed treatment regimen.

Anxiety. The diagnosis, as well as the necessity of long-term treatment and follow-up, are often distressing to the patient. Patients diagnosed as having tuberculosis may have many questions about the disease and its treatment. Allow time for the patient and family members to ask questions. In some instances, it may be necessary to refer the patient to other healthcare workers, such as a social service worker or the dietitian.

Noncompliance. Antitubercular drugs are given for a long time, and careful patient and family instruction and close medical supervision are necessary. Noncompliance can be a problem whenever a disease or disorder requires long-term treatment. The patient and family must understand that short-term therapy is of *no value* in treating this disease. Be alert to statements made by the patient or family that may indicate future noncompliance to the medication regimen necessary in controlling the disease.

■ *Patient and Family Teaching*
Review the dosage schedule and adverse effects associated with the prescribed drug with the patient and family.

Information applying to all patients taking these drugs includes the following:

- The results of drug therapy will be monitored at periodic intervals. Laboratory and diagnostic tests and visits to the physician's office or clinic are necessary.
- Take the drug exactly as directed on the prescription container. Do not omit, increase, or decrease a dose unless advised to do so by the physician.
- Avoid the use of nonprescription drugs, especially those containing aspirin, unless use has been approved by the physician.
- Discuss the drinking of alcoholic beverages with the physician. A limited amount of alcohol may be allowed, but excessive intake should usually be avoided.

The following information is also included when a specific antitubercular drug is prescribed:

- Aminosalicylate, ethambutol, ethionamide: Take these drugs with food or meals.
- Aminosalicylate: If aftertaste occurs, experiment with methods to eliminate this problem, for example, the use of sugarless gum, juice, or mouthwash.
- Cycloserine: This drug may cause drowsiness. Do not drive or perform other hazardous tasks if drowsiness occurs.
- Isoniazid: Take this drug 1 hour before or 2 hours after meals. If GI upset occurs, take the drug with food.
- Ethionamide: This drug may cause GI upset (nausea, vomiting, diarrhea), loss of appetite, a metallic taste in the mouth, or salivation. If these become bothersome or increase in severity, notify the physician. Management of diabetes may be more difficult when using ethionamide. Careful monitoring of blood glucose levels is necessary. Notify the physician of any changes in blood glucose levels.
- Ethambutol: Take this drug once a day at the same time each day. If a dose is missed, do *not* double the dose the next day. Notify the physician of any changes in vision or the occurrence of a skin rash.
- Pyrazinamide: Notify the physician if any of the following occurs: nausea, vomiting, loss of appetite, fever, malaise, visual changes, yellowish discoloration of the skin, or severe pain in the knees, feet, or wrists. (*Note:* Pain in these areas may be signs of active gout.)

■ *Expected Outcomes for Evaluation*
- Anxiety is reduced
- Adverse reactions are identified and reported to the physician

- Patient verbalizes an understanding of treatment modalities and importance of continued follow-up care
- Patient and family demonstrate understanding of drug regimen
- Patient complies to the prescribed drug regimen

Leprostatic Agents

Leprosy (Hansen's disease) is a chronic, communicable disease caused by the bacterium *mycobacterium leprae*. Although rare in colder climates, this disease may be seen in tropical and subtropical zones. Dapsone and clofazimine (Lamprene) are the two drugs currently used to treat leprosy.

ACTIONS OF THE LEPROSTATIC AGENTS

Dapsone is bactericidal and bacteriostatic against the *mycobacterium leprae*. Clofazimine is primarily bactericidal. The mode of action of these drugs is unknown.

USES OF THE LEPROSTATIC AGENTS

These drugs are used in the treatment of leprosy. Dapsone also may be used in the treatment of dermatitis herpetiformis, a chronic, inflammatory skin disease. The leprostatics are listed in Summary Drug Table 12-1.

ADVERSE REACTIONS ASSOCIATED WITH THE ADMINISTRATION OF THE LEPROSTATIC AGENTS

Dapsone. Administration may result in hemolysis (destruction of red blood cell), nausea, vomiting, anorexia, and blurred vision.

Clofazimine. May cause pigmentation of the skin, abdominal pain, diarrhea, nausea, and vomiting.

NURSING MANAGEMENT

These drugs are often given on an outpatient basis. Each time the patient is seen in the clinic or physician's office, perform a general physical examination, with particular attention to the affected areas.

Give leprostatics orally and with food to minimize GI upset. Antitubercular drugs, such as rifampin, may be given concurrently during initial therapy to minimize bacterial resistance to the leprostatic drug.

Nursing Process
The Patient Receiving a Leprostatic Agent

■ Assessment
A complete physical examination and history is performed before the institution of therapy. The involved areas are examined and described in detail on the patient's record to provide a database for comparison during therapy.

■ Nursing Diagnoses
Depending on the individual, one or more of the following nursing diagnoses may apply to the patient receiving a leprostatic:
- **Anxiety** related to diagnosis, long-term therapeutic regimen, other factors (specify)
- **Noncompliance** related to indifference, lack of knowledge, other factors
- **Risk for Ineffective Management of Therapeutic Regimen** related to indifference, lack of knowledge, other factors

■ Planning and Implementation
The patient's major goals may include a reduction in anxiety and an understanding of and compliance to the prescribed treatment regimen. More specific criteria may be added to make these goals more measurable.

Anxiety. Treatment with a leprostatic drug may require many years. These patients are faced with long-term medical and drug therapy and possibly severe disfigurement. The nurse must spend time with these patients, allowing them to verbalize their anxieties, problems, and fears.

Noncompliance. Be alert to patient statements regarding the long-term treatment regimen. Note factors such as depression or indifference that may be indicative of treatment noncompliance. Use a positive approach when doing patient and family teaching.

■ Patient and Family Teaching
To ensure compliance to the treatment regimen, explain the dosage schedule, the possible adverse effects, and the importance of scheduled follow-up visits to the patient and family members. In particular, emphasize the importance of adhering to the prescribed dosage schedule.

■ Expected Outcomes for Evaluation
- Anxiety is reduced
- Adverse reactions are identified and reported to the physician
- Patient verbalizes an understanding of treatment modalities and importance of continued follow-up care
- Patient and family demonstrate understanding of drug regimen
- Patient complies to the prescribed drug regimen

Chapter Summary

- Antitubercular drugs are used to treat active cases of tuberculosis and as a preventative treatment to decrease the spread of tuberculosis. Antitubercular drugs are classified as primary and secondary agents. The most effective treatment of active tuberculosis is the combination of three primary drugs (isoniazid, rifampin, and pyrazinamide) for 2 months followed by isoniazid and rifampin for 4 months. For patients who cannot take pyrazinamide, the physician may order a 9-month treatment program of isoniazid and rifampin. If laboratory studies reveal that the patient is resistant to isoniazid, the physician may order a combination of rifampin and ethambutol for a minimum of 12 months. Various other combinations may be used based on the results of laboratory tests indicating to which drugs the organism is sensitive.
- The secondary agents are used to treat extrapulmonary tuberculosis or drug-resistant organisms. The drugs used in the treatment of tuberculosis do not "cure" the disease but they render the patient noninfectious to others.
- Antitubercular agents are bacteriostatic against the *M. tuberculosis* bacillus. Most antitubercular agents cause hepatotoxicity. Patients should be monitored for abnormal liver function tests and signs of hepatitis. Other adverse reactions include nausea, vomiting, GI upsets, peripheral neuritis, and hypersensitivity reactions.
- One of the major concerns is that patient noncompliance to the drug regimen sometimes occurs over a 12-month period. To ensure that the patient is compliant to the drug regimen, DOT is used by various healthcare providers. In the DOT method, the healthcare provider observes or witnesses the patient taking the drug.

- The leprostatic agents are used to treat leprosy. Dapsone and clofazimine are the two drugs currently used to treat leprosy. Adverse reactions associated with dapsone include hemolysis, nausea, vomiting, anorexia, and blurred vision. Clofazimine causes pigmentation of the skin, abdominal pain, and GI disturbances. Leprostatics are given orally with food to minimize GI upset.

- Antitubercular agents and leprostatic agents are most often given on an outpatient basis. To insure compliance to the prescribed treatment regimen, the dosage schedule, possible adverse reactions, and scheduled follow-up visits are explained to the patient and family. The importance of adhering to the prescribed dosage schedule is emphasized.

Critical Thinking Exercises

1. Ms. Burns has been diagnosed with tuberculosis. She is concerned because her physician has informed her that the treatment regimen consists of two drugs, isoniazid and ethambutol, taken for at least 18 months. What rationales can the nurse give Ms. Burns for the use of two drugs and the need for long-term therapy in tuberculosis?

2. While Mr. Johnson is taking isoniazid, what instructions would the nurse give him concerning side effects? What symptoms would be important for Mr. Johnson to report?

13

Antiviral and Antifungal Drugs

Key Terms

Exacerbations
Fungicidal
Fungistatic
Fungus
Granulocytopenia
Mycotic infections
Photosensitivity
Remissions
Retinitis

Chapter Outline

Chapter Objectives

On completion of this chapter the student will:

- *Discuss the uses of antiviral drugs*
- *List adverse effects associated with the administration of antiviral drugs*
- *Use the nursing process when administering the antiviral drugs*
- *Discuss nursing management when administering the antiviral drugs*
- *Discuss the uses of antifungal drugs*
- *List some of the adverse reactions associated with the administration of antifungal drugs*
- *Use the nursing process when administering an antifungal drug*
- *Discuss nursing management when administering an antifungal drug*

Scherer JC, Roach S: INTRODUCTORY CLINICAL PHARMACOLOGY,
FIFTH EDITION © 1996 Lippincott-Raven Publishers

More than 200 viruses have been identified as capable of producing disease. Acute viruses, such as the common cold, have a rapid onset and quick recovery. Chronic viral infections, such as acquired immunodeficiency syndrome (AIDS) have recurrent episodes of *exacerbations* (increases in severity of symptoms of the disease) and *remissions* (periods of partial or complete disappearance of the signs and symptoms).

Fungal infections range from superficial skin infections to life-threatening systemic infections. Superficial infections include ringworm (tinea), athlete's foot, and yeast infections, such as those caused by *Candida albicans*. Systemic fungal infections are serious infections that occur when fungi gain entrance into the interior of the body.

Antiviral Drugs

Although viral infections are common, few drugs are available for their treatment. This stems from the fact that viruses can reproduce only within a living cell. A virus consists of either DNA or RNA surrounded by a protein shell. It is capable of reproducing only when it uses the body's cellular material. Agents toxic to the virus are often toxic to the cells of the body as well.

Acyclovir (Zovirax), amantadine (Symmetrel), didanosine, ganciclovir (Cytovene), ribavirin (Virazole), vidarabine (Vira-A), and zidovudine (AZT, Retrovir) are antiviral drugs presently in use.

ACTIONS OF ANTIVIRAL DRUGS

Acyclovir, didanosine, ganciclovir, ribavirin, zalcitabine, and zidovudine appear to inhibit viral replication. Amantadine prevents the virus from entering the cell. The exact mode of action of vidarabine is not completely understood.

USES OF ANTIVIRAL DRUGS

Although infections caused by a virus are common, antiviral drugs have limited use since they are only effective against a small number of specific viral infections.

Unlabeled uses are included for some of these drugs. Approval by the Food and Drug Administration (FDA) is necessary for a drug to be prescribed. On occasion the use of a drug for a specific disorder or condition may be under investigation or may be approved for use in another country. In this instance the drug may be prescribed by the physician for the condition under investigation. The use of the drug for a specific disorder or condition that is not officially approved by the FDA is called an "unlabeled use." Since there are very few effective antiviral drugs the physician may decide to prescribe a drug for an unlabeled use even though documentation of its effectiveness is lacking.

Acyclovir. Acyclovir is used for the initial and recurrent treatment of the herpes simplex virus (HSV-1 and HSV-2) and for the treatment of herpes zoster (shingles). Examples of the unlabeled uses of this drug include the treatment of infectious mononucleosis and varicella (chickenpox) pneumonia.

Amantadine. Amantadine is used for the prevention or treatment of respiratory tract illness caused by influenza A virus. This drug is also used in the treatment of Parkinson's disease.

Didanosine. Didanosine is used to treat advanced human immunodeficiency virus infection in patients who cannot tolerate zidovudine or who have exhibited decreased effectiveness with zidovudine therapy.

Ganciclovir. Ganciclovir is used in the treatment of *retinitis* (inflammation of the retina of the eye) caused by the cytomegalovirus in immunocompromised individuals, such as those with AIDS or those who have recently undergone bone marrow transplantation.

Ribavirin. Ribavirin is used to treat infants and young children with severe lower respiratory tract infections due to the respiratory syncytial virus. Unlabeled uses of this drug include treatment of influenza A and B (aerosol form), acute and chronic hepatitis, herpes genitalis, and measles (oral form).

Vidarabine. Vidarabine may be used in the treatment of herpes simplex virus encephalitis. An unlabeled use of this drug is the early treatment of herpes zoster in immunocompromised patients.

Zidovudine. Commonly known as AZT, zidovudine is used orally and intravenously in the treatment of patients with AIDS.

ADVERSE REACTIONS ASSOCIATED WITH THE ADMINISTRATION OF ANTIVIRAL DRUGS

The more common adverse reactions associated with the administration of these drugs are listed in Summary Drug Table 13-1.

Acyclovir. Acyclovir is available for use orally, topically, and parenterally (for IV use). Side effects when given orally include nausea, vomiting, diarrhea, headache, dizziness, and skin rashes. Topical administration causes transient burning, stinging, and pruritus. When given IV, acyclovir can cause phlebitis, lethargy, confusion, tremors, skin rashes, nausea, and crystalluria (presence of crystals in the urine).

Amantadine. Side effects of amantadine include gastrointestinal upsets with nausea, vomiting, constipation, depression, visual disturbances, psychosis, urinary retention, and orthostatic hypotension.

Didanosine. Side effects reported with didanosine include headache, peripheral neuropathy, rhinitis, cough, diarrhea, nausea, vomiting, anorexia, abnormal liver function tests, and pancreatitis.

Ribavirin. Ribavirin is given by inhalation and can cause worsening of respiratory status, hypotension, and ocular irritation including erythema (redness of skin), conjunctivitis, and blurred vision.

Zidovudine. Adverse reactions associated with zidovudine include headache, weakness, malaise, nausea, abdominal pain, and diarrhea. Hematologic changes include anemia and *granulocytopenia* (low levels of granulocytes, a type of white blood cell, in the blood).

NURSING MANAGEMENT

Give acyclovir, ganciclovir, vidarabine, and zidovudine IV. Never give these drugs intramuscularly or subcutaneously. Prepare according to the manufacturer's directions. The administration rate is ordered by the physician. Closely observe the injection site for signs of phlebitis.

Depending on the patient's symptoms, monitor vital signs every 4 hours or as ordered by the physician. Observe and notify the physician of any adverse drug reactions.

In addition to the general instructions mentioned above, the following are special considerations for specific drugs.

Acyclovir. Begin treatment with acyclovir as soon as symptoms of herpes simplex appear. Give with food or on an empty stomach. Maintain adequate hydration to prevent crystalluria by drinking 2000–3000 mL of fluid each day. Use a finger cot or glove for topical application to prevent spread of infection.

Amantadine. Protect capsules from moisture. Start therapy within 24 to 48 hours after symptoms begin. Be especially alert for signs of mental changes. Also monitor patients with a history of seizure disorder or congestive heart failure. Observe for signs of renal impairment, mottling of the skin, orthostatic hypotension, and visual disturbances.

Didanosine. Administer on an empty stomach. Tablets are not swallowed whole; they should be chewed or crushed and mixed thoroughly with at least 1 ounce of water. Mix buffered powder with four ounces of water (not juice), stir until dissolved, and give to drink immediately.

> **Nursing Alert**
>
> Patients receiving didanosine or other antiviral drugs for human immunodeficiency virus infections may continue to develop opportunistic infections and other complications of human immunodeficiency virus infection. Monitor all patients closely for signs of infection such as fever (even low grade fever), malaise, sore throat, or lethargy.

Monitor for symptoms of pancreatitis (nausea, vomiting, and abdominal pain). Observe for signs of peripheral neuropathy (numbness, tingling, or pain in the feet or hands).

Ribavirin. Give ribavarin by inhalation using the SPAG-2 aerosol generator. Discard and replace the solution every 24 hours. Treatment with ribavirin lasts for at least 3 days (but not more than 7) for 12 to 18 hours per day. Women of childbearing age should *not* administer this drug since there is evidence linking it to birth defects.

> **Nursing Alert**
>
> Sudden deterioration of respiratory status can occur in infants receiving ribavirin. Monitor respiratory function closely throughout therapy.

Summary Drug Table 13-1. Antiviral Drugs

Generic Name	Trade Name*	Uses	Adverse Reactions	Dose Ranges
acyclovir	Zovirax	Herpes simplex, herpes zoster	Nausea, vomiting, diarrhea, headache, dizziness	Oral: 200 mg q 4h while awake for a total of 5 capsules/d for 10 d; parenteral: 5 mg/kg IV q 8h for 5 d; topical: apply to all lesions q 3h for 7 d
amantadine	Symmetrel, *generic*	Prevention or treatment of influenza A	Nausea, dizziness, hypotension, lightheadedness, blurred vision	200 mg/d PO or 100 mg PO bid
didanosine	Videx	HIV infection	Headache, rhinitis, cough, diarrhea, nausea, vomiting, pancreatitis, granulocytopenia, peripheral neuropathy	≥ 60 kg 200 mg bid; <60 kg 125 mg bid
famciclovir	Famvir	Acute herpes zoster (shingles)	Fatigue, fever, nausea, vomiting, diarrhea, constipation, headache, sinusitis	500 mg q 8h for 7 d PO
ganciclovir sodium	Cytovene	Retinitis caused by cytomegalovirus	Hematologic changes, fever, rash	5 mg/kg IV, IM, SC q 12h for 14–21 d, then qd
ribavirin	Virazole	Severe lower respiratory tract infection (infants, young children)	Worsening of pulmonary status, bacterial pneumonia, hypotension, cardiac arrest	Administered by aerosol with special aerosol generator
vidarabine	Vira-A	Herpes simplex encephalitis, herpes zoster	Anorexia, nausea, vomiting	Herpes simplex encephalitis: 15 mg/kg/d IV for 10 d; herpes zoster: 10 mg/kg IV for 5 d
zalcitabine	HIVID	In combination with zidovudine for advanced HIV infection	Oral ulcers, peripheral neuropathy, headache, vomiting, diarrhea, CHF, cardiomyopathy	0.75 mg with 200 mg zidovudine q 8h
zidovudine (AZT)	Retrovir	HIV infection	Asthenia, headache, anorexia, diarrhea, nausea, GI pain, paresthesias, dizziness, insomnia, anemia, agranulocytosis	100–200 mg PO q4h; 1–2 mg/kg IV q4h

*The term, *generic,* indicates that the drug is available in generic form.

Zidovudine. Assess patient for increase in severity of symptoms of AIDS and for symptoms of opportunistic infections. Perform frequent blood counts to monitor for anemia and granulocytopenia. Protect capsules and syrup from light.

Nursing Process
The Patient Receiving an Antiviral Drug

■ *Assessment*
Assessment of the patient receiving an antiviral agent depends on the patient's symptoms or diagnosis. Record the patient's symptoms. Take and record vital signs. Additional assessments may be necessary in certain types of viral infections or in patients who are acutely ill.

■ *Nursing Diagnoses*
Depending on the reason for administration, one or more of the following nursing diagnoses may apply to a person receiving an antiviral agent:
- **Anxiety** related to diagnosis, symptoms of illness
- **Noncompliance** to therapeutic regimen
- **Risk for Ineffective Management of Therapeutic Regimen** related to indifference, lack of knowledge, other factors (specify)

■ Planning and Implementation
The major goals of the patient may include a reduction in anxiety and an understanding of and compliance to the prescribed treatment regimen. To make these goals measurable, more specific criteria must be added.

Anxiety. Because these drugs may be used in the treatment of certain types of severe and sometimes life-threatening viral infections, the patient may be concerned over his or her diagnosis and prognosis. Allow the patient time to talk and ask questions about methods of treatment, especially when the drug is given IV. Explain the prescribed treatment methods to the patient and family members.

■ Patient and Family Teaching
When an antiviral agent is given orally, explain the dosage regimen to the patient and family. Take the drug exactly as directed and for the full course of therapy. If a dose is missed, take as soon as remembered but do not double the dose at the next dosage time. Report any adverse reactions to the physician or the nurse.

Include the following information in the teaching plan of specific drugs:

- Acyclovir: This drug is not a cure for herpes simplex but will shorten the course of the disease and will promote healing of the lesions. The drug will not prevent the spread of the disease to others. Topical application should not exceed the frequency prescribed. Apply with a finger cot or gloves and cover all lesions. Instruct the patient with genital herpes to have no sexual contact while lesions are present.
- Amantadine: Do not drive a car or do work for which mental alertness is necessary until the effect of the drug is apparent because vision and coordination can be affected. Rise slowly from a prone to a sitting position to decrease the possibility of lightheadedness due to orthostatic hypotension. Report changes such as nervousness or depression.
- Didanosine: Take on an empty stomach since food decreases absorption. Follow the instructions for administration carefully. The drug is crushed and mixed with water. Discontinue the drug and notify physician if any numbness or tingling of the extremities is experienced. Report any signs of abdominal pain, nausea, or vomiting. Convey to the patient that didanosine is not a cure for AIDS and does not prevent the spread of the disease. However, it may decrease the symptoms of AIDS.
- Ribavirin: Explain the purpose and the route of administration, as well as the importance of receiving the medication for the full course of therapy. Blurred vision and *photosensitivity* (sensitivity to light) may be experienced during therapy.
- Zidovudine: This drug may cause dizziness. Avoid activities requiring alertness until drug response is known. This drug does not cure AIDS and does not prevent transmission to others. Notify physician if fever, sore throat, or signs of infection occur.

■ Expected Outcomes for Evaluation
- Anxiety is reduced
- Patient and family demonstrate understanding of drug regimen
- Patient verbalizes importance of complying with the prescribed treatment regimen

Antifungal Drugs

A *fungus* is a colorless plant lacking chlorophyll. Fungi that cause disease in humans may be yeast-like or moldlike and are called *mycotic infections* or *fungal infections*.

Mycotic infections may be one of two types: (1) superficial mycotic infections or (2) deep (systemic) mycotic infections. The superficial mycotic infections are those occurring on the surface of or just below the skin or nails. Deep mycotic infections are those occurring inside the body, such as in the lungs. Treatment for deep mycotic infection is often difficult and prolonged.

The various antifungal drugs are listed in Summary Drug Table 13-2.

ACTIONS OF ANTIFUNGAL DRUGS

Antifungal drugs may be *fungicidal* (able to destroy fungi) or *fungistatic* (able to slow or retard the multiplication of fungi).

Amphotericin B (Fungizone IV), miconazole (Monistat IV), nystatin (Mycostatin), and ketoconazole (Nizoral) are thought to have an effect on the cell membrane of the fungus, resulting in a fungicidal or fungistatic effect. The fungicidal or fungistatic effect of these drugs appears to be related to their concentration in body tissues. Fluconazole (Diflucan) has fungistatic activity, which appears to result from the depletion of sterols (a group of substances related to fats) in the fungus cells.

Summary Drug Table 13-2. Antifungal Drugs

Generic Name	Trade Name*	Uses	Adverse Reactions	Dose Ranges
amphotericin B	Fungizone	Active progressive fungal infections; Cryptococcosi, blastomycosis, disseminated moniliasis; Topically: treatment of superficial fungal infections	IV: fever, headache, anorexia, abnormal renal function, nausea, vomiting, malaise, shaking chills, joint and muscle pain, anemia	0.25–1.5 mg/kg/d IV; Topically: apply 2–4 times daily
itraconazole	Sporanox	Blastomycosis/histoplasmosis, aspergillosis	Rash, headache, hyperlesion, hepatic function abnormalities	Blastomycosis/histoplasmosis PO 200: mg/d; aspergillosis PO 200–400 mg/d
fluconazole	Diflucan	Oropharyngeal and esophageal candidiasis, cryptococcal meningitis	Nausea, vomiting, rash, headache	200–400 mg PO, IV first day followed by 100–200 mg/d PO, IV
flucytosine	Ancobon	Infections caused by strains of *Candida* or *Cryptococcus*	Nausea, vomiting, diarrhea, rash, anemia, leukopenia, thrombocytopenia	50–150 mg/kg/d PO in divided doses q6h
griseofulvin microsize, ultramicrosize	Grisactin, Grisactin Ultra, Fulvicin-U/F, Fulvicin-P/G, *generic*	Ringworm infections	Rash, urticaria, oral thrush, nausea, vomiting, headache, diarrhea	Microsize: 500 mg to 1 g/d PO; ultramicrosize: 330–750 mg/d PO
ketoconazole	Nizoral	Candidiasis, oral thrush, blastomycosis, histoplasmosis, coccidioidomycosis, chronic mucocutaneous candidiasis	Nausea, vomiting, headache, dizziness, abdominal pain, pruritus	200–400 mg/d PO
miconazole nitrate	Monistat 3 or 7, Micatin, Monistat-Derm	Vulvovaginal candidiasis, topical fungal infections (ringworm, athlete's foot)	Vaginal use: burning, itching, irritation; topical: irritation, burning	Vaginal cream: 1 applicator full daily at hs; vaginal suppository: 1 daily at hs; topical cream, powder, lotion: cover affected areas bid
miconazole (parenteral)	Monistat IV	Coccidioidomycosis, candidiasis, cryptococcosis	Phlebitis, pruritus, rash, nausea, vomiting, diarrhea, anorexia, febrile reactions, drowsiness, flushing of the skin	200–3600 mg/d IV infusion
nystatin (oral)	Mycostatin, *generic*	Intestinal candidiasis	Rare; epigastric distress, nausea, vomiting	500,000–1 million U PO tid
nystatin (topical)	Nilstat, Mycostatin	Cutaneous or mucocutaneous infections caused by Candida	Rare; local irritation	Apply 2–3 times/d
nystatin (vaginal)	Nilstat, Mycostatin, *generic*	Vulvovaginal candidiasis	Rare; local irritation	1 tablet/d intravaginally for 2 wk

*The term, *generic,* indicates that the drug is available in generic form.

Griseofulvin (Grisactin) is deposited in keratin precursor cells, which are then gradually lost (due to the constant shedding of top skin cells), and replaced by new, noninfected cells. The mode of action of flucytosine (Ancobon) is not clearly understood.

USES OF ANTIFUNGAL DRUGS

Antifungal drugs are used in the treatment of superficial and deep fungal infections. The specific uses of the antifungal drugs are given in Summary Drug Table 13-2. Amphotericin B is the most effective drug available for the treatment of most systemic fungal infection. Fungal infections of the skin or mucous membranes may be treated with topical or vaginal preparations.

ADVERSE REACTIONS ASSOCIATED WITH THE ADMINISTRATION OF ANTIFUNGAL DRUGS

When topical antifungal drugs are applied to the skin or mucous membranes, few adverse reactions are seen with these drugs. On occasion, a local reaction, such as irritation or burning, may occur with topical use.

Amphotericin B. Administration often results in serious reactions, which include fever, shaking, chills, headache, malaise, anorexia, joint and muscle pain, abnormal renal function, nausea, vomiting, and anemia. This drug is given parenterally, usually over several months. Its use is reserved for serious and potentially life-threatening fungal infections. Some of these adverse reactions may be lessened by aspirin, antihistamines, or antiemetics.

Flucytosine. Administration may result in nausea, vomiting, diarrhea, rash, anemia, leukopenia, and thrombocytopenia. Signs of renal impairment include elevated blood urea nitrogen and serum creatinine levels. Periodic renal function tests are usually performed during therapy.

Miconazole. Parenteral administration may result in phlebitis, pruritus, rash, nausea, vomiting, diarrhea, and anorexia. Febrile reactions, drowsiness, and flushing of the skin may also be seen. Vaginal use may result in burning, itching, and irritation. Adverse reactions associated with topical use are rare.

Fluconazole. Administration may result in nausea, vomiting, headache, diarrhea, and skin rash. Abnormal liver function tests may be seen and may require follow-up tests to determine if liver function has been affected.

Griseofulvin. Administration may result in a hypersensitivity-type reaction that includes rash and urticaria. Nausea, vomiting, oral thrush, diarrhea, and headache may also be seen.

Ketoconazole. This drug is usually well-tolerated but nausea, vomiting, headache, dizziness, abdominal pain, and pruritus may be seen. Most adverse reactions are mild and transient. On rare occasions, hepatic toxicity may be seen and the drug must be discontinued immediately. Monthly hepatic function tests are recommended.

Nystatin. This drug is usually well tolerated with few reported adverse reactions. Large oral doses have caused diarrhea, gastrointestinal distress, nausea, and vomiting.

NURSING MANAGEMENT

Observe the patient every 2 to 4 hours for adverse drug reactions when an antifungal agent is given by the oral or parenteral route. When these drugs are applied topically to the skin, inspect the area at the time of each application for localized skin reactions. When used vaginally, question the patient regarding any discomfort or other sensations experienced after insertion of the antifungal preparation. Evaluate and chart the response to therapy daily.

Specific areas of nursing management for some of the antifungal drugs are discussed below.

Amphotericin B. Administer this drug daily or every other day over several months. The patient is often acutely ill with a life-threatening deep fungal infection. Monitor vital signs every 2 to 4 hours depending on the patient's condition. Administer the IV infusion over 6 or more hours immediately after reconstitution. Protect the IV solution from exposure to light. A brown paper bag or aluminum foil may be wrapped around the infusion bottle after reconstitution of the powder and during administration of the solution. Some authorities believe that this maneuver is not necessary because the solution decomposes slowly. Consult the physician or hospital pharmacist regarding whether or not to use a protective covering for the infusion container. Check the IV infusion rate and the infusion site frequently during administration of the drug. This is especially important if the patient is restless or confused. Monitor the intake and output because this drug may be nephrotoxic (harmful to the kidneys). In some instances, hourly measurements of the urinary output may be necessary. Periodic laboratory tests are usually ordered to monitor the patient's response to therapy and to detect toxic drug reactions.

Nursing Alert

Renal damage is the most serious adverse reaction with the use of Amphotericin B. Renal impairment usually improves with modification of dosage regimen (reduction of dosage or increasing time between dosages). Serum creatinine levels and blood urea nitrogen levels are checked frequently during the course of therapy to monitor kidney function.

Flucytosine. Give flucytosine orally. The prescribed dose may range from two to six capsules per dose. To reduce the incidence of gastrointestinal distress, the capsules may be given one or two at a time over a 15-minute period. If gastrointestinal distress still occurs, notify the physician.

Miconazole. Give miconazole by IV infusion over 30 to 60 minutes. Fungal infections of the bladder are treated with IV administration of this drug and instillation of the IV form into the bladder. Fungal meningitis is also treated with an IV infusion of the drug and instillation of the drug into the subarachnoid space by means of a lumbar, cervical, or cisternal puncture. Monitor the vital signs every 2 to 4 hours depending on the patient's condition. Measure the intake and output and notify the physician if the oral intake is inadequate or there is a change in the intake and output ratio. If nausea and vomiting occurs, notify the physician because additional measures, such as giving the infusion over a longer time or administering an antiemetic, may be necessary.

Fluconazole. When administered IV, follow the manufacturer's directions regarding removal of the wrapping around the container. Do not remove the overwrap until the unit is ready for use. Do not administer solution that is cloudy or contains precipitate.

Nursing Process
The Patient Receiving an Antifungal Drug

■ *Assessment*
Information gathered before the administration of the first dose establishes a data base for comparison during therapy. Before administration of the first dose of an antifungal drug, assess the patient for signs of the infection. Inspect superficial fungal infections of the skin or skin structures (hair, nails) and describe on the patient's record. For other superficial and deep fungus infections, record the patient's signs and symptoms. Also take and record vital signs. Weigh the patient scheduled to receive amphotericin or flucytosine, because the dosage of the drug is determined according to the patient's weight.

■ *Nursing Diagnoses*
Depending on the drug, dose, and reason for administration, one or more of the following nursing diagnoses may apply to a person receiving an antifungal drug:
- **Anxiety** related to diagnosis, symptoms, treatment modalities, other factors (specify)
- **Noncompliance** related to indifference, lack of knowledge, length of treatment, other factors
- **Risk for Ineffective Management of Therapeutic Regimen** related to indifference, lack of knowledge, other factors (specify)

■ *Planning and Implementation*
The major goals of the patient may include a reduction in anxiety and an understanding of and compliance to the prescribed treatment regimen. To make these goals measurable, more specific criteria must be added.

Anxiety. Superficial and deep fungal infections respond slowly to antifungal therapy. Many patients experience anxiety and depression over the fact that therapy must continue for a prolonged time. Depending on the method of treatment, patients may be faced with many problems during therapy and therefore need time to talk about their problems as they arise. Examples of problems are the cost of treatment, hospitalization (when required), the failure of treatment to adequately control the infection, and loss of income.

Help the patient and the family to understand that therapy must be continued until the infection is under control, which in some cases may take weeks or months.

■ *Patient and Family Teaching*

If the patient is being treated with topical antifungal drugs include the following points in the teaching plan:

- Clean the involved area and apply the ointment or cream to the skin as directed by the physician.
- Do not increase or decrease the amount used or number of times the ointment or cream should be applied unless directed to do so by the physician.
- If the drug (cream or tablet) is administered vaginally, insert the drug high in the vagina using the applicator provided with the product.
- During treatment for a ringworm infection, keep towels and facecloths used for bathing separate from those of other family members to avoid the spread of the infection. The affected area is kept clean and dry.
- Flucytosine: Nausea and vomiting may occur with this drug and may be reduced or eliminated by taking a few capsules at a time over a 15-minute period. If nausea, vomiting, or diarrhea persists, notify the physician as soon as possible.
- Griseofulvin: Beneficial effects may not be noticed for some time; therefore, take the drug for the full course of therapy. Avoid exposure to sunlight and sunlamps because an exaggerated skin reaction (which is similar to a severe sunburn) may occur even after a brief exposure to ultraviolet light.
- Ketoconazole: Complete the full course of therapy as prescribed by the physician. Do not take this drug with an antacid. Avoid the use of nonprescription drugs unless use of a specific drug is approved by the physician. This drug may produce headache, dizziness, and drowsiness. If drowsiness or dizziness should occur, observe caution while driving or performing other hazardous tasks. Notify the physician if abdominal pain, fever, or diarrhea become pronounced.
- Miconazole: When a vaginal cream is prescribed, wear a sanitary napkin after insertion of the drug to prevent staining of the clothing and bed linen.
- Nystatin: Oral candidiasis—keep the liquid drug in the mouth as long as possible before swallowing. Avoid the use of commercial mouthwashes. Brush teeth immediately after eating.

■ *Expected Outcomes for Evaluation*

- Anxiety is reduced
- Adverse reactions are identified and reported to the physician
- Patient and family demonstrate understanding of drug regimen
- Patient verbalizes importance of complying with the prescribed treatment regimen

Chapter Summary

- Antiviral drugs are used to treat viral infections, which can be as mild and self-limiting as a common cold or as serious as AIDS. Although viral infections are common, only a few drugs are available for their treatment.
- Acyclovir is used for the treatment of herpes simplex virus and herpes zoster. Amantadine is used to treat respiratory illness caused by influenza A. Didanosine and zidovudine are used in the treatment of AIDS. Ribavirin is used in the treatment of severe lower respiratory tract infection caused by the respiratory syncytial virus. Antiviral drugs do not cure the disorder caused by a virus but they do decrease and lessen the symptoms, allowing the virus to run its course in a shorter time.
- Adverse reactions for the antiviral drugs include nausea, vomiting, diarrhea, orthostatic hypotension, and hemotologic changes. Patients may experience dizziness and should be warned against driving or engaging in activities that require alertness until the individual drug response is identified. Administered topically, these drugs cause transient burning, stinging, and pruritus.
- Ribavirin is given by inhalation and, even though used to treat respiratory infections, can cause worsening of the respiratory status. Respiratory status must be monitored throughout therapy. Patients should be monitored for signs and symptoms of infection before and throughout therapy. Skin lesions should be assessed daily. Evaluation of the effectiveness of therapy is evidenced by resolution of the signs and symptoms of the viral infection.
- Antifungal drugs are used to treat mycotic or fungal infections. Fungal infections of the skin and mucous membranes may be treated with topical drugs. Deep, systemic mycotic infections are treated most effectively with the antifungal agent amphotericin B.
- Most antifungal drugs have a fungicidal or fungistatic action. Adverse reactions when administered topically are few. Amphotericin B may cause renal impairment. Serum creatinine levels and blood urea nitrogen are monitored frequently during the course of therapy.
- Patients must be assessed for signs of infection throughout the course of therapy. Skin and mucous membranes must also be evaluated daily. When the drug is administered topically, a finger cot or gloves are used to prevent spread of infection. Signs and symptoms will diminish and le-

sions will heal as the infection resolves. However, deep mycotic infections may require weeks or months of therapy to heal.

Critical Thinking Exercises

1. A young mother is concerned because her 2-month-old daughter has been diagnosed with respiratory syncytial virus. The infant is receiving inhalation treatments with Ribavirin. The mother questions this treatment. How could the nurse explain treatment with Ribavirin to the mother? What possible effects could the drug have on the infant? on the mother?

2. A nurse is preparing to administer Amphotericin B to a patient with a systemic mycotic infection. This is the first time the nurse has administered Amphotericin B. What information should the nurse be aware of concerning the administration of this drug? Explain your answer.

14

Drugs Used in the Treatment of Parasitic Infections

Key Terms

Amebiasis
Anthelmintic
Cinchonism
Gametocytes
Helminthiasis
Helminths
Merozoites
Parasite
Scolex
Sporozoites

Chapter Outline

Chapter Objectives

On completion of this chapter the student will:

- *Discuss the use and major adverse effects of the drugs used in the treatment of helminth infections*
- *Use the nursing process when administering a drug used in the treatment of helminth infections*
- *Discuss the use and major adverse effects of the drugs used in the prevention and treatment of malaria*
- *Use the nursing process when administering a drug used in the prevention or treatment of malaria*
- *Discuss the use and major adverse effects of the drugs used in the treatment of amebiasis*
- *Use the nursing process when administering a drug used in the treatment of amebiasis*
- *Discuss the nursing implications to be considered when administering drugs used in the treatment of helminth infections, malaria, or amebiasis*

Scherer JC, Roach S: INTRODUCTORY CLINICAL PHARMACOLOGY,
FIFTH EDITION © 1996 Lippincott-Raven Publishers

A *parasite* is an organism that lives in or on another organism (the host) without contributing to the survival or well-being of the host. *Helminthiasis* (invasion of the body by *helminths* [worms]), *amebiasis* (invasion of the body by the ameba, *Entamoeba histolytica*) and malaria are worldwide parasitic health problems.

Pinworm is a helminth infection that is universally common, whereas helminthiasis and most other helminth infections are predominantly found in certain countries or areas of the world, particularly in areas lacking proper sanitary facilities.

Malaria is rare in the United States, but is sometimes seen in individuals who have traveled to or lived in areas where this disease is a health problem. The first antimalarial drug, quinine, is derived from the bark of the cinchona tree.

Amebiasis is seen throughout the world but is less common in developed countries where sanitary facilities prevent the spread of this organism.

Anthelmintic Drugs

Anthelmintic (against helminths) drugs are used to treat helminthiasis. Roundworms, pinworms, whipworms, hookworms, and tapeworms are examples of helminths. Table 14-1 lists the organisms causing helminth infections. The anthelmintic drugs are listed in Summary Drug Table 14-1.

ACTIONS AND USES OF ANTHELMINTIC DRUGS

Although the actions of anthelmintic drugs vary, their prime purpose is to kill the parasite.

Mebendazole. Mebendazole (Vermox) blocks the uptake of glucose by the helminth, resulting in a depletion of the helminth's own glycogen. Glycogen depletion results in a decreased formation of adenosine triphosphate, which is required by the helminth for reproduction and survival. This drug is used in the treatment of whipworm, pinworm, roundworm, American hookworm, and the common hookworm.

Niclosamide. The *scolex* (head) and proximal segments of the helminth are killed on contact with niclosamide (Niclocide). The head then becomes loosened from the intestinal wall and is passed in the feces. This results in death of the helminth. Niclosamide is used in the treatment of beef tapeworm, fish tapeworm, and dwarf tapeworm.

Table 14-1. Common Names and Causative Organisms of Parasitic Infections

Common Name	Causative Organism
roundworm	*Ascaris lumbricoides*
pinworm	*Enterobius vermicularis*
whipworm	*Trichuris trichiura*
threadworm	*Strongyloides stercoralis*
hookworm	*Ancylostoma duodenale, Necator americanus*
beef tapeworm	*Taenia saginata*
pork tapeworm	*Taenia solium*
fish tapeworm	*Diphyllobothrium latum*
dwarf tapeworm	*Hymenolepsis nana*

Piperazine. The action of piperazine against pinworms is unknown. When roundworms are present, this drug paralyzes the helminth, causing it to dislodge from the intestinal wall and be excreted in the feces. Piperazine is used in the treatment of pinworm and roundworm.

Pyrantel. The activity of pyrantel (Antiminth) is probably due to its ability to paralyze the helminth, which then releases its grip on the intestinal wall and is excreted in the feces. Pyrantel is used in the treatment of roundworm and pinworm.

Quinacrine. Quinacrine (Atabrine) decreases protein synthesis, which then results in the death of the helminth. This drug is used in the treatment of beef tapeworm, pork tapeworm, dwarf tapeworm, and fish tapeworm. It also may be used in the treatment of giardiasis, a protozoa infection caused by *Giardia lamblia*.

Thiabendazole. The exact mechanism of action of thiabendazole (Mintezol) is unknown. This drug appears to suppress egg or larval production and therefore may interrupt the life cycle of the helminth. Thiabendazole is used in the treatment of threadworm.

ADVERSE REACTIONS ASSOCIATED WITH THE ADMINISTRATION OF ANTHELMINTIC DRUGS

If they occur, the adverse reactions associated with the anthelmintic drugs are usually mild when the drug is used in the recommended dosage. Some pa-

Summary Drug Table 14-1. Anthelmintic Drugs

Generic Name	Trade Name*	Uses	Adverse Reactions	Dose Ranges
mebendazole	Vermox	Treatment of whipworm, pinworm, roundworm, common and American hookworm	Transient abdominal pain, diarrhea	100 mg PO morning and evening for 3 consecutive days; pinworm: 100 mg PO as a single dose
niclosamide	Niclocide	Treatment of beef, fish, and dwarf tapeworm	Nausea, vomiting, abdominal cramps, diarrhea, anorexia	Beef and fish tapeworm: 2 g PO as a single dose; dwarf tapeworm: 2 g PO once daily for 7 d
piperazine	*generic*	Treatment of pinworm and roundworm	Same as niclosamide	Pinworm: 65 mg/kg PO as a single daily dose for 7 consecutive days; roundworm: 3.5 g PO as a single daily dose for 2 consecutive days
pyrantel	Antiminth	Treatment of pinworm and roundworm	Same as niclosamide	11 mg/kg PO as a single dose
quinacrine hydrochloride	Atabrine HCl	Treatment of beef, pork, fish, and dwarf tapeworm and giardiasis	Headache, dizziness, GI complaints	Beef, pork, fish tapeworm: 4 doses of 200 mg PO 10 minutes apart; dwarf tapeworm: day 1—900 mg divided into 3 doses taken 20 min apart; days 2–4—100 mg PO tid; giardiasis: 100 mg PO tid for 5–7 d
thiabendazole	Mintezol	Treatment of threadworm	Hypersensitivity reactions, drowsiness, dizziness	Up to 1.5 mg/dose PO bid for 2 d

*The term, *generic*, indicates that the drug is available in generic form.

tients receiving niclosamide, piperazine, and pyrantel may experience gastrointestinal (GI) side effects, such as nausea, vomiting, abdominal cramps, or diarrhea. The most frequent adverse reactions seen with quinacrine include headache, dizziness, and GI complaints. Thiabendazole may cause hypersensitivity reactions, drowsiness, and dizziness.

NURSING MANAGEMENT

The method of administration of an anthelmintic drug may vary somewhat from the administration of other drugs. To achieve the desired results, it is most important that the drug be given as directed by the physician, drug label, or package insert.

- Mebendazole—Give tablets crushed and mixed with food or instruct the patient to chew the table or swallow it whole.

- Niclosamide—The tablets must be chewed thoroughly before swallowing. Only a small amount of water is to be used in swallowing the drug. If the patient is uncooperative, crush the tablet, then mix it with a small amount of water and spoonfeed to the patient.
- Piperazine—Give on an empty stomach, that is, 1 hour before or 2 hours after a meal.
- Pyrantel—Give any time without regard to meals or time of day. The drug can be given with milk or fruit juices.
- Quinacrine—Review the package insert or the physician's orders carefully for the directions regarding a special diet and enemas that usually are necessary before the drug is given for a helminth infection. When necessary, the tablets may be thoroughly crushed for ease in administration.
- Thiabendazole—Give the drug with food to minimize GI upset and distress.

Nursing Process
The Patient Receiving an Anthelmintic Drug

■ *Assessment*

The diagnosis of a helminth infection is made by examination of the stool for ova and all or part of the helminth. Several stool specimens may be necessary before the helminth is seen and identified. The patient history may also lead to a suspicion of a helminth infection, but some patients have no symptoms.

When a pinworm infection is suspected, examine and take a specimen from the anal area, preferably early in the morning before the patient gets out of bed.

Patients with massive helminth infections may or may not be acutely ill. The acutely ill patient requires hospitalization, but many individuals with helminth infections can be treated on an outpatient basis.

Obtain vital signs before the first dose of the anthelmintic drug is given. Weighing the patient may also be necessary if the drug's dosage is determined by weight or if the patient is acutely ill.

■ *Nursing Diagnoses*

Depending on the individual and the type of helminth infection, one or more of the following nursing diagnoses may apply to a patient receiving an anthelmintic drug:
- **Anxiety** related to diagnosis, treatment regimen
- **Risk for Ineffective Management of Therapeutic Regimen** related to insufficient knowledge of medication regimen, lack of knowledge of prevention of future infections

■ *Planning and Implementation*

The major goals of the patient may include a reduction in anxiety and an understanding of and compliance to the prescribed therapeutic regimen. To make these goals measurable, more specific criteria must be added.

Unless ordered otherwise, save all stools that are passed following administration of the drug. Visually inspect each stool for passage of the helminth. If stool specimens are to be saved for laboratory examination, follow the hospital procedure for saving the stool and transporting it to the laboratory. If the patient is acutely ill or has a massive infection, monitor vital signs every 4 hours and measure and record intake and output.

Observe the patient for adverse drug reactions, as well as severe episodes of diarrhea. Notify the physician if these occur.

Depending on hospital policy, as well as the type of helminth infection, linen precautions may be necessary. Wear gloves when changing bed linens, emptying bedpans, or obtaining or handling stool specimens. Wash hands thoroughly after removing the gloves. Instruct the patient to wash the hands thoroughly following personal care and use of the bedpan.

Anxiety. The diagnosis of a helminth infection is often distressing to patients and their family. Allow time to explain the treatment and future preventive measures, as well as to allow the patient or family members to discuss their concerns or ask questions.

■ *Patient and Family Teaching*

When an anthelmintic is prescribed on an outpatient basis, give the patient or a family member complete instructions about taking the drug, as well as household precautions that should be followed until the helminth is eliminated from the intestine.

Develop a teaching plan to include the following:
- Follow the dosage schedule exactly as printed on the prescription container. (See earlier section on administration for the directions specific for each drug.) It is absolutely necessary to follow the directions for taking the drug to eradicate the helminth.
- Follow-up stool specimens will be necessary because this is the only way to determine the success of drug therapy.
- To prevent reinfection and the infection of others in the household, change and launder bed linens and undergarments daily, separately from those of other members of the family.
- Daily bathing (showering is best) is recommended. Disinfect toilet facilities daily. Disinfect the bathtub or shower stall immediately after bathing. Use the disinfectant recommended by the physician or use chlorine bleach. Scrub the surfaces thoroughly and allow the disinfectant to remain in contact with the surfaces for several minutes.
- Wash the hands thoroughly after urinating or defecating and before preparing and eating food. It is important to clean under the fingernails daily and avoid putting fingers in the mouth and nail-biting.

■ *Expected Outcomes for Evaluation*
- Anxiety is reduced
- Patient verbalizes an understanding of therapeutic regimen modalities and importance of continued follow-up testing

- Describes or lists measures used to prevent the spread of infection to others
- Verbalizes importance of complying with the prescribed treatment regimen and preventive measures

Antimalarial Drugs

Malaria is transmitted by a certain species of the *Anopheles* mosquito. The four different protozoans causing malaria are *Plasmodium falciparum, Plasmodium malariae, Plasmodium ovale,* and *Plasmodium vivax.* Drugs that are used in treating or preventing malaria are called antimalarial drugs. Examples of antimalarial drugs in use today are listed in Summary Drug Table 14-2.

ACTIONS OF ANTIMALARIAL DRUGS

The plasmodium causing malaria must enter the mosquito to develop and reproduce. When the mosquito bites a person infected with malaria, it ingests the male and female forms (*gametocytes*) of the plasmodium. The gametocytes mate in the mosquito's stomach and ultimately form *sporozoites* (an animal reproductive cell) that make their way to the salivary glands of the mosquito. When the mosquito bites an individual, the sporozoites enter the individual's bloodstream and lodge in the liver and other tissues. These sporozoites undergo asexual cell division and reproduction, forming *merozoites* (cells formed as a result of asexual reproduction). The merozoites then divide asexually and enter the red blood cells of the individual where they form the male and female forms of the plasmodium. When the merozoites enter the individual's red blood cells, the symptoms of malaria (shaking, chills, and fever) appear.

Antimalarial drugs interfere with or are active against the life cycle of the plasmodium, primarily when it is present in the red blood cells. Destruction at this stage of the plasmodium life cycle prevents the development of the male and female forms of the plasmodium, which must then enter the mosquito (when the mosquito bites an infected individual) to begin its life cycle.

USES OF ANTIMALARIAL DRUGS

There are two terms used when discussing the use of antimalarial drugs: (1) *suppression,* the prevention of malaria, and (2) *treatment,* the management of a malarial attack.

Not all antimalarial drugs are effective in preventing (suppressing) or treating all four of the plasmodium causing malaria. In addition, resistant plasmodium strains have developed and some antimalarial drugs are no longer effective against some of these strains. The physician must select the antimalarial drug that reportedly is effective, at present, for the type of malaria the individual either has (treatment) or could be exposed to (prevention) in a specific area of the world.

Chloroquine hydrochloride (Aralen HCl) and chloroquine phosphate (Aralen Phosphate) also are used in the treatment of extraintestinal amebiasis (see next section). Hydroxychloroquine sulfate (Plaquenil) may be used in the treatment of lupus erythematosus and rheumatoid arthritis. Quinine also may be used for the prevention and treatment of nocturnal leg cramps.

ADVERSE REACTIONS ASSOCIATED WITH THE ADMINISTRATION OF ANTIMALARIAL DRUGS

Chloroquine and Hydroxychloroquine. The adverse reactions associated with the administration of chloroquine (Aralen HCl and phosphate) and hydroxychloroquine include hypotension, electrocardiographic changes, headache, nausea, vomiting, anorexia, diarrhea, and abdominal cramps. These drugs may impart a yellow color to the skin and urine.

Doxycycline. Doxycycline (Vibramycin) is an antibiotic belonging to the tetracycline group of antibiotics. The adverse reactions associated with this drug are discussed in Chapter 8.

Mefloquine. Mefloquine (Lariam) may cause vomiting, dizziness, a disturbed sense of balance, nausea, fever, headache, and visual disturbances.

Primaquine. Primaquine may cause nausea, vomiting, epigastric distress, and abdominal cramps.

Pyrimethamine. Nausea, vomiting, anorexia, and hematologic changes may be seen with the use of pyrimethamine (Daraprim). Hypersensitivity reactions may be seen, even when taken in low doses.

Quinacrine. Headache, dizziness, and GI complaints may occur with the use of quinacrine (Atabrine). Long-term therapy can result in aplastic anemia, hepatitis, and skin eruptions.

Summary Drug Table 14-2. Antimalarial Drugs

Generic Name	Trade Name*	Uses	Adverse Reactions	Dose Ranges
chloroquine hydrochloride	Aralen HCl	Treatment of malaria when oral therapy not feasible	Hypotension, ECG changes, headache, nausea, vomiting. anorexia, diarrhea, abdominal cramps	*Dose expressed as base.* 160–200 mg (4–5 mL) IM and repeat in 6 h if necessary
chloroquine phosphate	Aralen Phosphate	Treatment and prevention of malaria	Same as chloroquine hydrochloride	*Dose expressed as base.* Prevention: 300 mg PO weekly; treatment: initially 600 mg PO and 300 mg PO 6 h later then 300 mg/d PO for 2 d
doxycycline	Vibramycin, *generic*	Short-term prevention of malaria	Photosensitivity, anorexia, nausea, vomiting, superinfection, rash, diarrhea	100 mg PO once daily
hydroxychloroquine sulfate	Plaquenil Sulfate	Prevention and treatment of malaria	Same as chloroquine HCl	*Dose expressed as base.* Prevention: 310 mg PO weekly; treatment: initially 620 mg PO, and 310 mg 6 h later then 310 mg/d PO for 2 d
mefloquine hydrochloride	Lariam	Prevention and treatment of malaria	Vomiting, dizziness, disturbed sense of balance, nausea, fever, headache, visual disturbances	Prevention: 250 mg/week PO for 4 wk then 250 mg PO ever other week; treatment: 5 tablets PO as a single dose
primaquine phosphate	*generic*	Treatment of malaria	Nausea, vomiting, epigastric distress, abdominal cramps	*Dose expressed as base.* 15 mg PO daily for 14 d
pyrimethamine	Daraprim	Prevention of malaria	Nausea, vomiting, anorexia, hematologic changes	25 mg PO once weekly
quinacrine hydrochloride	Atabrine HCl	Prevention and treatment of malaria	Headache, dizziness, GI complaints	Prevention: 100 mg/d PO; treatment: 200 mg PO with sodium bicarbonate q6h for 5 doses then 100 mg PO tid for 6 d
quinine sulfate	Quinamm, *generic*	Treatment of malaria	Cinchonism, hematologic changes, vertigo, skin rash, visual disturbances	600–650 mg PO q8h for 5–7 d
sulfadoxine and pyrimethamine	Fansidar	Prevention and treatment of malaria	Hematologic changes, nausea, emesis, headache, hypersensitivity reactions, Stevens-Johnson syndrome	Prevention: 1 tablet PO weekly or 2 tablets every 2 wk; treatment: 3 tablets PO as a single dose

*The term, *generic*, indicates that the drug is available in generic form.

Quinine. The use of quinine can cause *cinchonism* at full therapeutic doses. Cinchonism is a group of symptoms associated with quinine. Symptoms of cinchonism include tinnitus, dizziness, headache, GI disturbances, and visual disturbances. These symptoms usually disappear when the dosage is reduced. Other adverse reactions include hematologic changes, vertigo, and skin rash.

Sulfadoxine and Pyrimethamine. Sulfadoxine (a sulfonamide) and pyrimethamine (an antimalarial) are combined in one tablet (Fansidar). The adverse reactions that may be seen with this drug combination include hematologic changes, nausea, emesis, headache, hypersensitivity reactions, and Stevens-Johnson syndrome (see Chap. 11).

NURSING MANAGEMENT

When an antimalarial drug is prescribed for the prevention (suppression) of malaria, thoroughly review the drug regimen with the patient. When the drug is to be taken once a week, advise patients to select a day of the week that will best remind them to take the drug. Emphasize the importance of taking the drug exactly as prescribed because failure to take the drug on an exact schedule will not give protection against malaria.

The doses of some antimalarial drugs are expressed as base. The drug label will identify the dose of the tablet and the dose of the tablet as base. An example of the drug label is 200 mg tablets equivalent to 155 mg base. The physician may order the drug dosage as the base equivalent or as the labeled dose of the tablet. If the drug order is stated as *620 mg base* and the tablets are labeled as 200 mg tablets equivalent to 155 mg base, 620 mg is divided by 155 mg. The correct dose would then be four 200 mg tablets.

Nursing Process
The Patient Receiving an Antimalarial Drug

■ *Assessment*

When an antimalarial drug is given to a hospitalized patient for treatment of malaria, the initial assessment includes vital signs and a summary of the nature and duration of the symptoms. Laboratory tests may be ordered for the diagnosis of malaria. Additional laboratory tests, such as a complete blood count, may be ordered to determine the patient's general health status.

■ *Nursing Diagnoses*

Depending on the reason for administration (prevention or treatment), one or more of the following nursing diagnoses may apply to a person receiving an antimalarial drug:

- **Noncompliance** related to indifference, lack of knowledge, other factors
- **Risk for Ineffective Management of Therapeutic Regimen** related to knowledge deficit of medication regimen, adverse drug effects, thera-

peutic modalities, importance of adhering to the medication regimen

■ *Planning and Implementation*

The major goals of the patient may include an understanding of and compliance to the prescribed therapeutic or prevention regimen. To make these goals measurable, more specific criteria must be added.

If the patient is hospitalized with malaria, take vital signs every 4 hours or as ordered by the physician. Observe the patient every 1 to 2 hours for the symptoms of malaria. Antipyretics may be ordered for fever. If the patient is acutely ill, measure and record the intake and output. In some instances, intravenous fluids may be required.

Administration. These drugs are given with food or meals. The exception is quinacrine, which is given after meals with a full glass of water, tea, or fruit juice.

■ *Patient and Family Teaching*

The patient must have a complete understanding of the therapeutic regimen. Review the drug dosage schedule with the patient and stress the importance of adhering to the prescribed dosage schedule.

When an antimalarial drug is used for prevention of malaria and taken once a week, the drug must be taken on the *same day* each week. The program of prevention is usually started 1 week before departure to an area where malaria is prevalent.

The following additional information is relevant to specific antimalarial drugs:

- Chloroquine and hydroxychloroquine—Take these drugs with food or milk. These drugs may cause diarrhea, loss of appetite, nausea, stomach pain, or vomiting. Notify the physician if these become pronounced. Also notify the physician if any of the following occur: visual changes, ringing in the ears, difficulty in hearing, fever, sore throat, unusual bleeding or bruising, unusual color (blue-black) of the skin, skin rash, or unusual muscle weakness.
- Quinacrine—Take this drug with food or meals. A yellow color to the skin or urine may be seen. Contact the physician promptly if any visual changes occur.
- Quinine—Take this drug with food or immediately after a meal. Do not drive or perform other hazardous tasks requiring alertness if blurred vision or dizziness occurs. If the tablet or capsule is difficult to swallow, do *not* chew the tablet or open the capsule because the drug is irritating to the stomach.

■ *Expected Outcomes for Evaluation*
- Patient verbalizes importance of complying with the prescribed therapeutic or prophylaxis regimen
- Patient verbalizes an understanding of the prophylaxis or treatment schedule

Amebicides

Amebicides (drugs that kill amebas) are used for the treatment of amebiasis caused by the parasite *E. histolytica*. An ameba is a one-celled organism found in soil and water. Examples of amebicides are listed in Summary Drug Table 14-3.

ACTIONS AND USES OF AMEBICIDES

These drugs are amebicidal (ie, they kill amebas). The two types of amebiasis are intestinal and extraintestinal. In the intestinal form, the ameba is confined to the intestine, and a drug effective for this form of amebiasis is selected. The extraintestinal form is present when the ameba is found outside of the intestine, such as in the liver. The extraintestinal form of amebiasis is more difficult to treat.

Chloroquine hydrochloride or phosphate (Aralen) is used in the treatment of extraintestinal amebiasis. Iodoquinol (Yodoxin), metronidazole (Flagyl), and paromomycin (Humatin) are used to treat intestinal amebiasis. Metronidazole and paromomycin are also used to treat infections caused by susceptible microorganisms and are discussed in Chapters 10 and 9, respectively.

ADVERSE REACTIONS ASSOCIATED WITH THE ADMINISTRATION OF AMEBICIDES

Chloroquine. Hypotension, electrocardiographic changes, headache, nausea, vomiting, anorexia, diarrhea, abdominal cramps, and psychic stimulation can occur with the use of chloroquine hydrochloride or phosphate.

Iodoquinol. Various types of skin eruptions, nausea, vomiting, fever, chills, abdominal cramps, vertigo, and diarrhea may occur with administration of iodoquinol.

Summary Drug Table 14-3. Amebicides				
Generic Name	Trade Name*	Uses	Adverse Reactions	Dose Ranges
chloroquine hydrochloride	Aralen HC1	Extraintestinal amebiasis when oral therapy not feasible	Hypotension, ECG changes, headache, nausea, vomiting, anorexia, diarrhea, abdominal cramps, psychic stimulation	*Dose expressed as base.* 160–200 mg IM daily for 10–12 d
chloroquine phosphate	Aralen Phosphate	Same as chloroquine hydrochloride	Same as chloroquine hydrochloride	*Dose expressed as base.* 600 mg PO daily for 2 d then 300 mg PO for 2–3 wk
iodoquinol	Vodoxin	Treatment of intestinal amebiasis	Skin eruptions, nausea, vomiting, fever, chills, abdominal cramps, vertigo, diarrhea	650 mg PO tid after meals for 20 d
metronidazole	Flagyl, *generic*	Treatment of intestinal amebiasis	Convulsive seizures, headache, nausea, peripheral neuropathy	750 mg PO tid for 5–10 d
paromomycin	Humatin	Treatment of intestinal amebiasis	Nausea, vomiting, diarrhea	25–35 mg/kg/d in three divided doses with meals for 5–10 d

*The term, *generic*, indicates that the drug is available in generic form.

Metronidazole. Convulsive seizures, headache, nausea, and peripheral neuropathy (numbness and tingling of the extremities) have been reported with the use of metronidazole.

Paromomycin. Nausea, vomiting, and diarrhea are the most common reactions seen with administration of paromomycin.

NURSING MANAGEMENT

The patient with amebiasis may or may not be acutely ill. Nursing management depends on the condition of the patient and the information obtained during the initial assessment.

If the patient is acutely ill or has vomiting and diarrhea, measure the intake and output and observe the patient closely for signs of dehydration. If dehydration is apparent, notify the physician. If the patient is or becomes dehydrated, oral or intravenous fluid and electrolyte replacement may be necessary. Take vital signs every 4 hours or as ordered by the physician.

Isolation is usually not necessary but hospital policy may require isolation procedures. Stool precautions are usually necessary. Wash the hands thoroughly after all patient care and the handling of stool specimens.

Nursing Process
The Patient Receiving an Amebicide

■ *Assessment*
Diagnosis of amebiasis is made by examination of the stool, as well as by the symptoms. Once the patient is diagnosed as having amebiasis, local health department regulations often require investigation into the source of infection. A thorough foreign travel history is necessary. If the patient has not traveled to a foreign country, further investigation of local travel, use of restaurants, the local water supply (especially well water), and so on may be necessary to identify the source of the infection. Immediate family members are usually tested for amebiasis.

Before administration of the first dose of an amebicide, record the patient's vital signs and weight. Evaluate the general physical status of the patient and look for evidence of dehydration, especially if severe vomiting and diarrhea have occurred.

■ *Nursing Diagnoses*
Depending on the type of amebiasis and the condition of the patient, one or more of the following nursing diagnoses may apply to a person receiving an amebicide:
- **Diarrhea** related to amebiasis
- **Risk for Fluid Volume Deficit** related to amebiasis
- **Anxiety** related to diagnosis, treatment regimen, other factors (specify)
- **Risk for Ineffective Management of Therapeutic Regimen** related to knowledge deficit of medication regimen, adverse drug effects, therapeutic modalities

■ *Planning and Implementation*
The major goals of the patient may include a reduction in anxiety, an absence of diarrhea, maintenance of an adequate intake of fluids, an understanding of the therapeutic regimen (hospitalized patients), and an understanding of and compliance to the prescribed therapeutic regimen (outpatients). To make these goals measurable, more specific criteria must be added.

Diarrhea, Fluid Volume Deficit. Record the number, character, and color of stools passed. Daily stool specimens may be ordered to be sent to the laboratory for examination. *Immediately* deliver to the laboratory all stool specimens saved for examination because the ameba dies (and therefore cannot be seen microscopically) when the specimen cools. Inform laboratory personnel that the patient has amebiasis because the specimen must be kept at or near body temperature until examined under a microscope.

Observe the patient with severe or frequent episodes of diarrhea for symptoms of a fluid volume deficit. Notify the physician if signs of dehydration become apparent because intravenous fluids may be necessary.

Anxiety. Explain to the patient and family the treatment measures and the necessary laboratory examination of stool specimens. Allow time for the patient and family members to discuss the diagnosis and ask questions about the treatment and future preventive measures.

■ *Patient and Family Teaching*
Stress the importance of completing the full course of treatment. Give patients receiving an amebicide on an outpatient basis the following information:

- Take the drug exactly as prescribed. Complete the *full* course of therapy to eradicate the ameba. Failure to complete treatment may result in a return of the infection.
- Prevention—Follow measures to control the spread of infection. Wash hands immediately before eating or preparing food and after defecation.
- Food handlers—Do not resume work until a full course of treatment is completed and stools are negative for the ameba.
- Chloroquine—Notify the physician if any of the following occurs: ringing in the ears, difficulty hearing, visual changes, fever, sore throat, unusual bleeding or bruising.
- Iodoquinol—Notify the physician if nausea, vomiting, or other GI distress becomes severe.
- Metronidazole—This drug may cause GI upset. Take this drug with food or meals. The use of alcohol, in any form, must be avoided until the course of treatment is completed. The ingestion of alcohol may cause a mild to severe reaction with symptoms of severe vomiting, headache, nausea, abdominal cramps, flushing, and sweating. These symptoms may be so severe that hospitalization may be required.
- Paromomycin—Notify the physician if any of the following occurs: vaginal or rectal itching, soreness of the mouth or tongue, fever, cough, or a black furry tongue.

■ *Expected Outcomes for Evaluation*
- Anxiety is reduced
- Bowel elimination is normal
- Patient verbalizes an understanding of therapeutic modalities and importance of continued follow-up care
- Patient verbalizes importance of complying with the prescribed therapeutic regimen

Chapter Summary

- A parasite is an organism that lives in or on another organism (the host) without contributing to the survival or well-being of the host.
- Malaria is rare in the United States but is sometimes seen in individuals who have traveled to or lived in areas where this disease is a health problem. Amebiasis is seen throughout the world but is less common in developed countries where sanitary facilities prevent the spread of this organism.
- Roundworms, pinworms, whipworms, hookworms, and tapeworms are examples of parasites that may be treated with anthelmintic drugs, which kill or interrupt the life cycle of the helminth.
- Malaria is transmitted by a certain species of the *Anopheles* mosquito. The four different protozoans causing malaria are *Plasmodium falciparum, Plasmodium malariae, Plasmodium ovale,* and *Plasmodium vivax.* Antimalarial drugs interfere with or are active against the life cycle of the plasmodium, primarily when it is present in the red blood cells.
- Not all antimalarial drugs are effective in preventing (suppressing) or treating all four of the plasmodium causing malaria. Resistant plasmodium strains have developed and some antimalarial drugs are no longer effective against some of these strains.
- Amebicides (drugs that kill amebas) are used for the treatment of amebiasis caused by the parasite *Entamoeba histolytica.* The two types of amebiasis are intestinal and extraintestinal. In the intestinal form, the ameba is confined to the intestine, and a drug effective for this form of amebiasis is selected. The extraintestinal form is present when the ameba is found outside of the intestine, such as in the liver. The extraintestinal form of amebiasis is more difficult to treat.

Critical Thinking Exercises

1. While living outside the country for 3 years Mr. Evans developed a helminth infection. The parasite has been identified and the appropriate drug prescribed. What points would you include in a teaching plan for this patient?
2. A child in a family of four children is found to have pinworms. What would you include in a teaching plan to prevent the spread of pinworms to other family members?

Drugs Used to Manage Pain

III

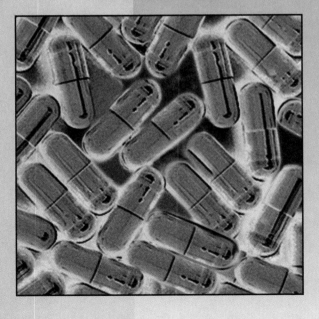

15

The Nonnarcotic Analgesics

Key Terms

Aggregation
Analgesic
Antipyretic
Glossitis
Jaundice
Methemoglobinemia
Nonsalicylate
Pancytopenia
Prostaglandin
Reye's syndrome
Salicylate
Salicylism
Tinnitus

Chapter Outline

Chapter Objectives

On completion of this chapter the student will:

- *Discuss the types, uses, and general drug actions of the nonnarcotic analgesics*
- *List the general adverse reactions associated with the administration of the nonnarcotic analgesics*
- *Discuss nursing management when administering a nonnarcotic analgesic*
- *Use the nursing process when administering a nonnarcotic analgesic*

The nonnarcotic *analgesics* are a group of drugs that are used to relieve pain. In addition to their use as *analgesics* (pain-relieving drugs), these drugs are also used as *antipyretics* (drugs that decrease body temperature) and some are used as antiinflammatory agents. Use of these drugs does not result in physical dependency, which can occur with the use of the narcotic analgesics.

The nonnarcotic analgesics can be divided into the *salicylates* and the *nonsalicylates*. The *salicylates* include aspirin (acetylsalicylic acid) and related drugs, such as magnesium salicylate and sodium salicylate. The *nonsalicylates* include drugs that are not related to the salicylates, such as acetaminophen.

Another group, the nonsteroidal antiinflammatory drugs (NSAIDs), also have antiinflammatory, analgesic, and antipyretic effects. These drugs have emerged as important drugs in the treatment of the pain and inflammation associated with disorders, such as rheumatoid arthritis or osteoarthritis. Examples of NSAIDs include ibuprofen (Advil) and naproxen (Naprosyn).

The Salicylates

The *salicylates* have analgesic, antipyretic, and antiinflammatory effects. All the salicylates are similar in pharmacologic activity; however, aspirin has a greater antiinflammatory effect than the other salicylates. Specific salicylates are listed in Summary Drug Table 15–1.

ACTIONS OF THE SALICYLATES

The manner in which salicylates relieve pain and reduce inflammation is not fully understood. It is thought that the antiinflammatory action of the salicylates is due to the inhibition of prostaglandins. *Prostaglandins* are fatty acid derivatives found in almost every tissue of the body and body fluid. Release of prostaglandin is thought to increase the sensitivity of peripheral pain receptors. Salicylates lower an elevated body temperature by dilating peripheral blood vessels, which, in turn, cools the body. Aspirin prolongs the bleeding time by inhibiting the *aggregation* (clumping) of platelets. When the bleeding time is prolonged, it takes a longer time for the blood to clot after a cut, surgery, or other injury to the skin or mucous membranes. The other salicylates do not have an effect on platelets and therefore do not affect the bleeding time.

USES OF THE SALICYLATES

The salicylate nonnarcotic analgesics are used for the following reasons:

- Relief of mild to moderate pain
- Reduction of elevated body temperature (fever)
- Treatment of inflammatory conditions, such as rheumatoid arthritis, osteoarthritis, and rheumatic fever
- Reduction of the risk of myocardial infarction in those with unstable angina—aspirin only
- Reduction of the risk of transient ischemic attacks or strokes in *males* who have had transient ischemia of the brain due to fibrin platelet emboli—aspirin only

ADVERSE REACTIONS ASSOCIATED WITH THE ADMINISTRATION OF THE SALICYLATES

Gastric upset, heartburn, nausea, vomiting, anorexia, and gastrointestinal (GI) bleeding may occur with salicylate use. Although these drugs are relatively safe when taken as recommended on the label or by the physician, their use can occasionally result in more serious reactions. Some individuals are allergic to aspirin and the other salicylates. Allergy to the salicylates may be manifested by hives, rash, angioedema, bronchospasm with asthmalike symptoms, and anaphylactoid reactions.

Salicylate toxicity produces a condition called *salicylism*. Mild *salicylism* usually occurs with repeated administration of large doses of a salicylate. The symptoms of salicylism include dizziness, *tinnitus* (a ringing sound in the ear), difficulty in hearing, nausea, vomiting, diarrhea, mental confusion, and lassitude. This condition is reversible with reduction of the dosage. Large doses of the salicylates may lead to respiratory depression and coma.

Loss of blood through the GI tract occurs with salicylate use. The amount of blood lost is insignificant when one normal dose is taken. Use of these drugs over a long period, however, even in normal doses, can result in a significant blood loss. Because the salicylates prolong bleeding time, they are contraindicated in those with bleeding disorders or bleeding tendencies. These include patients with GI bleeding

Summary Drug Table 15-1. Nonnarcotic Analgesics

Generic Name	Trade Name*	Uses	Adverse Reactions	Dose Ranges
SALICYLATES				
aspirin (acetyl-salicyclic acid)	Bayer, Ecotrin, Anacin, Empirin, Bufferin, *generic*	Analgesic, antipyretic, antiinflammatory	Nausea, vomiting, epigastric distress, GI bleeding, allergic and anaphylactic reactions, salicylism with overuse	325–650 mg PO with up to 8 g/d PO in divided doses for some disorders; 325–650 mg rectally
magnesium salicylate	Original Doan's Magan	Analgesic, antipyretic, antiinflammatory	Nausea, vomiting, epigastric distress, GI bleeding, allergic and anaphylactic reactions, salicylism with overuse	650 mg PO q4h and up to 4.8 g/d PO in divided doses for some disorders
sodium salicylate	*Generic*	Analgesic, antipyretic, antiinflammatory	Nausea, vomiting, epigastric distress, GI bleeding, allergic and anaphylactic reactions, salicylism with overuse	325–650 mg PO q4h
NONSALICYLATES				
acetaminophen	Anacin-3, Tylenol, Panadol, Datril *generic*	Analgesic, antipyretic	Rare when used as directed; skin eruptions; fever, hypo-glycemia, cyanosis, methe-moglobinemia, hemolytic anemia	325–650 mg PO q4–6h; 650 mg rectally

*The term, *generic*, indicates that the drug is available in generic form.

(due to any cause), blood dyscrasias, and those receiving anticoagulant or antineoplastic drugs.

NURSING MANAGEMENT

Give the salicylates with food or milk or a full glass of water to prevent gastric upset. If gastric distress occurs, notify the physician because other drug therapy may be necessary. An antacid may be prescribed to minimize GI distress.

Avoid the use of salicylates for at least 1 week before any type of major or minor surgery, including dental surgery, because of the possibility of postoperative bleeding. Do not use the salicylates following any type of surgery until complete healing has occurred. Acetaminophen or an NSAID may be used after surgery or a dental procedure when relief of mild pain is necessary.

Studies suggest that the use of salicylates (especially aspirin) may be involved in the development of *Reye's syndrome* in children with chickenpox or influenza. This rare but life-threatening disorder is characterized by vomiting and lethargy progressing to coma.

Nursing Alert

Use of salicylates in children with chickenpox, fever, or flulike symptoms is *not* recommended. Acetaminophen is recommended for the management of symptoms associated with these disorders.

Observe patients for adverse drug reactions. When high doses of salicylates are administered, for example to those with severe arthritic disorders, observe the patient for signs of salicylism. Should signs of salicylism occur, notify the physician because a reduction in dose or determination of the plasma salicylate level may be necessary.

Nursing Alert

Signs of salicylism: tinnitus, impaired hearing, nausea, vomiting, flushing, sweating, rapid deep breathing, thirst, headache, tachycardia, diarrhea, and drowsiness. Notify the physician before the next dose if any of these symptoms appear. Periodic monitoring of plasma salicylate levels may be ordered. Therapeutic levels are between 100 and 300 mcg/mL.

Tinnitus or impaired hearing probably indicates high blood salicylate levels. Hearing loss disappears gradually after the drug is discontinued.

Check the color of the stools. Black or dark stools or bright red blood in the stool may indicate GI bleeding. Any change in the color of the stool is reported to the physician.

The Nonsalicylates

The major drug classified as a nonsalicylate is acetaminophen (Tylenol, Datril, Panadol). Acetaminophen is the only drug of its kind available in the United States at this time. It is the most widely used aspirin substitute for patients who are allergic to aspirin or who suffer from extreme GI upset when taking aspirin. Acetaminophen is also the drug of choice for treating children with fever and flulike symptoms.

ACTIONS OF THE NONSALICYLATES

Acetaminophen is a nonsalicylate nonnarcotic analgesic whose mechanism of action is unknown. Like the salicylates, acetaminophen has analgesic and antipyretic activity. Acetaminophen does *not* possess antiinflammatory action and therefore is of no value in the treatment of inflammation or inflammatory disorders.

USES OF THE NONSALICYLATES

Acetaminophen is used to relieve mild to moderate pain and to reduce elevated body temperature (fever). This drug is particularly useful for those with aspirin allergy and with bleeding disorders such as bleeding ulcer or hemophilia; those on anticoagulant therapy; and those who have recently had minor surgical procedures. Although acetaminophen has *no* antiinflammatory action, it may be used to relieve the *pain and discomfort* associated with arthritic disorders.

ADVERSE REACTIONS ASSOCIATED WITH THE ADMINISTRATION OF THE NONSALICYLATES

Acetaminophen causes few adverse reactions when used as directed on the label or recommended by the physician. Adverse reactions associated with the use of acetaminophen usually occur with chronic use or when exceeding the recommended dosage. Adverse reactions to acetaminophen include skin eruptions; urticaria (hives); hemolytic anemia; hypoglycemia; cyanosis; *methemoglobinemia* (a condition in which a portion of the body's hemoglobin is unable to transport oxygen); *pancytopenia* (a reduction in all cellular components of the blood); *jaundice* (yellow discoloration of the skin); drowsiness; and *glossitis* (inflammation of the tongue). Hepatotoxicity (damaging to the liver) and hepatic failure have been seen in chronic alcoholics taking this drug.

NURSING MANAGEMENT

Assess overall health and alcohol usage prior to administration. Alcoholics or malnourished patients are at risk to develop hepatotoxicity (damage to the liver) with the use of acetaminophen.

Administer with a full glass of water. This drug may be taken with meals or on an empty stomach.

Symptoms of overdosage include: nausea, vomiting, diaphoresis, and generalized malaise. Acute overdosage may be treated with the administration of the drug acetylcysteine (Mucomyst) to prevent liver damage.

Report any signs of methemoglobinemia: bluish discoloration of the nailbeds or mucous membranes, dyspnea, headache, or dizziness.

The Nonsteroidal Antiinflammatory Drugs

Another type of nonnarcotic analgesic are the nonsteroidal antiinflammatory drugs (NSAIDs). This group of drugs includes fenoprofen (Nalfon), ibuprofen (Advil), naproxen (Naprosyn), and ketoprofen (Orudis). Like the salicylates, these drugs have antiinflammatory, antipyretic, and analgesic effects.

ACTIONS OF THE NONSTEROIDAL ANTIINFLAMMATORY DRUGS

The NSAIDs are so called because they do not belong to the steroid group of drugs, do not possess the adverse reactions associated with the steroids (see Chap. 42), and yet have antiinflammatory effects. In addition, they have analgesic and antipyretic properties. The exact mechanism of action is unknown.

USES OF THE NONSTEROIDAL ANTIINFLAMMATORY DRUGS

NSAIDs have a variety of uses that vary depending on the drug selected. The uses of individual NSAIDs are given in Summary Drug Table 15-2.

ADVERSE REACTIONS ASSOCIATED WITH THE ADMINISTRATION OF NONSTEROIDAL ANTIINFLAMMATORY DRUGS

There are many adverse reactions associated with the use of the NSAIDs. However, many patients take these drugs and experience few, if any, side effects. Some of the adverse reactions associated with the use of these drugs include the following:

GI tract—nausea, vomiting, diarrhea, constipation, epigastric pain, indigestion, abdominal distress or discomfort, intestinal ulceration, stomatitis, jaundice, bloating, anorexia, dry mouth
Central nervous system—dizziness, anxiety, lightheadedness, vertigo, headache, drowsiness, insomnia, confusion, depression, psychic disturbances
Cardiovascular—congestive heart failure, decrease or increase in blood pressure, cardiac dysrhythmias
Renal—hematuria, cystitis, elevated blood urea nitrogen, polyuria, dysuria, oliguria, acute renal failure in those with impaired renal function
Special senses—visual disturbances, blurred or diminished vision, diplopia, swollen or irritated eyes, photophobia, reversible loss of color vision, tinnitus, taste change, rhinitis
Hematologic—neutropenia, eosinophilia, leukopenia, pancytopenia, thrombocytopenia, agranulocytosis, aplastic anemia
Skin—rash, erythema, irritation, skin eruptions, exfoliative dermatitis, Stevens-Johnson syndrome, ecchymosis, purpura
Metabolic/endocrinologic—decreased appetite, weight increase or decrease, hyperglycemia, hypoglycemia, flushing, sweating, menstrual disorders, vaginal bleeding
Other—thirst, fever, chills, vaginitis

NURSING MANAGEMENT

Give these drugs with food, milk, or antacids. Observe the patient receiving an NSAID for adverse drug reactions throughout therapy. Because these drugs have many adverse reactions, inform the physician of *any* complaints the patient may have. GI reactions are the most common and can be severe and sometimes fatal, especially in those prone to upper GI disease. Withhold the next dose and notify the physician immediately if any GI symptoms, especially nausea, vomiting, diarrhea, evidence of GI bleeding (blood in stool, tarry stools), or abdominal pain occurs.

Nursing Alert

Serious GI toxicity can cause bleeding, ulceration, and perforation, and can occur at any time during therapy, with or without symptoms. While minor GI problems are common, remain alert for ulceration and bleeding in patients receiving long term therapy, even if no previous GI symptoms have been experienced.

Patients who do not respond therapeutically to one NSAID may respond to another. However, several weeks of treatment may be necessary to receive full therapeutic response.

Nursing Process
The Patient Receiving a Nonnarcotic Analgesic

■ *Assessment*

Assess the type, onset, and location of the pain. Determine if this problem is different in any way from previous episodes of pain or discomfort. If the patient is receiving a nonnarcotic analgesic for an arthritic or musculoskeletal disorder or soft tissue inflammation, examine the joints or areas involved. Note and record the appearance of the skin over the joint or affected area or any limitation of motion. Evaluate the patient's ability to carry out activities of daily living. Use this important information to develop a care plan, as well as to evaluate the response to drug therapy.

■ *Nursing Diagnoses*

Depending on the drug, dose, and reason for administration, one or more of the following nursing diagnoses may apply to a person receiving a nonnarcotic analgesic:

- **Risk for Altered Body Temperature: Hyperthermia** related to disease process (for example, infection or surgery)
- **Anxiety** related to pain, discomfort, other factors (specify)

Summary Drug Table 15-2. Nonsteroidal Antiinflammatory Drugs

Generic Name	Trade Name*	Uses	Adverse Reactions	Dose Ranges
diclofenac sodium	Voltaren	Signs and symptoms of rheumatoid arthritis and osteoarthritis, ankylosing spondylitis	Nausea, vomiting, diarrhea, constipation, gastric or duodenal ulcer formation, GI bleeding	Osteoarthritis: 100–150 mg/d PO in divided doses; rheumatoid arthritis: 150–200 mg/d PO in divided doses; ankylosing spondylitis: 100–125 mg/d PO in divided doses
fenoprofen calcium	Nalfon	Signs and symptoms of rheumatoid arthritis and osteoarthritis, long-term management of mild to moderate pain	Dizziness, visual disturbances, jaundice, nausea, vomiting, peptic ulcer	Rheumatoid and osteoarthritis: 300–600 mg PO tid, qid; pain: 200 mg PO q4–6h
flurbiprofen	Ansaid	Signs and symptoms of rheumatoid arthritis and osteoarthritis	Nausea, vomiting, diarrhea, constipation, gastric or duodenal ulcer formation, GI bleeding	Up to 300 mg/d PO in divided doses
ibuprofen	Advil, Nuprin, Motrin, Rufen, *generic*	Mild to moderate pain, rheumatoid disorders, painful dysmenorrhea	Nausea, vomiting, diarrhea, constipation, gastric or duodenal ulcer formation, GI bleeding	Arthritis disorders: 1.2–3.2 g/d PO in divided doses; pain: 400 mg PO q4–6h; dysmenorrhea: 400 mg PO q4h
indomethacin	Indocin	Rheumatoid arthritis, ankylosing spondylitis, moderate to severe osteoarthritis, acute painful shoulder, acute gouty arthritis	Nausea, vomiting, diarrhea, constipation, gastric or duodenal ulcer formation, GI bleeding, hematologic changes	Antiinflammatory and analgesic: 25–50 mg 2–3 times daily not to exceed 200 mg or 75 mg sustained release capsules not to exceed 150 mg SR/d
ketoprofen	Orudis	Mild to moderate pain, rheumatoid disorders, painful dysmenorrhea	Dizziness, visual disturbances, jaundice, nausea, constipation, vomiting, diarrhea, gastric or duodenal ulcer formation, GI bleeding	150–300 mg/d PO in divided doses; arthritic disorders: up to 300 mg/d PO in divided doses
ketorolac	Toradol	Short-term management of pain; osteoarthritis, rheumatoid arthritis	Dyspepsia, nausea, GI pain, pain at injection site, drowsiness	30–60 mg IM initially, followed by ½ the initial dose q6h prn
naproxen	Naprosyn	Management of inflammatory disorders including rheumatoid arthritis and osteoarthritis, management of mild to moderate pain, treatment of dysmenorrhea	Dizziness, visual disturbances, jaundice, nausea, constipation, vomiting, diarrhea, gastric or duodenal ulcer formation, GI bleeding	Pain, primary dysmenorrhea: up to 1.25 g/d PO in divided doses; arthritic disorders: 250–500 mg PO bid
piroxicam	Feldene	Mild to moderate pain, rheumatoid arthritis and osteoarthritis	Nausea, vomiting, diarrhea, drowsiness, gastric or duodenal ulcer formation, GI bleeding	20 mg/d PO as a single dose or 10 mg bid PO
sulindac	Clinoril	Mild to moderate pain, rheumatoid arthritis ankylosing spondylitis, osteoarthritis, gouty arthritis	Nausea, vomiting, diarrhea, constipation, gastric or duodenal ulcer formation, GI bleeding	150–200 mg PO bid X 1–2 wks, then reduce dose
tolmetin sodium	Tolectin	Mild to moderate pain, rheumatoid arthritis and osteoarthritis	Nausea, vomiting, diarrhea, constipation, gastric or duodenal ulcer formation, GI bleeding	400 mg PO tid or bid, not to exceed 2 g/d

*The term, *generic*, indicates that the drug is available in generic form.

- **Pain** related to physical disorder (name disorder)
- **Risk for Ineffective Management of Therapeutic Regimen** due to insufficient knowledge of medication regimen, other factors (specify)

■ *Planning and Implementation*

The major goals of the patient may include a reduction in anxiety, relief of pain, and an understanding of and compliance to the prescribed treatment regimen. To make these goals measurable, more specific criteria must be added. Additional strategies for implementation may be found under Nursing Management.

Anxiety. Anxiety related to pain or discomfort may be experienced by some patients, especially those with chronic mild to moderate pain. Anxiety may also occur because the patient is concerned about the ability of the drug to relieve pain. This is especially true in those having minor surgery or dental procedures.

Discuss the problem with the physician if the patient appears concerned about the ability of the drug to relieve pain or discomfort or if the drug fails to provide relief.

Pain and Fever. Notify the physician if a nonnarcotic analgesic fails to relieve pain or discomfort.

If the patient is receiving a nonnarcotic analgesic for reduction of elevated body temperature, check the temperature immediately before and 45 to 60 minutes after administration of the drug. If a suppository form of the drug is used, check the patient after 30 minutes for retention of the suppository. If the drug fails to lower an elevated temperature, notify the physician because other means of temperature control, such as a cooling blanket, may be necessary.

However, some physicians may not prescribe an antipyretic for the patient with an elevated temperature since there is evidence to suggest that fever activates the immune system to produce disease-fighting antibodies. The physician's decision to treat an elevated temperature with an antipyretic is an individual one, based on the cause of the fever and the patient's physical condition.

■ *Patient and Family Teaching*

In some instances, a nonnarcotic analgesic may be prescribed for a prolonged period, for example, when the patient has arthritis. Some patients may discontinue their medication, fail to take the medication at the prescribed or recommended intervals, increase the dose, or decrease the time interval between doses, especially if there is an increase or decrease in their symptoms. The patient and family must understand that the medication is to be taken even though symptoms have been relieved.

Develop a teaching plan to include the following:

General Points

- Take the drug exactly as prescribed by the physician. Do not increase or decrease the dosage. Do not take any over-the-counter (OTC) medications without first consulting the physician. Notify the physician or dentist if the pain is not relieved.
- Take the drug with food or a full glass of water unless indicated otherwise by a physician. If GI upset occurs, the drug should be taken with food or milk. If the problem persists, the physician should be contacted.
- Physicians or dentists must always be informed when these drugs are taken on a regular or occasional basis.
- If the drug is used to reduce fever, the physician should be contacted if the temperature continues to remain elevated for more than 24 hours.
- An OTC nonnarcotic analgesic should not be used consistently to treat chronic pain without first consulting a physician.
- Severe or recurrent pain or high or continued fever may indicate serious illness. If pain persists more than 10 days in adults or if fever persists more than 3 days consult a physician.

Salicylates

If taking a salicylate, the physician must be notified if any of the following symptoms occur: ringing in the ears, GI pain, nausea, vomiting, flushing, sweating, thirst, headache, diarrhea, episodes of unusual bleeding or bruising, or dark-colored stools.

- All drugs deteriorate with age. Salicylates often deteriorate at a more rapid rate than many other drugs. If there is a vinegar odor to the salicylate, the entire contents of the container must be discarded. Salicylates should be purchased in small amounts when used on an occasional basis. The container is kept tightly closed at all times because salicylates deteriorate rapidly when exposed to air, moisture, and heat.
- The ingredients of some OTC drugs contain aspirin. The name of the salicylate may not appear in the name of the drug but it is listed on the label. These products should not be used while taking a salicylate, especially during high-dose or long-term salicylate therapy. Consult the pharmacist about the product's ingredients if in doubt.
- If surgery or a dental procedure such as tooth extraction or gum surgery is anticipated, notify the

physician or dentist. Salicylates may be discontinued 1 week before the procedure because of the possibility of postoperative bleeding.

Nonsalicylates
- In the case of arthritis, do not change from aspirin to acetaminophen without consulting the physician, because acetaminophen lacks the antiinflammatory properties of aspirin.
- Notify the physician if any of the following adverse reactions occur: dyspnea, weakness, dizziness, bluish discoloration of the nailbeds, unexplained bleeding, bruising, sore throat.
- Avoid the use of alcoholic beverages.

Nonsteroidal Antiinflammatory Drugs
- Avoid the use of aspirin or other salicylates when taking an NSAID.
- The drug may take several days to produce an effect (relief of pain and tenderness). If some or all of the symptoms are not relieved after 2 weeks of therapy, continue the medication but notify the physician.
- These drugs may cause drowsiness, dizziness, or blurred vision. Caution should be exercised while driving or performing tasks that require alertness.
- Notify the physician if any of the following adverse reactions occur: skin rash, itching, visual disturbances, weight gain, edema, diarrhea, black stools, nausea, vomiting, or persistent headache.

■ Expected Outcomes for Evaluation
- Anxiety is reduced
- Pain is relieved; discomfort is reduced or eliminated
- Body temperature is normal
- Patient verbalizes importance of complying with the prescribed treatment regimen
- Patient demonstrates understanding of treatment regimen, adverse drug effects

Chapter Summary

- The nonnarcotic analgesics are drugs used primarily to relieve mild to moderate pain. In addition, they can also be used to reduce fever, and decrease inflammation. The nonnarcotic analgesics can be subdivided into the salicylates, the nonsalicylates, and the NSAIDs.
- The salicylates reduce inflammation and pain by inhibiting the production of prostaglandins.

The antipyretic action is due to vasodilation. Actions of the nonsalicylates and the NSAIDs are not clearly understood. Unlike the NSAIDs and the salicylates, the nonnarcotic nonsalicylate acetaminophen, does not have antiinflammatory effects.
- The nonnarcotic analgesics are used for mild to moderate pain, fever, and inflammatory conditions, such as rheumatoid arthritis and osteoarthritis. Aspirin and acetaminophen are available in many OTC drugs and are used for minor aches and pains, headaches, fever, and flulike symptoms. Acetaminophen may be used to treat the pain associated with arthritis but will have no effect on the inflammation. Aspirin is not given to children because of its association with *Reye's syndrome,* a life-threatening condition characterized by vomiting and lethargy progressing to coma. Acetaminophen is the drug of choice for children with fever.
- Examples of adverse reactions associated with the salicylates include gastric upset, nausea, vomiting, and GI bleeding. Salicylate toxicity or salicylism can occur with the administration of large doses of a salicylate. Symptoms of salicylism include dizziness, tinnitus, and difficulty hearing. Some adverse reactions with the NSAIDs include nausea, epigastric pain, intestinal ulceration, and skin rash. The more common adverse reactions occur within the GI system. Acetaminophen has few adverse reactions when taken as directed. Hepatic failure has been seen in alcoholics taking acetaminophen.
- If the drug is taken as an analgesic, the type, onset, location, and intensity of the pain must be assessed. If the patient is receiving one of the nonnarcotics for an arthritic condition or inflammation, the joints or affected areas are examined for signs of clinical improvement. When taken for the pain and inflammation associated with an arthritic condition, it may be several weeks before a full therapeutic effect is attained.
- An OTC nonnarcotic analgesic should not be used consistently to treat chronic or recurrent pain without first consulting a physician. If pain persists more than 10 days in an adult or if fever persists more than 3 days, the patient is instructed to consult a physician.

Critical Thinking Exercises

1. Mr. Nunn, aged 68, has been prescribed an NSAID for the treatment of arthritis and has been

taking the medication for 3 weeks. When keeping an outpatient appointment, Mr. Nunn tells you that he has noticed very little, if any, improvement in his arthritis and complains of nausea, constipation, and bloating. What steps might you take to investigate this problem? Give a reason for your answers.

2. On a visit to an outpatient clinic, Ms. Cain tells you that she takes aspirin daily for the minor aches and pains she experiences. What might you want to discuss with Ms. Cain to explore her use of this drug? What might you incorporate into the teaching plan to increase her knowledge of the drug and to prevent any complications?

16

The Narcotic Analgesics and the Narcotic Antagonists

Chapter Outline

Chapter Objectives

On completion of this chapter the student will:

* *Discuss the general drug action of the narcotic analgesics and the narcotic antagonists*
* *Describe the effects of a narcotic on organs and structures of the body*
* *List the uses of the narcotic analgesics and narcotic antagonists*
* *List the major adverse reactions associated with the administration of a narcotic analgesic and a narcotic antagonist*
* *Discuss nursing management when administering a narcotic analgesic and a narcotic antagonist*
* *Use the nursing process when administering a narcotic analgesic or narcotic antagonist*

Scherer JC, Roach S: INTRODUCTORY CLINICAL PHARMACOLOGY, FIFTH EDITION © 1996 Lippincott-Raven Publishers

Pain is a complex occurrence that is uniquely experienced by each individual. It has been defined as the emotional and sensory perceptions associated with real or potential tissue damage. Acute pain is a warning that something is not right in the body. Chronic pain is pain that persists beyond the expected time for healing. *Analgesics* are drugs that relieve pain. The narcotic analgesics are used to treat moderate to severe pain. One of the major adverse effects associated with the administration of the narcotic analgesics is the depressant effect on the central nervous system (CNS), particularly the respiratory system.

Drugs that counteract the effects of the narcotic analgesics are the narcotic antagonists. These drugs compete with the narcotics at the receptor sites and are used to reverse the depressant effects of the narcotic analgesics. Both types of drugs are discussed in this chapter.

The Narcotic Analgesics

The narcotic analgesics are divided into two classes: (1) the narcotic analgesics obtained from raw opium and (2) the synthetic narcotic analgesics.

The narcotics obtained from raw opium (also called the opiates, opioids, or opiate narcotics) include morphine, codeine, hydrochlorides of opium alkaloids (Pantopon), and camphorated tincture of opium (paregoric). Morphine, once extracted from raw opium and treated chemically, yields hydromorphone (Dilaudid), oxymorphone (Numorphan), and heroin. Heroin is an illegal narcotic in the United States and is not used in medicine.

Examples of synthetic narcotic analgesics are butorphanol (Stadol), levorphanol (Levo-Dromoran), and meperidine (Demerol). Additional synthetic narcotics are listed in Summary Drug Table 16-1.

ACTIONS OF THE NARCOTIC ANALGESICS

How the narcotic analgesics relieve pain is not completely understood. What is known is that the relief of pain is a complex physiologic and pharmacologic process.

When pain impulses are transmitted across afferent nerve fibers to the brain (which then interprets the sensation as pain), there is a release of two substances: *enkephalins* and *endorphins*. When released, enkephalins and endorphins occupy specific receptors (called opiate receptors) in the brain, brain stem, and spinal cord. When they occupy these receptors, they prevent the release of a neurotransmitter (neurohormone) from the afferent nerve fibers that carry pain impulses to the CNS. If a neurotransmitter is not released from nerve fibers, pain impulses cannot travel along these fibers and reach areas of the brain that interpret a sensation as pain.

Narcotic analgesics can be divided into two types: (1) those that are pure *agonists* and (2) those that have both *agonist-antagonist* properties. An *agonist* is a narcotic capable of occupying the same opiate receptors as do enkephalins and endorphins; therefore, it prevents the release of a neurotransmitter from the afferent nerve fibers carrying pain impulses to the brain. A narcotic possessing *agonist and antagonist* properties has two actions: (1) it acts like the pure narcotic agonists (agonist property) and (2) it blocks the activity of morphine, meperidine, and other opiates (antagonist property). Examples of narcotic agonist-antagonist analgesics are butorphanol (Stadol), nalbuphine (Nubain), and pentazocine (Talwin).

Administration of a narcotic analgesic elevates the pain threshold and alters the patient's perception of pain. The sedative action of the narcotic analgesics reduces the anxiety that accompanies pain, which appears to help the analgesic activity of the drug.

Morphine is considered the prototype or "model" narcotic, and the actions, uses, and ability to relieve pain of other narcotic analgesics are often compared with morphine. Morphine, as well as other narcotic analgesics, affects the following organs and structures of the body:

CNS—Drowsiness, euphoria, sedation, sleep, lethargy, and mental clouding often occur. The degree to which these occur usually depends on the drug and the dose.

Eye—Morphine and the other opiate narcotics cause constriction of the pupil (miosis). Codeine and the synthetic narcotics have a lesser miotic effect on the pupil.

Respiratory—The respiratory rate and depth are decreased by morphine and, to a varying degree, by the other opiates. Synthetic narcotics also depress the respiratory rate and depth.

Cough reflex—Morphine and other opiates have an antitussive (depression of the cough reflex) action because of their ability to depress the cough center in the medulla. Codeine has the most noticeable effect on the cough reflex and occasionally is used as an antitussive agent, as well as an analgesic.

Summary Drug Table 16-1. Narcotic Analgesics

Generic Name	Trade Name*	Uses	Adverse Reactions	Dose Ranges†
OPIATE NARCOTICS				
camphorated tincture of opium	Paregoric	Diarrhea	Same as morphine but may vary depending on dose	5–10 mL PO up to 4 times/d
codeine	*generic*	Mild to moderate pain; antitussive	Respiratory depression, sedation, nausea, vomiting, anorexia, constipation, dry mouth, hypotension, rash, drug dependency with continued use	Analgesic: 15–60 mg PO, IM, IV, SC; antitussive: 10–20 mg PO
hydromorphone hydrochloride	Dilaudid, *generic*	Moderate to severe pain	CNS depression, lightheadedness, dizziness, anorexia, sedation, vomiting, constipation‡	2–4 mg PO; 2 mg SC, IM; may also be given by slow IV injection; 3 mg rectally
morphine sulfate	*generic*	Severe pain, preoperatively for sedation, dyspnea associated with acute left ventricular failure and pulmonary edema	CNS depression, lightheadedness, dizziness, anorexia, sedation, vomiting, constipation,	10–30 mg PO; 5–20 mg IM, SC; 4–10 mg IV; 10–20 mg rectally
oxymorphone hydrochloride	Numorphan	Moderate to severe pain, preoperative sedation, obstetric analgesia	CNS depression, lightheadedness, dizziness, anorexia, sedation, nausea vomiting, constipation‡	0.5 mg IV; 1–1.5 mg SC, IM; 5 mg rectally
SYNTHETIC AND SEMISYNTHETIC NARCOTICS				
buprenorphine hydrochloride	Buprenex	Moderate to severe pain	Sedation, dizziness, vertigo, hypotension, nausea, vomiting, sweating, headache	0.3–0.6 mg IM or slow IV
butorphanol tartrate	Stadol	Mild to moderate pain, preoperatively to support anesthesia	Sedation, nausea, sweating, headache, vertigo, confusion	1–4 mg IM, 0.5–2 mg IV
fentanyl	Sublimaze	Analgesia before, during, or after anesthesia	CNS depression, lightheadedness, dizziness, anorexia, sedation, nausea, vomiting, constipation‡	Preanesthesia: 0.05–0.1 mg IM; postoperative: 0.05–0.1 mg IM; anesthesia: administered by anesthesiologist
fentanyl transdermal system	Duragesic	Chronic pain	Drowsiness, confusion, dizziness, constipation, nausea, vomiting	25–100 mcg/hr
levorphanol tartrate	Levo-Dromoran	Moderate to severe pain, preoperatively to relieve apprehension, provide prolonged analgesia, and reduce thiopental requirements	CNS depression, lightheadedness, dizziness, anorexia, sedation, nausea, vomiting, constipation‡	2–3 mg PO, SC
meperidine hydrochloride	Demerol, *generic*	Moderate to severe pain, preoperative to relieve anxiety and support anesthesia	CNS depression, lightheadedness, dizziness, anorexia, sedation, nausea, vomiting, constipation‡	50–150 mg IM, SC, PO
methadone hydrochloride	Dolophine HCL, *generic*	Severe pain, maintenance and treatment of heroin addiction	CNS depression, lightheadedness, dizziness, anorexia, sedation, nausea, vomiting, constipation‡	Pain: 2.5–10 mg IM, SC, PO; heroin addiction: 15–120 mg PO

(continued)

Summary Drug Table 16-1 (Continued)

Generic Name	Trade Name*	Uses	Adverse Reactions	Dose Ranges
nalbuphine hydrochloride	Nubain, *generic*	Moderate to severe pain and supplement in balanced anesthesia	Sedation, nausea, vomiting, dizziness, dry mouth	10–20 mg IM, SC, IV
pentazocine	Talwin	Moderate to severe pain, preoperative or pre-anesthetic medication	Nausea, dizziness, vomiting, euphoria, lightheadedness	50–100 mg PO; up to 60 mg IM, SC; up to 30 mg IV
propoxyphene hydrochloride	Darvon, Pulvules, Dolene, *generic*	Mild to moderate pain	Dizziness, weakness, sedation, nausea, vomiting	65 mg PO
propoxyphene napsylate	Darvon-N	Mild to moderate pain	Dizziness, weakness, sedation, nausea, vomiting	100 mg PO

*The term, *generic*, indicates that the drug is available in a *generic* form.
†Doses may be administered whenever needed (prn) with intervals depending on the dose and reason for use.
‡The adverse reactions of some narcotics are basically similar to those of morphine but some of these reactions may be less severe or intense than those seen with morphine.

Medulla—When the *chemoreceptor trigger zone* located in the medulla is stimulated, nausea and vomiting can occur. To a varying degree, narcotic analgesics may stimulate the chemoreceptor trigger zone, resulting in nausea and vomiting. The narcotic analgesics also depress the chemoreceptor trigger zone; therefore, nausea and vomiting may or may not occur when these drugs are given.

Gastrointestinal tract—The opiate narcotics slow peristalsis in the stomach, duodenum, and small and large intestines. After ingestion of food, the emptying time of the stomach is delayed and movement of food through the digestive tract is slowed. Gastric, pancreatic, and biliary secretions are decreased. These drug actions can result in anorexia and constipation.

Gallbladder and common bile duct—Spasm of the biliary tract may occur in some patients after administration of morphine. Other narcotic analgesics have a lesser effect on the biliary tract.

Genitourinary tract—Narcotic analgesics may induce spasms of the ureter. Urinary urgency may also occur due to the action of these drugs on the detrusor muscle of the bladder. Some patients may experience difficulty in voiding due to contraction of the bladder sphincter.

USES OF THE NARCOTIC ANALGESICS

The ability of a narcotic analgesic to relieve pain depends on several factors, such as the drug, the dose, the route of administration, the type of pain, the patient, and the length of time the drug has been administered. Morphine is an effective drug for moderately severe to severe pain. Other narcotics are effective for moderate to severe pain. For mild to moderate pain, the physician may order a narcotic, such as codeine or pentazocine.

Some narcotic analgesics may be used as part of a preoperative medication to lessen anxiety and sedate the patient. Patients who are relaxed and sedated when anesthesia is given are easier to anesthetize (and therefore require a smaller dose of an induction anesthetic) as well as to maintain under anesthesia.

In addition to the relief of pain, specific narcotic analgesics may be used for the following reasons:

- Treatment of severe diarrhea and intestinal cramping—camphorated tincture of opium
- Relief of severe, persistent cough—codeine
- Dyspnea associated with acute left ventricular failure and pulmonary edema—morphine
- Obstetric analgesia—oxymorphone

Although codeine has the ability to depress the cough reflex, use of the drug for this reason has declined.

Methadone, a synthetic narcotic, may be used for the relief of pain but it is also used in the detoxification and maintenance treatment of those addicted to narcotics. Detoxification involves withdrawing the patient from the narcotic while at the same time preventing the abstinence syndrome (see Chap. 51). Maintenance therapy is designed to reduce the patient's desire to return to the drug that caused addiction, as well as to prevent the abstinence syndrome. The dosages used vary with the patient, the length of time the individual has been addicted, and the average amount of drug used each day.

Patients enrolled in an outpatient methadone program for detoxification or maintenance therapy on methadone must continue to receive methadone when hospitalized.

ADVERSE REACTIONS ASSOCIATED WITH THE ADMINISTRATION OF THE NARCOTIC ANALGESICS

One of the major hazards of narcotic administration is respiratory depression with a decrease in the respiratory rate and depth. The most frequent adverse reactions include lightheadedness, dizziness, sedation, constipation, anorexia, nausea, vomiting, and sweating. When these effects occur, the physician may lower the dose in an effort to either eliminate or decrease the intensity of the adverse reaction. Other adverse reactions that may be seen with the administration of an *agonist* narcotic analgesic include the following:

CNS—euphoria, weakness, headache, pinpoint pupils, insomnia, agitation, tremor, impairment of mental and physical tasks
Gastrointestinal—dry mouth, biliary tract spasms
Cardiovascular—flushing of the face, peripheral circulatory collapse, tachycardia, bradycardia, palpitations
Genitourinary—spasms of the ureters and bladder sphincter, urinary retention or hesitancy
Allergic—pruritus, rash, urticaria
Other—physical dependence, pain at injection site, local tissue irritation

Administration of a narcotic *agonist-antagonist* may result in symptoms of narcotic withdrawal in those addicted to narcotics. Other adverse reactions associated with the administration of a narcotic agonist-antagonist include sedation, nausea, vomiting, sweating, headache, vertigo, dry mouth, euphoria, and dizziness.

PATIENT-CONTROLLED ANALGESIA

Patient-controlled analgesia (PCA) allows patients to administer their own analgesic by means of an intravenous (IV) pump system (Fig. 16-1). The dose and the time interval permitted between doses is programmed into the device to prevent accidental overdosage.

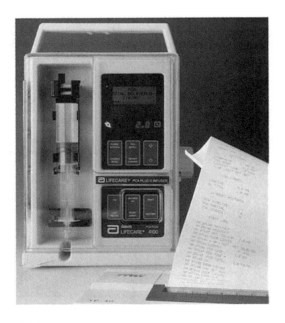

Figure 16-1

LifeCare PCA Plus II Infuser for pain management. (From Weinstein, SM. *Principles and Practices of Intravenous Therapy,* 5th ed. Philadelphia: JB Lippincott, 1993)

Many postoperative patients require *less* narcotics when they are able to self-administer a narcotic for pain. Because the self-administration system is under control of the nurse, who adds the medication to the infusion pump and sets the time interval (or lockout interval) between doses, the patient cannot receive an overdose of the drug.

EPIDURAL PAIN MANAGEMENT

Administration of certain narcotic analgesics, specifically morphine and fentanyl, by the *epidural* route has provided an alternative to the intramuscular or oral route. *Epidural* administration offers several advantages over other routes. Lower total dosages of the drug used, fewer adverse reactions, and greater patient comfort are all benefits seen with epidural administration.

Access to the epidural route is made through the use of a percutaneous epidural catheter. The epidural catheter is placed into the space between the dura mater and the vertebral column (Fig. 16-2). Medication injected through the catheter spreads freely throughout all the tissues in the space, interrupting pain conduction at the points where sensory fibers exit from the spinal cord. The administration

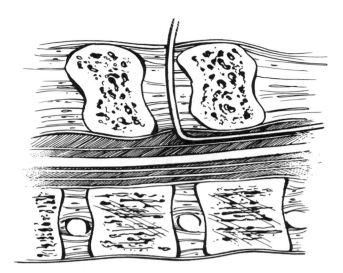

Figure 16-2

Epidural catheter placement. (Adapted from Weinstein, SM. *Plumer's Principles and Practices of Intravenous Therapy*, 5th ed. Philadelphia: JB Lippincott, 1993)

of the narcotic is either by bolus or by continuous infusion pump.

This type of pain management is used for postoperative pain, labor pain, and cancer pain. The most serious adverse reaction associated with the administration of narcotics by the epidural route is respiratory depression. The patient may also experience sedation, confusion, nausea, pruritis, or urinary retention. Fentanyl is increasingly used as an alternative to morphine sulfate because patients experience fewer adverse reactions.

Nursing care includes close monitoring of the patient immediately after insertion of the epidural catheter and throughout therapy for respiratory depression. Vital signs are taken every 30 minutes, apnea monitors are used, and a narcotic antagonist, such as naloxone, is readily available.

Policies and procedures for administering, monitoring, and documenting drugs given through the epidural route must be specific to the Nurse Practice Act in each state and in accordance with federal and state regulations. This type of analgesia is most often managed by registered nurses with special training in the care and management of epidural catheters.

NURSING MANAGEMENT

Review the patient's health history, allergy history, and past and present drug therapies before the ad-

ministration of a narcotic analgesic. This is especially important when a narcotic is given for the first time because data may be obtained during the initial history and physical assessment that require contacting the physician. For example, the patient may state that nausea and vomiting occurred when he or she was given a pain medication several years ago. Further questioning of the patient is necessary since this information may influence the physician regarding administration of a specific narcotic drug. A thorough drug history, as well as physical assessment, may raise a question of drug dependency. Notify the physician of any suspicion of drug dependency.

Nursing Alert

Administration of a narcotic with agonist-antagonist properties can result in withdrawal symptoms in those addicted to a narcotic. Careful monitoring by the nurse is necessary. Restlessness, an increase in body temperature, or an increase in pulse and respiratory rate are reported to the physician.

Each time the patient requests a narcotic analgesic, determine the exact location of the pain, obtain a description of the pain (eg, sharp, dull, stabbing), and an estimate of when the pain began. Further questioning and more detailed information about the pain is necessary if the pain is of a different type than the patient had been experiencing previously, or if it is in a different area. Nursing judgment must be exercised because not all instances of a change in pain type, location, or intensity require notifying the physician. For example, if a patient recovering from recent abdominal surgery experiences pain in the calf of the leg, the physician should be notified immediately. On the other hand, the physician need not be contacted for pain that is slightly worse because the patient has been moving in bed.

In addition, determine if any controllable factors (eg, uncomfortable position, cold room, drafts, bright lights, noise, thirst) may be decreasing the patient's tolerance to pain. If these factors are present, correct them as soon as possible, but do not deny pain medication or make the patient wait for the drug.

Administration

Assess the blood pressure, pulse, and respiratory rate immediately before preparing a narcotic analgesic for administration.

Depending on clinical circumstances and nursing judgment, additional factors may require withholding the drug and contacting the physician. Notify the physician immediately if the pain is in a different area, if the pain is more intense, or if the character or type of the pain has changed.

When an opiate is used as an antidiarrheal agent, record each bowel movement, as well as appearance, color, and consistency of each stool. Notify the physician immediately if diarrhea is not relieved, if diarrhea becomes worse, or if severe abdominal pain or blood in the stool is noted.

Adverse Drug Effects

Obtain the blood pressure, pulse, and respiratory rate 15 to 30 minutes after the drug is administered intramuscularly or subcutaneously, 30 or more minutes if the drug is given orally, and in 5 to 10 minutes if the drug is given IV. Report any significant change in these vital signs to the physician immediately. If the respiratory rate is 10 per minute or below, monitor the patient at frequent intervals and notify the physician immediately. Administration of a narcotic antagonist may be ordered by the physician if the respiratory rate continues to fall.

Narcotics may depress the cough reflex. Encourage patients receiving a narcotic on a regular basis, even for a few days, to cough and breathe deeply every 2 hours. This task prevents the pooling of secretions in the lungs, which can lead to hypostatic pneumonia and other lung problems.

Notify the physician of any nausea and vomiting. A different analgesic or an antiemetic may be necessary.

Nursing Process
The Patient Receiving a Narcotic Analgesic

■ *Assessment*
Assess the type, location, and intensity of pain prior to and following administration of the narcotic analgesic. Monitor blood pressure, pulse, and respiratory rate before and after the patient receives the narcotic analgesic. Assess bowel function throughout drug therapy.

■ *Nursing Diagnoses*
Depending on factors such as the reason for administration (pain, obstetrical analgesia, diarrhea) and the patient's diagnosis, one or more of the following nursing diagnoses may apply to a person receiving a narcotic analgesic:
- **Pain** related to medical or surgical disorder
- **Anxiety** related to pain
- **Risk for Injury** related to effect of narcotic on the CNS
- **Constipation** related to the effects of the narcotics on the gastrointestinal system
- **Altered Nutrition: Less than body requirements** related to anorexia secondary to effects of the narcotic
- **Risk for Ineffective Management of Therapeutic Regimen** related to lack of knowledge of medication regimen, adverse drug effects, PCA infusion pump

■ *Planning and Implementation*
The major goals of the patient may include a relief of pain, reduction in anxiety, absence of injury, an adequate nutrition intake, an understanding of the use of the PCA device (when applicable), and an understanding of and compliance to the prescribed treatment regimen. To make these goals measurable, more specific criteria must be added. Implementation of nursing measures described under Nursing Management can be used to assist in meeting these goals.

Pain. Assess the patient for relief of pain approximately 30 minutes after a narcotic analgesic is given. Notify the physician if the analgesic is ineffective because a higher dose or a different narcotic analgesic may be required.

Perform nursing tasks, such as getting the patient out of bed, and encourage therapeutic activities, such as deep breathing, coughing, and leg exercises (when ordered), when the drug is producing its greatest analgesic effect, which is usually 1 to 2 hours after the narcotic is administered.

When a narcotic is used for obstetric analgesia, observe the neonate closely for CNS and respiratory depression at the time of birth and for 4 to 6 hours afterward.

Anxiety. Pain causes anxiety. Anxiety, in some instances, can intensify pain. The analgesic effect of narcotic analgesics is best obtained when a narcotic is given *before* the patient experiences intense pain. This not only keeps the patient more comfortable but also reduces anxiety.

Injury. Narcotics may produce orthostatic hypotension which, in turn, results in dizziness. Assist the patient with ambulatory activities and with rising slowly from a sitting or lying position.

Miosis (pinpoint pupils) may occur with the administration of some narcotics, and is most pronounced with morphine, hydromorphone, and hydrochlorides of opium alkaloids. Miosis decreases the ability to see in dim light. Therefore, keep the room well-lighted during daytime hours and advise the patient to seek assistance when getting out of bed at night.

Constipation. Check the bowel elimination pattern daily because constipation can occur with repeated doses of a narcotic. Keep a daily record of bowel movements and inform the physician if constipation appears to be a problem. A stool softener, enema, or other means of relieving constipation may be ordered by the physician.

Nutrition. When a narcotic is prescribed for a prolonged time, anorexia (loss of appetite) may occur. Those receiving a narcotic for the relief of pain due to terminal cancer often have severe anorexia, due to the disease as well as the narcotic. Assess food intake after each meal. When anorexia is prolonged, weigh the patient weekly or as ordered by the physician. Notify the physician of continued weight loss and anorexia.

Chronic Severe Pain. Morphine is the most widely used drug in the management of chronic severe pain, such as is seen in terminal cancer patients. The fact that this drug can be given orally, subcutaneously, intramuscularly, intravenously, and rectally in the form of a suppository allows tremendous versatility. Most cancer patients can be managed on 30 to 60 mg of morphine orally every 4 hours. Respiratory depression is less likely to occur when given orally.

Fentanyl transdermal is a transdermal system that is effective in the management of the severe pain associated with cancer. The transdermal system allows for a timed release patch containing the drug fentanyl to be activated over a 72-hour period. A small number of patients may require systems applied every 48 hours. Adverse effects are monitored in the same manner as other narcotic analgesics (eg, the physician is notified if the respiratory rate is less than 10/min).

On rare occasions, when pain is not relieved by the narcotic analgesics alone, a mixture of an oral narcotic and other drugs may be used to obtain relief. The term *Brompton's mixture* is commonly used to identify these solutions. In addition to the narcotics, such as morphine or methadone, other drugs may be used in the solution, including antidepressants, stimulants, and tranquilizers. The pharmacist prepares the solution according to the physician's instructions.

It is necessary to monitor for the adverse reactions of each drug contained in the solution. The time interval for administration varies. Some physicians may order the mixture on an as needed basis; others may order it given at regular intervals.

Drug Dependence. Drug dependence can occur when a narcotic is administered over a long period. If dependence appears to occur, discuss the problem with the physician. For some patients, such as those who are terminally ill and in severe pain, drug addiction is not considered a problem because the most important task is to keep the patient as comfortable as possible for the time he or she has remaining.

When a patient does not have a painful terminal illness, drug dependence must be avoided. Signs of drug dependence may include occurrence of an abstinence syndrome (see Chap. 51) when the narcotic is discontinued; requests for the narcotic at frequent intervals around the clock; personality changes if the narcotic is not given immediately; and constant complaints of pain and failure of the narcotic to relieve pain. While these behaviors can have other causes, drug dependence should be considered. Although dependence is a possibility, most patients receiving the narcotic analgesics for medical purposes do *not* develop dependence.

Drug dependence can also occur in a newborn whose mother was dependent on opiates during pregnancy. Withdrawal symptoms usually appear during the first few days of life. Symptoms include irritability, excessive crying, yawning, sneezing, increased respiratory rate, tremors, fever, vomiting, and diarrhea.

■ *Patient and Family Teaching*

Inform the patient that the medication he or she is receiving is for pain. Additional information such as how often the medication can be given and the name of the drug being given is also included.

Instruction on the use of the PCA must be given to patients receiving drugs through the PCA infusion pump. Include the following in the explanation and demonstration given to the patient:

- Description of how the unit works, including, for example, the location of the control button that activates the administration of the drug
- Differentiation between the control button for the PCA and the button to call the nurse (when both are similar in appearance and feel)
- Reassurance that the machine regulates the dose of the drug as well as the time interval between doses
- Reassurance that if the patient uses the control button too soon after the last dose, the machine will not deliver the medication until the correct time
- Reassurance that pain relief should occur shortly after pushing the button
- Instruction to call the nurse if pain relief does not occur after two successive doses

Narcotics for outpatient use may be prescribed in the oral form or as a timed release transdermal patch. In certain cases, such as when terminally ill patients are being cared for at home, the family may receive instruction in the parenteral administration of the drug. When a narcotic has been prescribed, the following points are included in a teaching plan:

- This drug may cause drowsiness, dizziness, and blurring of vision. Caution should be used when driving or performing tasks requiring alertness.
- Avoid the use of alcoholic beverages unless use has been approved by the physician. Alcohol may intensify the action of the drug and cause extreme drowsiness or dizziness. In some instances, the use of alcohol and a narcotic can have extremely serious and even life-threatening consequences that may require emergency medical treatment.
- Take the drug as directed on the container label. The prescribed dose should *not* be exceeded. Contact the physician if the drug is not effective.
- If gastrointestinal upset occurs, take the drug with food.
- Notify the physician if nausea, vomiting, and constipation become severe.
- To administer the transdermal system, remove the system from the package and immediately apply to the skin of the upper torso. To assure

complete contact with the skin surface press for 10 to 20 seconds with the palm of the hand. After 72 hours, the system is removed and if continuous therapy is prescribed, a new system is applied.

■ *Expected Outcomes for Evaluation*

- Pain is relieved
- Anxiety is reduced
- No evidence of injury
- Body weight is maintained
- Diet is adequate
- Patient and family demonstrate understanding of drug regime
- Patient demonstrates ability to effectively use PCA

The Narcotic Antagonists

Specific antagonists have been developed to reverse the respiratory depression associated with the opiates. The two narcotic antagonists in use today are *naloxone* (Narcan) and *naltrexone* (Re Via; Summary Drug Table 16-2). Naloxone is capable of restoring respiratory function within 1 to 2 minutes after administration. Naltrexone is used primarily for the treatment of narcotic dependence to block the effects of the opiates, especially the euphoric effects experienced in opiate dependence.

ACTIONS OF THE NARCOTIC ANTAGONISTS

Naloxone. Administration of naloxone prevents or reverses the effects of the opiates. The exact mechanism of action is not fully understood but it is believed that naloxone reverses opioid effects by competing for opiate receptor sites (see Actions of the Narcotic Analgesics). If the individual has taken or received an opiate, the effects of the opiate are reversed. If the individual has *not* taken or received an opiate, naloxone has no drug activity.

Naltrexone. Naltrexone completely blocks the effect of IV opiates, as well as drugs with agonist-antagonist actions (butorphanol, nalbuphine, and pentazocine). The mechanism of action appears to be the same as for naloxone.

Summary Drug Table 16-2. Narcotic Antagonists

Generic Name	Trade Name*	Uses	Adverse Reactions	Dose Ranges
nalmefene	Revex	Complete or partial reversal of opioid effects	Nausea, vomiting, tachycardia, hypertension, return of post operative pain, fever, dizziness	Initial dose 0.25 mcg/kg followed by 0.25 mcg/kg at 2 to 5 minute intervals IV; 1 mg IM or SC
naloxone hydrochloride	Narcan	Narcotic overdose, postoperative narcotic depression	Abrupt reversal of narcotic depression may result in nausea, vomiting, sweating, increased blood pressure, tachycardia	0.4–2 mg IV initially with additional doses repeated at 2–3 min intervals; smaller doses used for postoperative narcotic depression
naltrexone hydrochloride	Re Via	Narcotic addiction, alcohol dependence	Anxiety, difficulty sleeping, abdominal cramps, nasal congestion, joint and muscle pain, nausea, vomiting, dizziness, irritability	Maintenance treatment: 50 mg PO daily and 100 mg PO on Saturdays, or 100 mg every other day, or 150 mg PO every third day

USES OF NARCOTIC ANTAGONISTS

Naloxone. This drug is used for complete or partial reversal of narcotic depression, including respiratory depression. Drugs causing narcotic depression and responding to naloxone administration include the natural and synthetic opiates, propoxyphene, methadone, nalbuphine, butorphanol, and pentazocine. Narcotic depression may be due to intentional or accidental overdose (self-administration by an individual), accidental overdose by medical personnel, and drug idiosyncrasy. It may also be used for diagnosis of a suspected acute opioid overdosage.

Naltrexone. Naltrexone is used in the treatment of persons formerly dependent on opioids. Patients receiving naltrexone have been detoxified and are enrolled in a program for treatment of narcotic addiction. Naltrexone, along with other methods of treatment (counseling, psychotherapy), is used to maintain an opioid-free state. Patients taking naltrexone on a scheduled basis will not experience any *narcotic* drug effects should they use an opioid.

ADVERSE REACTIONS ASSOCIATED WITH THE ADMINISTRATION OF THE NARCOTIC ANTAGONISTS

Naloxone. Although not a true adverse reaction, abrupt reversal of narcotic depression may result in nausea, vomiting, sweating, tachycardia, increased blood pressure, and tremors.

Nursing Alert

The postoperative patient who receives naloxone for a narcotic overdose may have a reversal of the analgesic effect of the narcotic. This results in a sudden return of pain (for which the narcotic was given) and, in some cases, excitement, hypotension or hypertension, ventricular tachycardia and fibrillation, and pulmonary edema.

Naltrexone. Administration of naltrexone may result in anxiety, difficulty in sleeping, abdominal cramps, nasal congestion, joint and muscle pain, nausea, vomiting, dizziness, irritability, depression, fatigue, and drowsiness.

NURSING MANAGEMENT

Before the administration of naloxone, obtain the blood pressure, pulse, and respiratory rate and review the record for the drug suspected of causing the overdosage. If there is sufficient time, review the initial health history, allergy history, and current treatment modalities.

Depending on the patient's condition, cardiac monitoring, artificial ventilation (respirator), and other drugs may be used during and after the administration of naloxone. A patent airway must be maintained. Suction equipment must be readily available because abrupt reversal of narcotic depression may cause vomiting. If naloxone is given by IV infusion, the physician orders the IV fluid and amount, the drug dosage, and the infusion rate. Giving the drug by IV infusion requires use of a secondary line or IV piggyback.

Before and after administration of naloxone, monitor the blood pressure, pulse, and respiratory rate at frequent intervals, usually every 5 minutes, until the patient responds. After the patient has shown response to the drug, monitor vital signs every 5 to 15 minutes. Notify the physician if any adverse drug reactions occur, because additional medical treatment may be needed.

> ### Nursing Alert
>
> The effects of some narcotics may last longer than the effects of naloxone. A repeat dose of naloxone may be ordered by the physician if results obtained from the initial dose are unsatisfactory. The duration of close patient observation depends on the patient's response to the administration of the narcotic antagonist.

Maintain a patent airway and suction the patient as needed. Monitor the intake and output and notify the physician of any change in the intake-output ratio. Contact the physician if there is any sudden change in the patient's condition.

Nursing Process
The Patient Receiving a Narcotic Antagonist for Respiratory Depression

■ Assessment
Assess respiratory rate, rhythm, and depth, pulse, blood pressure, and level of consciousness until effects of narcotics wear off.

■ *Nursing Diagnosis*
- **Ineffective Airway Clearance** related to administration of a narcotic (specify overdose, drug idiosyncrasy, or other cause)

■ *Planning and Implementation*
The major goal of the patient with respiratory depression is a normal respiratory rate, rhythm, and depth. To make these goals measurable, more specific criteria must be added. Specific implementation strategies are identified in the Nursing Management section.

■ *Expected Outcomes for Evaluation*
- Respiratory rate, rhythm, and depth are normal
- Clear airway is maintained

Nursing Process
The Patient Receiving a Narcotic Antagonist for Treatment of Opioid Dependency

■ *Assessment*
Obtain a complete drug history. Perform a complete physical examination and psychological evaluation before initiation of therapy. The extent of the pretreatment assessment is usually based on the guidelines set up by the clinic or agency dispensing the drug.

■ *Nursing Diagnoses*
- **Anxiety** related to dependency history, effectiveness of treatment program, other factors (specify)
- **Noncompliance** related to anxiety, difficulty in staying drug-free, other factors (specify)
- **Risk of Ineffective Management of Therapeutic Regimen** related to indifference, requirements of treatment program, other factors (specify)

■ *Planning and Implementation*
The major goals of the person formerly dependent on opioids may include reducing anxiety, complying with the treatment program, and remaining drug-free. To make these goals measurable, more specific criteria must be added.

Anxiety, Noncompliance. Entering a program for drug dependency may cause great anxiety due to many factors. Examples of possible causes of anxiety include the socioeconomic impact of drug dependency, the effectiveness of the treatment program, and concern over remaining drug-free. Individuals vary in their ability to communicate their fears and concerns. At times, identification of those situations causing anxiety and exploration of the possible solutions to the many problems faced by these patients may be possible.

One of the greatest problems associated with former drug dependency is remaining drug-free. The administration techniques of the drug treatment program must be followed precisely. Some people find it difficult to break away from situations, individuals, or pressures that promote drug use. Because of this, some opioid users entering a drug rehabilitation program may, in time, not report to the program or agency to receive their drug and thus are more apt to return to the use of an opiate.

All staff members of the rehabilitation program should work to encourage adherence to the medication regimen, and attempt to identify those situations that may encourage a return to drug use.

■ *Patient and Family Teaching*

Instruct patients under treatment for narcotic addiction to wear or carry identification indicating that they are receiving naltrexone. If the patient is taking naltrexone and requires hospitalization, it is important that all medical personnel be aware of therapy with this drug. Narcotics administered to these patients have no effect and therefore do not relieve pain. Patients receiving naltrexone obviously may pose a problem if they develop acute pain. The physician must decide what methods must be used to control pain in these patients.

Teach the patient taking naltrexone the impact of therapy. While taking the drug, any use of heroin or other opiate results in no effect. Large doses of heroin or other opiates can overcome the drug's effect and result in coma or death.

■ *Expected Outcomes for Evaluation*

- Factors causing anxiety are identified
- Anxiety is reduced
- Patient complies to the prescribed treatment regimen
- Patient remains drug-free
- Patient demonstrates understanding of the therapeutic regimen and requirements of the rehabilitation program

Chapter Summary

- Narcotic analgesics are drugs used in the management of moderate to severe pain. In addition to the relief of pain, these drugs can be used to treat diarrhea, to relieve severe cough, to treat dyspnea associated with left ventricular failure, to relieve preoperative anxiety, and as an adjunct to balanced anesthesia. The narcotic methadone is used in the detoxification and maintenance treatment of those addicted to narcotics.
- Morphine is the prototype or model narcotic and the drug to which all other narcotics are compared. Morphine, as well as the other narcotic analgesics, affects all major organ systems of the body. The most profound effect is on the CNS, particularly the respiratory system. The most common adverse reactions associated with the administration of the narcotic analgesics are light-headedness, dizziness, sedation, constipation, anorexia, nausea, and vomiting.
- Prior to the administration of a narcotic analgesic, the exact location of the pain must be determined and a description of the pain must be obtained. In addition to assessing the pain the patient is experiencing, the blood pressure, pulse, and respiratory rate must be evaluated. The narcotic is withheld and the physician contacted if the respiratory rate is below 10/min; if there is a significant decrease in the pulse rate or change in the pulse quality; or if the systolic pressure is below 100 mm Hg.
- The narcotic antagonists, naloxone and naltrexone, are capable of reversing the depressant effects of the narcotics. Naloxone reverses the opioid effects by competing for opiate receptor sites. Naloxone is used to reverse the respiratory depressant effects of the narcotic analgesics and to diagnose acute opioid overdosage. Naltrexone is used in the treatment of narcotic addiction.

Critical Thinking Exercises

1. Ms. Taylor is receiving meperidine for postoperative pain management. In assessing Ms. Taylor approximately 20 minutes after receiving an injection of meperidine, the nurse discovers Ms. Taylor's vital signs as blood pressure 100/50, pulse rate 100, respiratory rate 10. What action, if any, should the nurse take?
2. Mr. Talley, a 64-year-old retired schoolteacher, has cancer and is to receive morphine through a PCA infusion pump. His wife is eager to help but Mr. Talley is very independent and refuses any assistance from her. Formulate a teaching plan for Mr. Talley that includes the use of PCA, adverse reactions to expect, and what adverse reactions to report. What methods might the nurse use to include Ms. Talley in the care of her husband?

Drugs That Affect the Nervous System

IV

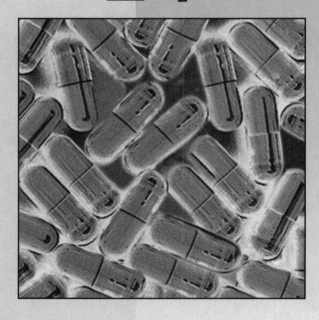

17

Adrenergic Drugs

Key Terms

Autonomic nervous
system
Central nervous system
Neurotransmitter
Parasympathetic nervous
system
Peripheral nervous system
Somatic nervous system
Sympathetic nervous
system
Vasopressor

Chapter Outline

Chapter Objectives

On completion of this chapter the student will:

- *Discuss the types, uses, and general drug actions of the adrenergic drugs*
- *List some of the adverse reactions associated with the administration of adrenergic drugs*
- *Use the nursing process when administering an adrenergic drug*
- *Discuss the nursing implications to be considered when administering adrenergic drugs*

The adrenergic drugs are drugs that produce pharmacologic effects similar to the effects that occur in the body when the adrenergic nerves or the medulla is stimulated. The primary effects of these drugs are found on the heart, the blood vessels, and smooth muscles, such as the bronchi. A basic knowledge of the nervous system is necessary to understanding these drugs and how they work in the body.

THE NERVOUS SYSTEM

The nervous system is a complex part of the human body concerned with the regulation and coordination of body activities such as movement, the digestion of food, sleep, and the elimination of waste products. The nervous system has two main divisions: the *central nervous system* and the *peripheral nervous system*. Figure 17-1 illustrates the divisions of the nervous system.

The *central nervous system (CNS)* consists of the brain and the spinal cord and receives, integrates, and interprets nerve impulses. The *peripheral nervous system (PNS)* is the term used to describe all nerves outside of the brain and spinal cord. The PNS serves to connect all parts of the body with the CNS.

The PNS is further divided into the *somatic nervous system* and the *autonomic nervous system*. The *somatic* part (branch) of the PNS is concerned with sensation and voluntary movement. The sensory part of the somatic nervous system sends messages to the brain concerning the internal and external environment, for example, sensations of heat, pain, cold, and pressure. The voluntary part of the somatic nervous system is concerned with (voluntary) movement of skeletal muscles, for example, walking, chewing food, or writing a letter. The *autonomic* part (branch) of the PNS is concerned with those functions essential to the survival of the organism. Functional activity of the autonomic nervous system is not consciously controlled (ie, the activity is automatic). This system controls blood pressure, heart rate, gastrointestinal activity, and glandular secretions.

The autonomic nervous system is divided into the *sympathetic* and the *parasympathetic nervous system*. The *sympathetic nervous system* (sympathetic branch of the autonomic nervous system) tends to regulate the expenditure of energy and is operative when the organism is confronted with stressful situations, such as danger, intense emotion, or severe illness. The *parasympathetic nervous system* (parasympathetic branch of the autonomic nervous system) works to help conserve body energy and is partly responsible for such activities as slowing the heart rate, digesting food, and eliminating body wastes.

Neurotransmitters are chemical substances called neurohormones released at the nerve endings that facilitate the transmission of nerve impulses. There are two neurohormones (neurotransmitters) of the sympathetic nervous system: *epinephrine* and *norepinephrine*. Epinephrine is secreted by the adrenal medulla. Norepinephrine is secreted mainly at nerve endings of sympathetic (also called adrenergic) nerve fibers.

Adrenergic Drugs

Adrenergic drugs act like or mimic the activity of the sympathetic nervous system and are also called *sympathomimetic drugs*. Epinephrine and norepinephrine are neurohormones produced naturally by the body. Synthetic preparations of these two neurohormones, which are identical to those naturally produced by the body, are used in medicine. Adrenergic drugs such as metaraminol (Aramine), isoproterenol (Isuprel), and ephedrine are synthetic adrenergic drugs.

ACTIONS OF ADRENERGIC DRUGS

Generally, adrenergic drugs produce one or more of the following responses in varying degrees:

Central nervous system—wakefulness; quick reaction to stimuli; quickened reflexes

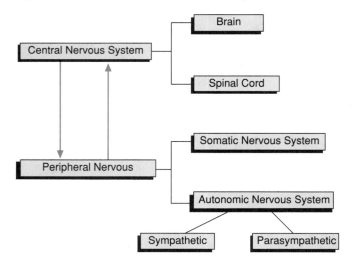

Figure 17-1

The nervous system.

Peripheral nervous system—relaxation of the smooth muscles of the bronchi; constriction of blood vessels, sphincters of the stomach; dilatation of coronary blood vessels; decrease in gastric motility
Heart—increase in the heart rate
Metabolism—increased use of glucose (sugar) plus liberation of fatty acids from adipose tissue

Adrenergic nerve fibers have either alpha- or beta-receptors. Adrenergic drugs may act on alpha-receptors only, beta-receptors only, or both alpha- and beta-receptors. For example, phenylephrine (Neo-Synephrine) acts chiefly on alpha-receptors; isoproterenol acts chiefly on beta-receptors; and epinephrine acts on both alpha- and beta-receptors. Whether an adrenergic drug acts on alpha-, beta-, or alpha- and beta-receptors accounts for the variation of responses for this group of drugs. Table 17-1 gives the action of the autonomic nervous system on the body along with the type of adrenergic nerve fiber receptor for each.

Alpha- and beta-receptors can be further divided into alpha-1 and alpha-2 adrenergic receptors and beta-1 and beta-2 adrenergic receptors. Table 17-2 indicates the effects in the body when stimulation of these receptors occurs.

USES OF ADRENERGIC DRUGS

Adrenergic drugs have a wide variety of uses and may be given as all or part of the treatment for the following:

Table 17-1. Action of the Autonomic Nervous System on Body Organs and Structures

Organs or Structures	Sympathetic (Adrenergic) Effects	Type of Sympathetic (Adrenergic) Receptor	Parasympathetic (Cholinergic) Effects
Heart	Increase in heart rate, heart muscle contractility, increase in speed of atrioventricular conduction	Beta	Decrease in heart rate, decrease in heart muscle contractility
Blood vessels			
1. Skin, mucous membranes	Constriction	Alpha	
2. Skeletal muscle	Usually dilatation	Cholinergic,* beta	
Bronchial muscles	Relaxation	Beta	Contraction
Gastrointestinal			
1. Muscle motility, tone decrease		Beta	Increase
2. Sphincters	Usually contraction	Alpha	Usually relaxation
3. Gallbladder	Relaxation		Contraction
Urinary bladder			
1. Detrusor muscle	Relaxation	Beta	Contraction
2. Trigone, sphincter muscles	Contraction	Alpha	Relaxation
Eye			
1. Radial muscle of iris	Contraction (pupil dilates)	Alpha	
2. Sphincter muscle of iris			Contraction (pupil constricts)
3. Ciliary muscle			Contraction
Skin			
1. Sweat glands	Increased activity in localized areas	Cholinergic*	
2. Pilomotor muscles	Contraction (gooseflesh)	Alpha	
Uterus	Relaxation	Beta	
Salivary glands	Thickened secretions	Alpha	Copious, watery secretions
Liver	Glycogenolysis	Beta	
Lacrimal and nasopharyngeal glands			Increased secretion
Male sex organs	Emission	Alpha	Erection

*Cholinergic transmission, but nerve cell chain originates in the thoracolumbar part of the spinal cord, and is therefore sympathetic.

Table 17-2. Effects of the Adrenergic Receptors

Receptor	Site	Effect
Alpha 1	Peripheral blood vessles	Vasoconstriction of peripheral blood vessels
Alpha 2	Presynaptic neuron	Regulates release of neurotransmitters, decreases tone, motility, and secretions of GI tract
Beta 1	Myocardium	Increased heart rate, increased force of myocardial contraction
Beta 2	Peripheral blood vessels	Vasodilation of peripheral vessels
	Bronchial smooth muscles	Bronchodilation

- Moderately severe to severe episodes of hypotension
- Control of superficial bleeding during surgical and dental procedures of the mouth, nose, throat, and skin
- Bronchial asthma
- Cardiac arrest
- Allergic reactions (anaphylactic shock, angioneurotic edema)
- Temporary treatment of heart block
- Ventricular arrhythmias (under certain conditions)
- Nasal congestion (applied topically)
- In conjunction with local anesthetics to prolong anesthetic action in medicine and dentistry

It should be noted that a specific adrenergic agent is selected as all or part of the treatment for any one of the above situations.

ADVERSE REACTIONS ASSOCIATED WITH THE ADMINISTRATION OF ADRENERGIC DRUGS

The adverse reactions associated with the administration of adrenergic drugs depend on the drug used, the dose administered, and individualized patient response. Some of the adverse reactions for specific adrenergic agents are listed in Summary Drug Table 17-1. Some of the more common adverse reactions include cardiac dysrhythmias such as bradycardia and tachycardia, headache, insomnia, nervousness, anorexia, and an increase in blood pressure (which may reach dangerously high levels).

NURSING MANAGEMENT

The major goal of nursing management is to perform the appropriate procedures for drug administration and to competently observe the patient for drug response. Management of the patient receiving an adrenergic agent varies and depends on the drug used, the reason for administration, and the patient's individual response to the drug. In most instances, adrenergic drugs are potent and potentially dangerous. Great care must be exercised in the calculation and preparation of these drug for administration. Report all adverse effects to the physician as soon as possible, but again, nursing judgment is necessary. Some adverse effects, such as the development of cardiac arrhythmias, must be reported immediately, regardless of the time of day or night. Other adverse effects, such as anorexia, should be reported but usually are not of an emergency nature. Report and record any complaint the patient may have (subjective data) using judgment regarding the seriousness of the complaint.

Although adrenergic drugs are potentially dangerous, proper supervision and management before, during, and after administration aids in minimizing the occurrence of any serious problems.

When the patient has marked hypotension and requires administration of a *vasopressor* (a drug that raises the blood pressure because of its ability to constrict blood vessels), the physician determines the cause of the hypotension and then selects the best method of treatment. Some hypotensive episodes require the use of a less potent vasopressor such as metaraminol, whereas at other times a more potent vasopressor such as dopamine (Intropin) or norepinephrine (Levophed) is necessary.

Summary Drug Table 17-1. Adrenergic Drugs

Generic Name	Trade Name*	Uses	Adverse Reactions	Dose Ranges
dobutamine	Dobutrex	Short-term treatment of cardiac decompensation	Increased heart rate, blood pressure, anginal and nonspecific chest pain and palpitations	IV 250 mg in 250–500 ml of diluent; 2.5–15 mcg/kg/min (up to 40 mcg/kg/min)
dopamine	Intropin, *generic*	Severe hypotension episodes	Ectopic beats, nausea, vomiting, anginal pain	2–50 mcg/kg/min IV
ephedrine sulfate	*generic*	Acute hypotensive episodes; as systemic bronchodilator and decongestant	Palpitations, tachycardia, headache, insomnia, nausea, vomiting	Hypotension: 25–50 mg IM, SC, slow IV; systemic bronchodilator, decongestant: 25–50 mg IM, SC, IV
epinephrine	Adrenalin, *generic*	Cardiac arrest, anaphylactic shock, angioneurotic edema, acute asthma, topically to control capillary bleeding	Elevation of blood pressure, headache, anxiety, palpitations, cardiac dysrhythmias	Cardiac arrest: 5–10 mL of 1:10,000 solution IV; acute asthma: 0.3–0.5 mL of 1:1000 SC, IM; anaphylactic shock, angioneurotic edema: same as acute asthma
isoproterenol hydrochloride	Isuprel, *generic*	Cardiac arrest, some cardiac arrhythmias, Adams-Stokes syndrome, shock; as systemic bronchodilator	Tachycardia, insomnia, nervousness, restlessness, tremor, palpitations	2 mg in 500 mL of diluent by IV infusion; 0.1–0.2 mg by IV injection; 0.02–1 mg IM; 0.15–0.2 mg SC; 5–50 mg sublingually; 5–50 mg rectally
metaraminol bitartrate	Aramine, *generic*	Hypotension	Tachycardia or other cardiac dysrhythmias, headache, flushing	2–10 mg IM, SC; 15–100 mg in 500 mL sodium chloride or 5% dextrose by IV infusion; 0.05–5 mg by direct IV injection
norepinephrine (levarterenol)	Levophed	Acute hypotensive states	Bradycardia, headache, hypertension (due to overdose)	Up to 4 mL in 5% dextrose IV only
phenylephrine hydrochloride	Neo-Synephrine	Hypotensive episodes; topically as a nasal decongestant	Headache, reflex bradycardia, cardiac arrhythmias	1–10 mg IM, SC; 0.1–0.5 mg IV; 10 mg in 500 mL dextrose or sodium chloride by IV infusion

*The term, *generic*, indicates that the drug is available in a *generic* form.

Consider the following points when administering the potent vasopressors, dopamine and norepinephrine:

1. Use an electronic infusion pump to administer these drugs.
2. Do not mix dopamine with other drugs, especially sodium bicarbonate or other alkaline intravenous (IV) solutions. Check with the hospital pharmacist before adding a second drug to an IV solution containing this drug.
3. Norepinephrine and dopamine are administered *only* by the IV route. Dilute these drugs in an IV solution before administration. The physician orders the IV solution, the amount of drug added to the solution, and the initial rate of infusion.
4. Monitor the blood pressure and pulse rate at frequent intervals, usually every 5 to 15 minutes, during the administration of these drugs.
5. Adjust the rate of administration according to the patient's blood pressure. Readjustment of the rate of flow of the IV solution is often necessary. The frequency of adjustment will depend on the patient's response to the vasopressor.

6. Inspect the needle site and surrounding tissues at frequent intervals for leakage (extravasation, infiltration) of the solution into the subcutaneous tissues surrounding the needle site.

7. Do not allow intravenous solutions containing either of these drugs to extravasate or infiltrate into the subcutaneous tissues surrounding the needle site. If either situation occurs, establish another IV line immediately, discontinue the IV containing the vasopressor, and notify the physician.

8. Increase or decrease the rate of administration of the IV solution to maintain the patient's blood pressure at the systolic level ordered by the physician.

9. Do not leave unattended the patient receiving these drugs.

The less potent vasopressors, such as metaraminol, also require close supervision during administration. Follow the same procedure as that for norepinephrine and dopamine. Blood pressure and pulse determinations may be taken at less frequent intervals, usually every 15 to 30 minutes. Use sound clinical judgment in determining the frequency because there is no absolute minimum or maximum time limit between determinations.

Other adrenergic agents have specific uses. Isoproterenol may be used in the treatment of some cardiac arrhythmias, cardiac arrest, shock, Adams-Stokes syndrome, or as a systemic bronchodilator. Epinephrine may be used to treat bronchial asthma, anaphylactic shock, and other allergic reactions. Epinephrine may be used topically to control capillary bleeding, or may be used with a local anesthetic to control bleeding, as well as to prolong local anesthetic action. The uses of various adrenergic agents are given in Summary Drug Table 17-1.

Remember the following points before, during, and after the administration of an adrenergic agent:

1. Assess the patient's symptoms, problems, or needs before the administration of the drug. Record any subjective or objective data on the patient's chart. In emergency situations, assessments must be made quickly and accurately.

2. Observe the patient for the effect of the drug. For example, is the breathing of the asthmatic patient improved? Is the blood pressure responding to the administration of the vasopressor?

3. Evaluate and record the effect of the drug. Comparison of assessments made before and after administration may help the physician

determine future use of the drug for this patient.

4. Observe and report any adverse drug reactions to the physician as soon as possible. Do not administer the next dose of the drug until the physician has been contacted.

Nursing Process
The Patient Receiving an Adrenergic Drug

■ Assessment

Assessment of the patient receiving an adrenergic drug differs depending on the drug, the patient, and the reason for administration. For example, assessment of the patient in shock who is to be treated with norepinephrine is different from that for the patient receiving nose drops containing phenylephrine. Both are receiving adrenergic agents, but the circumstances are different.

When a patient is to receive an adrenergic agent for shock, obtain the blood pressure, pulse rate and quality, and respiratory rate and rhythm. This information provides an important data base that is used during treatment. A general survey of the patient is also necessary. Look for additional symptoms of shock such as cool skin, cyanosis, diaphoresis, and a change in the level of consciousness. Other assessments may be necessary if the hypotensive episode is due to trauma, severe infection, or blood loss. When a patient is to have nose drops instilled for nasal congestion, examine the nasal passages and describe the type of secretions present in the nose. Obtain the blood pressure as well, because nose drops that contain adrenergic agents are not given to those with high blood pressure.

■ Nursing Diagnoses

Depending on the drug, dose, and reason for administration, one or more of the following nursing diagnoses may apply to a person receiving an adrenergic drug:

• **Anxiety** related to seriousness of disorder (shock, impending or borderline shock), activity of medical personnel in managing the disorder, invasive procedures (insertion of IV or intraarterial lines), actual or perceived threat to biologic integrity, other factors

• **Risk for Altered Body Temperature: Hyperthermia** related to infection secondary to invasive procedures

- **Risk for Infection** related to invasive procedures
- **Risk for Ineffective Management of Therapeutic Regimen** related to insufficient knowledge of regimen, other factors (specify)

■ *Planning and Implementation*

The major goals of the patient will depend on the reason for administration of an adrenergic agent. Patient goals may include a normal body temperature, an absence of infection, a reduction in anxiety, and an understanding of why the drug is being given. To make these goals measurable, more specific criteria must be added. Additional strategies for implementation are found in the Nursing Management section of this chapter.

Anxiety. Depending on the clinical situation, some anxiety and fear may be experienced by the patient receiving an adrenergic drug for a serious disorder, such as shock or bronchial asthma. Invasive procedures (eg, establishing IV or intraarterial lines) also create anxiety.

Explain all treatments and procedures to the patient or family members. The type and length of explanation will depend on the clinical situation. Reassure the patient and family members that care is being exercised in performing treatments or procedures and that the patient will be closely observed while the drug is being administered.

Altered Body Temperature and Infection. When the patient is receiving an adrenergic drug by the IV route, monitor the temperature every 4 hours or as ordered. A temperature greater than 101°F (38.3°C.) or any decrease in body temperature less than normal is reported to the physician.

Inspect the entrance point of IV or intraarterial line for signs of infection, namely redness, streaking, or drainage from the site.

■ *Patient and Family Teaching*

Some adrenergic drugs, such as the vasopressors, are given only by medical personnel. The nurse's responsibility for teaching involves explaining the drug to the patient or family. Depending on the situation, teaching may include facts such as how the drug will be given (eg, the route of administration) and what results are expected from the administration of the drug. The nurse must use judgment regarding some of the information given to the patient or family regarding administration of an adrenergic drug in life-threatening situations because certain facts, such as the seriousness of the patient's condition, are usually best given by the physician.

When a nasal decongestant (drops or spray) containing an adrenergic drug has been recommended or prescribed, show the patient or family member the correct method of instillation. Explain possible adverse effects and the importance of an adherence to the dose regimen prescribed or recommended by the physician. Because many nasal decongestants are over-the-counter drugs, advise patients using them that these drugs are contraindicated in those with high blood pressure and that overuse can *increase* nasal congestion (rebound congestion).

If an adrenergic drug, such as ephedrine or isoproterenol, has been prescribed as a bronchodilator, explain the drug regimen to the patient. Stress the importance of reporting adverse reactions to the physician as soon as possible. If the drug is prescribed in sublingual form, demonstrate the technique of placing the drug under the tongue. Warn the patient not to use any nonprescription (over-the-counter) drug unless use has been approved by the physician. Encourage patients receiving a bronchodilator to contact their physician if the drug fails to produce at least partial relief of their symptoms.

■ *Expected Outcomes for Evaluation*

- Anxiety is reduced
- Body temperature is normal
- Localized infection at venipuncture or arterial puncture site is not present
- Patient verbalizes an understanding of treatment modalities and importance of continued follow-up care

Chapter Summary

- Adrenergic drugs mimic the activity of the sympathetic nervous system. Because of this, they are also called sympathomimetic drugs. Epinephrine and norepinephrine are neurotransmitters produced naturally by the sympathetic nervous system. Synthetic preparations of these two neurohormones are used medically.
- Adrenergic drugs are used to treat hypotensive episodes, bronchial asthma, cardiac arrest, heart block, ventricular arrhythmias, and allergic reactions, and to control superficial bleeding during surgical and dental procedures. Adrenergic drugs applied topically can be used to relieve nasal congestion.

- The more common adverse reactions associated with the administration of adrenergic drugs include: cardiac arrhythmias such as bradycardia and tachycardia, headache, insomnia, nervousness, anorexia, and an increase in blood pressure.
- Management of the patient receiving an adrenergic agent varies and depends on the drug used, the reason for administration, and the patient's individual response to the drug. In most instances, adrenergic drugs are potentially dangerous and great care must be taken in preparation and administration. The patient is observed for adverse drug reactions and these are reported to the physician as soon as possible.

Critical Thinking Exercise

1. Mr. Cole is receiving dopamine for the treatment of severe hypotension. In planning the care for Mr. Cole what would be the most important aspects of nursing management? Explain your answers.

18

Adrenergic Blocking Agents

Key Terms

Alpha-adrenergic blocking agents

Alpha / beta-adrenergic blocking agents

Antiadrenergic agents

Beta-adrenergic blocking agents

Cardiac dysrhythmia

Orthostatic hypotension

Pheochromocytoma

Postural hypotension

Chapter Outline

Chapter Objectives

On completion of this chapter the student will:

- *Discuss the types, uses, and general drug actions of the adrenergic blocking agents*
- *List the general adverse reactions associated with the administration of the various types of adrenergic blocking agents*
- *Describe the nursing actions that may be taken to minimize orthostatic or postural hypotension*
- *Discuss nursing management when administering an adrenergic blocking agent*
- *Use the nursing process when administering an adrenergic blocking agent*

Adrenergic blocking agents, also called sympathomimetic blocking drugs, may be divided into four groups:

Alpha-adrenergic blocking agents—drugs that block alpha-adrenergic receptors
Beta-adrenergic blocking agents—drugs that block beta-adrenergic receptors
Antiadrenergic agents—drugs that block adrenergic nerve fibers
Alpha/beta-adrenergic blocking agents—drugs that block both alpha- and beta-adrenergic receptors

Alpha-Adrenergic Blocking Agents

Alpha-adrenergic blocking agents produce their greatest effect on alpha receptors of adrenergic nerves that control the vascular system.

ACTIONS OF THE ALPHA-ADRENERGIC BLOCKING AGENTS

Stimulation of alpha-adrenergic fibers results in vasoconstriction (see Table 17-1). If stimulation of these alpha-adrenergic fibers is interrupted or blocked, the result will be vasodilatation, which is the direct opposite of the effect of an adrenergic drug having mainly alpha activity. Phentolamine (Regitine) is an example of an alpha-adrenergic blocking agent.

USES OF THE ALPHA-ADRENERGIC BLOCKING AGENTS

Phentolamine is used for its vasodilating effect on peripheral blood vessels, and therefore may be beneficial in the treatment of hypertension due to *pheochromocytoma*, a tumor of the adrenal gland that produces excessive amounts of epinephrine and norepinephrine.

ADVERSE REACTIONS ASSOCIATED WITH THE ADMINISTRATION OF ALPHA-ADRENERGIC BLOCKING AGENTS

Administration of an alpha-adrenergic blocking agent may result in *cardiac arrhythmias* (abnormal rhythm of the heart), hypotension, and tachycardia.

Beta-Adrenergic Blocking Agents

Beta-adrenergic blocking agents produce their greatest effect on beta-receptors of adrenergic nerves, primarily the beta-receptors of the heart.

ACTIONS OF THE BETA-ADRENERGIC BLOCKING AGENTS

Stimulation of beta-receptors of the heart results in an increase in the heart rate. If stimulation of these beta-adrenergic fibers is interrupted or blocked, the heart rate decreases. Examples of beta-adrenergic blocking agents are metoprolol (Lopressor), esmolol (Brevibloc), propranolol (Inderal), and nadolol (Corgard).

Beta-adrenergic blocking agents when used topically as ophthalmic drops appear to reduce the production of aqueous humor in the anterior chamber of the eye.

USES OF THE BETA-ADRENERGIC BLOCKING AGENTS

These drugs are primarily used in the treatment of hypertension (Summary Drug Table 18-1; see Chap. 34) and certain cardiac arrhythmias. Some of these drugs have additional uses, such as the use of propranolol for migraine headaches and nadolol for angina pectoris.

Beta-adrenergic blocking agents as ophthalmic eye drops, for example, timolol (Timoptic) and betaxolol (Betoptic), are used in the treatment of glaucoma. Glaucoma is a narrowing or blockage of the drainage channels (canals of Schlemm) between the anterior and posterior chambers of the eye, which then results in a buildup of pressure (increased intraocular pressure) in the eye. If glaucoma is not treated, blindness may occur.

ADVERSE REACTIONS ASSOCIATED WITH THE ADMINISTRATION OF BETA-ADRENERGIC BLOCKING AGENTS

Some of the adverse reactions observed with the administration of beta-adrenergic blocking agents include bradycardia, dizziness, vertigo, bronchospasm

Summary Drug Table 18-1. Adrenergic Blocking Agents

Generic Name	Trade Name*	Uses	Adverse Reactions	Dose Ranges
ALPHA-ADRENERGIC BLOCKING DRUGS				
phentolamine	Regitine	Hypertension due to pheochromocytoma	Hypotension, tachycardia, cardiac arrhythmias	5 mg IM, IV
BETA-ADRENERGIC BLOCKING DRUGS				
acebutolol hydrochloride	Sectral	Hypertension, ventricular arrhythmias	Bradycardia, dizziness, vertigo, rash, hyperglycemia, bronchospasm, hypotension, agranulocytosis	400–1200 mg/d PO in divided doses
atenolol	Tenormin	Hypertension, angina pectoris; acute myocardial infarction	Bradycardia, dizziness, fatigue, weakness, hypotension	50–150 mg/d PO; 5 mg IV
betaxolol hydrochloride	Kerlone	Hypertension	Dizziness, nervousness, bradycardia, impotence	10 mg/d PO may increase to 20 mg/d
betaxolol (ophthalmic)	Betoptic	Glaucoma	Brief discomfort, tearing	1–2 drops/d
esmolol hydrochloride	Brevibloc	Supraventricular tachycardia	Dizziness, headache, nausea, hypotension, phlebitis	25–200 mcg/kg/min IV
metoprolol tartrate	Lopressor	Hypertension, angina pectoris, acute myocardial infarction	Fatigue, weakness, depression, bradycardia	100–450 mg/d PO in single or divided doses; 5 mg IV
nadolol	Corgard	Angina pectoris, hypertension	Fatigue, weakness, bradycardia, nausea, vomiting	Angina: 40–240 mg/d PO; hypertension: 40–320 mg/d PO
pindolol	Visken	Hypertension	Bradycardia, dizziness, vertigo, rash, hyperglycemia, bronchospasm, hypotension, agranulocytosis	10–60 mg/d in divided doses
propranolol hydrochloride	Inderal, *generic*	Cardiac arrhythmias, hypertrophic subaortic stenosis, pheochromocytoma, migraine, angina pectoris, myocardial infarction, hypertension	Bradycardia, dizziness, vertigo, rash, hyperglycemia, bronchospasm, hypotension, agranulocytosis	Arrhythmias: 10–30 mg PO tid, qid; hypertension: 40–640 mg/d PO in divided doses; angina: 10–320 mg/d PO in divided doses; aortic stenosis: 20–40 mg/d PO in divided doses; pheochromocytoma: preoperative 60 mg/d PO in divided doses and inoperable tumor 30 mg/d PO in divided doses; life-threatening dysrhythmias: up to 1 mg/min IV; migraine: 160–240 mg/d PO in divided doses
timolol maleate	Blocadren	Hypertension, myocardial infarction	Fatigue, weakness, insomnia, peripheral vasoconstriction, diarrhea, nausea, vomiting	Hypertension: 20–60 mg/d PO in divided doses; myocardial infarction: 10 mg PO bid
timolol (ophthalmic)	Timoptic	Glaucoma	Ocular irritation, headache, dizziness, bradycardia	1–2 drops/d
ANTIADRENERGIC DRUGS				
Centrally Acting				
clonidine hydrochloride	Catapres TTS-1	Hypertension	Dry mouth, drowsiness, anorexia, rash, malaise, constipation, dizziness, sedation	0.2–2.4 mg/d PO in divided doses
methyldopa	Aldomet	Hypertension	Sedation, bradycardia, vomiting, rash	250 mg to 3 g/d PO in divided doses

(continued)

Summary Drug Table 18-1 (Continued)

Generic Name	Trade Name*	Uses	Adverse Reactions	Dose Ranges
BETA-ADRENERGIC BLOCKING DRUGS				
Peripherally Acting				
guanethidine monosulfate	Ismelin	Hypertension	Dizziness, weakness, fluid retention, anorexia, orthostatic hypotension	10–50 mg/d PO
ALPHA/BETA ADRENERGIC BLOCKING AGENTS				
labetolol hydrochloride	Normodyne	Hypertension	Fatigue, headache, nausea, vomiting, weakness, diarrhea, drowsiness	100 mg to 1.2 g PO bid; 20–50 mg IV; 50–300 mg IV infusion

*The term, *generic*, indicates that the drug is available in *generic* form.

(especially in those with a history of asthma), hyperglycemia, nausea, vomiting, and diarrhea. Many of these reactions are mild and may disappear with therapy.

Examples of adverse reactions associated with the use of beta-adrenergic ophthalmic preparations include headache, depression, cardiac arrhythmias, and bronchospasm.

Antiadrenergic Agents

The *antiadrenergic agents* are drugs that block the adrenergic nerve fibers within the central nervous system or within the peripheral nervous system. They are used primarily to treat hypertension.

ACTIONS OF THE ANTIADRENERGIC AGENTS

One group of antiadrenergic drugs inhibits the release of norepinephrine (a neurohormone of the sympathetic nervous system; see Chap 17) from certain adrenergic nerve endings in the peripheral nervous system. This group is called a *peripherally acting* (ie, acting on peripheral structures) antiadrenergic drug. An example of a peripherally acting antiadrenergic drug is guanethidine (Ismelin). The other antiadrenergic drugs are called *centrally acting* antiadrenergic drugs because they act on the central nervous system rather than on the peripheral ner-

vous system. This group affects specific central nervous system centers, thereby decreasing some of the activity of the sympathetic nervous system in this part of the nervous system. Although the action of both types of antiadrenergic drugs is somewhat different, the results are basically the same. An example of a centrally acting antiadrenergic drug is clonidine (Catapres-TTS-1).

USES OF THE ANTIADRENERGIC AGENTS

Antiadrenergic agents are used mainly for the treatment of certain cardiac arrythmias and hypertension. The uses of some of the available antiadrenergic agents are given in Summary Drug Table 18-1.

ADVERSE REACTIONS ASSOCIATED WITH THE ADMINISTRATION OF ANTIADRENERGIC AGENTS

Some of the adverse reactions associated with administration of a centrally acting antiadrenergic agent include dry mouth, drowsiness, sedation, anorexia, rash, malaise, and weakness. Adverse reactions associated with the administration of the peripherally acting antiadrenergic agents include hypotension, weakness, lightheadedness, and bradycardia.

Alpha/Beta-Adrenergic Blocking Agents

Alpha/beta adrenergic blocking agents act on both alpha and beta nerve fibers. Only one drug is in this category: labetalol (Normodyne).

ACTIONS OF THE ALPHA/BETA-ADRENERGIC BLOCKING AGENTS

Alpha/beta adrenergic blocking agents block the stimulation of alpha and beta adrenergic receptors resulting in peripheral vasodilatation.

USES OF THE ALPHA/BETA-ADRENERGIC BLOCKING AGENTS

Labetalol is the only drug in this category that is available. It is used in the treatment of hypertension, either as a single agent or in combination with another agent such as a diuretic.

ADVERSE REACTIONS ASSOCIATED WITH THE ADMINISTRATION OF ALPHA/BETA-ADRENERGIC BLOCKING AGENTS

Most adverse effects of labetalol are mild and do not require discontinuation of therapy. Examples of the adverse reactions are fatigue, headache, diarrhea, dyspnea, and skin rash.

NURSING MANAGEMENT

The major goals of nursing management are to observe the patient for the results of drug therapy, to detect adverse drugs reactions, to reduce patient anxiety, and to develop and implement an effective teaching plan.

Assessment and evaluation are planned, carried out continuously during drug therapy, and primarily based on the disease or condition treated. Some patients may experience one or more adverse drug reactions. As with any drug, report adverse reactions to the physician and record them on the patient's chart. Nursing judgment in this matter is necessary because some adverse reactions are serious or potentially serious in nature; in these cases, withhold the next dose of the drug and contact the physician immediately. Adverse reactions that pose no serious threat to the patient's well-being, such as dry mouth or mild constipation, are reported to the physician but may have to be tolerated by the patient. In some instances, these less serious reactions disappear or lessen in intensity after a time. However, even minor adverse drug reactions can be distressing to the patient, especially when the reactions persist for a long time.

Whenever possible, minor adverse reactions are relieved with simple nursing measures. For example, a dry mouth can often be relieved by giving frequent sips of water or allowing a piece of hard candy to dissolve in the mouth (provided that the patient is not a diabetic or on a special diet that limits sugar intake). Constipation can often be relieved by increasing the fluid intake, unless extra fluids are contraindicated. The physician may also order a laxative or stool softener. Maintain a daily record of bowel elimination.

Hypertension

During therapy with an adrenergic blocking agent for hypertension, take the blood pressure before each dose is given. Some patients have an unusual response to the drugs, and some drugs may, in some individuals, decrease the blood pressure at a more rapid rate than other drugs.

> **Nursing Alert**
>
> If there is a significant decrease in the blood pressure since the last dose was given, withhold the drug and notify the physician immediately. If there is a significant rise in the blood pressure, give the drug but notify the physician immediately because additional drug therapy may be necessary.

Monitor the blood pressure on both arms and in the sitting, standing, and lying down positions for the first week or more of therapy. Once the patient's blood pressure has stabilized, take the blood pressure before each drug administration using the *same* arm and position for each reading. Make a notation on the Kardex or care plan about the position and arm used for blood pressure determinations.

Cardiac Arrhythmia

Some adrenergic blocking agents are used to treat *cardiac arrhythmias*. Ongoing assessment and nursing management of these patients depend on the type of arrhythmia and the method of treatment. Some arrhythmias, such as ventricular fibrillation, are life-threatening and require immediate attention. Other arrhythmias are serious and require treatment but are not immediately life-threatening.

The patient with a life-threatening arrhythmia may receive an adrenergic blocking drug, such as propranolol, by the intravenous route. When these drugs are given intravenously, cardiac monitoring is necessary. Patients not in a specialized unit, such as a coronary care unit, are usually transferred to one as soon as possible. Administering these drugs for a life-threatening arrhythmia requires constant patient supervision, frequent monitoring of the blood pressure and respiratory rate, and cardiac monitoring. Frequent communication with the physician about the patient's response to the drug is necessary. When propranolol is given orally for a less serious cardiac arrhythmia, cardiac monitoring is usually not necessary. Monitor the blood pressure and pulse rate and rhythm at varying intervals depending on the length of treatment and the patient's response to the drug. If propranolol is given for angina, ask the patient about the relief of symptoms and record responses on the patient's chart. If the angina worsens or does not appear to be controlled by the drug, contact the physician immediately.

Glaucoma

The patient with glaucoma who is using a beta-adrenergic blocking ophthalmic preparation, such as timolol, requires periodic follow-up examination by the ophthalmologist. At the time of the examination, the intraocular pressure is obtained to determine the effectiveness of drug therapy.

Nursing Process
The Patient Receiving an Adrenergic Blocking Agent

■ *Assessment*
As with most drugs, assessment depends on the drug, the patient, and the reason for administration. Establish an accurate data base *before* any adrenergic blocking agent is administered for the first time.

If, for example, the patient has a peripheral vascular disease, note the subjective and objective symptoms of the disorder during the initial assessment. Once drug therapy is started, evaluation of the effects of therapy can be made by comparing the patient's present symptoms with the symptoms experienced before therapy was initiated.

Patients with hypertension must have their blood pressure and pulse taken on both arms in sitting, standing, and lying down positions before therapy is begun. If the patient has a cardiac arrhythmia, take the pulse rate and determine the pulse rhythm during the initial assessment, and note the patient's general appearance. Obtain subjective data (ie, the patient's complaints or description of symptoms) at this time. The physician usually orders an electrocardiogram. Additional diagnostic studies and laboratory tests may also be ordered.

■ *Nursing Diagnoses*
Depending on the drug, dose, and reason for administration, one or more of the following nursing diagnoses may apply to a person receiving an adrenergic blocking drug:
- **Anxiety** related to symptoms of disorder, diagnosis, other factors (specify)
- **Risk for Injury** related to vertigo secondary to orthostatic hypotension
- **Altered Health Maintenance** related to inability to comprehend drug regimen
- **Risk for Ineffective Management of Therapeutic Regimen** related to lack of knowledge, negative side effects of drug therapy, anxiety, other factors (specify)

■ *Planning and Implementation*
The major goals of the patient depend on the reason for administration of an adrenergic blocking agent but may include an optimal response to drug therapy, a reduction in anxiety, absence of adverse drug reactions, absence of injury, and an understanding of and compliance to the prescribed treatment regimen. To make these goals measurable, more specific criteria must be added. Additional strategies for implementation may be found under Nursing Management.

Anxiety. Some patients may experience anxiety because of their diagnosis, treatment regimen, or the appearance of adverse drug reactions. Explain the treatment regimen thoroughly to the patient and inform the patient of possible adverse drug reactions. Explain that most drug reactions are mild, transient in nature, and may disappear in time.

Adverse Reactions. Observe the patient continually for the appearance of adverse drug reactions. Report all drug reactions to the physician. Some adverse reactions are mild, while others such as diarrhea may cause a problem especially if the patient is elderly or debilitated.

Risk for Injury. On occasion, patients receiving an adrenergic blocking agent may experience *orthostatic* or *postural hypotension. Postural hypotension* is characterized by a feeling of lightheadedness and dizziness when *suddenly* changing from a lying to a sitting or standing position or from a sitting to a standing position. *Orthostatic hypotension* is characterized by principally the same symptoms as postural hypotension when the patient changes or shifts position after standing in one place for a long period. These adverse reactions can be minimized as follows:

- Instruct patients to rise slowly from a sitting or lying position.
- Provide assistance for patients when getting out of a bed or a chair if symptoms of postural hypotension are severe. Place the call light nearby and instruct patients to ask for assistance each time they get in and out of a bed or a chair.
- Assist bed patients to a sitting position and have them sit on the edge of the bed for about 1 minute before standing. Help patients sitting in a chair to a standing position and instruct them to stand in one place for about 1 minute before ambulating. Remain with patients while they are standing in one place as well as during ambulation.
- Instruct patients to avoid standing in one place for prolonged periods. This is rarely a problem in the hospital but should be included in the patient and family teaching plan.

Often, symptoms of postural or orthostatic hypotension lessen with time, and the patient may be allowed to get out of a bed or chair slowly without assistance. Good judgment must be exercised in this matter. Allowing the patient to rise from a lying or sitting position without help is done only when the determination has been made that the symptoms have lessened and ambulation poses no danger of falling.

■ Patient and Family Teaching

Some patients do not adhere to the prescribed drug regimen for a variety of reasons such as failure to comprehend the regimen, cost of drug therapy, and failure to understand the importance of continued and uninterrupted therapy. If the patient departs from the prescribed drug regimen, investigate the possible cause of the problem. In some instances, financial assistance may be necessary; in other instances, patients need to know *why* they are taking a drug and *why* therapy must be continuous to attain and maintain an optimal state of health and wellbeing.

Stress the importance of continued and uninterrupted therapy when teaching the patient who is prescribed an adrenergic blocking drug.

The Patient With Hypertension, Cardiac Arrhythmia, or Angina. If a beta-adrenergic blocking drug has been prescribed for hypertension, cardiac arrhythmia, angina, or other cardiac disorders, the patient must have a full understanding of the treatment regimen. In some instances, the physician may advise the hypertensive patient to lose weight or eat a special diet such as a diet low in salt. A special diet may also be recommended for the patient with angina or a cardiac arrhythmia. When appropriate, stress the importance of diet and weight loss in the therapy of hypertension.

Include the following additional points in the teaching plan for the patient with hypertension, angina, or a cardiac arrhythmia:

- Do not stop abruptly except on the advice of a physician.
- Notify the physician promptly if adverse drug reactions occur.
- Observe caution while driving or performing other hazardous tasks because these drugs (beta-adrenergic blocking agents) may cause drowsiness, dizziness, or lightheadedness.
- Do not use any nonprescription drug unless approved by the physician.
- Inform dentists and other physicians of therapy with this drug.
- Keep all appointments with the physician because close monitoring of therapy is essential.
- Check with a physician or pharmacist to determine if the drug is to be taken with food or on an empty stomach.

When an adrenergic blocking drug is prescribed for hypertension, the physician may want the patient to monitor blood pressure between office visits. If this is recommended, teach the patient and a family member how to take a blood pressure reading. Supervise the patient and a family member during several trial blood pressure readings to ensure accuracy of their measurements. Suggest to the patient that the same arm and body position be used each time the blood pressure is taken. Patients should also understand that the blood pressure can vary slightly with emotion, the time of day, the position of the body, and so on. A slight change in readings is normal but if a drastic change in either or both the systolic or diastolic readings occurs, the physician should be contacted as soon as possible.

The Patient With Glaucoma. Demonstrate the technique of eye drop instillation and explain the prescribed treatment regimen to the patient. Stress the importance of adhering to the instillation schedule because omitting or discontinuing the drug without approval of the physician may result in a marked increase in intraocular pressure, which can lead to blindness.

■ *Expected Outcomes for Evaluation*
• Anxiety is reduced
• Adverse reactions are identified and reported to the physician
• No evidence of injury
• Patient complies to the prescribed drug regimen
• Patient and family demonstrate understanding of drug regimen

Chapter Summary

• Adrenergic blocking agents, also called sympathomimetic blocking drugs, are divided into four groups: (1) the alpha-adrenergic blocking agents, (2) the beta-adrenergic blocking agents, (3) the antiadrenergic agents and the (4) alpha/beta-adrenergic blocking agents.
• The alpha-adrenergic blocking agents block the effects of the alpha-adrenergic receptors thereby inhibiting the normal excitatory response of epinephrine and norepinephrine. These drugs are used to treat the hypertension associated with pheochromocytoma, a tumor of the adrenal gland that produces excessive amounts of epinephrine and norepinephrine.
• The beta-adrenergic blocking agents block beta-adrenergic receptors, resulting in a decrease in the heart rate. These drugs are used to treat hypertension, cardiac arrhythmias, angina pectoris, and glaucoma. Some adverse reactions seen with the use of these drugs include: bradycardia, dizziness, vertigo, and bronchospasm.
• The antiadrenergic agents inhibit the release of norepinephrine from certain adrenergic nerve endings in the nervous system. These drugs may act peripherally or centrally to produce basically the same effect: to suppress the activity of the sympathetic nervous system. The antiadrenergic drugs are used primarily to treat hypertension and cardiac arrhythmias.
• Only one drug belongs to the alpha/beta-adrenergic blocking agent group: labetalol. This drug is used to treat hypertension. Most adverse reactions of labetalol are mild and include headache, fatigue, and skin rash.
• Patients treated with the adrenergic blocking agents must have their blood pressure and pulse monitored throughout therapy. These drugs may cause postural hypotension. Advise the patient to rise slowly from a lying to a sitting position. Assistance may be needed for ambulation. Any position change should be made slowly to minimize postural hypotension.

Critical Thinking Exercise

1. Ms. Martin has been prescribed propanolol for hypertension. When keeping an outpatient clinic appointment, Ms. Martin tells you she is having episodes of dizziness and at times feels as if she is going to faint. How would you investigate this problem and what information could you give Ms. Martin that might help her?

19

Cholinergic Drugs

Chapter Outline

Chapter Objectives

On completion of this chapter the student will:

* *Discuss the uses and drug actions of the cholinergic drugs*
* *Identify adverse reactions associated with the administration of cholinergic drugs*
* *Discuss nursing management when administering cholinergic drugs*
* *Use the nursing process when administering a cholinergic drug*

Cholinergic drugs mimic the activity of the parasympathetic nervous system. They are also called *parasympathomimetic drugs.*

The parasympathetic nervous system is a part of the autonomic nervous system; it helps conserve body energy. It is partly responsible for activities such as slowing the heart rate, digesting food, and eliminating body wastes.

Electron microscopic study reveals an incalculably small space between nerve endings and the effector organ (eg, the muscle, cell, or gland) that is innervated (or controlled) by a nerve fiber. For a nerve impulse to be transmitted from the nerve ending (motor end plate) across the space to the effector organ, a neurohormone is needed.

There are two neurohormones (neurotransmitters) of the parasympathetic nervous system: *acetylcholine* (ACh) and *acetylcholinesterase* (AChE). These two neurohormones are released at nerve endings of parasympathetic nerve fibers; at some nerve endings in the sympathetic nervous system; and at nerve endings of skeletal muscles. These parasympathetic neurohormones are believed to be manufactured by special cells located in the nerve ending. When a parasympathetic nerve fiber is stimulated, the nerve fiber releases ACh, and the nerve impulses pass (travel) from the nerve fiber to the effector organ or structure. After the impulse has crossed over to the effector organ or structure, ACh is inactivated (destroyed) by the neurohormone AChE. When the next nerve impulse is ready to travel along the nerve fiber, ACh is again released and then inactivated by AChE.

Cholinergic Drugs

Cholinergic drugs have limited usefulness in medicine, in part because of the adverse reactions that may occur during administration. In some diseases or conditions, however, cholinergic drugs are either definitely indicated or may be of value. These drugs are particularly useful in the treatment of glaucoma, myasthenia gravis, and postoperatively to treat urinary retention.

ACTIONS OF CHOLINERGIC DRUGS

Cholinergic drugs may act like the neurohormone ACh, or they may inhibit the release of the neurohormone AChE. Cholinergic drugs that act like ACh are called *direct-acting* cholinergics. If a cholinergic drug inhibits the body's release of AChE, it prolongs the activity of the ACh produced by the body. Cholinergic drugs that prolong the activity of ACh by inhibiting the release of AChE are called *indirect-acting* cholinergics. Although a specific cholinergic drug may act in either of these two ways, the results of drug action are basically the same.

USES OF CHOLINERGIC DRUGS

Glaucoma, a disorder of the eye, may be treated by topical application (eg, eye drops) of a cholinergic agent, such as carbachol or pilocarpine (Isopto Carpine). Treatment of glaucoma with a cholinergic agent produces miosis (constriction of the iris), which then opens the blocked channels and allows the normal passage of fluid between the anterior and posterior chamber, thus reducing intraocular pressure.

Myasthenia gravis is a disease that involves rapid fatigue of skeletal muscles due to the lack of ACh released at the nerve endings of parasympathetic nerve fibers; it responds to the administration of a cholinergic agent. Drugs used in the treatment of this disorder include ambenonium (Mytelase) and pyridostigmine (Mestinon).

Urinary retention may be treated with bethanechol chloride (Urecholine), provided the retention is not caused by a mechanical obstruction, such as a stone in the bladder or an enlarged prostate. The parasympathetic nervous system partly controls the process of *micturation* (voiding of urine), which is both a voluntary and involuntary act, by constricting the detrusor muscle and relaxing the bladder sphincter (see Table 17-1). Administration of this drug may result in the spontaneous passage of urine.

ADVERSE REACTIONS ASSOCIATED WITH THE ADMINISTRATION OF CHOLINERGIC DRUGS

Unless applied topically, as in the treatment of glaucoma, cholinergic agents are not selective in action. Therefore, they may affect many organs and structures of the body, causing a variety of adverse effects. Oral or parenteral administration can result in nausea, diarrhea, abdominal cramping, salivation, flushing of the skin, cardiac arrhythmias, and muscle weakness. Topical administration usually produces few adverse effects, but a temporary reduction of visual acuity (sharpness) and headache may occur. Summary Drug Table 19-1 lists the adverse reactions that may be seen with specific cholinergic drugs.

Summary Drug Table 19-1. Cholinergic Drugs

Generic Name	Trade Name*	Uses	Adverse Reactions	Dose Ranges
ambenonium	Mytelase	Myasthenia gravis	Increased bronchial secretions, cardiac arrhythmias, muscle weakness	5–75 mg PO tid, qid
bethanecol chloride	Urecholine, *generic*	Acute nonobstructive urinary retention, neurogenic atony of urinary bladder with retention	Abdominal discomfort, diarrhea, nausea, vomiting, salivation, urgency, flushing, sweating	10–50 mg PO bid to qid; 2.5–5 mg SC tid to qid
carbachol, topical	Isopto Carbachol	Glaucoma	Temporary reduction of visual acuity, headache	1–2 drops in eye up to 4 times/d
pilocarpine hydrochloride	Isopto Carpine, Pilocar, *generic*	Glaucoma	Temporary reduction of visual acuity, headache	1 drop in eye 1–6 times/d
pilocarpine ocular therapeutic system	Ocusert Pilo-20, Ocusert Pilo-40	Elevated intraocular pressure	Temporary reduction of visual acuity, headache	1 unit placed in the conjunctival sac, replaced as directed by the physician (usually every 7 d)
neostigmine *generic*	Prostigmin	Myasthenia gravis	Cardiac arrhythmias, vomiting, bowel cramps, increased peristalsis, urinary frequency, flushing, weakness, diaphoresis, nausea, diarrhea, salivation	Myasthenia gravis: maintenance dose 150–375 mg/d
pyridostigmine bromide	Mestinon	Myasthenia gravis	Increased bronchial secretions, cardiac arrhythmias, muscle weakness	Average dose is 600 mg/d PO at spaced intervals, with doses as low as 60 mg/d and as high as 1500 mg/d

*The term, *generic*, indicates the drug is available in generic form.

NURSING MANAGEMENT

Nursing management varies depending on the reason the drug is given. As in the administration of any drug, identification of adverse drug effects and accurate assessment of the results of drug therapy are of utmost importance.

Glaucoma

Check the physician's order and the drug label carefully when instilling any ophthalmic preparation. The drug label must indicate that the preparation is for *ophthalmic* use. In addition, carefully check the name of the drug and the drug dosage or strength as stated on the label against the physician's orders. Instill the drug in the lower conjunctival sac unless the physician orders a different method of instillation. Support the hand holding the eyedropper against the patient's forehead. The tip of the dropper must never touch the eye.

In some instances, the patient may have been using an ophthalmic preparation for glaucoma for a long time, and the physician may allow the hospitalized patient to instill his or her own eye drops. When this is so stated on the patient's order sheet, the medication can be left at the patient's bedside. Even though the drug is self-administered, check the patient at intervals to be sure that the medication is instilled at the prescribed time using the correct technique for ophthalmic instillation.

If the pilocarpine ocular system is prescribed for the hospitalized patient, check the cheek and eye area several times a day because the system can become displaced from the eye. Most patients are usually aware of displacement of the system, but some patients, the elderly in particular, may not realize that the system has come out of the eye. If displacement does occur, insert a new system and inform the physician of the problem. On occasion, patients cannot insert the system by themselves or cannot retain the system in the eye for the required time. When this occurs, notify the physician because the ocular system should remain in place until it is time for it to be changed.

Change the pilocarpine ocular system every 7 days unless the physician orders otherwise. When this system is used to treat glaucoma, check the eye and the area around the eye daily for evidence of redness, inflammation, and excessive secretions. If secretions are present around the eye, remove them with a cotton ball or gauze soaked in normal saline or other cleansing solution recommended by the physician. If patients have a problem retaining the system, placing the system in the upper conjunctival cul-de-sac is preferable. The system can be gently manipulated from the lower to the upper conjunctival cul-de-sac using gentle massage through the eyelid. Contact the physician if the symptoms of glaucoma increase, if the patient is unable to retain the ocular system, or if redness, eye irritation, or excessive secretions are noted.

Because drug-induced myopia (nearsightedness) may occur after instillation of a cholinergic ophthalmic drug for the treatment of glaucoma, assist the patient in getting out of bed or ambulating. Keep the patient's room dimly lit at night because night vision may be decreased. Place obstacles that may hinder ambulation or result in falls, such as slippers, chairs, and tables, out of the way, especially during the night.

Myasthenia Gravis

In the beginning, determining the dosage that will control symptoms may be difficult. In many cases, the dosage must be adjusted upward or downward until optimal drug effects are obtained.

Nursing Alert

Because of the need to make frequent dosage adjustments, observe the patient closely for symptoms of drug overdosage or underdosage. Signs of drug overdosage include muscle rigidity and spasm, salivation, and clenching of the jaw. Signs of drug underdosage are signs of the disease itself, namely, rapid fatigability of the muscles, drooping of the eyelids, and difficulty breathing. If symptoms of drug overdosage or underdosage develop, contact the physician immediately because a change in dosage is usually necessary.

In the case of overdosage, an antidote, such as atropine, and other treatment may also be necessary.

Assess the patient for the presence or absence of the symptoms of myasthenia gravis *before* each drug dose. In patients with severe myasthenia gravis, these assessments may be carried out between drug doses, as well as immediately before drug administration. Document each symptom, as well as the patient's response or lack of response to drug therapy.

Assessment is important because the dosage frequently has to be increased or decreased early in therapy depending on the patient's response. Regulation of dosage is important in keeping the symptoms of myasthenia gravis from incapacitating the patient. For many patients, the symptoms are fairly well-controlled with drug therapy once the optimal drug dose is determined.

Urinary Retention

Voiding usually occurs in 5 to 15 minutes after subcutaneous drug administration and 30 to 90 minutes after oral administration. Place the call light and any other items the patient might need, such as the urinal or the bedpan, within easy reach. Some patients, however, are not able to reach or handle these aids easily and thus require prompt answering of their call light. Measure and record intake and output. Notify the physician if the patient fails to void after drug administration.

If a cholinergic drug is ordered for the prevention of urinary retention, measure and record intake and output. If the amount of each voiding is insufficient or the patient fails to void, palpate the bladder to determine its size and notify the physician.

Adverse Drug Effects

When a cholinergic drug is given by the oral or parenteral route, adverse drug effects may be related to many systems of the body, such as the heart, respiratory and gastrointestinal tracts, and the central nervous system. Observe the patient closely for the appearance of adverse drug effects, such as a change in vital signs, or an increase in symptoms. Document any complaints the patient may have and notify the physician as soon as possible.

Nursing Process
The Patient Receiving a Cholinergic Drug

■ *Assessment*
Assessment depends on the drug and the reason for administration.

Glaucoma. Before therapy for glaucoma is started, the physician thoroughly examines the eye. Review the physician's diagnosis and comments, take a general patient health history, and evaluate the patient's ability to carry out the activities of daily living, especially if the patient is elderly or has limited vision.

Myasthenia Gravis. When a cholinergic drug is given to a patient with myasthenia gravis, the patient has a complete neurologic assessment before the therapy is begun, usually performed by the physician. Once therapy is underway, the nurse must document any problems (any increase in the symptoms of the disease or adverse drug reactions) before giving each dose of the drug.

When performing such an assessment, look for signs of muscle weakness such as drooling (ie, the lack of ability to swallow); inability to chew and swallow; drooping of the eyelids; inability to perform repetitive movements, such as walking, combing hair, using eating utensils; difficulty breathing; and extreme fatigue.

Urinary Retention. If a patient receives a cholinergic drug for the treatment of urinary retention, palpate the bladder to determine its size and take the blood pressure and pulse rate. Closely monitor intake and output.

■ *Nursing Diagnoses*
Depending on the drug, dose, and reason for administration, one or more of the following nursing diagnoses may apply to a person receiving a cholinergic drug:
- **Altered Health Maintenance** related to inability to comprehend drug regimen, inability to handle the prescribed drug regimen
- **Risk for Ineffective Management of Therapeutic Regimen** related to indifference, lack of knowledge, other factors

■ *Planning and Implementation*
The major goals of the patient may include an absence of adverse drug effects and an understanding of and compliance to the prescribed therapeutic regimen. To make these goals measurable, more specific criteria must be added. Specific nursing strategies for implementation may be found in the Nursing Management section.

Patients required to take a drug over a long period may incur lapses in their medication schedule. For some, it is a matter of occasionally forgetting to take a medication but for others it may be caused by other factors such as failure to understand the importance of drug therapy, inability to instill an eye medication (when the drug is prescribed for glaucoma), the cost of the drug, or unfamiliarity with the consequences associated with discontinuing the drug therapy.

■ *Patient and Family Teaching*
When developing a teaching plan for the patient and family, emphasize the importance of uninterrupted drug therapy. Allow the patient and family time to ask questions. Explore any problems that appear to be associated with the prescribed drug regimen in depth and then report to the physician. Review the purpose of the drug therapy with the patient and family, as well as the adverse effects that may be seen.

Glaucoma. When a cholinergic drug is prescribed for glaucoma, instruct the patient and a family member in instillation of the eye drops. If a family member is to instill the drug, allow time for instruction as well as supervised practice of the procedure. Warn the patient that the eye drops may sting when instilled into the eye and that this is a normal but often temporary discomfort. Advise the patient to observe caution while driving or performing any task that requires visual acuity.

Include the following points in the teaching plan for a patient using a liquid eye medication:
- Keep the bottle tightly closed.
- Do not wash the tip of the dropper.
- Do not lay the dropper on a table or other surface.
- Place the dropper back in the bottle immediately after use.
- Tilt the head back and instill the prescribed number of drops in the inner lower eyelid (lower conjunctival sac).
- Apply light finger pressure to the inner corner of the eye (lacrimal sac) for about 1 minute after instillation (teaching the use of this maneuver should be approved by the physician).
- If unable to instill eye drops, contact the physician immediately.

If the pilocarpine ocular system is prescribed, the patient's ability to insert and remove the system must be evaluated by the physician or nurse. A package insert is provided with the system and is reviewed with the patient. Instruct the patient to remove and replace the system every 7 days or as instructed by the physician. Replacement is best done at bedtime (unless the physician orders otherwise) because there is some impairment of vision for a short time after insertion. Tell the patient to check for unit placement before retiring at night and in the morning on arising. The physician is notified if eye secretions are excessive or irritation occurs.

Myasthenia Gravis. Many patients with myasthenia gravis learn to adjust their drug dosage according to their needs, since dosages may vary slightly from day to day. Teach the patient and family members to recognize symptoms of overdosage and underdosage, as well as what steps the physician wishes them to take if either occurs. Explain the dosage regimen and how to adjust the dosage upward or downward. Give the patient a written or printed description of the signs and symptoms of drug overdosage or underdosage. Instruct the patient to keep a record of the response to drug therapy (eg, time of day, increased or decreased muscle strength, fatigue) and to bring this to each physician or clinic visit until the symptoms are well-controlled and the drug dosage is stabilized. Instruct these patients to wear or carry identification (such as Medic-Alert) indicating that they have myasthenia gravis.

■ *Expected Outcomes for Evaluation*
- Adverse reactions are identified and reported to the physician
- Patient verbalizes importance of complying with the prescribed treatment regimen
- Patient complies to the prescribed drug regimen
- Patient and family demonstrate understanding of drug regimen

- Cholinergic drugs are used in treating myasthenia gravis and glaucoma, and to induce voiding in patients with urinary retention. Adverse reactions of the cholinergic drugs include nausea, diarrhea, abdominal cramping, flushing of the skin, cardiac arrhythmias, and muscle weakness. Topical application may cause a temporary reduction in visual acuity.
- Nursing management varies depending on the reason the drug is given. As in the administration of any drug, identification of adverse drug effects and accurate assessment of the results of drug therapy are of utmost importance.
- When a cholinergic drug is prescribed for glaucoma, the patient is instructed in instillation of the eye drops or insertion of the ocular system. The patient is warned that the eye drops may sting when instilled into the eye and that this discomfort often disappears after a short time. If the pilocarpine ocular system is prescribed, the patient's ability to insert and remove the system must be evaluated by the physician or nurse.
- For patients with myasthenia gravis, determining the dosage that will control symptoms may be difficult in the beginning. In many cases, the dosage must be adjusted upward or downward until optimal drug effects are obtained. Because of the need to make frequent dosage adjustments, observe the patient closely for symptoms of drug overdosage or underdosage. Signs of drug overdosage include muscle rigidity and spasm, salivation, and clenching of the jaw. Signs of drug underdosage are signs of the disease itself, namely, rapid fatigability of the muscles. If symptoms of drug overdosage or underdosage develop, contact the physician immediately because a change in dosage is usually necessary.

Chapter Summary

- Cholinergic drugs mimic the activity of the parasympathetic nervous system. This system is the part of the autonomic nervous system that helps conserve energy and is responsible for slowing of the heart rate, digesting food, and eliminating body wastes. Cholinergic drugs act directly by prolonging the action of the neurohormone ACh or indirectly by preventing the breakdown of ACh by inhibiting the release of AChE.

Critical Thinking Exercise

1. Mr. Johnson, aged 78, has glaucoma and is prescribed the pilocarpine ocular system. On a visit to the outpatient clinic, Mr. Johnson tells you that he is having problems retaining the ocular system. You notice that his right eye is very red and inflamed. How can you investigate this problem further with Mr. Johnson? What suggestions can you make that will help Mr. Johnson to retain the system?

20

Cholinergic Blocking Drugs

Key Terms

Anticholinergics
Cholinergic blocking drugs
Cycloplegia
Mydriasis
Parasympathomimetic blocking drugs
Photophobia

Chapter Outline

Chapter Objectives

On completion of this chapter the student will:

- *Discuss the uses and general drug actions of the cholinergic blocking drugs*
- *List some of the adverse reactions seen with the administration of cholinergic blocking drugs*
- *Discuss nursing management when administering a cholinergic blocking drug*
- *Use the nursing process when administering a cholinergic blocking drug*

Cholinergic blocking drugs are also called *anti-cholinergics* or *parasympathomimetic blocking drugs*. Like adrenergic blocking agents, this group of drugs has an effect on the autonomic nervous system. Cholinergic blocking drugs, for example, atropine and scopolamine, may be derived from natural sources (eg, plants) but most drugs in this group are produced synthetically.

Cholinergic Blocking Drugs

ACTIONS OF THE CHOLINERGIC BLOCKING DRUGS

Cholinergic blocking drugs *inhibit* the activity of acetylcholine in parasympathetic nerve fibers. See Chapter 19 for a description of the role of acetylcholine in the transmission of nerve impulses across parasympathetic nerve fibers. When the activity of acetylcholine is inhibited, nerve impulses traveling along parasympathetic nerve fibers cannot pass from the nerve fiber to the effector organ or structure. These drugs are also capable of reversing the action of cholinergic drugs.

Because of the wide distribution of parasympathetic nerves, these drugs affect many organs and structures of the body including the eyes, the respiratory and gastrointestinal tracts, the heart, and the bladder (see Table 17-1). Cholinergic blocking agents produce the following responses:

Central nervous system (CNS)—dreamless sleep, drowsiness; atropine may produce mild stimulation in some patients
Eye—*mydriasis* (dilatation of the pupil), *cycloplegia* (paralysis of accommodation or inability to focus the eye)
Respiratory tract—drying of the secretions of the mouth, nose, throat, bronchi, relaxation of smooth muscles of the bronchi resulting in slight bronchodilatation
Gastrointestinal tract—decrease in secretions of the stomach, decrease in gastric and intestinal movement (motility)
Cardiovascular system—increase in pulse rate (most pronounced with atropine administration)
Urinary tract—Dilatation of smooth muscles of the ureters and kidney pelvis, contraction of the detrusor muscle of the bladder

These responses to administration of a cholinergic drug may vary and often depend on the drug and the dose used. Occasionally, scopolamine may cause ex-

citement, delirium, and restlessness, which is thought to be a drug idiosyncrasy.

The synthetic cholinergic blocking drugs generally produce the same response as the natural agents. However, the intensity of their effect on one or more body systems is often less than those produced by the natural agents.

USES OF THE CHOLINERGIC BLOCKING DRUGS

Because of their widespread effect on many organs and structures of the body, cholinergic blocking drugs have a variety of uses. For example, some of the uses of atropine include treatment of pylorospasm, peptic ulcer, ureteral and biliary colic, vagal-induced bradycardia, parkinsonism, and preoperatively to reduce secretions of the upper respiratory tract before the administration of a general anesthetic. Other cholinergic blocking agents have a more selective action, that is, they affect principally one structure of the body. An example of this type of drug is clidinium bromide (Quarzan), which is used only in the treatment of peptic ulcer. Summary Drug Table 20-1 lists the uses of specific cholinergic blocking drugs.

ADVERSE REACTIONS ASSOCIATED WITH THE ADMINISTRATION OF CHOLINERGIC BLOCKING DRUGS

Dryness of the mouth with difficulty in swallowing, blurred vision, and *photophobia* (aversion to bright light) may be seen with the administration of a cholinergic blocking agent. The severity of many adverse reactions is often dose dependent, that is, the larger the dose, the more intense the adverse reaction. Even in normal doses, some degree of dryness of the mouth almost always occurs.

Constipation, which is due to a decrease in intestinal motility, may occur in those taking one of these drugs on a regular basis, for example, the patient under treatment for a peptic ulcer. Drowsiness may occur with the use of these drugs but there are times when this adverse reaction is desirable, such as when atropine is used as a preoperative medication to reduce the production of secretions in the respiratory tract.

Other adverse reactions that may be seen with the administration of a cholinergic blocking agent include the following:

Summary Drug Table 20-1. Cholinergic Blocking Drugs

Generic Name	Trade Name*	Uses	Adverse Reactions	Dose Ranges
anisotropine methylbromide	Valpin 50, *generic*	Peptic ulcer	Urinary hesitancy or urgency, blurred vision, dry mouth, nausea, vomiting, palpitation, headache, flushing, drowsiness	50 mg PO tid
atropine sulfate	*generic*	Pylorospasm, reduction of bronchial and oral secretions, excessive vagal-induced bradycardia, ureteral and biliary colic	Drowsiness, blurred vision, tachycardia, dry mouth, urinary hesitancy	0.4–0.6 mg PO; 0.4–1 mg IM, SC, IV
belladonna alkaloids	*generic*	Adjunctive therapy for peptic ulcer, digestive disorders, diverticulitis, pancreatitis, diarrhea	Drowsiness, blurred vision, tachycardia, dry mouth, urinary hesitancy	0.25–0.5 mg PO tid, qid
clidinium bromide	Quarzan	Peptic ulcer	Confusion, dry mouth, constipation, hesitancy, urinary retention, blurred vision	2.5–5 mg PO tid, qid ac and hs
glycopyrrolate	Robinul, *generic*	Oral: peptic ulcer; parenteral: in conjunction with anesthesia to reduce bronchial and oral secretions; to block cardiac vagal inhibitory reflexes during induction of anesthesia and intubation	Drowsiness, blurred vision, tachycardia, dry mouth, urinary hesitancy	Oral: 1–2 mg bid, tid; Parenteral: peptic ulcer 0.1–0.2 mg IM, IV tid, qid; preanesthesia: 0.002 mg/lb IM; intraoperative: 0.1 mg IV
L-hyoscyamine sulfate	Levsin, Anaspaz, Cysto-Spaz	Peptic ulcer, acute rhinitis, renal colic, cystitis, parkinsonism, preoperatively to reduce bronchial and oral secretions	Confusion, dry mouth, constipation, hesitancy, urinary retention, blurred vision	Oral: 0.125–0.25 mg tid, qid; parenteral: 0.25–0.5 mg SC, IM, IV q6h
propantheline bromide	Pro-Banthine, *generic*	Adjunctive therapy for peptic ulcer	Confusion, dry mouth, constipation, hesitancy, urinary retention, blurred vision	15 mg PO 30 min ac and 30 mg PO hs
scopolamine hydrobromide (hyoscine hydrobromide)	*generic*	Preanesthetic sedation	Confusion, dry mouth, constipation, hesitancy, urinary retention, blurred vision	0.32–0.65 mg SC, IM, and IV when diluted with sterile water for injection

*The term, *generic*, indicates that the drug is available in generic form.

Central nervous system—headache, flushing, nervousness, drowsiness, weakness, insomnia, nasal congestion, fever

Eyes—blurred vision, mydriasis, photophobia, cycloplegia, increased ocular tension

Gastrointestinal tract—nausea, vomiting, difficulty in swallowing, heartburn

Urinary tract—urinary hesitancy and retention, dysuria

Cardiovascular system—palpitations, bradycardia (following low doses of atropine), tachycardia (after higher doses of atropine)

Other—urticaria, anaphylactic shock, other skin manifestations

When these drugs are given to elderly patients, confusion or excitement may be seen even with small doses. Those receiving a cholinergic blocking agent during the hot summer months should be observed for signs of heat prostration (fever, tachycardia, flushing, warm dry skin, mental confusion) because these drugs decrease sweating.

Administration of these drugs can result in urinary retention. Patients with an enlarged prostate are given these drugs with great caution because urinary retention may occur. This caution applies to some over-the-counter preparations available for the relief of allergy and cold symptoms and as aids to induce sleep in those who have difficulty falling asleep. Some of these products contain atropine, scopolamine, or other cholinergic blocking agents, and although this warning is given on the container or package, many users fail to read the fine print on drug labels.

Cholinergic blocking agents are also contraindicated in those with glaucoma because use of these drugs may lead to an attack of acute glaucoma. Unfortunately, glaucoma in its early stages may have few, if any, symptoms and the individual is unaware of this disorder until he or she has an eye examination. The lack of symptoms of early glaucoma plus the fact that many individuals fail to read drug labels can have serious consequences.

NURSING MANAGEMENT

Daily assessment and close observation of the patient are necessary when administering a cholinergic blocking agent. Nursing management includes checking vital signs, observing for adverse drug reactions, and evaluating the symptoms and complaints related to the patient's diagnosis. For example, question the patient with a peptic ulcer regarding current symptoms, then compare these symptoms to the symptoms present before the start of therapy. Report any increase in the severity of symptoms to the physician immediately.

The Patient With Heart Block

Place the patient receiving atropine for third degree heart block on a cardiac monitor, both during and after administration of the drug. Watch the monitor for a change in pulse rate or rhythm. Report tachycardia, other cardiac arrhythmias, or failure of the drug to increase the heart rate to the physician immediately because other drugs or medical management may be necessary.

The Patient Receiving a Preoperative Medication

If a cholinergic blocking agent is administered as a preoperative medication, instruct the patient to void before the drug is given. Inform the patient that his

or her mouth will become extremely dry, that this is normal, and that fluid is not to be taken. Raise the side rails of the bed and instruct the patient to remain in bed following administration of the preoperative medication.

> **Nursing Alert**
>
> Preoperative medication is administered at the exact time prescribed because the cholinergic blocking agent must be allowed to produce the greatest effect (ie, the drying of upper respiratory and oral secretions) before the administration of a general anesthetic. Notify the anesthesiologist if the preoperative medication is given late.

Adverse Drug Reactions

Since this group of drugs may have widespread effects, closely observe all patients for the appearance of adverse drug reactions.

Observe the elderly patient receiving a cholinergic blocking agent at frequent intervals for excitement, agitation, mental confusion, drowsiness, urinary retention, or other adverse effects. If any of these should occur, withhold the next dose of the drug and contact the physician. Ensure patient safety until these adverse reactions disappear. Cholinergic blocking agents are usually not included in the preoperative medication of patients over 60 years of age because of the effects of these agents on the eye and the central nervous system.

In hot weather, sweating may decrease and may be followed by heat prostration. Observe the patient at frequent intervals for signs of heat prostration (see Adverse Reactions), especially if the patient is elderly or debilitated. Withhold the next dose of the drug and contact the physician immediately if heat prostration is suspected.

Nursing Process
The Patient Receiving a Cholinergic Blocking Drug

■ *Assessment*

Before administration of a cholinergic blocking agent for the first time, obtain a thorough health history as well as a history of the signs and symptoms of the present disorder. The focus of the initial physical assessment depends on the reason for administering the drug. In most instances, the blood pressure, pulse, and respiratory rate are obtained. Additional assessments may include checking the stool of the patient who has a peptic ulcer for color and signs of occult blood; determining visual acuity in the patient with glaucoma; or looking for signs of dehydration and weighing the patient if prolonged diarrhea is one of the patient's symptoms.

■ *Nursing Diagnoses*

Depending on the drug, dose, and reason for administration, one or more of the following nursing diagnoses may apply to a person receiving a cholinergic blocking drug:

- **Anxiety** related to diagnosis, drug regimen, other factors (specify)
- **Altered Oral Mucous Membranes** related to drug action on mucous membranes
- **Risk for Injury** related to effect of drug
- **Altered Health Maintenance** related to inability to comprehend drug regimen
- **Risk for Ineffective Management of Therapeutic Regimen** related to indifference, lack of knowledge, other factors (specify)

■ *Planning and Implementation*

The major goals of the patient may include maintenance of oral mucous membrane integrity and an understanding of and compliance to the prescribed therapeutic regimen. To make these goals measurable, more specific criteria should be added. Additional implementation strategies can be found in the Nursing Management section.

Anxiety. Some patients may experience anxiety for reasons such as their diagnosis, impending surgery (when a preoperative cholinergic blocking agent is given as part of the preoperative medication), or necessity for prolonged drug therapy. Formulating an effective teaching plan, explaining the adverse drug effects that may need to be tolerated, and listening to the concerns of the patient can help to reduce anxiety.

Altered Oral Mucous Membranes. When taking these drugs on a daily basis, mouth dryness may be severe and extremely uncomfortable in some patients. The patient may have moderate to extreme difficulty swallowing oral drugs and food. Encouraging the patient to take a few sips of water before, as well as while, taking an oral medication and sipping water at intervals during meals may help this problem. If allowed, hard candy slowly dissolved in the mouth and frequent sips of water during the day may help relieve persistent oral dryness. Check the oral cavity daily for soreness or ulcerations.

Risk for Injury. These drugs may cause drowsiness, dizziness, and blurred vision. The patient (especially the elderly) may require assistance with ambulation. For elderly patients, as well as those experiencing visual difficulties, place items of furniture (eg, footstools, chairs, stands) that obstruct ambulatory areas against the wall. Those with photophobia may be more comfortable in a semidarkened room, especially on sunny days. Use overhead lights as little as possible. Mydriasis and cycloplegia, if they occur, may interfere with reading, watching television, and similar activities. If these drug effects upset the patient, discuss the problem with the physician. At times, these visual impairments will have to be tolerated because drug therapy cannot be changed or discontinued. Attempt to find other forms of diversional therapy such as interaction with other patients, listening to the radio, and so on.

Noncompliance and Altered Health Maintenance. In some instances, a cholinergic blocking agent may be prescribed for a prolonged period. Some patients may discontinue their medication especially if their original symptoms have been relieved. The patient and family must understand that the prescribed medication is to be taken even though symptoms have been relieved.

■ *Patient and Family Teaching*

When a cholinergic blocking drug is prescribed for outpatient use, make the patient aware of the more common adverse reactions associated with these drugs, such as dry mouth, drowsiness, dizziness, and visual impairments. Warn the patient that if drowsiness, dizziness, or blurred vision occurs, caution must be observed while driving or performing other tasks requiring alertness and good vision.

At times, some of the adverse reactions associated with the cholinergic blocking agents may be uncomfortable or distressing. Encourage the patient to discuss these problems with the physician. Suggestions to lessen the intensity of some of these adverse reactions can be made. Below is a list of adverse reactions that can be included in the teaching plan with the measures that may lessen their intensity or allow the patient to perform tasks at times when these adverse reactions are least likely to occur.

- *Photophobia*—Wear sunglasses when outside, even on cloudy days; keep rooms dimly lit; Close curtains or blinds if there is bright sunlight in the room; soft indirect lighting is usually more comfortable; schedule outdoor activities (when necessary) before the first dose of the drug is taken, such as early in the morning.

- *Dry mouth*—Take frequent sips of cool water during the day; several sips of water can be taken before oral medications; sip water frequently during meals; chew gum or dissolve hard candy in the mouth.
- *Constipation*—Drink plenty of fluids during the day; exercise if approved by physician; include foods high in fiber in the diet.
- *Heat prostration*—Avoid going outside on hot, sunny days; use fans to cool the body if the day is extremely warm; sponge the skin with cool water if other cooling measures are not available; wear loose-fitting clothes in warm weather.
- *Drowsiness*—Schedule tasks requiring alertness during times when drowsiness does not occur, such as early in the morning before the first dose of the drug is taken.

The Patient Receiving a Preoperative Medication. When one of these drugs is administered preoperatively, give the patient an explanation of the preoperative medication, that is, why the drug is being given, when the drug will be given, and when he or she is going to surgery. Allow sufficient time for the patient to void before the preoperative medication is administered. Instruct the patient to remain in bed after the preoperative medication has been given. Inform the patient and family members present at this time that drowsiness and extreme dryness of the mouth and nose will occur about 20 to 30 minutes after the drug is given. Stress the importance of remaining in bed with the side rails raised after the drug is administered.

The Patient With a Peptic Ulcer. Give the patient with a peptic ulcer a full explanation of the treatment regimen, which may include drugs and a special diet. Instruct the patient to take the drug exactly as prescribed by the physician (eg, 30 minutes before meals or between meals) to obtain the desired results. Discuss the importance of diet in the treatment of peptic ulcer. Provide a full explanation of the special diet (when ordered).

The Elderly Patient. Advise the family of an elderly patient of possible visual and mental impairments (blurred vision, confusion, agitation) that may occur during therapy with these drugs. Objects or situations that may cause falls such as throw rugs, footstools, and wet or newly waxed floors should be removed or avoided whenever possible. Alert the family of the dangers of heat prostration and what steps to take to avoid this problem. Observe the patient closely during the first few days of therapy, and notify the physician if mental changes occur.

■ *Expected Outcomes for Evaluation*
- Anxiety is reduced
- Oral mucous membranes appear normal
- Patient complies to the prescribed drug regimen
- No evidence of injury
- Patient and family demonstrate understanding of drug regimen
- Patient verbalizes importance of complying with the prescribed therapeutic regimen

Chapter Summary

- Cholinergic blocking drugs are also called anticholinergic drugs or parasympathomimetic blocking drugs. These drugs inhibit the activity of acetylcholine in parasympathetic nerve fibers. Cholinergic blocking drugs are capable of reversing the action of the cholinergic drugs. Some effects of the cholinergic blocking agents include: drowsiness, mydriasis, cycloplegia, drying of the secretions of the respiratory tract, a decrease in the secretions of the gastrointestinal tract, and an increase the pulse rate (most pronounced with atropine). The response to administration of a cholinergic drug will vary and often depends on the drug and the dose used.
- Anticholinergic drugs are useful in the treatment of peptic ulcers, as well as in the treatment of pylorospasm, renal colic, and for preanesthetic sedation. Atropine is useful in vagal-induced bradycardia and preoperatively to reduce secretions of the upper respiratory tract prior to general anesthesia.
- Some of the adverse reactions associated with the administration of the cholinergic blocking agents include: dryness of the mouth with difficulty swallowing, blurred vision, photophobia, constipation, and drowsiness. The severity of the adverse reactions are dose dependent.
- When these drugs are given to the elderly, confusion or excitement may be seen even with small doses. Those receiving a cholinergic blocking drug during the summer should be observed for signs of heat prostration because these drugs decrease sweating. These drugs can cause urinary retention. For this reason, they are given with great caution to patients with an enlarged prostate gland. These drugs are also not given to patients with glaucoma because they increase intraocular pressure and can lead to an attack of acute glaucoma.

• Daily assessment and observation of the patient receiving a cholinergic blocking agent are necessary and include checking vital signs, observing for adverse drug reactions, and evaluating the symptoms and complaints related to the patient's diagnosis. At times, some of the adverse reactions associated with the cholinergic blocking agents may be uncomfortable or distressing. Encourage the patient to discuss these problems with the physician. Suggestions to lessen the intensity of some of these adverse reactions can be made by the nurse.

Critical Thinking Exercises

1. Mr. Anthony is prescribed a cholinergic blocking drug for the treatment of peptic ulcer. In planning patient teaching for Mr. Anthony before dismissal from the hospital, what information must be included to prevent complications in therapy?

2. A nurse assistant asks you what is the purpose of preoperative medication and why patients cannot get out of bed after receiving a preoperative medication? How would you explain this to the nurse assistant?

21

Sedatives and Hypnotics

Key Terms

Hypnotic
Sedative
Soporifics

Chapter Outline

Chapter Objectives

On completion of this chapter the student will:

- *Differentiate between a sedative and a hypnotic*
- *Discuss the general drug actions of the barbiturate and nonbarbiturate sedatives and hypnotics*
- *List the general adverse reactions that may be seen with the administration of a sedative or hypnotic*
- *Describe how the nurse may assess the patient's need for a sedative or hypnotic*
- *Discuss the nursing management of a patient given a sedative or hypnotic*
- *Use the nursing process when administering a sedative or hypnotic*

Scherer JC, Roach S: INTRODUCTORY CLINICAL PHARMACOLOGY,
FIFTH EDITION © 1996 Lippincott-Raven Publishers

A *sedative* is a drug that produces a relaxing, calming effect. Sedatives are usually given during daytime hours and although they may make the patient drowsy, they usually do not produce sleep.

A *hypnotic* is a drug that induces sleep, that is, it allows the patient to fall asleep and stay asleep. Hypnotics may also be called *soporifics*. Hypnotics are given at night or hour of sleep (hs).

Sedatives and Hypnotics

Sedatives and hypnotics may be divided into two classes:

1. Barbiturates

   a. *Ultrashort-acting* (eg, thiamylal [Surital], thiopental [Pentothal]). The ultrashort-acting barbiturates are used as anesthetic agents (see Chap. 27). Single doses have a duration of 20 minutes or less.

   b. *Short-acting* (eg, secobarbital [Seconal], pentobarbital [Nembutal]). The average duration of action of the short-acting barbiturates is 3 to 4 hours.

   c. *Intermediate-acting* (eg, amobarbital [Amytal], aprobarbital [Alurate], butabarbital [Butisol]). The average duration of action of the intermediate-acting barbiturates is 6 to 8 hours.

   d. *Long-acting* (eg, phenobarbital, mephobarbital [Mebaral]). The average duration of action of the long-acting barbiturates is 10 to 16 hours.

   Summary Drug Table 21-1 gives examples of the short-, intermediate- and long-acting barbiturate sedatives and hypnotics.

2. Nonbarbiturates
   The nonbarbiturates consist of a group of nonrelated drugs and a second group called the benzodiazepines. Examples of the nonrelated group of drugs include ethchlorvynol (Placidyl) and zolpidem (Ambien). Examples of the benzodiazepines include estazolam (ProSom), flurazepam (Dalmane), and quazepam (Doral). The nonbarbiturate sedatives and hypnotics are listed in Summary Drug Table 21-2.

ACTIONS OF THE SEDATIVES AND HYPNOTICS

Barbiturates

All the barbiturates have essentially the same mode of action. Depending on the dose given, these drugs are capable of producing central nervous system (CNS) depression and mood alteration ranging from mild excitation to mild sedation, hypnosis (sleep), and deep coma. These drugs are also respiratory depressants with the degree of depression usually depending on the dose given. When used as hypnotics, the respiratory depressant effect is usually similar to that occurring during sleep.

Sleep induced by a barbiturate reduces the amount of time spent in the rapid eye movement (REM) stage (the dreaming stage) of sleep. Dreams appear to be a necessary part of sleep. When an individual is deprived of dreaming for a prolonged period, a psychosis can develop. Use of the barbiturates over time deprives an individual of the dreaming phase of sleep.

The sedative or hypnotic effects of the barbiturates diminishes after approximately 2 weeks. Persons taking these drugs for periods longer than 2 weeks may have a tendency to increase the dose to produce the desired effects (eg, sleep, sedation). Physical and psychological dependence may occur especially after prolonged use of high doses. Discontinuing a barbiturate after prolonged use may result in severe and sometimes fatal withdrawal symptoms.

Nonbarbiturates

Most of the nonbarbiturates have essentially the same mode of action as the barbiturates, that is, they depress the CNS. The nonbarbiturates have a varying effect on the respiratory rate and the time spent in rapid eye movement sleep.

The sedative or hypnotic effects of the nonbarbiturates diminishes after approximately 2 weeks. Persons taking these drugs for periods longer than 2 weeks may have a tendency to increase the dose to produce the desired effects (eg, sleep, sedation). Physical and psychological dependence may occur, especially after prolonged use of high doses; however, their addiction potential appears to be somewhat less than that of the barbiturates. Discontinuing a nonbarbiturate after prolonged use may result in mild to severe withdrawal symptoms.

Summary Drug Table 21-1. Sedatives and Hypnotics: The Barbiturates

Generic Name	Trade Name*	Uses	Adverse Reactions	Dose Ranges
amobarbital sodium	Amytal Sodium	Sedative, hypnotic, pre-anesthetic sedation	Respiratory and CNS depression, nausea, vomiting, constipation, diarrhea, bradycardia, hypotension, syncope, hypersensitivity reactions, headache	Sedative: 30–50 mg IM; hypnotic: 65–200 mg IM. May be given IV when other routes not feasible
aprobarbital	Alurate	Sedative, hypnotic	Same as amobarbital sodium	Sedative: 40 mg PO tid; hypnotic 40–160 mg PO
butabarbital	Butibel Sodium, *generic*	Sedative, hypnotic, preoperative sedation	Same as amobarbital sodium	Sedative: 15–30 mg PO tid, qid; hypnotic: 50–100 mg PO; preoperative sedation: 50–100 mg PO 60–90 min before surgery
mephobarbital	Mebaral	Sedative	Same as amobarbital sodium	32–100 mg PO tid, qid
pentobarbital sodium	Nembutal Sodium *generic*	Sedative, hypnotic	Same as amobarbital sodium	Sedative: 20 mg PO, IM tid, qid; hypnotic: 100 mg PO, IM
phenobarbital	Solfoton, Luminal Sodium, *generic*	Sedative, hypnotic, preoperative sedation	Same as amobarbital sodium	Sedative: 30–120 mg/d PO, IM, IV in 2–3 divided doses; hypnotic: 100–200 mg PO, IM, IV; preoperative sedation: 100–200 mg IM
secobarbital sodium	*generic*	Hypnotic, preoperative sedation	Same as amobarbital sodium	Hypnotic: 100–200 mg IM, 50–250 mg IV; preoperative sedation: 1 mg/kg IM, IV

*The term, *generic*, indicates the drug is available in generic form.

USES OF THE SEDATIVES AND HYPNOTICS

The primary use of the sedatives and hypnotics is to provide sedation or sleep. Sedative doses, usually given during daytime hours, may be used in the treatment of anxiety and apprehension. Patients with chronic disease may require sedation, not only to reduce anxiety, but also as adjuncts in the treatment of their disease. Although the use of barbiturates and nonbarbiturates for sedation has largely been replaced by the tranquilizers (see Chap. 25), they occasionally may be used to provide sedation before certain types of procedures, such as the administration of a local or general anesthesia or cardiac catheterization.

When a barbiturate or nonbarbiturate is used as a hypnotic, a dose larger than that required to pro-

duce sedation is given. Elderly patients may require a smaller hypnotic dose, and, in some instances, a sedative dose produces sleep. Helping the patient sleep is an important part of the management of illness. The patient is in an unfamiliar surrounding that is unlike his or her home situation. There are noises and lights at night, which often interfere with or interrupt sleep. Sleep deprivation may interfere with the healing process; therefore, a hypnotic may be given during hospitalization. These drugs may also be prescribed for short-term use as hypnotics after discharge from the hospital.

Barbiturates and nonbarbiturates are detoxified by the liver. All drugs entering the body ultimately leave the body. Some leave virtually unchanged, whereas others are transformed into other chemicals or compounds before they are eliminated. The liver is the organ that changes these and many other

Summary Drug Table 21-2. Sedatives and Hypnotics: The Nonbarbiturates

Generic Name	Trade Name*	Uses	Adverse Reactions	Dose Ranges
chloral hydrate	Noctec, *generic*	Hypnotic, sedative	Disorientation, gastric irritation, nausea, vomiting, delirium, light-headedness, vertigo, hypersensitivity reactions	Sedative: 250 mg PO tid; hypnotic 500 mg to 1 g PO
ethchlorvynol	Placidyl	Hypnotic	Vomiting, gastric upset, dizziness, blurred vision, hypotension	500–750 mg PO
ethinamate	Valmid Pulvules	Hypnotic	Paradoxical excitement, GI symptoms, skin rash	500–1000 mg PO
glutethimide	Doriden, *generic*	Hypnotic	Drowsiness, skin rash, vertigo, headache, depression, dizziness	250–500 mg PO
paraldehyde	Paral, *generic*	Sedative, hypnotic, delirium tremens	Strong, unpleasant breath	Sedative: 5–10 mL PO, rectal; hypnotic: 4–8 mL PO, 10–20 mL rectal; delirium tremens: 10–35 mL PO
propiomazine hydrochloride	Largon	Sedation: preoperative, during surgery, during labor	Dry mouth, moderate rise in blood pressure	Preoperative, during labor: 20–40 mg IM, IV; during surgery: 10–20 mg
zolpidem tartrate	Ambien	Hypnotic	Drowsiness, amnesia, dizziness, nausea, vomiting, diarrhea	5–10 mg PO
Benzodiazepines				
estazolam	ProSom	Hypnotic	Headache, heartburn, palpitations, somnolence, weakness, rash, body and joint pain, nausea, vomiting	1–2 mg PO
flurazepam	Dalmane, *generic*	Hypnotic	Same as estazolam	15–30 mg PO
quazepam	Doral	Hypnotic	Same as estazolam	7.5–15 mg PO
temazepam	Restoril, *generic*	Hypnotic	Same as estazolam	15–30 mg PO

drugs into compounds that are ultimately excreted by the kidney. Patients with liver disease are given these drugs with great caution.

In preparation for surgery, a hypnotic may be given the night before the operation. On the day of surgery, a barbiturate or nonbarbiturate may be used either alone or with other drugs as part of the preoperative medication. The anesthesiologist or surgeon selects a drug that is tailored to the patient's needs.

Paraldehyde, a nonbarbiturate, may be used in the treatment of delirium tremens and other psychiatric conditions. The barbiturates that are used as anticonvulsants are discussed in Chapter 23.

ADVERSE REACTIONS ASSOCIATED WITH THE ADMINISTRATION OF SEDATIVES AND HYPNOTICS

Barbiturates

Adverse reactions associated with barbiturate administration include the following:

CNS—somnolence, agitation, confusion, CNS depression, ataxia, nightmares, lethargy, residual sedation (drug hangover), hallucinations, paradoxical excitement

Respiratory—hypoventilation, apnea, respiratory depression, bronchospasm, laryngospasm

Gastrointestinal—nausea, vomiting, constipation, diarrhea, epigastric pain

Cardiovascular—bradycardia, hypotension, syncope

Hypersensitivity—rash, angioneurotic edema, fever, urticaria

Other—headache, liver damage

Nonbarbiturates

Adverse reactions associated with administration of the nonbarbiturates vary depending on the drug used. Some of the adverse reactions that may be seen with nonbarbiturate administration are listed in Summary Drug Table 21-2.

NURSING MANAGEMENT

Before administering a prn (whenever necessary) hypnotic, the nurse must assess the following patient needs:

1. Is the patient uncomfortable? If the reason for discomfort is pain, an analgesic rather than a hypnotic may be required.
2. Is it too early for the patient to receive the drug? Is a later hour preferred?
3. On previous nights, has the drug helped the patient sleep? If not, a different drug or dose may be needed, and the physician is consulted regarding the drug's ineffectiveness.
4. Does the patient receive a narcotic analgesic every 4 to 6 hours? A hypnotic may not be necessary because a narcotic analgesic is also capable of causing drowsiness and sleep.
5. Are there disturbances in the environment that may keep the patient awake and decrease the effectiveness of the drug?

Barbiturates have little or no analgesic action, and therefore are not given if the patient has pain and cannot sleep.

Nursing Alert

Because narcotic analgesics depress the CNS (see Chap. 16), a barbiturate or nonbarbiturate is not administered approximately 2 hours before or after administration of a *narcotic analgesic or other CNS depressant*. If the time interval between administration of a narcotic analgesic and a sedative or hypnotic is less than 2 hours, the patient may experience severe respiratory depression, bradycardia, and unresponsiveness.

If the patient has an order for a prn narcotic analgesic or other CNS depressant *and* a hypnotic, consult the physician regarding the time interval between administration of these drugs. Usually at least 2 hours should elapse between administration of a hypnotic and any other CNS depressant but this interval may vary depending on factors such as the patient's age and diagnosis.

If the patient is receiving one of these drugs for daytime sedation, assess the patient's general mental state and level of consciousness. If the patient appears sedated and difficult to awaken, withhold the drug and contact the physician as soon as possible.

Nursing Process
The Patient Receiving a Sedative or Hypnotic

■ *Assessment*

Assessment of the patient receiving a sedative or hypnotic drug depends on the reason for administration and whether the drug is given routinely or prn. Before administering a barbiturate or nonbarbiturate, the patient's blood pressure, pulse, and respiratory rate are taken and recorded.

■ *Nursing Diagnoses*

Depending on the drug, dose, and reason for administration, one or more of the following nursing diagnoses may apply to a person receiving a sedative or hypnotic drug:

● **Risk for Injury** related to sedative or hypnotic effects of drug
● **Anxiety** related to inability to sleep, other factors (specify)
● **Noncompliance** related to indifference, lack of knowledge, failure of the drug to produce sedation or sleep, other factors
● **Risk for Ineffective Management of Therapeutic Regimen** related to lack of knowledge of medication regimen, adverse drug effects, warnings regarding use of the drug

■ *Planning and Implementation*

The major goals of the patient may include sedation or sleep, reduction in anxiety, and an understanding of and compliance with the postdischarge medication regimen (when applicable). To make these goals measurable, more specific criteria must be added.

Administration. Never leave hypnotics and sedatives at the patient's bedside to be taken at a later hour. This applies to all drugs except for those specifically ordered to be left at the patient's bedside. Hypnotics and sedatives are controlled substances (see Chap. 1). Do not leave these drugs unattended in the nurses' station, hallway, or other areas to which patients, visitors, or hospital personnel have direct access. If these drugs are prepared in advance, place them in a locked cupboard until the time of administration.

Following assessment of the patient, make a decision regarding administration of the drug. This is especially true when one of these drugs is ordered to be given prn. Withhold the drug and notify the physician if any one or more vital signs significantly varies from the data base, if the respiratory rate is 10 per minute or below, or if the patient appears lethargic. In addition, determine if there are any factors (eg, noise, lights, pain, discomfort) that would interfere with sleep and whether these may be controlled or eliminated.

When giving these drugs orally, encourage the patient to drink a full glass of water with the medication. When barbiturates are administered intramuscularly, give the drug in the gluteus maximus or vastus lateralis or other areas where there is little risk of encountering a nerve trunk or major artery. Injection near or into peripheral nerves may result in permanent nerve damage. When giving oral paraldehyde, mix the drug with cold orange or tomato juice to eliminate some of the pungent taste.

When paraldehyde is ordered for rectal administration, the dose of the drug, which is usually 10 to 20 mL, is dissolved in one to two parts of oil or isotonic sodium chloride and given as a retention enema.

Risk for Injury. After administration of a hypnotic, raise the side rails and advise the patient to remain in bed and call for assistance if it is necessary to get out of bed. Patients receiving sedative doses may or may not require this safety measure, depending on the patient's response to the drug. Assess the patient receiving a sedative dose and determine what safety measures must be taken. Assess the patient receiving a hypnotic 1 to 2 hours after the drug is given to evaluate the effect of the drug.

Adverse Drug Reactions. Observe the patient for adverse drug reactions. Check elderly and debilitated patients for marked excitement, CNS depression, and confusion. If excitement or confusion occurs, observe the patient at frequent intervals (as often as every 5 to 10 minutes may be necessary) for the duration of this occurrence and institute safety measures to prevent injury. Notify the physician if the patient fails to sleep, awakens one or more times during the night, or develops an adverse drug reaction. In some instances, supplemental doses of a hyp-

notic may be ordered if the patient awakens during the night.

Excessive drowsiness and headache the morning after a hypnotic has been given ("drug hangover") may occur in some patients. Report this problem to the physician because a smaller dose or a different drug may be necessary.

Drug Dependency. If a barbiturate or nonbarbiturate has been taken for a long time, drug dependency may develop. These drugs must *never* be suddenly discontinued when there is a question of possible dependency. Symptoms of withdrawal, especially barbiturate withdrawal, can result in serious consequences, especially in those with existing diseases or disorders.

Anxiety. Many hospitalized patients find it difficult to sleep. The inability to fall asleep or stay asleep often results in varying degrees of anxiety. Reassure the patient that in most instances the drug being given will help them sleep.

Noncompliance. Sedatives and hypnotics are subject to abuse when taken on an outpatient basis. The most common abuses are increasing the dose of the drug and drinking an alcohol beverage shortly before, with, or shortly after taking the sedative or hypnotic. Sedatives and hypnotics can become less effective after they are taken for a period of time; thus, there may be a tendency to increase the dose without consulting the physician. Alcohol is a CNS depressant, as are the sedatives and hypnotics. When alcohol and a sedative or hypnotic are taken together, there is an additive effect and an increase in CNS depression, which has, on occasion, resulted in death.

To ensure compliance to the treatment regimen, emphasize the importance of *not* increasing or decreasing the dose unless a change in dosage is recommended by the physician. In addition, stress the importance of *not* repeating the dose during the night if sleep is interrupted or sleep only lasted a few hours unless the physician has approved of taking the drug more than once per night.

Emphasize the importance of not drinking alcohol while taking this drug. Stress the fact that the use of alcohol and any one of these drugs can result in serious effects. Deaths have been reported with the consumption of alcohol either with the drug or several hours before or after the drug is taken.

■ *Patient and Family Teaching*

The patient and family are given an explanation of the prescribed drug and dosage regimen, as well as situations that should be avoided.

Develop a teaching plan to include one or more of the following:

- Do not drink any alcoholic beverage 2 hours before, with, or 8 hours after taking the drug.
- If the drug appears to be ineffective, contact the physician. Do *not* increase the dose unless advised to do so by the physician.
- Notify the physician if any adverse drug reactions occur.
- The physician usually prescribes these drugs for short-term use only.
- When taken as a sedative, be aware that the drug can impair the mental and physical abilities required for performing potentially dangerous tasks, such as driving a car or operating machinery.
- Observe caution when getting out of bed at night after taking a drug for sleep. Keep the room dimly lit and remove any obstacles that may result in injury when getting out of bed. Never attempt to drive or perform any hazardous task after taking a drug intended to produce sleep.
- Over-the-counter cold, cough, or allergy medications cannot be used while taking this drug unless their use has been approved by the physician. Some of these products contain antihistamines or other drugs that also may cause mild to extreme drowsiness. Others may contain an adrenergic drug, which is a mild stimulant, and therefore will defeat the purpose of the drug.

■ *Expected Outcomes for Evaluation*

- Anxiety is reduced
- Patient obtains optimal benefit from the drug
- No evidence of injury
- Patient and family demonstrate understanding of drug regimen
- Patient verbalizes importance of complying with the prescribed therapeutic regimen
- Patient verbalizes understanding of things to avoid while taking the drug

Chapter Summary

- A *sedative* is a drug that produces a relaxing, calming effect and is usually given during daytime hours. A *hypnotic* is a drug that induces sleep.
- All the barbiturates have essentially the same mode of action. Depending on the dose given, these drugs are capable of producing CNS depression and mood alteration ranging from mild excitation to mild sedation, hypnosis (sleep), and deep coma. These drugs are also respiratory depressants with the degree of depression usually depending on the dose given.
- Most of the nonbarbiturates have essentially the same mode of action as the barbiturates.
- The primary use of the sedatives and hypnotics is to provide sedation or sleep.
- Adverse reactions associated with barbiturate administration include CNS and respiratory depression, nausea, vomiting, bradycardia, and hypersensitivity reactions. Adverse reactions associated with administration of the nonbarbiturates vary depending on the drug used.
- Before administering a prn hypnotic, the nurse must assess the following patient needs, as well as determine if other controllable factors could be interfering with sleep.
- Because narcotic analgesics depress the CNS (see Chap. 16), a barbiturate or nonbarbiturate is not administered shortly before or after administration of a narcotic analgesic or other CNS depressant.

Critical Thinking Exercises

1. Ms. Parker's husband was killed in an automobile accident and she has had trouble coping with her loss. She complains of being unable to sleep for more than an hour before she wakes. The physician prescribes a hypnotic, one capsule per night for use over the next 3 weeks. In 2 weeks she calls the physician's office and asks for a refill of her medication. What questions would you ask Ms. Parker?
2. Mr. Davidson, who is 67 years old, is to be discharged after major bowel surgery. The physician gives him a prescription for a 21 tablets of zolpidem (Ambien). When reading Mr. Davidson's chart you note that he works part time on weekends as a bartender. What would you emphasize when explaining the prescription to Mr. Davidson?
3. Mr. Allen, who is hospitalized in CCU with a myocardial infarction, is restless and tells you that although he has been able to sleep other nights while in the hospital, he is unable to sleep tonight. Although he has an order for flurazepam (Dalmane) 30 mg hs, what would you investigate prior to making a decision regarding administration of the hypnotic?

22

Central Nervous System Stimulants

Key Terms

Analeptics
Anorexiants

Chapter Outline

Chapter Objectives

On completion of this chapter the student will:

- *List the actions and uses of central nervous system stimulants*
- *Discuss the nursing implications to be considered when administering a central nervous system stimulant*
- *Use the nursing process when administering a central nervous system stimulant*

Central nervous system stimulants include the *analeptics*, drugs that stimulate the respiratory center of the central nervous system (CNS); the amphetamines; and the *anorexiants*, drugs used to suppress the appetite.

Central Nervous System Stimulants

ACTIONS OF CENTRAL NERVOUS SYSTEM STIMULANTS

Analeptics

Doxapram (Dopram) and caffeine, as caffeine and sodium benzoate, are the two analeptics used in medicine. Doxapram increases the depth of respirations by stimulating special receptors located in the carotid arteries and upper aorta. These special receptors (called chemoreceptors) are sensitive to the amount of oxygen in arterial blood. Stimulation of these receptors results in an increase in the depth of the respirations. In larger doses, doxapram increases the respiratory rate by stimulating the medulla.

Caffeine is a mild to potent CNS stimulant with the degree of its stimulating effect dependent on the dose administered. Caffeine stimulates the CNS at all levels including the cerebral cortex, the medulla, and the spinal cord. Caffeine has mild analeptic (respiratory stimulating) activity. Other actions include cardiac stimulation (which may produce tachycardia); dilatation of coronary and peripheral blood vessels; constriction of cerebral blood vessels; and skeletal muscle stimulation. Caffeine also has mild diuretic activity.

Amphetamines

The amphetamines, for example, amphetamine, dextroamphetamine (Dexedrine), and methamphetamine (Desoxyn), are sympathomimetic (ie, adrenergic) drugs that stimulate the CNS (see Chap. 17). Their drug action results in an elevation of blood pressure, wakefulness, and an increase or decrease in pulse rate. The ability of these drugs to act as anorexiants and suppress the appetite is thought to be due to their action on the appetite center in the hypothalamus.

Anorexiants

The anorexiants, for example, phentermine and phendimetrazine, are nonamphetamine drugs pharmacologically similar to the amphetamines. Like the amphetamines, their ability to suppress the appetite is thought to be due to their action on the appetite center in the hypothalamus.

USES OF CENTRAL NERVOUS SYSTEM STIMULANTS

The CNS stimulants have limited use in medicine. Examples of CNS stimulants are given in Summary Drug Table 22-1.

Analeptics

Doxapram is used in the treatment of drug-induced respiratory depression and for temporary treatment of respiratory depression in chronic pulmonary disease. This drug may also be used during the postanesthesia period when respiratory depression is due to anesthesia. It is also used to stimulate deep breathing in the postanesthesia patient.

Caffeine and sodium benzoate are administered intramuscularly or intravenously as part of the treatment of respiratory depression due to CNS depressants, such as narcotic analgesics and alcohol. Because caffeine also has other effects, such as constriction of cerebral arteries and stimulation of skeletal muscles, the use of caffeine for this purpose has largely been replaced by narcotic antagonists for respiratory depression due to narcotic overdose or other drugs with greater analeptic activity (eg, doxapram). Orally, caffeine, either as a beverage (coffee, tea) or in nonprescription tablet form, may be used by some individuals to relieve fatigue. Caffeine also may be included in some nonprescription analgesics.

Amphetamines

Amphetamines may be used in the short-term treatment of exogenous obesity, for example, obesity due to a persistent calorie intake that is greater than needed by the body. Long-term use of these drugs for obesity is not recommended because amphetamines

Summary Drug Table 22-1. Central Nervous System Stimulants

Generic Name	Trade Name*	Uses	Adverse Reactions	Dose Ranges
ANALEPTICS				
caffeine and sodium benzoate	*generic*	Respiratory depression due to overdoses of CNS depressants (alcohol, narcotics)	Tachycardia, palpitations, nausea, vomiting	500 mg to 1 g IM or slow IV injection
doxapram hydrochloride	Dopram	Drug-induced postanesthesia respiratory depression, drug-induced respiratory depression	Dizziness, headache, apprehension, disorientation, nausea, vomiting, cough, dyspnea, urinary retention	0.5–2 mg/kg IV
AMPHETAMINES				
amphetamine sulfate	*generic*	Narcolepsy, attention deficit disorder with hyperactivity, exogenous obesity	Insomnia, tachycardia, nervousness, headache, anorexia, dizziness, excitement	Narcolepsy: 5–60 mg/d PO in divided doses; attention deficit disorder: up to 40 mg/d PO; obesity; 5–30 mg/d PO in divided doses
dextroamphetamine sulfate	Dexedrine, *generic*	Same as amphetamine sulfate	Same as amphetamine sulfate	Same as amphetamine sulfate
methamphetamine hydrochloride	Desoxyn	Attention deficit disorder with hyperactivity, exogenous obesity	Same as amphetamine sulfate	Attention deficit disorder: up to 25 mg/d PO once or twice per day
ANOREXIANTS				
Diethylpropion hydrochloride	Tenuate, Tepanil, *generic*	Exogenous obesity	Same as amphetamine	25 mg PO tid ac or 2 mg PO once daily before lunch
fenfluramine hydrochloride	Pondimin	Same as diethylpropion hydrochloride	Same as amphetamine	20–40 mg PO tid ac
phentermine hydrochloride	Fastin, *generic*	Same as diethylpropion hydrochloride	Same as amphetamine	8 mg PO tid ac or 15–37.5 mg as single dose before breakfast

*The term, *generic*, indicates the drug is available in generic form.

have addiction potential. Amphetamines are also subject to abuse and because of this, their use in treating exogenous obesity has declined. These drugs may also be helpful in the management of narcolepsy, which is a disorder manifested by an uncontrollable desire to sleep during normal waking hours even though the individual has a normal nighttime sleeping pattern. Amphetamines are also used in the management of attention deficit disorder in children. This disorder is characterized by a short attention span, hyperactivity, impulsiveness, and emotional lability. How the amphetamines, which are CNS stimulants, calm the hyperactive child is unknown.

Anorexiants

Phendimetrazine and phentermine are chemically related to the amphetamines and are used for *short-term* treatment of exogenous obesity. These drugs are available only by prescription and have addiction and abuse potential. Some nonprescription diet aids contain phenylpropanolamine, an adrenergic agent that has actions similar to the adrenergic agent ephedrine. These diet aids are not true anorexiants, and those containing phenylpropanolamine have limited appetite-suppressing ability when compared to the anorexiants. Phenylpropanolamine also has little abuse potential and has no addiction potential.

ADVERSE REACTIONS ASSOCIATED WITH THE ADMINISTRATION OF CENTRAL NERVOUS SYSTEM STIMULANTS

The adverse reactions associated with the administration of doxapram include excessive CNS stimulation, symptoms of which may include headache, dizziness, apprehension, disorientation, and hyperactivity. Other adverse reactions include nausea, vomiting, cough, dyspnea, urinary retention, and variations in the heart rate. Administration of caffeine and sodium benzoate may result in tachycardia, palpitations, nausea, and vomiting.

One of the chief adverse reactions associated with the amphetamines and anorexiants is overstimulation of the CNS, which may result in a variety of adverse reactions such as insomnia, tachycardia, nervousness, headache, anorexia, dizziness, and excitement. In some instances, the intensity of these reactions are dose dependent but some individuals may experience an intense degree of these symptoms even with low doses. Other individuals experience few symptoms of CNS stimulation.

Nursing Alert

The amphetamines and anorexiants are known to have abuse and addiction potential.

The amphetamines and anorexiants are recommended only for short-term use in selected patients for the treatment of exogenous obesity. When used for treatment of attention deficit disorders in children, long-term use must be followed by gradual withdrawal of the drug.

Long-term use of amphetamines for obesity may result in tolerance to the drug and a tendency to increase the dose. Extreme psychological dependency may also occur.

NURSING MANAGEMENT

Respiratory depression can be a serious event requiring administration of a respiratory stimulant. When an analeptic is administered, note and record the rate, depth, and character of the respirations prior to administration of the drug to provide a data base for evaluation of the effectiveness of drug therapy. Oxygen is usually ordered for before and after administration of a respiratory stimulant. Following

administration, monitor the respirations closely and record the effects of therapy.

Nausea and vomiting may occur with the administration of an analeptic, therefore, a suction machine is kept nearby should vomiting occur. Urinary retention may be seen with the administration of doxapram; therefore, measure intake and output and notify the physician if the patient is unable to void or the bladder appears distended on palpation.

Nursing Process
The Patient Receiving a Central Nervous System Stimulant

■ *Assessment*
Assessment of the patient receiving a CNS stimulant depends on the drug, the patient, and the reason for administration.

Analeptics. When a CNS stimulant is prescribed for respiratory depression, initial assessments will include the blood pressure, pulse, and respiratory rate. It is important to note the depth of the respirations and any pattern to the respiratory rate, such as shallow respirations or alternating deep and shallow respirations. Also review of recent laboratory tests (if any), such as arterial blood gas studies. Before administration of the drug, an adequate airway is necessary. Oxygen is usually administered before, during, and after drug administration.

Amphetamines. When an amphetamine is prescribed for any reason, weigh the patient and take and record the blood pressure, pulse, and respiratory rate before starting drug therapy.

The child with attention deficit disorder should be initially observed for the various patterns of abnormal behavior. Record a summary of the behavior pattern in the patient's chart to provide a comparison with future changes that may occur during therapy.

Anorexiants. When an anorexiant or amphetamine is used as part of the treatment of obesity, the drug is usually prescribed for outpatient use. Obtain and record the blood pressure, pulse, respiratory rate, and weight before therapy is started.

■ *Nursing Diagnoses*
Depending on the drug, dose, and reason for administration, one or more of the following nursing diagnoses may apply to a person receiving a CNS stimulant:
- **Anxiety** related to adverse drug reactions, other factors (specify)

- **Risk for Ineffective Management of Therapeutic Regimen** related to inadequate knowledge of medication regimen

■ *Planning and Implementation*

The major goals of the patient may include a reduction in anxiety and an understanding of the medication regimen. To make these goals measurable, more specific criteria must be added.

Respiratory Depression. After administration of an analeptic, closely monitor the respiratory rate and pattern until the respirations return to normal. Monitor the level of consciousness, the blood pressure, and pulse rate at 5- to 15-minute intervals or as ordered by the physician. Arterial blood gases may be drawn at intervals to determine the effectiveness of the analeptic, as well as the need for additional drug therapy. Observe the patient for adverse drug reactions and report their occurrence immediately to the physician.

Attention Deficit Disorder. If the child is hospitalized, enter a daily summary of the child's behavior in the patient's record. This provides a record of the results of therapy.

Narcolepsy. Observe the patient with narcolepsy during daytime hours. If periods of sleep are noted, record the time of day they occur and their length. Because most of these individuals are outpatients, instruct the patient and family members to keep a record of the periods of sleep.

Weight Loss. When an amphetamine or anorexiant is prescribed for obesity, obtain the patient's weight and vital signs at the time of each outpatient visit.

Adverse Drug Reactions. The adverse drug reactions that may occur with the use of an amphetamine, such as insomnia and a significant increase in blood pressure and pulse rate, may be serious enough to require discontinuation of the drug. In some instances, the adverse drug effects are mild and may even disappear during therapy. Inform the physician of all adverse reactions.

Anxiety. Some patients or family members, for example, the patient with narcolepsy or parents of the child with an attention deficit disorder, may have concern over the prescribed drug therapy and the ability of the drug to control symptoms. Allow the patient or family member time to ask questions and to discuss the planned therapeutic regimen. If anxiety appears to be drug related, discuss this problem with the physician because it may be necessary to decrease the dosage or prescribe another drug.

■ *Patient and Family Teaching*

Explain the therapeutic regimen and adverse drug reactions to the patient and family. The type of information included in the teaching plan will depend on the drug and the reason for use. Emphasize the importance of following the recommended dosage schedule. Additional teaching points may include the following.

- Attention deficit disorder: Write a daily summary of the child's behavior including periods of hyperactivity, general pattern of behavior, socialization with others, attention span, and so on. Bring this record to each physician or clinic visit because this record may help the physician determine future drug dosages or additional treatment modalities.
- Narcolepsy: Keep a record of the number of times per day that periods of sleepiness occur, and bring this record to each physician or clinic visit.
- Amphetamines and anorexiants: These drugs are taken early in the day to avoid insomnia. Do not increase the dose or take more frequently except on the advice of a physician. These drugs may impair the ability to drive or perform hazardous tasks and may mask extreme fatigue. If dizziness, lightheadedness, anxiety, nervousness, or tremors occur, contact the physician. The use of coffee, tea, and carbonated beverages containing caffeine are avoided or taken in small amounts.
- Caffeine (oral, nonprescription): Avoid the use of oral caffeine-containing products to stay awake if there is a history of heart disease, high blood pressure, or stomach ulcers. These products are intended for occasional use and should be discontinued if heart palpitations, dizziness, or lightheadedness occurs.

■ *Expected Outcomes for Evaluation*

- Anxiety is reduced
- Patient complies to the prescribed drug regimen
- Patient and family demonstrate understanding of drug regimen
- Patient verbalizes importance of complying with the prescribed therapeutic regimen

Chapter Summary

- Central nervous system stimulants include the analeptics, drugs that stimulate the respiratory center of the CNS; the amphetamines; and the anorexiants, drugs that suppresses the appetite. The CNS stimulants have limited use in medicine.

- Doxapram (Dopram) and caffeine, as caffeine and sodium benzoate, are the two analeptics used in medicine. Doxapram increases the respiratory rate by stimulating special receptors located in the carotid arteries and upper aorta. Caffeine is a mild to potent CNS stimulant with the degree of its effect dependent on the dose administered. Caffeine stimulates the CNS at all levels.
- The amphetamines are sympathomimetic (ie, adrenergic) drugs that stimulate the CNS.
- The anorexiants are nonamphetamine drugs pharmacologically similar to the amphetamines. Like the amphetamines, their ability to suppress the appetite is thought to be due to their action on the appetite center in the hypothalamus.
- Doxapram is used in the treatment of drug-induced respiratory depression; for temporary treatment of respiratory depression in chronic pulmonary disease; during the postanesthesia period when respiratory depression is due to anesthesia; and to stimulate deep breathing in the postanesthesia patient.
- Caffeine and sodium benzoate is used in the treatment of respiratory depression due to CNS depressants, such as narcotic analgesics and alcohol. Orally, caffeine may be used to relieve fatigue.

Caffeine also may be included in some nonprescription analgesics.
- Amphetamines may be used in the short-term treatment of exogenous obesity, in the management of narcolepsy, and the management of attention deficit disorder in children. Anorexiants are used for *short-term* treatment of exogenous obesity.
- One of the chief adverse reactions associated with CNS stimulants is overstimulation of the CNS resulting in a variety of adverse reactions, such as insomnia, tachycardia, nervousness, anorexia, dizziness, and excitement.

Critical Thinking Exercises

1. Ms. Stone is given a special diet and prescribed an anorexiant to help her lose 20 pounds prior to reconstructive knee surgery. What instructions would you include in a teaching plan for this patient?
2. Mr. Trent has narcolepsy and is prescribed amphetamine 10 mg per day. What questions would you ask Mr. Trent when he returns to the clinic for evaluation following 1 month of therapy?

23

Anticonvulsant Drugs

Key Terms

Anticonvulsants
Ataxia
Convulsion
Epilepsy
Gingival hyperplasia
Nystagmus
Seizure
Status epilepticus
Tonic-clonic seizure

Chapter Outline

Chapter Objectives

On completion of this chapter the student will:

- *Describe the general drug action of anticonvulsant drugs*
- *List some of the adverse reactions associated with the administration of anticonvulsant drugs*
- *Discuss nursing management when administering an anticonvulsant drug*
- *Use the nursing process when administering an anticonvulsant drug*

The terms *convulsion* and *seizure* are often used interchangeably and basically have the same meaning. A *seizure* may be defined as a periodic attack of disturbed cerebral function. A *seizure* may also be described as an abnormal disturbance in the electrical activity in one or more areas of the brain. Seizures may be classified as partial or generalized. Partial seizures arise from a localized area in the brain and cause specific symptoms. Each different type of seizure disorder is characterized by a specific pattern of events, as well as a different pattern of motor or sensory manifestations. A partial seizure can spread to the entire brain and cause a generalized seizure. Manifestations of a generalized *tonic-clonic seizure* include alternate contraction (tonic phase) and relaxation of muscles (clonic phase), a loss of consciousness, and abnormal behavior.

Seizure disorders are generally categorized as idiopathic or acquired. Idiopathic seizures have no known cause; acquired seizure disorders have a known cause. The causes of acquired seizures include high fever, electrolyte imbalances, uremia, hypoglycemia, hypoxia, brain tumors, and some drug withdrawal reactions. Once the cause is removed (if it can be removed), the seizures theoretically cease.

Epilepsy may be defined as a permanent, recurrent seizure disorder. Examples of the known causes of epilepsy include brain injury at birth, head injuries, and inborn errors of metabolism. In some patients, the cause of epilepsy is never determined.

Anticonvulsant Drugs

Drugs used for the management of convulsive disorders are called *anticonvulsants*. Most anticonvulsants have specific uses, that is, they are of value only in the treatment of certain types of seizure disorders.

The types of anticonvulsants included in this chapter are the barbiturates, the benzodiazepines, the hydantoins, the oxazolidinediones, the succinimides, and miscellaneous anticonvulsant preparations.

ACTIONS OF THE ANTICONVULSANT DRUGS

Generally, the anticonvulsants reduce the excitability of the neurons (nerve cells) of the brain. When neuron excitability is decreased, the seizures are theoretically reduced in intensity and frequency of occurrence or, in some instances, are virtually eliminated. For some patients, only partial control of the seizure disorder may be obtained with anticonvulsant drug therapy.

USES OF THE ANTICONVULSANT DRUGS

The more common types of seizures responding to a specific anticonvulsant drug are given in Summary Drug Table 23-1. In some cases, the patient does not respond well to one drug, and another drug or a combination of anticonvulsant drugs must be tried. Dosage increases and decreases are often necessary during the initial period of treatment. Dosage adjustment may also be necessary during times of stress, severe illness, or when other drugs are being taken for treatment of conditions other than a seizure disorder. There also may be undetermined circumstances that require a dosage adjustment or a change in the anticonvulsant drug.

Occasionally, *status epilepticus* (an emergency situation characterized by continual seizure activity with no interruptions) can occur. Diazepam (Valium) is most often the initial drug prescribed for this condition. However, because the effects of diazepam last less than 1 hour, a longer lasting anticonvulsant, such as phenytoin or phenobarbital, must be given as well to control the seizure activity.

ADVERSE REACTIONS ASSOCIATED WITH ADMINISTRATION OF ANTICONVULSANT DRUGS

The Barbiturates

The most common adverse reaction associated with mephobarbital (Mebaral) and phenobarbital is sedation, which can range from mild sleepiness or drowsiness to somnolence. These drugs may also cause nausea, vomiting, constipation, bradycardia, hypoventilation, skin rash, headache, fever, and diarrhea. Agitation, rather than sedation, may occur in some patients. Some of these adverse effects may be reduced or eliminated as therapy continues. Occasionally, a slight dosage reduction, without reducing the ability of the drug to control the seizures, will reduce or eliminate some of these adverse reactions.

Summary Drug Table 23-1. Anticonvulsants

Generic Name	Trade Name*	Uses	Adverse Reactions	Dose Ranges
BARBITURATES				
mephobarbital	Mebaral	Tonic-clonic (grand mal) epilepsy, absence seizures (petit mal)	Somnolence, agitation, nausea, vomiting, constipation, bradycardia, headache, fever, diarrhea, hypoventilation, rash, drowsiness	Adult: 400–600 mg/d PO Pediatric: 16–64 mg/d PO
phenobarbital	*generic*	Status epilepticus, generalized tonic-clonic and cortical focal seizures	Somnolence, agitation, nausea, vomiting, constipation, bradycardia, headache, fever, diarrhea, hypoventilation, rash, drowsiness	Adult: 60–250 mg PO bid, tid Pediatric: 1–6 mg/kg PO bid, tid
phenobarbital sodium	Luminal *generic*	Symptomatic control of acute convulsions	Somnolence, agitation, nausea, vomiting, constipation, bradycardia, headache, fever, diarrhea, hypoventilation, rash, drowsiness	Adult: 120–800 mg IV, IM per dose with a maximum of 1–2 g/24 h Pediatric: 6–20 mg/kg IV with a maximum of 40 mg/kg/24 h
BENZODIAZEPINES				
clonazepam	Klonopin	Absence seizures, variant, akinetic, and myoclonic seizures	Drowsiness, depression, lethargy, apathy, diarrhea, constipation, dry mouth, bradycardia, tachycardia, fatigue, visual disturbances, urticaria, anorexia, rash, pruritus	Adult: 1.5–20 mg/d PO Pediatric: 0.05–0.2 mg/kg d PO in divided doses
clorazepate dipotassium	Tranxene, *generic*	Partial seizures	Dizziness, drowsiness, lethargy, rash, blurred vision, nausea, vomiting	Adult: up to 90 mg/d PO in divided doses Pediatric: up to 60 mg/d PO in divided doses
diazepam	Valium, *generic*	Adjunct in treatment of convulsive disorders	Dizziness, drowsiness, rash, lethargy, blurred vision, nausea, vomiting	Adult: 2–10 mg PO bid to qid, 15–30 mg extended release once daily Pediatric: 1–2.5 mg PO tid, qid
HYDANTOINS				
ethotoin	Peganone	Tonic-clonic, psychomotor seizures	Nystagmus, ataxia, mental confusion, thrombocytopenia, leukopenia, agranulocytosis, granulocytopenia hepatotoxicity, slurred speech, nausea, vomiting, rash	Adult: initial—1 g/d or less PO in 4–6 divided doses; maintenance—2–3 g/d PO Pediatric: initial—up to 750 mg/d PO in 4–6 divided dose; maintenance—500 mg to 3 g/d PO in divided doses
mephenytoin	Mesantoin	Tonic-clonic, jacksonian, and psychomotor seizures	Nystagmus, ataxia, mental confusion, dizziness, drowsiness, thrombocytopenia, leukopenia, agranulocytosis, granulocytopenia, slurred speech, rash, hepatotoxicity	Adult: initial—1 g/d or less PO in 4–6 divided doses; maintenance—2–3 g/d PO Pediatric: initial—up to 750 mg/d PO in 4–6 divided doses; maintenance—500 mg to 3 g/d PO in divided doses
phenytoin	Dilantin	Tonic-clonic, psychomotor seizures	Nystagmus, ataxia, mental confusion, dizziness, drowsiness, leukopenia, thrombocytopenia, agranulocytosis, pancytopenia, granulocytopenia, slurred speech, rash, gingival hyperplasia, hepatotoxicity	Adult: 100–600 mg/d PO in divided doses Pediatric: 4–8 mg/kg d PO in divided doses
phenytoin sodium, extended	Dilantin, Kapseals, *generic*	Tonic-clonic psychomotor seizures	Same as phenytoin	300 mg PO taken once a day

(continued)

Summary Drug Table 23-1 (Continued)

Generic Name	Trade Name*	Uses	Adverse Reactions	Dose Ranges
phenytoin sodium, parenteral	Dilantin, *generic*	Status epilepticus of grand mal type, prevention and treatment of seizures during neurosurgery	Same as phenytoin	Status epilepticus: 15–25 mg/kg rate not to exceed 25–50 mg/min IV; neurosurgery: 100–200 mg IM q 4h
OXAZOLIDINEDIONES				
paramethadione	Paradione	Absence seizures	Aplastic anemia, nephrosis, rash, diplopia, vomiting, hematologic changes, changes in blood pressure	Adult: 900 mg to 2.4 g/d PO in 3–4 divided doses Pediatric: 300–900 mg/d PO in 3–4 divided doses
trimethadione	Tridione	Absence seizures	Aplastic anemia, nephrosis, rash, diplopia, vomiting, hematologic changes, changes in blood pressure	Adult: 900 mg to 2.4 g/d PO in 3–4 divided doses Pediatric: 300–900 mg/d PO in 3–4 divided doses
SUCCINIMIDES				
ethosuximide	Zarontin	Absence seizures	Nausea, vomiting, gastric cramps, anorexia, confusion, pruritus, urinary frequency, weight loss, hematologic changes, urticaria	Adult: 500 mg/d PO up to 1–5 g/d Pediatric: 250 mg/d up to 1 g/d
methsuximide	Celontin Kapseals	Absence seizures	Nausea, vomiting, gastric cramps, anorexia, confusion, pruritus, urinary frequency, weight loss, hematologic changes, urticaria	300 mg to 1.2 g/d PO
phensuximide	Milontin Kapseals	Absence seizures	Nausea, vomiting, gastric cramps, anorexia, confusion, pruritus, urinary frequency, weight loss, hematologic changes, urticaria	1–3 g/d PO in divided doses
MISCELLANEOUS PREPARATIONS				
acetazolamide	Diamox, *generic*	Absence seizures, unlocalized seizures, adjunct in tonic-clonic seizures	Paresthesias, fever, rash, crystalluria, acidotic state, anorexia, nausea, vomiting	250–1000 mg/d PO in divided doses
carbamazepine	Tegretol, *generic*	Partial seizures, tonic-clonic seizures, mixed seizure patterns	Dizziness, drowsiness, nausea, vomiting, aplastic anemia, and other blood cell abnormalities	200–1200 mg/d PO in divided doses
lamotrigine	Lamictal	Epilepsy	Dizziness, diplopia, ataxia, blurred vision, nausea, vomiting, headache	No more than 150 mg day bid
magnesium sulfate	*generic*	Prevention and control of seizures in preeclampsia or eclampsia and convulsions associated with epilepsy	High magnesium blood levels with flushing, sweating, depressed reflexes, hypotension, cardiac and CNS depression	1–5 g of 25–50% solution IM; 1–4 g of 10–20% solution IV; 4 g in 250 mL of 5% dextrose by IV infusion
phenacemide	Phenurone	Severe epilepsy	GI disturbances, headache, drowsiness, dizziness, insomnia, weight loss	Adult: 2–3 g/d PO in divided doses; starting dose may be lower Pediatric: ½ the adult dose
primidone	Mysoline, *generic*	Psychomotor, focal, tonic-clonic seizures	Ataxia, vertigo, nausea, anorexia, vomiting, drowsiness, headache	Adult: 100–250 mg PO 1–4 times/d Pediatric: 50–250 mg PO 1–3 times/d
valproic acid	Depakene, *generic*	Simple and complex absence seizures, multiple seizure types	Nausea, vomiting, sedative effects, rash, indigestion, nystagmus, diplopia	15–60 mg/kg/d PO in single or divided doses

*The term, *generic,* indicates that the drug is available in generic form.

The Benzodiazepines

As with the barbiturates, the most common adverse reaction seen with the use of clonazepam (Klonopin), clorazepate (Tranxene), and diazepam (Valium) is sedation in varying degrees. Additional adverse effects may include anorexia, constipation, or diarrhea. Some adverse reactions are dose-dependent, whereas others may diminish in intensity or cause few problems after several weeks of therapy.

The Hydantoins

Many adverse reactions are associated with the use of ethotoin (Peganone), mephenytoin (Mesantoin), and phenytoin (Dilantin). Phenytoin is the most commonly prescribed anticonvulsant. The adverse reactions most often seen with the hydantoins are related to the central nervous system and *nystagmus* (constant, involuntary movement of the eyeball); *ataxia* (loss of control of voluntary movements, especially gait); slurred speech; and mental changes. Other adverse reactions that may be seen include various types of skin rashes, nausea, vomiting, *gingival hyperplasia* (overgrowth of gum tissue), hematologic changes (changes relating to the blood or blood-forming tissue), and hepatotoxicity. Some of these adverse reactions diminish with continuous use of the hydantoins.

The Oxazolidinediones

Paramethadione (Paradione) and trimethadione (Tridione) administration may result in hematologic changes, such as pancytopenia, leukopenia, aplastic anemia, and thrombocytopenia. Also reported are various types of skin rashes, diplopia (double vision), vomiting, changes in blood pressure, and fatal nephrosis. Because these drugs have been associated with fetal malformations and serious adverse reactions, they should be used only when other less toxic drugs are not effective in controlling seizures.

The Succinimides

Gastrointestinal symptoms occur frequently with the administration of ethosuximide (Zarontin), methsuximide (Celontin Kapseals), and phensuximide (Milontin Kapseals). Mental confusion and

other personality changes, pruritus, urticaria, urinary frequency, weight loss, and hematologic changes may also be seen.

Miscellaneous Anticonvulsant Drugs

The adverse reactions seen with the various miscellaneous anticonvulsants are given in Summary Drug Table 23-1.

NURSING MANAGEMENT

Anticonvulsants control but do not cure epilepsy. The dosage of the anticonvulsant may require frequent adjustments during the initial treatment period. Dosage adjustments are based on the patient's response to therapy (eg, the control of the seizures), as well as the occurrence of adverse reactions. Depending on the patient's response to therapy, a second anticonvulsant may be added to the therapeutic regimen or one anticonvulsant may be changed to another. Observations related to the patient's seizures, as well as response to drug therapy, are of utmost importance when a hospitalized patient is receiving an anticonvulsant. Careful documentation of each seizure with regard to the time of occurrence, the length of the seizure, and the psychic or motor activity occurring before, during, and after the seizure is essential. Most seizures occur without warning and the nurse may not see the patient until after the seizure begins or after the seizure is over. Any observations made during and after the seizure are important and may aid in the diagnosis of the type of seizure, as well as assist the physician in evaluating the effectiveness of drug therapy.

Do not miss or omit a dose of an anticonvulsant drug (except by order of the physician). An abrupt interruption in therapy may result in a recurrence of the seizures. In some instances, abrupt withdrawal of an anticonvulsant can result in *status epilepticus*, which is a state of continuous seizures that can become life-threatening. Continuity of anticonvulsant administration is aided by making a notation on the care plan, as well as by informing all health team members of the importance of the medication.

ADMINISTRATION

To prevent gastric upset, give oral anticonvulsant drugs with food or soon after eating. Oral suspensions are shaken well before measuring. Caution is used when giving an oral preparation if the patient appears drowsy because aspiration of the tablet, capsule, or liquid may occur. Test the swallowing ability of the patient by offering *small* sips of water before giving the drug. Withhold the drug and notify the physician as soon as possible if the patient has difficulty in swallowing. If this occurs, a different route of administration may be necessary.

The Barbiturates

The barbiturate phenobarbital (Luminal) is commonly use in the treatment of convulsive disorders. When administering the barbiturates by the intravenous (IV) route, do not exceed at rate of 60 mg per minute and administer within 30 minutes of preparation. Monitor blood pressure and respirations frequently. The barbiturates can produce a hypersensitivity rash. Should a skin rash occur, notify the physician immediately.

The Benzodiazepines

The dosage of the benzodiazepines is highly individualized and must be increased cautiously to avoid adverse reactions, particularly in elderly and debilitated patients.

Intravenous diazepam may bring seizures quickly under control. However, patients may have a return of seizure activity due to the short duration of the effects of the drug. Be prepared to readminister the drug. Do not mix diazepam with other drugs and give by IV push only. Inject IV diazepam slowly, allowing at least 1 minute for each 5 mg of drug. The IV route is the preferred route for the convulsing patient but the drug may be given intramuscularly as well.

The Hydantoins

The hydantoin, phenytoin is the most commonly prescribed anticonvulsant due to its effectiveness and relatively low toxicity. However, a genetically linked limitation to metabolize phenytoin has been identified. For this reason, serum concentrations of the drug must be monitored on a regular basis to detect signs of toxicity.

Nursing Alert

Monitor continuously for the following signs of drug toxicity with the administration of phenytoin: slurred speech, ataxia, lethargy dizziness, nausea, and vomiting. Phenytoin plasma levels between 10 and 20 mcg/mL give optimal anticonvulsant effect. Levels greater than 20 mcg/mL are associated with toxicity.

Monitor the vital signs daily or as ordered. Observe and report any adverse drug reactions or signs of toxicity to the physician immediately.

Abrupt withdrawal of any anticonvulsant drug may precipitate status epilepticus. The dosage must be gradually withdrawn or another anticonvulsant substituted gradually.

Be alert to the signs of blood dyscrasias, such as sore throat, fever, general malaise, bleeding of the mucous membranes, epistaxis (bleeding from the nose), and easy bruising. Report these reactions to the physician immediately.

Hypersensitivity reactions and Stevens-Johnson syndrome (a serious, sometimes fatal inflammatory disease) have been reported. Therefore, notify the physician immediately if a skin rash occurs.

The hydantoins have an effect on the blood glucose levels. These drugs can have an inhibitory effect on the release of insulin in the body, causing hyperglycemia. Blood glucose levels should be monitored closely, particularly in diabetic patients. Report any abnormalities to the physician.

The Oxazolidinediones

The oxazolidinediones are used only when other less toxic drugs have not been effective in controlling the seizure disorder since they have been associated with fetal abnormalities and serious adverse reactions. Leukopenia, thrombocytopenia, pancytopenia, and agranulocytosis have occurred. The following adverse reactions must be reported to the physician immediately: sore throat, fever, malaise, easy bruising, or epistaxis (bleeding from the nose).

Since photosensitivity can occur, keep the patient out of the sun and use sunscreen and protective clothing until individual effects of the drug are known.

The Succinimides

The succinimides are easily absorbed in the gastrointestinal tract and are effective in controlling absence or petit mal seizures.

These drugs are given with food to prevent gastrointestinal upset. Be alert for signs of blood dyscrasias, such as the presence of fever, sore throat, and general malaise. Report any of these symptoms immediately since fatal blood dyscrasias have occurred.

Symptoms of overdosage include confusion, sleepiness, unsteadiness, flaccid muscles, slow shallow respirations, nausea, vomiting, hypotension, absent reflexes, and CNS depression leading to coma; symptoms should be reported to the physician immediately. Therapeutic serum blood levels of ethosuximide (Zarontin) range from 40 to 100 mcg per mL.

Miscellaneous Anticonvulsant Drugs

Valproic acid (Depakene) is unrelated chemically to the other anticonvulsants. This drug is absorbed rapidly when taken orally. Tablets should not be chewed but swallowed whole to avoid irritation to the mouth and throat. The capsules may be opened and the drug sprinkled on a small amount of food, such as pudding or applesauce. This mixture must be swallowed whole immediately and *not* chewed.

Nursing Process
The Patient Receiving an Anticonvulsant Drug

■ *Assessment*
Seizures that occur in the outpatient are almost always seen first by family members or friends rather than by a member of the medical profession. The occurrence of abnormal behavior patterns or convulsive movements usually prompts the patient to visit the physician's office or a neurologic clinic. A thorough patient history is necessary to identify the type of seizure disorder. Information obtained from those who have observed the seizure should include the following:
- A description of the seizures (the motor or psychic activity occurring during the seizure)
- The frequency of the seizures (approximate number per day)
- The average length of a seizure

- A description of an aura (a subjective sensation preceding a seizure) if any has occurred
- A description of the degree of impairment of consciousness
- A description of what, if anything, appears to bring on the seizure

Additional patient information should include a family history of seizures (if any) and recent drug therapy (all drugs being presently used). Depending on the type of seizure disorder, other information may also be needed, for example, a history of a head injury or a thorough medical history.

Take vital signs at the time of the initial assessment to provide baseline data. The physician may order many laboratory and diagnostic tests, such as an electroencephalogram, computed tomographic scan, complete blood count, and hepatic and renal function tests to confirm the diagnosis and identify a possible cause of the seizure disorder, as well as to provide a baseline during therapy with anticonvulsant drugs.

■ *Nursing Diagnoses*
Depending on the patient and type of seizure disorder, one or more of the following nursing diagnoses may apply to a person receiving an anticonvulsant drug:
- **Anxiety** related to diagnosis, lifetime medication, other factors
- **Risk for Injury** related to seizure disorder, adverse drug reactions (drowsiness, ataxia)
- **Altered Oral Mucous Membranes** related to adverse drug reactions (hydantoins)
- **Risk for Ineffective Management of Therapeutic Regimen** related to indifference, lack of knowledge, other factors

■ *Planning and Implementation*
The major goals of the patient may include a reduction in anxiety, absence of injury, normal oral mucous membranes, and an understanding of and compliance to the prescribed therapeutic regimen. To make these goals measurable, more specific criteria must be added.

Anxiety. The patient and family members are often distressed when epilepsy is first diagnosed. In addition, the development of a seizure disorder due to a known cause, for example, uremia, causes apprehension for the patient and family. Patients and their families need time to adjust to the diagnosis, as well as the opportunity to discuss treatment, expected results of treatment, and long-term management (epilepsy).

Assure the patient and the family that epilepsy is controllable when drug therapy is managed properly. Most patients are able to maintain a normal life-style with few modifications.

Altered Oral Mucous Membranes. Long-term administration of the hydantoins can cause gingivitis and gingival hyperplasia (overgrowth of gum tissue). Periodically inspect the teeth and gums of patients in a hospital or long-term clinical setting who are receiving one of these drugs. Report any changes in the gums or teeth to the physician. Give oral care after each meal.

Risk for Injury. Drowsiness is common, especially early in therapy. Assist the patient with all ambulatory activities. Take precautions to prevent falls and other injuries until seizures are controlled by medication. Injury may also occur when the patient has a seizure.

■ *Patient and Family Teaching*

If the patient is diagnosed as having epilepsy, understanding and assistance in adjusting to the diagnosis are need by the patient and the family.

Instruct family members in the care of the patient before, during, and after a seizure. Explain the importance of restricting some activities until the seizures are controlled by medication. Restriction of activities often depend on the age, sex, and occupation of the patient. For example, advise the mother with a seizure disorder and a newborn infant to have help when caring for her child. Another example would be to warn the carpenter about climbing ladders or using power tools. For some patients, the restriction of activities may create a problem with employment, management of the home environment, caring for children, and so on. If a problem is recognized, a referral may be needed to a social service worker, discharge planning coordinator, or public health nurse.

Review the adverse drug reactions associated with the prescribed anticonvulsant with the patient and family members. If any adverse reactions occur, instruct the patient and family members to contact the physician before the next dose of the drug is due. The drug is not stopped until the problem is discussed with the physician.

Some patients, once their seizures are under control (eg, stop occurring or occur less frequently), may have a tendency to stop their medication abruptly or begin to omit a dose occasionally. The patient and the family need to understand that the medication

must *never* be abruptly discontinued or doses omitted. If the patient experiences drowsiness during initial therapy, a family member should be responsible for administration of the medication.

Include the following points in a patient and family teaching plan:

• Do *not* omit, increase, or decrease the prescribed dose.
• Stress the importance of having anticonvulsant blood levels monitored at regular intervals even if the seizures are well controlled.
• Never abruptly discontinue this drug except when recommended by the physician.
• If the physician finds it necessary to stop the drug, another drug usually is prescribed and should be started immediately, for example, at the time the next dose of the previous drug was due.
• This drug may cause drowsiness or dizziness. Observe caution when performing hazardous tasks.
• Avoid the use of alcohol unless use has been approved by the physician.
• Carry identification, such as Medic-Alert, indicating medication use and the type of seizure disorder.
• Do *not* use *any* nonprescription drug unless use of a specific drug has been approved by the physician.
• Inform the dentist and other physicians of use of this drug.
• Brush and floss the teeth after each meal and make periodic dental appointments for oral examination and care. (Note: this should be emphasized when the hydantoins are prescribed.)
• Keep a record of all seizures (date, time, length), as well as any minor problems (such as drowsiness, dizziness, lethargy, and so on) and bring this information to each clinic or office visit.
• Contact the local branches of agencies, such as the Epilepsy Foundation of America, for information and assistance with problems such as legal matters, insurance, driver's license, low cost prescription services, and job training or retraining.

■ *Expected Outcomes for Evaluation*

• Anxiety is reduced
• No evidence of injury
• Oral mucous membranes appear normal
• Patient verbalizes importance of complying with the prescribed treatment regimen
• Patient verbalizes an understanding of treatment modalities and importance of continued follow-up care
• Patient and family demonstrate understanding of drug regimen

Chapter Summary

- A seizure or convulsion is defined as an abnormal disturbance in the electrical activity in one or more areas of the brain. Seizures may be classified as partial or generalized. Partial seizures arise from a localized area in the brain and cause specific symptoms. Each different type of seizure disorder is characterized by a specific pattern of events, as well as a different pattern of motor or sensory manifestations. Partial seizure activity can spread to the entire brain and cause a generalized seizure. Epilepsy may be defined as a permanent, recurrent seizure disorder.

- Anticonvulsants drugs are prescribed for the management of seizures. The goal of anticonvulsant therapy is to control or prevent seizures. For some patients, anticonvulsants must be taken throughout their entire lives. Types of anticonvulsants include: the **barbiturates,** the **benzodiazepines,** the **hydantoins,** the **oxazolidinediones,** the **succinimides,** and **miscellaneous anticonvulsant preparations.**

- The anticonvulsants act to reduce the excitability of the nerve cells of the brain, thereby reducing the seizure activity in both intensity and frequency of occurrence. In some instances, seizures are virtually eliminated. For some patients, only partial control of the seizure disorder may be obtained with anticonvulsant drug therapy.

- The dosage of the anticonvulsant is highly individualized and based on the patient's response and the occurrence of adverse reactions. Frequent adjustments during the initial treatment period may be necessary. During the course of therapy, frequent monitoring of plasma blood levels of the drug is necessary to maintain a therapeutic level. Signs of toxicity with the hydantoins include: slurred speech, ataxia, lethargy, dizziness, nausea, and vomiting. Phenytoin plasma levels between 10 and 20 mcg/mL give optimal anticonvulsant effects. Levels greater that 20 mcg/mL are associated with toxicity.

- Patients receiving the anticonvulsants are monitored closely for response to the drug regimen, the appearance of any adverse reactions, seizure activity, and signs of toxicity. Patient and family teaching is important and focuses on helping the patient understand the diagnosis and the drug regimen. Family members are instructed in the care of the patient before, during, and after a seizure. Most patients can maintain a normal lifestyle with strict adherence to the medication regimen.

Critical Thinking Exercises

1. Ms. Taylor tells you that since she has been taking Dilantin she has had no seizures. In fact, she states that she has omitted one or two doses over the last month because she is "doing so well." What is your response to Ms. Taylor's statement?

2. Mr. Parks, age 32, has recently been diagnosed with epilepsy. He has been taking the anticonvulsant carbamazepine, but his seizures are not yet under control. Mr. Parks asks you how long it will take to "cure" his epilepsy. How would you respond to Mr. Parks?

24

Antiparkinsonism Drugs

Key Terms

Blood-brain barrier
Choreiform movements
Dystonic movements
Parkinson's disease
Parkinsonism

Chapter Outline

Chapter Objectives

On completion of this chapter the student will:

- *Define the terms Parkinson's disease and parkinsonism*
- *List the major adverse reactions associated with the administration of antiparkinsonism drugs*
- *Discuss nursing management when administering an antiparkinsonism drug*
- *Use the nursing process when administering an antiparkinsonism drug*

Parkinson's disease, also called paralysis agitans, is thought to be due to a deficiency of dopamine and an excess of acetylcholine within the central nervous system. This disease is characterized by fine tremors, and rigidity of some muscle groups and weakness of others. As the disease progresses, speech becomes slurred. There is a masklike and emotionless expression of the face and the patient may have difficulty chewing and swallowing. The patient may have a shuffling and unsteady gait and the upper part of the body is bent forward. The fine tremors begin in the fingers with a pill-rolling movement, increase with stress, and decrease with purposeful movement.

There is no cure for Parkinson's disease but the antiparkinsonism drugs are used to relieve the symptoms and assist in maintaining the patient's mobility and functioning capability as long as possible.

Antiparkinsonism Drugs

Parkinsonism is a term that refers to the symptoms of Parkinson's disease, as well as the Parkinson-like symptoms that may be seen with the use of certain drugs, head injuries, and encephalitis. Drugs used to treat the symptoms associated with parkinsonism are called antiparkinsonism drugs.

ACTIONS OF ANTIPARKINSONISM DRUGS

Levodopa (Larodopa). The symptoms of parkinsonism are due to a depletion of dopamine in the central nervous system. Although not clearly understood, the *blood-brain barrier* is a term used to describe the apparent ability of the nervous system to prohibit large and potentially harmful molecules from crossing into the brain. Dopamine, when given orally, does not cross the blood-brain barrier and therefore is ineffective. Levodopa, the metabolic precursor of dopamine, does cross the blood-brain barrier and is then converted to dopamine. This has important implications for drug therapy because some drugs are able to pass through the blood-brain barrier more easily than others. The pharmacologic effect of levodopa on Parkinson's disease is possible because levodopa is able to cross the blood-brain barrier.

Carbidopa (Lodosyn). Carbidopa is used with levodopa and has no effect when given alone. Administration of carbidopa with levodopa makes more levodopa available to cross the blood-brain barrier, thus reducing the dosage of levodopa.

Drugs with Anticholinergic Activity. Drugs with anticholinergic activity inhibit acetylcholine (a neurohormone produced in excess in Parkinson's disease) in the central nervous system. Drugs with anticholinergic activity are generally less effective than levodopa. Examples of drugs with anticholinergic activity include procyclidine (Kemadrin) and trihexyphenidyl (Artane).

Amantadine (Symmetrel) and Selegiline (Eldepryl). The mechanism of action of these drugs in the treatment of parkinsonism is not fully understood.

USES OF ANTIPARKINSONISM DRUGS

As the term indicates, antiparkinsonism drugs are used in the treatment of parkinsonism. As with some other types of drugs, it may be necessary to change from one antiparkinsonism drug to another or to increase or decrease the dosage until maximum response is obtained (Summary Drug Table 24-1). Carbidopa is always given with levodopa, either as one medication or as two separate drugs. When it is necessary to titrate the dose of carbidopa, both carbidopa and levodopa may be given *at the same time* but as separate drugs. Selegiline is given to those being treated with carbidopa and levodopa but who have had a decreased response to therapy with these two drugs. Amantadine is also used as an antiviral agent (see Chap. 13)

ADVERSE REACTIONS ASSOCIATED WITH THE ADMINISTRATION OF ANTIPARKINSONISM DRUGS

Levodopa. The most serious and frequent adverse reactions seen with levodopa include *choreiform movements* (involuntary muscular twitching of the limbs or facial muscles), and *dystonic movements* (muscular spasms most often affecting the tongue, jaw, eyes, and neck). Less frequent but serious reactions include mental changes, such as depression, psychotic episodes, paranoia, and suicidal

Summary Drug Table 24-1. Antiparkinsonism Drugs

Generic Name	Trade Name*	Uses	Adverse Reactions	Dose Ranges
DRUGS WITH ANTICHOLINERGIC ACTIVITY				
benztropine mesylate	Cogentin, *generic*	Adjunctive treatment in all forms of Parkinsonism	Skin rash, urticaria, dry eyes, dry mouth, blurred vision, urinary retention, dysuria, muscle weakness, confusion	0.5–6 mg/d PO in divided doses, IV, IM, initially 2 mg, then 1–2 mg PO bid
biperiden	Akineton	Adjunctive treatment in all forms of Parkinsonism, drug-induced, extrapyramidal effects	Skin rash, urticaria, dry eyes, dry mouth, blurred vision, urinary retention, dysuria, muscle weakness, confusion	2 mg PO 1–4 times/d not to exceed 16 mg/d, 2 mg IM, IV
diphenhydramine	Benadryl, *generic*	Parkinsonism, drug-induced extrapyramidal reactions	Drowsiness, dry mouth, anorexia, blurred vision, dysuria, palpitations	25–50 mg PO 3–4 times/d; 10–100 mg IM, IV
ethopropazine hydrochloride	Parsidol	Adjunctive treatment in all forms of Parkinsonism	Skin rash, urticaria, dry eyes, dry mouth, blurred vision, urinary retention, dysuria, muscle weakness, confusion	50–600 mg/d PO in single or divided doses
procyclidine	Kemadrin	Parkinsonism, drug-induced extrapyramidal effects	Skin rash, urticaria, dry eyes, dry mouth, blurred vision, urinary retention, dysuria, muscle weakness, confusion	2.5–5 mg PO tid
trihexyphenidyl hydrochloride	Artane, *generic*	Adjunctive treatment in all forms of Parkinsonism	Skin rash, urticaria, dry eyes, dry mouth, blurred vision, urinary retention, dysuria, muscle weakness, confusion	1–15 mg/d PO in divided

(continued)

tendencies. Frequent and less serious adverse reactions include anorexia, nausea, vomiting, abdominal pain, dry mouth, difficulty in swallowing, increased hand tremor, headache, and dizziness.

Carbidopa. In recommended doses, carbidopa has no drug activity unless it is given with levodopa. The only adverse reactions seen with this drug are those seen with levodopa.

Drugs With Anticholinergic Activity. Frequently seen adverse reactions to drugs with anticholinergic activity include dry mouth, blurred vision, dizziness, mild nausea, and nervousness. These may become less pronounced as therapy progresses. Other adverse reactions may include skin rash, urticaria (hives), urinary retention, dysuria, tachycardia, muscle weakness, disorientation, and confu-

sion. If any of these reactions are severe, the drug may be discontinued for several days and restarted at a lower dosage or a different antiparkinsonism agent may be prescribed.

Amantadine. The most frequent serious adverse reactions to amantadine are depression, congestive heart failure, orthostatic hypotension, psychosis, urinary retention, convulsions, leukopenia, and neutropenia. Less serious reactions include hallucinations, confusion, anxiety, anorexia, nausea, and constipation. This drug may be given alone or in combination with an antiparkinsonism agent with anticholinergic activity.

Selegiline. Nausea, hallucinations, confusion, depression, loss of balance, and dizziness may be seen with the use of this drug.

Summary Drug Table 24-1 (Continued)

Generic Name	Trade Name*	Uses	Adverse Reactions	Dose Ranges
OTHER DRUGS				
amantadine hydrochloride	Symmetrel, *generic*	All forms of parkinsonism; influenza A respiratory tract illness	Depression, congestive heart failure, orthostatic hypotension, psychosis, urinary retention, confusion, nausea, ataxia	Parkinsonism: 100–400 mg/d PO in divided doses; influenza: 100 mg bid
carbidopa	Lodosyn	Given with levodopa for all forms of parkinsonism	None; adverse reactions when used with levodopa	Maximum daily dose 200 mg PO; used as a single agent when individualized titrations of carbidopa and levodopa are necessary
carbidopa and levodopa	Sinemet 10/100, Sinemet 25/100, Sinemet 25/250	Parkinsonism	Due to levodopa (see below)	1 tablet 3–4 times/d PO
levodopa	Dopar, Larodopa, *generic*	Parkinsonism	Choreiform or dystonic movements, anorexia, nausea, vomiting, abdominal pain, dysphagia, dry mouth, mental changes, headache, dizziness, increased hand tremor	0.5–8 g/d PO in divided doses
pergolide mesylate	Permax	Adjunctive treatment to carbidopa and levodopa therapy	Nausea, dyskinesia, dizziness, hallucinations, somnolence, insomnia, peripheral edema, constipation	Up to 5 mg/d PO in divided doses
selegiline hydrochloride	Eldepryl	Parkinson patients being treated with carbidopa and levodopa who have a decreased response to these drugs	Nausea, hallucinations, confusion, depression, loss of balance, dizziness	10 mg/d PO in divided doses; dose may be reduced if response is adequate

*The term, *generic*, indicates that the drug is available in a generic form.

NURSING MANAGEMENT

Effective management of the patient with parkinsonism requires careful monitoring of the drug therapy, physiological support, and a strong emphasis on patient and family teaching.

Evaluate the patient's response to drug therapy by neurologic observations. Compare the neurologic observations to the data obtained during the initial physical assessment. Although drug response may occur slowly in some patients, these observations aid the physician in adjusting the dosage of the drug upward or downward to obtain the desired therapeutic results.

These drugs are used to treat the parkinsonism that may occur with the administration of some of the psychotherapeutic drugs (see Chap. 25). When used for this purpose, the antiparkinsonism drugs

may exacerbate mental symptoms and precipitate a psychosis. Observe the patient's behavior at frequent intervals and if sudden behavioral changes are noted, withhold the next dose of the drug and immediately notify the physician.

Nursing Alert

Observe patients receiving levodopa or carbidopa *and* levodopa, for the occurrence of choreiform and dystonic movements, such as facial grimacing, protruding tongue, exaggerated chewing motions and head movements, and jerking movements of the arms and legs. If these occur, withhold the next dose of the drug and notify the physician because it may be necessary to reduce the dosage of levodopa or discontinue the drug.

The "on-off phenomenon" may occur in patients taking levodopa. This is a condition where the patient may suddenly alternate between improved clinical status and loss of therapeutic effect. Should this occur, the physician may order a "drug holiday" which includes complete withdrawal of levodopa for 5 to 14 days, followed by gradually restarting the drug at a lower dose.

Adverse Drug Reactions

Observe the patient daily for the development of adverse reactions. Report all adverse reactions to the physician because a dosage adjustment or change to a different antiparkinsonism drug may be necessary with the occurrence of the more serious adverse reactions. Some adverse reactions, although not serious, may be uncomfortable. An example of a less serious but uncomfortable adverse reaction is dryness of the mouth, which may be relieved by offering frequent sips of water, ice chips, or hard candy (if allowed).

Some patients with parkinsonism communicate poorly and do not tell the physician or nurse that problems are occurring. Observe the patient with parkinsonism for outward changes that may indicate one or more adverse reactions. For example, a sudden change in the facial expression or changes in posture may indicate abdominal pain or discomfort, which may be due to urinary retention, paralytic ileus, or constipation. Sudden changes in behavior may indicate hallucinations, depression, or other psychotic episodes. Visual difficulties (eg, adverse reactions of blurred vision, diplopia, and so on) may be evidenced by the patient's sudden refusal to read or watch television or by bumping into objects when ambulating. Any sudden changes in the patient's behavior or activity are carefully evaluated and then reported to the physician.

Nursing Process
The Patient Receiving an Antiparkinsonism Drug

■ Assessment

Because of memory impairment and alterations in thinking in some patients with parkinsonism, a history obtained from the patient may be unreliable. When necessary, obtain the history from a family member or relative and be sure to include information regarding the symptoms of the disorder; the

length of time the symptoms have been present; the ability of the patient to carry on activities of daily living; and the patient's present mental condition (eg, impairment in memory, signs of depression or withdrawal, and so on).

Before starting drug therapy; perform a physical assessment to provide a baseline for future evaluations of drug therapy. Include an evaluation of the patient's neurologic status. The neurologic evaluation includes observation for the following:

- Tremors of the hands or head while the patient is at rest
- A masklike facial expression
- Changes (from the normal) in walking
- The type of speech pattern (halting, monotone)
- Postural deformities
- Muscular rigidity
- Drooling, difficulty in chewing or swallowing
- Changes in thought processes
- Ability of the patient to carry out any or all of the activities of daily living (bathing, ambulating, dressing, and so on)

■ Nursing Diagnoses

Depending on the degree of severity and the individual, one or more of the following nursing diagnoses may apply to the patient receiving an antiparkinsonism drug:

- **Anxiety** related to diagnosis, therapeutic regimen, other factors
- **Risk for Injury** related to parkinsonism, adverse drug reactions (dizziness, lightheadedness, loss of balance)
- **Risk for Ineffective Management of Therapeutic Regimen** related to lack of knowledge, indifference, inability to assume responsibility for the prescribed drug therapy, other factors

■ Planning and Implementation

The major goals of the patient may include a reduction in anxiety, absence of injury, and an understanding of and compliance to the prescribed therapeutic regimen. More specific criteria must be added to make these goals measurable. Additional strategies for implementation may be found under Nursing Management.

Anxiety. The patient with early signs of Parkinson's disease may exhibit anxiety over the diagnosis, as well as the ability of medication to control symptoms. Allow patients time to discuss the prescribed medication regimen and ask questions about their drug therapy. Assure patients that the physician will closely monitor their drug therapy and that it may be several weeks or more before a relief of symptoms occur.

Risk for Injury. The patient with parkinsonism may have difficulty in ambulating. Adverse reactions such as dizziness, muscle weakness, and ataxia (lack of muscular coordination) may further increase difficulty with ambulatory activities. Assist the patient in getting out of the bed or a chair, walking, and other self-care activities; these individuals are especially prone to falls and other accidents due to their disease process and possible adverse drug reactions.

■ *Patient and Family Teaching*

Evaluate the patient's ability to understand the therapeutic drug regimen, ability to care for himself or herself in the home environment, and ability to comply with the prescribed drug therapy. If any type of assistance is needed, provide a referral to the discharge planning coordinator or social service worker.

If the patient requires supervision or help with daily activities and his or her medication regimen, encourage the family to create a home environment that is least likely to result in accidents or falls. Changes such as removing throw rugs, installing a handrail next to the toilet, and moving obstacles that can result in tripping or falling can be made at little or no expense to the family.

Include the following in a patient and family teaching plan:
* Take this drug as prescribed. Do not increase, decrease, or omit a dose or stop taking the drug unless advised to do so by the physician. If gastrointestinal upset occurs, take the drug with food.
* If dizziness, drowsiness, or blurred vision occurs, avoid driving or performing other tasks that require alertness.
* Avoid the use of alcohol unless use has been approved by the physician.
* Relieve dry mouth by hard candy (unless the patient is a diabetic) or frequent sips of water.
* Consult a dentist if dryness of the mouth interferes with wearing, inserting, or removing dentures or causes other dental problems.
* Notify the physician if any of these problems occur: severe dry mouth, inability to chew or swallow food, inability to urinate, feelings of depression, severe dizziness or drowsiness, rapid heartbeat, abdominal pain, and unusual (new) movements of the head, eyes, arms, legs, feet, mouth, or tongue.
* Keep all physician or clinic appointments because close monitoring of therapy is necessary.
* When taking levodopa, avoid vitamin B_6 (pyridoxine) since this vitamin may interfere with the action of levodopa.

■ *Expected Outcomes for Evaluation*
* Anxiety is reduced
* No evidence of injury
* Adverse reactions are identified and reported to the physician
* Patient verbalizes an understanding of treatment modalities, adverse reactions, and importance of continued follow-up care
* Patient and family demonstrate understanding of drug regimen

Chapter Summary

* Parkinson's disease is a progressive disease of the nervous system thought to be caused by a deficiency of dopamine and an excess of acetylcholine within the central nervous system. Symptoms include fine tremors; rigidity of some muscle groups and weakness of others; slurred speech; a mask-like and emotionless expression of the face; and a shuffling, unsteady gait.
* Parkinsonism is a term that refers to the symptoms of Parkinson's disease. Antiparkinsonism drugs are used in the treatment of parkinsonism. The most effective drug in the treatment of parkinsonism is levodopa. Levodopa crosses the blood-brain barrier where it is converted to dopamine. The drug carbidopa is given with levodopa to facilitate the passage of levodopa across the blood-brain barrier, thus reducing the amount of levodopa needed to produce a therapeutic effect. Carbidopa is given with levodopa either as one medication or as two separate drugs.
* The most serious and frequent adverse reactions seen with levodopa include choreiform and dystonic movements, such as facial grimacing, protruding tongue, exaggerated chewing motions and head movements, and jerking movements of the arms and legs. The patient is observed daily for the development of adverse drug reactions. All adverse reactions must be reported to the physician because a dosage adjustment or change to a different antiparkinsonism drug may be necessary.

- The nurse must evaluate the patient's ability to understand the therapeutic drug regimen, their ability to care for themselves in the home environment, and their ability to comply with the prescribed drug therapy. If any type of assistance is needed, the nurse must provide appropriate teaching and/or refer to the discharge planning coordinator or social service worker.

Critical Thinking Exercise

1. Ms. Dennis, aged 89, has Parkinson's disease and is taking the drug amantadine daily. In discussing her care with the family, what information would you include in the teaching plan? What information would be most important for the family to understand? Explain your answer.

25

Psychotherapeutic Drugs

Chapter Objectives

On completion of this chapter the student will:

- *Name the types of psychotherapeutic drugs*
- *List the general adverse reactions associated with the administration of the psychotherapeutic drugs*
- *Discuss nursing management when administering a psychotherapeutic drug*
- *Use the nursing process when administering a psychotherapeutic drug*

By definition, a *psychotherapeutic drug* is one that is used to treat disorders of the mind. A drug that affects the mind is called a *psychotropic drug.* Narcotics, sedatives and hypnotics, alcohol, hallucinogens, and psychotherapeutic drugs are examples of psychotropic agents.

The types of psychotherapeutic drugs used in the treatment of mental illness are the *antianxiety drugs* (tranquilizers), the *antidepressant drugs,* and the *antipsychotic drugs.* Summary Drug Tables 25-1, 25-2, and 25-3 give a brief overview of these drugs. Miscellaneous psychotherapeutic drugs are reviewed in Summary Drug Table 25-4.

Antianxiety Drugs

Anxiety is a feeling of apprehension, worry, or uneasiness that may or may not be based on reality. Anxiety may be seen in many types of situations ranging from the anxiety that may accompany one's employment to the acute anxiety that may be seen during withdrawal from alcohol. While a certain amount of anxiety is normal, excess anxiety interferes with day-to-day functioning and can cause undue stress in the lives of certain individuals. Drugs used to treat anxiety are called *antianxiety drugs.* Another term that refers to the antianxiety drugs is *anxiolytics.*

ACTIONS OF THE ANTIANXIETY DRUGS

Antianxiety drugs act on subcortical (beneath the cortex) areas of the brain. Their exact mechanism of action is not fully understood but it is believed that their effect on areas such as the limbic system and the reticular formation results in a reduction of anxiety. Examples of antianxiety drugs include oxazepam (Serax), chlordiazepoxide (Librium), diazepam (Valium), and buspirone (BuSpar).

USES OF THE ANTIANXIETY DRUGS

Antianxiety drugs are used in the short-term treatment of the symptoms of anxiety. Long-term use of these drugs is usually not recommended because prolonged therapy can result in drug dependence and serious withdrawal symptoms.

A few of these drugs may have additional uses. For example, clorazepate (Tranxene) and diazepam are also used as anticonvulsants (see Chap 23). Additional uses of the individual antianxiety drugs are given in Summary Drug Table 25-1.

ADVERSE REACTIONS ASSOCIATED WITH THE ADMINISTRATION OF THE ANTIANXIETY DRUGS

Drowsiness and sedation are common adverse reactions seen during initial therapy with antianxiety drugs. Depending on the severity of anxiety or other circumstances, it may be desirable to allow some degree of sedation to occur during early therapy. Other adverse reactions include constipation, diarrhea, dry mouth, nausea, vomiting, visual disturbances, and incontinence. Some adverse reactions may only be seen when higher dosages are used.

Long-term use of antianxiety drugs may result in physical drug dependence. These drugs must never be discontinued abruptly because withdrawal symptoms, which can be extremely severe, may occur.

Antidepressant Drugs

Depression is one of the most common psychiatric disorders. It is characterized by feelings of intense sadness, helplessness, worthlessness, and impaired functioning. Those experiencing a major depressive episode exhibit physical and psychological symptoms, such as appetite disturbances, sleep disturbances, and loss of interest in job, family, and other activities usually enjoyed. Depression is treated with the use of antidepressant drugs. There are three types of antidepressants: the tricyclic antidepressants, the monoamine oxidase inhibitors (MAOIs), and a group of miscellaneous, unrelated drugs.

ACTIONS OF THE ANTIDEPRESSANT DRUGS

The tricyclic antidepressants, for example, amitriptyline (Elavil) and doxepin (Sinequan) block the reuptake of the endogenous neurohormones, norepinephrine (see Chap. 17) and serotonin, which then results in stimulation of the central nervous system (CNS).

Summary Drug Table 25-1. Antianxiety Drugs

Generic Name	Trade Name*	Uses	Adverse Reactions	Dose Ranges
alprazolam	Xanax	Anxiety disorders, symptoms of anxiety, panic attacks, adjunct in the treatment of depression	Sedation, sleepiness, dizziness, lethargy, constipation, pruritus, diarrhea, apathy, urticaria, fever, hiccups, visual disturbances, nausea, vomiting	0.25–0.5 mg PO tid increased to 4 mg/d if required
buspirone hydrochloride	BuSpar	Anxiety disorders	Dizziness, drowsiness, nervousness, headache, fatigue, nausea, dry mouth	Up to 60 mg/d PO in divided doses
chlordiazepoxide	Librium, *generic*	Anxiety disorders, acute alcohol withdrawal, preoperative anxiety	Dizziness, drowsiness, hangover, headache, nausea, vomiting	Anxiety: 5–25 mg PO tid, qid; alcohol withdrawal: 50–100 mg PO, IM, IV; preoperative anxiety: 5–10 mg PO on day before surgery, 50–100 mg IM 1 h before surgery
clorazepate dipotassium	Tranxene	Anxiety disorders, acute alcohol withdrawal, partial seizures	Dizziness, drowsiness, lethargy, nausea, vomiting, blurred vision	Anxiety: 15–60 mg PO in divided doses; alcohol withdrawal: 30 mg initially then 15 mg PO bid, qid; anticonvulsant: up to 90 mg/d
diazepam	Valium, *generic*	Anxiety disorders, acute alcohol withdrawal, partial seizures	Dizziness, drowsiness, lethargy, rash, blurred vision, nausea, vomiting	Anxiety: 2–10 mg PO 2–4 times/d; acute alcohol withdrawal: 5–10 mg PO tid, qid; muscle relaxant: 2–10 mg PO bid, qid, 5–10 mg IV or IM up to 30 mg in 1 hr
halazepam	Paxipam	Anxiety disorders	Dizziness, drowsiness, lethargy	20–40 mg PO tid, qid
hydroxyzine	Atarax, Vistaril *generic*	Anxiety disorders, pruritus, preoperative and postoperative sedation, nausea, vomiting, psychiatric and emotional emergencies, prepartum and postpartum adjunctive therapy	Dry mouth, drowsiness, hypersensitivity reactions, pain at IM injection site	Anxiety: 50–100 mg PO qid; pruritus: 25 mg PO tid, qid; preoperative and postoperative: 25–100 mg IM; psychiatric emergencies: 100 mg IM; nausea, vomiting: 25–100 mg IM; prepartum and postpartum: 25–100 mg PO
lorazepam	Ativan, *generic*	Anxiety disorders, preanesthetic sedation	Dizziness, drowsiness, lethargy, hangover, paradoxical excitation, blurred vision	Anxiety: 2–10 mg/d PO in divided doses; preoperative sedation: up to 4 mg IM or 2 mg IV
meprobamate	Equanil, Miltown, *generic*	Anxiety disorders	Drowsiness, ataxia, nausea, vomiting, diarrhea, palpitations, tachycardia, rash, slurred speech, dizziness	1200–2400 mg/d PO in divided doses
oxazepam	Serax, *generic*	Anxiety disorders	Dizziness, drowsiness, lethargy, hangover, paradoxical excitation, blurred vision	10–30 mg PO tid, qid

*The term, *generic,* indicates that the drug is available in generic form.

Summary Drug Table 25-2. Antidepressants

Generic Name	Trade Name*	Uses	Adverse Reactions	Dose Ranges
amitriptyline hydrochloride	Elavil, Endep, *generic*	Depression	Sedation, confusion, nasal congestion, fatigue, blurred vision, hypotension, lethargy, dry mouth, dry eyes, orthostatic hypotension, nausea, vomiting	Up to 300 mg/d PO in divided doses, 20–30 mg IM qid
amoxapine	Asendin, *generic*	Depression accompanied by anxiety	Drowsiness, lethargy, sedation, fatigue, hypotension, dry mouth, dry eyes, constipation	Up to 400 mg/d PO in divided doses
bupropion hydrochloride	Wellbutrin	Depression	Agitation, dry mouth, insomnia, headache, nausea, vomiting, tremor, constipation, weight loss, anorexia, seizures (with doses exceeding 450 mg/d)	200–450 mg/d PO in divided doses
clomipramine hydrochloride	Anafranil	Obsessions and compulsions in those with with obsessive-compulsive disorders (OCD)	Sedation, drowsiness, lethargy, weakness, constipation, dry eyes, dry mouth, blurred vision	25–250 mg/d PO
doxepin hydrochloride	Adapin, Sinequan, *generic*	Anxiety or depression, emotional symptoms accompanying organic disease	Sedation, drowsiness, lethargy, weakness, constipation, dry eyes, dry mouth, blurred vision	10–300 mg/d PO in single or divided doses
fluoxetine hydrochloride	Prozac	Depression	Anxiety, nervousness, insomnia, drowsiness, fatigue, asthenia, tremor, sweating, dizziness, light-headedness, anorexia, nausea, diarrhea, headache	20 mg/d PO in the morning or 40–80 mg/d PO in divided doses
imipramine hydrochloride or pamoate	Tofranil, *generic*	Depression	Sedation, drowsiness, lethargy, weakness, constipation, dry eyes, dry mouth, blurred vision	75–200 mg/d PO, IM in divided doses
maprotiline hydrochloride	Ludiomil, *generic*	Depressive neurosis, manic-depressive illness, anxiety associated with depression	Sedation, drowsiness, lethargy, weakness, constipation, dry eyes, dry mouth, blurred vision	75–225 mg/d PO in single or divided dose
nefazodone	Serzone	Depression	Headache, dry mouth, asthenia, nausea, infection, constipation, diarrhea, blurred vision	Initially 200 mg/d in divided doses, may increase to 300–600 mg/d PO
nortriptyline hydrochloride	Aventyl	Depression	Sedation, drowsiness, lethargy, weakness, constipation, dry eyes, dry mouth, blurred vision	25 mg PO tid, qid
trazodone hydrochloride	Desyrel, *generic*	Depression	Drowsiness, skin conditions, tinnitus, anger, hostility, anemia, hypertension, blurred vision, abdominal/gastric disorder, hypotension, dry mouth, nausea, vomiting, diarrhea	150–600 mg/d PO in divided doses
MAOI ANTIDEPRESSANTS				
isocarboxazid	Marplan	Neurotic or atypical depression	Orthostatic hypotension, dizziness, vertigo, nausea, constipation, dry mouth, diarrhea, headache, restlessness, blurred vision	10–30 mg/d PO in single or divided doses

(continued)

Summary Drug Table 25-2 (Continued)

Generic Name	Trade Name*	Uses	Adverse Reactions	Dose Ranges
phenelzine	Nardil	Neurotic or atypical depression	Orthostatic hypotension, dizziness, vertigo, nausea, constipation, dry mouth, diarrhea, headache, restlessness, blurred vision	Up to 60 mg/d PO in divided doses
tranylcypromine	Parnate	Neurotic or atypical depression	Orthostatic hypotension, dizziness, vertigo, nausea, constipation, dry mouth, diarrhea, headache, restlessness, blurred vision	Up to 30 mg/d PO in divided doses

*The term, *generic,* indicates that the drug is available in generic form.

Drugs classified as MAOIs inhibit the activity of monoamine oxidase—a complex enzyme system that is responsible for breaking down amines. This results in an increase in endogenous epinephrine, norepinephrine, and serotonin in the nervous system. An increase in these neurohormones results in CNS stimulation.

The mechanism of action of most of the miscellaneous antidepressants is not clearly understood. Examples of this group of drugs include fluoxetine (Prozac) and bupropion (Wellbutrin).

USES OF THE ANTIDEPRESSANT DRUGS

Antidepressant drugs are used in the management of various types of depression or depression accompanied by anxiety. The uses of individual antidepressants are given in Summary Drug Table 25-2.

ADVERSE REACTIONS ASSOCIATED WITH THE ADMINISTRATION OF ANTIDEPRESSANT DRUGS

Sedation and dry mouth are the most common adverse reactions seen with the tricyclic antidepressants. Tolerance to these effects develops with continued use. Orthostatic hypotension, hypertension, mental confusion, disorientation, rash, nausea, vomiting, visual disturbances, and nasal congestion may also be seen.

Orthostatic hypotension is a common adverse reaction seen with the administration of the MAOIs. Other common adverse reactions include dizziness, vertigo, nausea, constipation, dry mouth, diarrhea, headache, and overactivity.

One serious adverse reaction associated with the use of the MAOIs is hypertensive crisis (extremely high blood pressure), which may occur when foods containing tyramine are eaten. Examples of foods containing tyramine (an amino acid present in some foods) are aged cheeses, beef or chicken livers, some meats, meat tenderizer, some sausages, imported beers and ales, red wine, figs, bananas, raisins, soy sauce, and avocados.

One of the earliest symptoms of hypertensive crisis is headache (usually occipital) followed by other symptoms such as a stiff or sore neck, nausea, vomiting, sweating, fever, chest pain, dilated pupils, and bradycardia or tachycardia. If a hypertensive crisis occurs, immediate medical intervention is necessary to reduce the blood pressure. Strokes (cerebrovascular accidents) and death have been reported.

Fluoxetine administration may result in headache, activation of mania or hypomania, insomnia, anxiety, nervousness, nausea, vomiting, and sexual dysfunction.

Antipsychotic Drugs

Antipsychotic drugs are also called *neuroleptic drugs.* These drugs are given to patients with a psychotic disorder, such as schizophrenia. A psychotic disorder is characterized by extreme personality dis-

Summary Drug Table 25-3. Antipsychotic Drugs

Generic Name	Trade Name*	Uses	Adverse Reactions	Dose Ranges
chlorpromazine hydrochloride	Thorazine, *generic*	Psychotic disorders, nausea, vomiting, intractable hiccups	Hypotension, postural hypotension, tardive dyskinesia, photophobia, urticaria, nasal congestion, dry mouth, akathisia, dystonia, pseudo-parkinsonism, behavioral changes, headache, photosensitivity	Psychiatric disorders: up to 800 mg/d PO in divided doses, 25–400 mg IM; nausea and vomiting: 10–25 mg PO, 25–50 mg IM, 50–100 mg rectal; hiccups: 25–50 mg PO, IM
chlorprothixene	Taractan	Psychotic disorders	Drowsiness, extrapyramidal effects, dystonia, akathisia, hypotension	Up to 600 mg/d PO in divided doses; 25–50 mg IM tid, qid
clozapine	Clozaril	Severely ill schizophrenic patients not responding to other therapies	Drowsiness, sedation, akathisia, seizures, dizziness, syncope, tachycardia, hypotension, nausea, vomiting	Up to 900 mg/d PO in divided doses
fluphenazine hydrochloride	Permitil, Prolixin	Psychotic disorders	Drowsiness, extrapyramidal effects, dystonia, akathisia, hypotension	0.5–10 mg/PO in divided doses; 2.5–10 mg/d IM in divided doses
haloperidol	Haldol	Psychotic disorders; Tourette's disorder	Extrapyramidal symptoms, akathisia, dystonia, tardive dyskinesia, drowsiness, headache, dry mouth, orthostatic hypotension	0.5–5 mg PO bid, tid with dosages up to 100 mg/d in divided doses; 2–5 mg IM
lithium	Eskalith, Lithane, *generic*	Manic episodes of manic-depressive illness	Headache, drowsiness, tremors, nausea, polyuria (see Table 25-1)	Based on lithium serum levels; average dose range is 900–1200 mg/d PO in divided doses
loxapine	Loxitane	Psychotic disorders	Extrapyramidal symptoms, akathisia, dystonia, tardive dyskinesia, drowsiness, headache, dry mouth, orthostatic hypotension	60–250 mg/d PO in divided doses; 12.5–50 mg IM
molindone hydrochloride	Moban	Schizophrenia	Sedation, extrapyramidal reactions, tardive dyskinesia, constipation, dry mouth	50–225 mg/d PO in divided doses
perphenazine	Trilafon, *generic*	Psychotic disorders, nausea and vomiting	Hypotension, postural hypotension, tardive dyskinesia, akathisia, dystonia, photophobia, urticaria, nasal congestion, dry mouth, pseudo-parkinsonism, behavioral changes, headache, photosensitivity	Psychotic disorders: 8–16 mg PO bid to qid, 5–10 mg IM; nausea, vomiting: 8–16 mg/d PO in divided doses
pimozide	Orap	Tourette's disorder	Parkinson-like symptoms, motor restlessness, dystonia, oculogyric crisis, tardive dyskinesia, dry mouth, diarrhea, headache, rash, drowsiness	Initial dose: 1–2 mg/d PO; maintenance dose: up to 10 mg/d PO
prochlorperazine	Compazine, Chlorazine, *generic*	Acute psychosis, nausea, vomiting	Extrapyramidal effects, sedation, tardive dyskinesia, dry eyes, blurred vision, constipation, dry mouth, photosensitivity	Psychotic disorders: up to 150 mg/d PO, 10–20 mg IM; nausea, vomiting: 15–40 mg/d in divided doses
promazine hydrochloride	Sparine, *generic*	Psychotic disorders	Drowsiness, extrapyramidal effects, dystonia, akathisia, hypotension	10–200 mg PO, IM q4–6h

(continued)

Summary Drug Table 25-3 (Continued)

Generic Name	Trade Name*	Uses	Adverse Reactions	Dose Ranges
thioridazine hydrochloride	Mellaril, *generic*	Psychotic disorders and agitation, depressed mood, tension, fears, sleep disturbances, anxiety in the elderly	Drowsiness, sedation, extrapyramidal effects, dystonia, hypotension, akathisia, constipation, photosensitivity	Psychotic disorders: up to 800 mg/d PO in divided doses; elderly: 20–200 mg/d PO in divided doses
trifluoperazine hydrochloride	Stelazine *generic*	Psychotic disorders	Drowsiness, extrapyramidal effects, dystonia, akathisia, hypotension	1–5 mg PO bid and up to 40 mg/d PO in divided doses; up to 6 mg/d IM in divided doses

*The term, *generic,* indicates that the drug is available in generic form.

organization and the loss of contact with reality. Hallucinations (a false perception having no basis in reality) or delusions (false beliefs that cannot be changed with reason) are usually present. Lithium is considered an antimanic drug. It is useful in treating the manic phase of a bipolar disorder and in preventing the wide mood swings characteristic of the disorder.

neurohormone dopamine and an increase in the firing of nerve cells in certain areas of the brain. These effects may be responsible for the ability of these drugs to suppress the symptoms of certain psychotic disorders. Examples of antipsychotic drugs include chlorpromazine (Thorazine), thioridazine (Mellaril), haloperidol (Haldol), and lithium.

ACTIONS OF THE ANTIPSYCHOTIC DRUGS

The exact mechanism of action of antipsychotic drugs is not well understood. The effects of these drugs include an alteration or inhibition of the release of the

USES OF THE ANTIPSYCHOTIC DRUGS

Antipsychotic drugs are used in the management of acute and chronic psychoses. Clomipramine (Anafranil) is used for the treatment of obsessive-

Summary Drug Table 25-4. Miscellaneous Psychotherapeutic Drugs

Generic Name	Trade Name*	Uses	Adverse Reactions	Dose Ranges
methylphenidate hydrochloride	Ritalin, Ritalin SR, *generic*	Attention deficit hyperactive disorders (ADHD), narcolepsy	Nervousness, insomnia, rash, anorexia, nausea, palpitations, tachycardia	ADHD: children less than 6 yrs 5 mg before breakfast and lunch; increase 5–10 mg/wk, not to exceed 60 mg/d; Narcolepsy: PO 10 mg bid-tid, may increase to 60 mg/d
pemoline	Cylert	Attention deficit hyperactive disorder	Insomnia, restlessness, nausea, rash, anorexia, dyskinetic movements of tongue, lips, and face	Children less than 6 yrs 32.5 mg in A.M. increase by 18.75 mg/wk, not to exceed 112.5 mg/d
tacrine	Cognex	Mild to moderate dementia associated	Elevated transaminases, nausea, vomiting, diarrhea, dyspepsia, anorexia, ataxia	40–80 mg/d in divided doses four times/d

*The term, *generic,* indicates that the drug is available in generic form.

compulsive disorders. Lithium is effective in the management of bipolar (manic-depressive) illness. More specific uses of these drugs are given in Summary Drug Table 25-3.

ADVERSE REACTIONS ASSOCIATED WITH THE ADMINISTRATION OF ANTIPSYCHOTIC DRUGS

Administration of these drugs may result in a wide variety of adverse reactions. The adverse reactions seen with the use of some of these drugs may include sedation, hypotension, postural hypotension, dry mouth, nasal congestion, photophobia, urticaria, photosensitivity (abnormal response or sensitivity when exposed to light), behavior changes, and headache.

Among the most significant adverse reactions associated with the antipsychotic drugs are the *extrapyramidal effects*. The term extrapyramidal effects refers to a group of adverse reactions occurring on the extrapyramidal portion of the nervous system as a result of antipsychotic drugs. This part of the nervous system affects body posture and promotes smooth and uninterrupted movement of various muscle groups. Antipsychotics disturb the function of the extrapyramidal portion of the nervous system, causing abnormal muscle movement. Extrapyramidal effects include: Parkinson-like symptoms (see Chap. 24), akathisia, and dystonia. Parkinson-like symptoms include the following: fine tremors, muscle rigidity, masklike appearance of the face, slowness of movement, slurred speech, and unsteady gait. *Akathisia* is exhibited by extreme restlessness and increased motor activity. *Dystonia* is manifested by facial grimacing and twisting of the neck into unnatural positions. Extrapyramidal effects usually diminish with a reduction in the dosage of the antipsychotic agent. The physician may also prescribe an antiparkinsonism drug, such as benztropine, to reduce the incidence of Parkinson-like symptoms.

Tardive dyskinesia may be observed in patients receiving an antipsychotic or after discontinuation of the antipsychotic. The highest incidence is found in those patients receiving an antiparkinson drug for extrapyramidal effects along with the antipsychotic drug. *Tardive dyskinesia* is characterized by rhythmic, involuntary movements of the tongue, face, mouth, or jaw, and sometimes the extremities. The tongue may protrude and there may be chewing movements, puckering of the mouth, and facial grimacing. When these symptoms occur during the course of therapy, the drug must be discontinued. Depending on the severity of the condition being treated, the physician may slowly taper the drug dose because abrupt discontinuation may result in a return of the psychotic symptoms.

Behavioral changes may also occur with the use of the antipsychotics. These changes include a catatonic-like state, an increase in the intensity of the psychotic symptoms, lethargy, hyperactivity, paranoid reactions, agitation, and confusion. A decrease in dosage may eliminate some of these symptoms but it also may be necessary to try another drug.

Lithium carbonate is rapidly absorbed after oral administration. The most common adverse reactions include tremors, nausea, vomiting, thirst, and polyuria. Toxic reactions may be seen when serum lithium levels reach greater than 1.5 mEq/L (Table 25-1). Because some of these toxic reactions are potentially serious, lithium blood levels are usually drawn during therapy and the dosage of lithium adjusted according to the results.

Miscellaneous Psychotherapeutic Drugs

Methylphenidate (Ritalin), pemoline (Cylert), and tacrine HCL (Cognex) are miscellaneous psychotherapeutic drugs.

Methylphenidate and pemoline are mild CNS stimulants used in the treatment of attention deficit hyperactivity disorder in children with moderate to severe hyperactivity and short attention span. Children with attention deficit hyperactivity disorder have learning or behavior problems that affect every area of their lives, particularly their ability to perform and learn in the classroom. Treatment with these drugs may greatly reduce the symptoms associated with attention deficit hyperactivity disorder.

Methylphenidate is also used to treat narcolepsy, a syndrome characterized by the individual experiencing an uncontrollable desire to sleep. Episodes occur without warning and may last several minutes to several hours. The mild stimulating effect of methylphenidate on the CNS is often effective in preventing the attacks.

Tacrine (Cognex) is used to treat the dementia associated with Alzheimer's disease. Alzheimer's disease is a progressive deterioration of mental, physical, and cognitive abilities. Specific pathological changes occur in brain tissue thought to be associated with deficiencies of one or more of the neurohormones, such as acetylcholine or norepinephrine. This drug acts to increase the level of acetylcholine in the CNS by inhibiting its breakdown. However,

Table 25-1. Signs of Lithium Toxicity

Lithium Level	Signs of Toxicity
1.5–2 mEq/L	Diarrhea, vomiting, nausea, drowsiness, muscular weakness, lack of coordination (early signs of toxicity)
2–3 mEq/L	Giddiness, ataxia, blurred vision, tinnitus, vertigo, increasing confusion, slurred speech, blackouts, myoclonic twitching or movement of entire limbs, choreo-athetoid movements, urinary or fecal incontinence, agitation or manic-like behavior, hyperreflexia, hypertonia, dysarthria
> 3 mEq/L	May produce a complex clinical picture involving multiple organs and organ systems including: seizures (generalized and focal), arrhythmias, hypotension, peripheral vascular collapse, stupor, muscle group twitching, spasticity, coma

the disease is progressive and tacrine does not alter the progress of the disease.

Adverse effects of the miscellaneous psychotherapeutic drugs are listed in Summary Drug Table 25-4.

NURSING MANAGEMENT

Many psychotherapeutic agents are administered for a long time. The exception is the antianxiety agents, which are not recommended for long-term use. The nurse plays an important role in the administration of these drugs in both the psychiatric and nonpsychiatric setting for several reasons: (1) the patient's response to drug therapy on an inpatient basis requires around-the-clock assessments because frequent dosage adjustments may be necessary during therapy; and (2) accurate assessments for the appearance of adverse drug effects assume a greater importance when the patient may not be able to verbalize physical changes to the physician or nurse.

Hospitalized Patients

Develop a nursing care plan to meet the patient's individual needs. Monitor vital signs at least daily. In some instances, such as when hypotensive episodes occur, monitor the vital signs more often. Report any significant change in the vital signs to the physician.

Behavioral records are written at periodic intervals, with their frequency depending on hospital or unit guidelines. An accurate description of the patient's behavior aids the physician in planning therapy, and, thus, becomes an important part of nursing management. Patients responding poorly to drug therapy may require dosage changes, a change to

another psychotherapeutic drug, or the addition of other therapies to the treatment regimen.

Drug Administration

When given parenterally, these drugs are given intramuscularly in a large muscle mass such as the gluteus muscle. Keep the patient lying down (when possible) for about 30 minutes after the drug is given.

Oral administration requires great care because some patients have difficulty swallowing (due to a dry mouth or other causes). Other patients may refuse to take their medication. *Never* force a patient to take an oral medication. If the patient refuses his or her medication, contact the physician regarding this problem because parenteral administration of the drug may be necessary.

After administration of an oral medication, inspect the patient's oral cavity to be sure the medication has been swallowed. If the patient resists having his or her oral cavity checked, report this refusal to the physician.

Adverse Drug Reactions

During initial therapy or whenever the dosage is increased or decreased, observe the patient closely for adverse drug reactions and *any* behavioral changes. Report any change in behavior or the appearance of adverse reactions to the physician because a further increase or decrease in dosage may be necessary or the drug may need to be discontinued.

Some adverse reactions, such as dry mouth, episodes of postural hypotension, and drowsiness, may need to be tolerated because drug therapy must continue. Nursing interventions to relieve some of these reactions may include offering frequent sips of water, assisting the patient out of the bed or chair, and supervising all ambulatory activities.

Antianxiety Drugs

Administer these drugs with food or meals to decrease the possibility of gastrointestinal upset. Sugarless gum, hard candy, or frequent sips of water may be used to reduce discomfort from dry mouth.

Check blood pressure prior to administration. If systolic pressure drops 20 mm Hg, do not administer the drug and notify physician.

Abrupt discontinuation of the antianxiety agents after 3 to 4 months of therapy may cause withdrawal symptoms: irritability, nervousness, insomnia, dry mouth, tremors, or convulsions.

Antidepressant Drugs

Full therapeutic effect may not be attained for 2 to 3 weeks. Patients with suicidal tendencies must be monitored closely. Report any expressions of guilt, hopelessness, helplessness, insomnia, weight loss, and direct or indirect threats of suicide.

Patients receiving MAOIs require strict dietary control because foods containing tyramine should not be eaten. Ask family members and visitors not to bring food to the patient and explain why this is important. Close observation of the patient when eating in a community setting may be necessary so that food is not taken or accepted from other patients.

> ### Nursing Alert
>
> Complaints of a headache (especially an occipital headache) may indicate the occurrence of a hypertensive crisis. Take the blood pressure and if elevated, notify the physician immediately. Monitor the blood pressure at 30-minute intervals. Notify the physician of any further symptoms of hypertensive crisis.

Antipsychotic Drugs

Antipsychotic drugs may be given orally as a single daily dose and be just as effective as when given several times a day. Full response to the antipsychotics takes several weeks. When administering the antipsychotic drugs, observe the patient for extrapyramidal effects: muscular spasms of the face and neck, the inability to sleep or sit still, tremors, rigidity, or involuntary rhythmic movements. Notify the physician because the occurrence of these symptoms may indicate a need for dosage adjustment.

Since there is no known treatment for tardive dyskinesia and because it is irreversible in some patients, symptoms must be reported.

> ### Nursing Alert
>
> Report any of the following signs and symptoms of tardive dyskinesia immediately to the physician: rhythmic, involuntary movements of the tongue, face, mouth, jaw, or the extremities.

Lithium toxicity can occur even when administered at therapeutic doses. Toxic symptoms may be seen with serum lithium levels of 1.5 or greater. Levels should not exceed 2 mEq/L (see Table 25-1). Therefore, patients taking lithium must be continually monitored for signs of toxicity such as: diarrhea, vomiting, nausea, drowsiness, muscular weakness, and lack of coordination. For early symptoms, the physician may order a dosage reduction or discontinue the drug for 24 to 48 hours, and then gradually restart the drug at a lower dosage.

For patients receiving lithium, increase the oral fluid intake to about 3000 mL/d. Have fluids readily available and offer extra fluids throughout waking hours. If there is any question regarding the oral fluid intake, monitor the intake and output. Lithium is contraindicated in pregnancy. Women of childbearing age may be placed on contraceptives while taking lithium.

Miscellaneous Psychotherapeutic Drugs

Administer methylphenidate and pemoline in divided doses two or three times daily. Give the last daily dose early in the evening preferably before 6:00 P.M. to avoid insomnia. These drugs may also mask symptoms of fatigue, impair physical coordination, or produce dizziness. Notify the physician if nervousness, insomnia, palpitations, or vomiting occur. Enter a daily summary of the child's behavior in the patient's record. This provides a record of the results of therapy. For prolonged therapy, behavior summaries may be made on a weekly basis.

For the patient with narcolepsy receiving methylphenidate or pemoline, close observation is necessary, particularly during the daytime hours. If periods of sleep occur, record the time of day and their length. Since most of these individuals are outpatients, the family members are instructed to keep a record of the periods of sleep.

When administering tacrine, transaminase levels must be monitored weekly for at least the first 18 weeks of treatment and every 3 months thereafter.

Alanine aminotransferase is found predominately in the liver. Disease or injury to the liver causes a release of this enzyme into the bloodstream, resulting in elevated alanine aminotransferase levels and indicating liver dysfunction. Any alanine aminotransferase level greater than five times the upper level of normal must be reported to the physician immediately. The physician may discontinue the drug because of the danger of hepatotoxicity. However, abrupt discontinuation may cause a decline in cognitive functioning.

The Outpatient

At the time of each physician's office or clinic visit, observe the patient for a response to therapy. In some instances, the patient or a family member may be questioned about the response to therapy. The type of questions asked depends on the patient and the diagnosis and may include questions such as "How are you feeling?", "Do you seem to be less nervous?", or "Would you like to tell me how everything is going?" Many times questions may need to be rephrased or the conversation directed toward other subjects until these patients feel comfortable and are able to discuss their therapy.

Ask the patient or a family member about adverse drug reactions or any other problems occurring during therapy. Bring these reactions or problems to the attention of the physician. Document a general summary of the patient's outward behavior and any complaints or problems in the patient's record. These notations are then compared to previous notations and observations.

Nursing Process
The Patient Receiving a Psychotherapeutic Drug

■ *Assessment*

A patient receiving a psychotherapeutic drug may be treated in the hospital or in an outpatient setting. The patient's mental status is assessed prior to and periodically throughout therapy. The presence of hallucinations, delusions, or suicidal thoughts must be noted and documented accurately in the patient's record.

Before starting therapy for the hospitalized patient, obtain a complete psychiatric and medical history. In the case of mild depression or anxiety, patients may (but sometimes may not) give a reliable history of their illness. When a severe psychosis is present, obtain the psychiatric history from a family member or friend. During the time the history is taken, observe the patient for any behavior patterns that appear to be deviations from normal. Examples of deviations are poor eye contact, failure to answer questions completely, inappropriate answers to questions, a monotone speech pattern, and inappropriate laughter, sadness, or crying.

Physical assessments should include the blood pressure on both arms and in a sitting position, pulse, respiratory rate, and weight.

The hospitalized patient may ultimately be discharged from the psychiatric setting. There are also patients, such as those with mild anxiety or depression, who do not require inpatient care. These patients are usually seen at periodic intervals in the physician's office or in a psychiatric outpatient setting.

The initial assessments of the outpatient are basically the same as those for the hospitalized patient. Obtain a complete medical history and a history of the symptoms of the mental disorder from the patient, a family member, or the patient's hospital records. During the initial interview, observe the patient for what appear to be deviations from a normal behavior pattern. The initial physical assessment should also include vital signs and weight.

■ *Nursing Diagnoses*

Depending on the drug, dose, and reason for administration, one or more of the following nursing diagnoses may apply to a person receiving a psychotherapeutic drug. Additional nursing diagnoses pertaining to the patient's mental and physical status may need to be added.
- **Risk for Injury** related to an adverse drug reaction (eg, drowsiness or ataxia)
- **Risk for Ineffective Management of Therapeutic Regimen** related to indifference, lack of knowledge, adverse reactions, other factors

■ *Planning and Implementation*

The major goals of the patient may include an absence of injury and a knowledge of and compliance to the prescribed therapeutic regimen. To make these goals measurable, more specific criteria must be added. Additional implementation strategies may be found in the Nursing Management section.

Risk for Injury. Provide total assistance with activities of daily living to the patient experiencing extreme sedation, including help with eating, dressing, and ambulating. On the other hand, extremely hyperactive patients must be protected from injury to themselves or others.

■ *Patient and Family Teaching*

Noncompliance is a problem with some patients once they are discharged to the home setting. Evaluate the patient's ability to assume responsibility for taking medications at home. The administration of psychotherapeutic drugs becomes a family responsibility if the outpatient appears to be unable to manage his or her own drug therapy.

Any adverse reactions that may occur with a specific psychotherapeutic drug are explained and the patient or family member is encouraged to contact the physician immediately if a serious drug *reaction* occurs.

If the patient is prescribed a MAOI, give and review a list of foods containing tyramine. Emphasis is placed on not eating *any* of the foods on the list.

Include the following points in a teaching plan for the patient or family member:

* Take the drug exactly as directed. Do *not* increase, decrease, or omit a dose or discontinue this drug unless directed to do so by the physician.
* Do not drive or perform other hazardous tasks if drowsiness occurs.
* Do not take *any* nonprescription drug unless use of a specific drug has been approved by the physician.
* Inform physicians, dentists, and other medical personnel of therapy with this drug.
* Do not drink alcoholic beverages unless approval is obtained from the physician.
* If dizziness occurs when changing position, rise slowly when getting out of bed or a chair. If dizziness is severe, always have help when changing positions.
* If dryness of the mouth occurs, it may be relieved by taking frequent sips of water, sucking on hard candy, or chewing gum (preferably sugarless).
* Antipsychotics—Report to the physician immediately if the following adverse reactions occur: restlessness, inability to sit still, muscle spasms, masklike expression, rigidity, tremors, drooling, or involuntary rhythmic movements of the mouth, face, or extremities. Advise the patient to avoid exposure to the sun. If exposure is unavoidable wear sunblock, keep arms and legs covered, and wear a sun hat.
* Lithium—Drink at least 10 large glasses of fluid each day and add extra salt to food. If any of the following occurs, do not take the next dose and notify the physician immediately: diarrhea, vomit-

ing, tremors, drowsiness, lack of muscle coordination, muscle weakness.
* Tacrine—Emphasize the importance of monitoring the alanine aminotransferase at intervals prescribed by the physician. Advise the caregiver to notify the physician if nausea, vomiting, diarrhea, dyspepsia, or anorexia occur
* Methylphenidate—Notify physician if nervousness, insomnia, palpitations, vomiting, fever, or skin rash occur.
* Keep all physician or clinic appointments because close monitoring of therapy is essential.
* Report any unusual changes or physical effects to the physician.

■ *Expected Outcomes for Evaluation*

* Patient verbalizes an understanding of treatment modalities and importance of continued follow-up care
* Patient verbalizes importance of complying with the prescribed therapeutic regimen
* Patient and family demonstrate understanding of drug regimen
* Adverse reactions are identified and reported to the physician
* No evidence of injury

Chapter Summary

* A psychotherapeutic drug is one that is used to treat disorders of the mind. Three types of psychotherapeutic drugs used in the treatment of mental illness are the antianxiety drugs (tranquilizers), the antidepressant drugs, and the antipsychotic drugs.
* Antianxiety drugs are used in the short-term treatment of the symptoms of anxiety. Long-term therapy is not recommended because prolonged therapy can result in drug dependency. Drowsiness and sedation are common adverse reactions seen during initial therapy, along with constipation, dry mouth, and visual disturbances. These drugs must never be discontinued abruptly because withdrawal symptoms may occur.
* Antidepressants are used to treat those suffering from depression. There are three types of antidepressants: the tricyclic antidepressants, the monoamine oxidase inhibitors (MAOIs), and a group of miscellaneous, unrelated drugs. One serious side effect associated with the use of the MAOIs is hypertensive crisis, which may occur when foods containing the amino acid tyramine

are eaten. Examples of foods containing tyramine are: aged cheeses, imported beer and ales, and beef or chicken livers. Hypertensive crisis is manifested by severe headache, stiff or sore neck, nausea, or vomiting. Immediate medical intervention is necessary to reduce the blood pressure.

- Antipsychotic drugs are also called neuroleptic drugs. These drugs are used in the management of acute and chronic psychoses. Among the most significant adverse reactions associated with the administration of the antipsychotic drugs are the extrapyramidal effects. Extrapyramidal effects include parkinsonism-like symptoms, akathisia, and dystonia. Extrapyramidal effects usually diminish with a reduction in the dosage of the antipsychotic drug. The physician may also prescribe an antiparkinsonism drug to reduce the incidence of Parkinson-like symptoms. Tardive dyskinesia may be observed in patients receiving an antipsychotic drug. Tardive dyskinesia is characterized by rhythmic, involuntary movements of the tongue, face, mouth, or jaw. When these symptoms occur, the drug must be discontinued. There is no known treatment for tardive dyskinesia and the manifestations can be permanent.
- Lithium carbonate is used to treat the manic phase of bipolar disorder. Lithium toxicity can occur even when administered at therapeutic doses. Signs of toxicity include: diarrhea, vomiting, drowsiness, muscular weakness, and lack of coordination. For early symptoms, the physician may order a dosage reduction or discontinue the drug for 24 to 48 hours then gradually restart the drug at a lower dosage. Lithium drug levels are usually drawn during drug therapy and the dosage of lithium adjusted according to the results.

Critical Thinking Exercises

1. Ms. Brown comes to the mental health clinic for a follow-up visit. She is taking lithium to control a bipolar disorder. In talking with Ms. Brown she tells you that she is concerned because her "hands are always shaking" and "Sometimes I walk like I have been drinking alcohol." How would you explore this problem with Ms. Brown?
2. As a nurse on the psychiatric unit you are assigned to discuss extrapyramidal effects at a team conference. How would you present and explain this topic? What points would you stress?
3. Ms. Fleming, age 79, is diagnosed with narcolepsy and prescribed methylphenidate (Ritalin). Ms. Fleming lives alone and refuses to move in with her daughter, even for a short while. How would you explore this problem with both Ms. Fleming and her daughter? What assessments would be most important to make concerning this situation?

26

Antiemetic and Antivertigo Drugs

Key Terms

Antiemetic
Antivertigo
Chemoreceptor trigger zone
Vertigo
Vestibular neuritis

Chapter Outline

Chapter Objectives

On completion of this chapter the student will:

* *Define the terms antiemetic and antivertigo*
* *Describe the actions, uses, and adverse reactions of antiemetic and antivertigo drugs*
* *Discuss the nursing management of a patient receiving an antiemetic or antivertigo drug*
* *Use the nursing process when administering an antiemetic or antivertigo drug*

Scherer JC, Roach S: INTRODUCTORY CLINICAL PHARMACOLOGY, FIFTH EDITION © 1996 Lippincott-Raven Publishers

An *antiemetic* drug is used to treat or prevent nausea or vomiting. An *antivertigo* drug is used to treat or prevent *vertigo* (a feeling of a spinning or rotation-type motion) that may occur with motion sickness, Ménière's disease of the ear, middle and inner ear surgery, and other disorders.

Vomiting due to drugs, radiation, and metabolic disorders usually occurs because of stimulation of the *chemoreceptor trigger zone* (CTZ), a group of nerve fibers located on the surface of the fourth ventricle of the brain. When these fibers are stimulated by chemicals such as drugs or toxic substances, impulses are sent to the vomiting center located in the medulla. The vomiting center may also be directly stimulated by disorders, such as gastrointestinal irritation, motion sickness, and *vestibular neuritis,* inflammation of the vestibular nerve.

Antiemetic and Antivertigo Drugs

ACTIONS OF ANTIEMETIC AND ANTIVERTIGO DRUGS

These drugs appear to act primarily by inhibition of the CTZ or by depressing the sensitivity of the vestibular apparatus of the inner ear. Those that act on the vestibular apparatus of the inner ear are more effective for motion sickness and middle and inner ear surgeries, whereas those that act on the CTZ are more effective for vomiting due to stimulation of the CTZ.

Dronabinol (Marinol) is the psychoactive substance found in marijuana; consequently, it has a potential for abuse and dependence. The mechanism of action of dronabinol is unknown.

USES OF ANTIEMETIC AND ANTIVERTIGO DRUGS

Antiemetic Drugs

An antiemetic is used for the prevention (prophylaxis) or treatment of nausea and vomiting. An example of prophylactic use is the administration of an antiemetic before surgery to prevent vomiting in the immediate postoperative period when the patient is recovering from anesthesia. Another example is giving an antiemetic before administration of one or a

combination of antineoplastic drugs (drugs used in the treatment of cancer; see Chap. 47), which have a high incidence of vomiting following administration.

Other causes of nausea and vomiting that may be treated with an antiemetic include radiation therapy for a malignancy, bacterial and viral infections, nausea and vomiting due to drugs, Ménière's disease and other ear disorders, and neurological diseases and disorders. Some of these drugs are also of use in the treatment of the nausea and vomiting seen with motion sickness. Some antiemetics are also antivertigo agents (Summary Drug Table 26-1).

Antivertigo Drugs

An antivertigo drug is used in the treatment of vertigo, which is usually accompanied by lightheadedness, dizziness, and weakness. The individual often has difficulty walking. Some of the causes of vertigo include a high alcohol consumption over a short time, certain drugs, inner ear disease, and postural hypotension. Motion sickness (sea sickness, car sickness) has similar symptoms but is caused by repetitive motion as may be seen in riding in an airplane, boat, or car. Both vertigo and motion sickness may result in nausea and vomiting.

Antivertigo drugs are essentially antiemetics since many of these preparations, whether used for motion sickness or vertigo, also have direct or indirect antiemetic properties. They prevent the nausea and vomiting that occur because of stimulation of the vestibular apparatus in the ear. Stimulation of this apparatus results in vertigo, which is often followed by nausea and vomiting.

ADVERSE REACTIONS ASSOCIATED WITH THE ADMINISTRATION OF ANTIEMETIC AND ANTIVERTIGO DRUGS

The most common adverse reactions seen with these drugs are varying degrees of drowsiness. Additional adverse reactions for each drug are listed in Summary Drug Table 26-1.

NURSING MANAGEMENT

If vomiting is severe, observe the patient for signs and symptoms of electrolyte imbalance (see Chap. 48). Monitor the blood pressure, pulse, and respira-

Summary Drug Table 26–1. Antiemetic and Antivertigo Drugs

Generic Name	Trade Name*	Uses	Adverse Reactions	Dose Ranges
chlorpromazine hydrochloride	Thorazine *generic*	Control of nausea and vomiting, intractable hiccoughs	Drowsiness, hypotension, postural hypotension, hypertension, bradycardia, hypersensitivity reactions, dry mouth, nasal congestion	Nausea and vomiting: 10–25 mg PO q4–6h prn; 50–100 mg rectal suppository q6–8h prn, 25–50 mg IM q3–4 prn; hiccoughs: 25–50 mg PO, IM, slow IV infusion
dimenhydrinate	Dramamine, Dramoject, Marmine, *generic*	Prevention and treatment of nausea, vomiting, dizziness, vertigo of motion sickness	Dizziness, confusion, nervousness, restlessness nausea, vomiting, diarrhea, blurred vision, palpitations	50–100 mg PO q4–6h prn, 50 mg IM as needed, 50 mg IV
diphenhydramine hydrochloride	Benadryl, *generic*	Prevention and treatment of motion sickness	Dizziness, sedation, epigastric distress, dizziness, faintness, allergic reactions, urinary frequency, thickening of bronchial secretions	25–50 mg PO tid, qid, 10–50 mg IM, IV
diphenidol	Vontrol	Vertigo and associated nausea and vomiting, Ménière's disease, middle and inner ear surgery, control of nausea and vomiting in postoperative period, malignancies, and inner ear disturbances	Auditory and visual hallucinations, disorientation, drowsiness, dry mouth, nausea, skin rash	25–50 mg PO q4th
dronabinol	Marinol	Treatment of nausea and vomiting due to antineoplastic drug therapy, appetite stimulant in AIDS patients with weight loss	Palpitations, tachycardia, nausea, vomiting, euphoria, dizziness, paranoid reaction, somnolence, hallucinations	Antiemetic: 5–15 mg/m² 1–3 hr prior to chemotherapy, then q2–4h after chemotherapy for a total of 4–6 doses/d; appetite stimulant: 2.5 mg PO bid ac lunch and supper
granisetron hydrochloride	Kytril	Treatment of nausea and vomiting due to antineoplastic drug therapy	Headache, weakness, somnolence, diarrhea, constipation	10 mcg/kg infused IV over 5 min, 30 min before chemotherapy
meclizine	Antivert, Antivert/25 Antivert/50, *generic*	Vertigo, prevention and treatment of nausea and vomiting due to motion sickness	Drowsiness, restlessness, rash, urticaria, dry mouth, nose and throat, anorexia, hypotension	Vertigo: 25–100 mg/d PO in divided doses; nausea and vomiting: 25–50 mg PO 1 h before travel and repeat every 24 hr prn
metoclopramide	Reglan, *generic*	Prevention of nausea and vomiting due to antineoplastic drug therapy	Restlessness, drowsiness, fatigue, lassitude, dizziness, nausea, diarrhea	1–2 mg/kg IV 15–30 min before chemotherapy
ondansetron hydrochloride	Zofran	Prevention of nausea and vomiting due to antineoplastic drug therapy, prevention of postoperative nausea and vomiting	Diarrhea, headache, fever, weakness, dry mouth, drowsiness, sedation	Chemotherapy: Three doses of 0.15 mg/kg IV or 8 mg PO 30 min before and 4 and 8 hr after chemotherapy; postoperative nausea and vomiting: 4 mg IV after induction of anesthsia

(continued)

Summary Drug Table 26-1 (Continued)

Generic Name	Trade Name*	Uses	Adverse Reactions	Dose Ranges
perphenazine	Trilafon	Control of nausea and vomiting, intractable hiccoughs	Same as chlorpromazine hydrochloride	8–16 mg/d PO in divided doses, 5 mg IM, IV q6h prn
prochlorperazine hydrochloride	Compazine, *generic*	Control of nausea and vomiting	Same as chlorpromazine hydrochloride	5–10 mg PO tid, qid, 5–10 mg IM, 25 mg rectal suppository bid
promethazine hydrochloride	Phenergan, *generic*	Treatment of motion sickness, prevention of nausea and vomiting associated with anesthesia and surgery	Same as diphenhydramine hydrochloride	Motion sickness: initial dose 25 mg PO ½ hr before travel and repeat in 8–12 hr, then 25 mg PO bid, 12.5–25 mg IM, IV; nausea and vomiting: 12.5–25 mg PO, IM, IV
transdermal scopolamine	Transderm-Scop	Prevention of nausea and vomiting due to motion sickness	Drowsiness, dry mouth, blurred vision	One system applied at least 4 hr before effect is required; repeat in 3d if needed
trimethobenzamide hydrochloride	Tigan, *generic*	Control of nausea and vomiting	Hypersensitivity reactions, hypotension (IM use), Parkinson-like symptoms, blurred vision, drowsiness, dizziness	250 mg PO tid, qid, 200 200 mg IM, rectal suppository tid, qid

*The term, *generic,* indicates that the drug is available in generic form.

tory rate every 2 to 4 hours or as ordered by the physician. Measure the intake and output (urine, emesis) until vomiting ceases and the patient is able to take oral fluids in sufficient quantity. Describe the emesis in the patient's chart and notify the physician if there is blood in the emesis or if vomiting suddenly becomes more severe.

Daily to weekly weights may also be indicated in those with prolonged and repeated episodes of vomiting, for example, those receiving chemotherapy for malignant disease.

Nursing Alert

Many of these drugs cause variable degrees of drowsiness. Advise the patient to seek help when getting out of bed if drowsiness occurs.

When an antiemetic is prescribed prior to administration of an antineoplastic drug, give the drug at the prescribed time to effectively relieve nausea and vomiting following chemotherapy.

Nursing Process
The Patient Receiving an Antiemetic or Antivertigo Drug

■ *Assessment*
Assess patients receiving one of these drugs for nausea and vomiting for signs of fluid and electrolyte imbalances. Estimate the number of times the patient has vomited and the approximate amount of fluid lost. Before starting therapy, take vital signs.

■ *Nursing Diagnoses*
Depending on the severity of symptoms and the reason for administration, one or more of the following nursing diagnoses may apply to the patient receiving an antiemetic or antivertigo drug:
● **Risk for Fluid Volume Deficit** related to nausea and vomiting
● **Risk for Injury** related to adverse drug effects of drowsiness
● **Anxiety** related to nausea, vomiting, other symptoms (vertigo, dizziness, if present)
● **Risk for Ineffective Management of Therapeutic Regimen** related to knowledge deficit of

medication regimen, adverse drug effects, treatment modalities

■ Planning and Implementation

The major goals of the patient may include a reduction in anxiety, absence of symptoms, a normal fluid and electrolyte balance, absence of injury, and an understanding of the medication regimen. To make these goals measurable, more specific criteria must be added.

Administration. If the patient is unable to retain the oral form of the drug, give it parenterally or as a rectal suppository (if the prescribed drug is available in these forms). If only the oral form has been ordered and the patient is unable to retain the medication, contact the physician regarding an order for a parenteral or suppository form of this or another antiemetic drug.

Assess the patient at frequent intervals for the effectiveness of the drug to relieve symptoms (eg, nausea, vomiting, or vertigo). Notify the physician if the drug fails to relieve or diminish symptoms.

Granisetron (Kytril), ondansetron (Zofran), and dronabinol are newer antiemetics that are used to prevent nausea and vomiting following cancer (antineoplastic) chemotherapy; administer them on the day the chemotherapy is given. Granisetron and ondansetron may be given intravenously. Mix these drugs according to manufacturer's directions and give them approximately 30 minutes before administration of an antineoplastic drug. Ondansetron may be given orally 30 minutes before antineoplastic therapy, as well as for 1 to 2 days after to prevent or relieve nausea and vomiting. Give dronabinol, which has abuse potential, orally 1 to 3 hours prior to administration of an antineoplastic drug, then every 2 to 4 hours after chemotherapy. These drugs have been shown to be effective in relieving or eliminating nausea and vomiting after antineoplastic therapy.

Fluid and Electrolyte Imbalance. Observe the patient for signs of dehydration, which include poor skin turgor, dry mucous membranes, decrease in or absence of urinary output, concentrated urine, restlessness, irritability, increased respiratory rate, and confusion. In addition, observe the patient for signs of electrolyte imbalance, particularly sodium and potassium deficits.

If signs of dehydration or electrolyte imbalance are noted, contact the physician because parenteral administration of fluids or fluids with electrolytes may be necessary. These observations are particularly important in the aged or chronically ill patient in whom severe dehydration may develop in a short time. If the patient is able to take and retain small amounts of oral fluids, offer sips of water at frequent intervals.

Risk for Injury. Administration of these drugs may result in varying degrees of drowsiness. To prevent accidental falls and other injuries, assist the patient who is allowed out of bed with ambulatory activities. If extreme drowsiness is noted, instruct the patient to remain in bed and provide a call light for assistance.

Anxiety. Nausea, vomiting, vertigo, and dizziness are disagreeable sensations. The patient with one or more of these problems additionally experiences anxiety and concern over these symptoms. Change the bedding and patient clothing or gown as needed because the odor of vomitus may only intensify the symptoms. Provide the patient with an emesis basin, check the basin at frequent intervals, and empty it as needed. Give the patient a damp washcloth and a towel to wipe the hands and face as needed. Offer mouthwash or frequent oral rinses to remove the disagreeable taste that accompanies vomiting.

■ Patient and Family Teaching

When an antiemetic or antivertigo drug is prescribed for outpatient use, include the following information in a patient teaching plan:

- Drowsiness may occur with use. Avoid driving or performing other hazardous tasks when taking this medication.
- If nausea, vomiting, or vertigo persist or become worse, contact the physician.
- Use only as directed. Do not increase the dose or frequency of use unless told to do so by the physician.
- Avoid the use of alcohol and other sedative-type drugs unless use has been approved by the physician.
- Motion sickness: Take the medication about 1 hour before travel.
- Administration of granisetron (Kytril), dronabinol (Marinol), or ondansetron (Zofran) prior to antineoplastic chemotherapy: The drug will be given (oral, intravenous) approximately 30 minutes before the chemotherapy treatment. After the treatment, take the prescribed antiemetic at the time recommended by the physician or printed on the drug container.
- Transdermal scopolamine: Review with the patient the directions for application that are sup-

plied with the drug. The system is applied behind the ear. Following application of the system, wash the hands *thoroughly* with soap and water and dry them. The disc will last approximately 3 days at which time another disc may be applied, if needed. Discard the used disc and thoroughly wash and dry the hands and previous application site. Apply the new disc behind the opposite ear and again wash and thoroughly dry the hands. Thorough handwashing is necessary to prevent any traces of the drug from coming in contact with the eyes. Use only one disc at a time. Dizziness, dry mouth, and blurred vision may occur with the use of this system. Observe caution when driving or performing hazardous tasks.

■ *Expected Outcomes for Evaluation*
- Anxiety is reduced
- No evidence of a fluid volume deficit or electrolyte imbalance
- No evidence of injury
- Patient verbalizes importance of complying with the prescribed treatment regimen
- Demonstrates understanding of drug regimen

Chapter Summary

- An antiemetic is a drug used to treat or prevent nausea or vomiting. An antivertigo drug is used to treat or prevent vertigo that may occur with motion sickness, Ménière's disease of the ear, and middle and inner ear surgery.
- These drugs appear to act primarily by inhibiting the CTZ or by depressing the sensitivity of the vestibular apparatus of the inner ear.
- An antiemetic is used for the prevention (prophylaxis) or treatment of nausea and vomiting. An an-

tivertigo drug is used in the treatment of vertigo, which is usually accompanied by lightheadedness, dizziness, weakness, and difficulty walking.
- Many of these drugs cause variable degrees of drowsiness. Advise the patient to seek help when getting out of bed if drowsiness occurs.
- If vomiting is severe, the patient is observed for signs and symptoms of electrolyte imbalance. The blood pressure, pulse, and respiratory rate are monitored every 2 to 4 hours or as ordered by the physician. The intake and output (urine, emesis) is measured until vomiting ceases and the patient is able to take oral fluids in sufficient quantity. The emesis is described in the patient's chart and the physician is notified if there is blood in the emesis or vomiting suddenly becomes more severe.
- When an antiemetic is prescribed prior to administration of an antineoplastic drug, give the drug at the prescribed time to effectively relieve nausea and vomiting following chemotherapy.
- When these drugs are taken on an outpatient basis, the patient requires full instruction for their use.

Critical Thinking Exercises

1. Ms. Davis was prescribed meclizine (Antivert-50) 50 mg for motion sickness. Upon return from a long car ride she tells you that the medicine did not help. What questions would you ask to determine if Ms. Davis followed the prescribed drug regimen?
2. Mr. Collins is prescribed transdermal scopolamine to relieve motion sickness. What rationale would you give him to stress the importance of washing his hands after applying or removing the transdermal system?

27

Anesthetic Agents

Key Terms

Analgesia
Brachial plexus block
Conduction block
Epidural block
General anesthesia
Local anesthesia
*Local infiltration
anesthesia*
Neuroleptanalgesia
Preanesthetic agent
Regional anesthesia
Spinal anesthesia
Transsacral block

Chapter Outline

Chapter Objectives

On completion of this chapter the student will:

- *State the uses of local and general anesthetics*
- *List and briefly describe the four stages of general anesthesia*
- *Discuss the nursing responsibilities when a local or general anesthetic is given*

*Scherer JC, Roach S: INTRODUCTORY CLINICAL PHARMACOLOGY,
FIFTH EDITION © 1996 Lippincott-Raven Publishers*

There are two types of anesthesia: *local anesthesia* and *general anesthesia*. Local anesthesia, as the term implies, is the provision of a pain-free state in a specific area (or region). When a local anesthetic is given, the patient is fully awake but does not feel pain in the area that has been anesthetized. Some procedures done under local anesthesia may require the patient to be sedated, and although not fully awake, patients may hear what is going on around them. When a general anesthetic is given, the patient loses consciousness and feels no pain. Reflexes, such as the swallowing and gag reflexes, are lost during deep general anesthesia.

Local Anesthetics

The various methods of administering a local anesthetic include topical application, local infiltration, or regional anesthesia.

TOPICAL ANESTHESIA

Topical anesthesia involves the application of the anesthetic agent to the surface of the skin, open area, or mucous membrane. The anesthetic agent may be applied with a cotton swab or sprayed on the area. This type of anesthesia may be used to desensitize the skin or mucous membrane to the injection of a deeper local anesthetic. In some instances, topical anesthetics may be applied by the nurse.

LOCAL INFILTRATION ANESTHESIA

Local infiltration anesthesia is the injection of a local anesthetic agent into tissues. This type of anesthesia may be used for dental procedures, the suturing of small wounds, or making an incision into a small area, such as that which is required for removing a superficial piece of tissue for biopsy.

REGIONAL ANESTHESIA

Regional anesthesia is the injection of a local anesthetic agent around nerves so that the area supplied by these nerves will not send pain signals to the brain. The anesthetized area is usually larger than the area affected by local infiltration anesthesia. Spinal anesthesia and conduction blocks are two types of regional anesthesia.

Spinal Anesthesia

Spinal anesthesia is a type of regional anesthesia that involves the injection of a local anesthetic agent into the subarachnoid space of the spinal cord usually at the level of the second lumbar vertebra. There is a loss of feeling (anesthesia) and movement in the lower extremities, lower abdomen, and perineum.

Conduction Blocks

A *conduction block* is a type of regional anesthesia produced by injection of a local anesthetic agent into or near a nerve trunk. Examples of a conduction block include an *epidural block* (injection of a local anesthetic into the space surrounding the dura of the spinal cord); a *transsacral* (caudal) *block* (injection of a local anesthetic into the epidural space at the level of the sacrococcygeal notch); and *brachial plexus block* (injection of a local anesthetic into the brachial plexus). Epidural and transsacral blocks are often used in obstetrics with the epidural block being more common. A brachial plexus block may be used for surgery of the arm or hand.

PREPARING THE PATIENT FOR LOCAL ANESTHESIA

Depending on the procedure performed, preparation for local anesthesia may or may not be similar to preparing the patient for general anesthesia. For example, the administration of a local anesthetic for dental surgery or the suturing of a small wound may require an explanation of how the anesthetic will be administered, an allergy history, and, when applicable, preparation of the area, such as cleaning the area with an antiseptic or shaving the area. Other local anesthetic procedures may require the patient to be in a fasting state because a sedative may also be administered. An intravenous sedative such as diazepam (Valium), a tranquilizer (see Chap. 25), may be administered during some local anesthetic procedures, such as cataract surgery or surgery performed under spinal anesthesia.

ADMINISTRATION OF LOCAL ANESTHESIA

A local injectable anesthetic is administered by a physician or dentist. Table 27-1 lists the more commonly used local anesthetics.

NURSING MANAGEMENT

When applicable, the nurse may be responsible for applying a dressing to the area. Depending on the reason for using local anesthesia, the nurse also may be responsible for observing the area for bleeding, oozing, or other problems after the administration of the anesthetic.

Preanesthetic Agents

A *preanesthetic agent* is a drug given prior to the administration of anesthesia. A preanesthetic agent is most commonly given prior to the administration of general anesthesia but on occasion it may be given prior to injection of the local anesthetic drug to sedate the patient.

The preanesthetic agent may consist of one drug or a combination of drugs. The general purpose of the preanesthetic agent is to prepare the patient for anesthesia. The more specific purposes of these agents are the following:

• Narcotic or tranquilizer—To decrease anxiety and apprehension immediately before surgery. The patient who is calm and relaxed can be anesthetized more quickly; usually requires a smaller dose of an induction agent; may require less anesthesia during surgery; and may have a smoother anesthesia recovery period (awakening from anesthesia).

• Cholinergic blocking agent—To decrease secretions of the upper respiratory tract. Some anesthetic gases and volatile liquids are irritating to the lining of the respiratory tract and thereby increase mucus secretions. The cough and swallowing reflexes are lost during general anesthesia and excessive secretions can pool in the lungs, resulting in pneumonia or atelectasis during the postoperative period. The administration of a cholinergic blocking agent, such as glycopyrrolate (Robinul) dries up secretions of the upper respiratory tract and lessens the possibility of excessive mucus production.

• Antiemetic—To lessen the incidence of nausea and vomiting during the immediate postoperative recovery period.

Preanesthetic agents may be omitted in those 60 years or older because many of the medical disorders for which these drugs are contraindicated are seen in older individuals. For example, atropine and glycopyrrolate, drugs that can be used to decrease secretions of the upper respiratory tract, are contraindicated in certain medical disorders, such as prostatic hypertrophy, glaucoma, and myocardial ischemia. Other preanesthetic agents that depress the central nervous system, such as narcotics, barbiturates, tranquilizers with or without antiemetic properties, may be contraindicated in the older individual.

The preanesthetic agent is usually selected by the anesthesiologist and may consist of one or more drugs (Table 27-2). A narcotic (see Chap. 16), tranquilizer (see Chap. 25), or barbiturate (see Chap. 21) may be given to relax or sedate the patient. Barbiturates are used only occasionally; narcotics are usually preferred for sedation. A cholinergic blocking drug (see Chap. 20) is given to dry secretions in the upper respiratory tract. Scopolamine and glycopyrrolate also have mild sedative properties and atropine may or may not produce some sedation. Tranquilizers have sedative action; when combined with a narcotic, they allow for a lowering of the narcotic dosage because they also have the ability to potentiate the sedative action of the narcotic. Diazepam (Valium), a tranquilizer, is one of the more commonly used tranquilizers for preoperative sedation.

In some hospitals, the anesthesiologist examines the patient the day or evening before surgery, although this may not be possible in emergency situations. The patient's physical status is evaluated and

Table 27-1. Local Anesthetics

Generic Name	Trade Name*
bupivacaine hydrochloride	Marcaine HCl, *generic*
chloroprocaine hydrochloride	Nesacaine, Nescaine-MPF
etidocaine hydrochloride	Duranest HCl
lidocaine hydrochloride	Dilocaine, Xylocaine, *generic*
mepivacaine hydrochloride	Carbocaine, Isocaine HCl
prilocaine hydrochloride	Citanest HCl
procaine hydrochloride, injectable	Novocain, *generic*
tetracaine hydrochloride	Pontocaine HC1

*The term, *generic,* indicates that the drug is available in generic form.

Table 27-2. Preanesthetic Agents

Generic Name	Trade Name*
NARCOTICS	
droperidol	Inapsine
fentanyl	Sublimaze, *generic*
meperidine hydrochloride	Demerol, *generic*
morphine sulfate	Duramorph, *generic*
BARBITURATES	
pentobarbital	Nembutal Sodium, *generic*
secobarbital	*generic*
CHOLINERGIC BLOCKING DRUGS	
atropine sulfate	*generic*
glycopyrrolate	Robinul, *generic*
scopolamine	*generic*
TRANQUILIZERS WITH ANTIEMETIC PROPERTIES	
hydroxyzine	Vistaril, Atarax, *generic*
TRANQUILIZERS	
chlordiazepoxide	Librium, *generic*
diazepam	Valium, *generic*
midazolam	Versed

*The term, *generic,* indicates that the drug is available in generic form.

an explanation of the anesthesia is given. Some hospitals use members of the operating room or postanesthesia recovery room staff to visit the patient the night before or the morning of surgery to explain certain facts, such as the time of surgery, the effects of the preanesthetic agent, preparations for surgery, and the postanesthesia recovery room. Proper explanation of anesthesia, the surgery itself, and the events that may occur in preparation for surgery, as well as care after surgery require a team approach. The nurse's responsibilities are as follows:

- To describe or explain the preparations for surgery ordered by the physician. Examples of preoperative preparations include fasting from midnight (or the time specified by the physician), enemas, shaving of the operative site, a hypnotic for sleep the night before, and the preoperative injection approximately 30 minutes before going to surgery.
- To describe or explain immediate postoperative care, such as the postanesthesia recovery room or a special postoperative surgical unit and the activities of the physicians and nurses during this period. The patient is told that his or her vital signs will be monitored frequently, and that other equipment, such as intravenous fluids and monitors, may be used.

- To describe, explain, and demonstrate postoperative patient activities, such as deep breathing, coughing, and leg exercises.

The preoperative explanations given by the nurse are tailored to fit the type of surgery scheduled. Not all of the above teaching points may be included in every explanation.

General Anesthetics

The administration of general anesthesia requires the use of one or more agents. The choice of anesthetic agents depends on many factors including the following:

- The general physical condition of the patient
- The area, organ, or system being operated on
- The anticipated length of the surgical procedure

The anesthesiologist selects the anesthetic agent or agents that will produce safe anesthesia, *analgesia* (absence of pain), and, in some surgeries, effective skeletal muscle relaxation.

AGENTS USED FOR GENERAL ANESTHESIA

Methohexital, Thiamylal, and Thiopental. Methohexital (Brevital), thiamylal (Surital), and thiopental (Pentothal), which are ultra–short-acting barbiturates, are used for the following: induction of anesthesia, short surgical procedures with minimal painful stimuli, and in conjunction with or as a supplement to other anesthetics. Thiopental may also be used for the control of convulsive states. These agents have a rapid onset and a short duration of action. They depress the central nervous system to produce hypnosis and anesthesia but do not produce analgesia. Recovery after a small dose is rapid.

Etomidate. Etomidate (Amidate), a nonbarbiturate, is used for induction of anesthesia. Etomidate may also be used to supplement other anesthetics, such as nitrous oxide, for short surgical procedures. It is a hypnotic without analgesic activity.

Propofol. Propofol (Diprivan) is used for induction and maintenance of anesthesia. It also may be used for sedation during diagnostic procedures and procedures that use a local anesthetic. This drug also is used for continuous sedation of intubated or respiratory controlled patients in intensive care units.

Midazolam. Midazolam (Versed), a short-acting benzodiazepine central nervous system depressant, is used as a preanesthetic agent to relieve anxiety, for induction of anesthesia, for conscious sedation before minor procedures, such as endoscopic procedures, and to supplement nitrous oxide and oxygen for short surgical procedures. When used for induction anesthesia, the patient gradually loses consciousness over a period of 1 to 2 minutes.

Alfentanil. Alfentanil (Alfenta) is a narcotic analgesic that may be used as a preanesthetic agent, as well as for induction and maintenance of anesthesia.

Sufentanil. Sufentanil (Sufenta) is a narcotic analgesic that may be used to relieve pain. It also may be used as an anesthetic agent for induction and maintenance of anesthesia for major surgical procedures.

Ketamine. Ketamine (Ketalar) is a rapid-acting general anesthetic. It produces an anesthetic state characterized by profound analgesia, cardiovascular and respiratory stimulation, normal or enhanced skeletal muscle tone, and occasionally mild respiratory depression. Ketamine is used for diagnostic and surgical procedures that do not require relaxation of skeletal muscles; for induction of anesthesia before the administration of other anesthetic agents; and as a supplement to other anesthetic agents.

Cyclopropane. An anesthetic gas, cyclopropane has a rapid onset of action and may be used for induction and maintenance of anesthesia. Skeletal muscle relaxation is produced with full anesthetic doses. Cyclopropane is supplied in orange cylinders. Disadvantages of cyclopropane are difficulty in detecting the planes of anesthesia, occasionally laryngospasm, cardiac arrhythmias, and postanesthesia nausea, vomiting, and headache. Cyclopropane and oxygen mixtures are explosive, which limits the use of this gas anesthetic.

Ethylene. Ethylene is an anesthetic gas with a rapid onset of action and a rapid recovery from its anesthetic effects. It provides adequate analgesia but has poor muscle-relaxant properties. The advantages of ethylene include minimal bronchospasm, laryngospasm, and postanesthesia vomiting. A disadvantage of ethylene is hypoxia. This gas is supplied in red cylinders. Mixtures of ethylene and oxygen are flammable and explosive.

Nitrous Oxide. Nitrous oxide is a commonly used anesthetic gas. It is a weak anesthetic and is usually used in combination with other anesthetic agents. It does not cause skeletal muscle relaxation. The chief danger in the use of nitrous oxide is hypoxemia. Nitrous oxide is nonexplosive and is supplied in blue cylinders.

Enflurane. Enflurane (Ethrane) is a volatile liquid (a liquid that evaporates on exposure to air) anesthetic that is delivered by inhalation. Induction and recovery from anesthesia are rapid. Muscle relaxation for abdominal surgery is adequate, but greater relaxation may be necessary and may require the use of a skeletal muscle relaxant. Enflurane may produce mild stimulation of respiratory and bronchial secretions when used alone. Hypotension may occur when anesthesia deepens.

Halothane. Halothane (Fluothane) is a volatile liquid given by inhalation for induction and maintenance of anesthesia. Induction and recovery from anesthesia are rapid and the depth of anesthesia can be rapidly altered. Halothane does not irritate the respiratory tract and an increase in tracheobronchial secretions usually does not occur. Halothane produces moderate muscle relaxation, but skeletal muscle relaxants may be used in certain types of surgeries. This anesthetic may be given with a mixture of nitrous oxide and oxygen.

Isoflurane. Isoflurane (Forane) is a volatile liquid given by inhalation. It is used for induction and maintenance of anesthesia.

Methoxyflurane. Methoxyflurane (Penthrane), a volatile liquid, provides analgesia and anesthesia. It is usually used in combination with nitrous oxide but may also be used alone. It does not produce good muscle relaxation and a skeletal muscle relaxant may be required.

Desflurane. Desflurane (Suprane), a volatile liquid, is used for induction and maintenance of anesthesia. A special vaporizer is used to deliver this anesthetic agent because delivery by mask results in irritation of the respiratory tract.

Fentanyl and Droperidol. The narcotic analgesic fentanyl (Sublimaze) and the neuroleptic (major tranquilizer) droperidol (Inapsine) may be used together as a single agent called Innovar. The combination of these two drugs results in *neuroleptanalgesia*, which is characterized by general quietness, reduced motor activity, and profound analgesia. Complete loss of consciousness may not occur unless other anesthetic agents are used. A fentanyl and droperidol combination may be used to produce tranquilization and analgesia for surgical and diagnostic procedures. It may also be used as a preanesthetic medication for the induction of anesthesia and in the maintenance of general anesthesia.

Droperidol may be used as a single agent to produce tranquilization, to reduce nausea and vomiting during the immediate postanesthesia period, as an induction agent, and as an adjunct to general anesthesia. Fentanyl may be used alone as a supplement to general or regional anesthesia. It may also be administered as a single agent or with other agents as a preoperative medication and as an analgesic in the immediate postoperative (recovery room) period.

SKELETAL MUSCLE RELAXANTS

The various skeletal muscle relaxants that may be used during general anesthesia are listed in Table 27-3. These drugs are administered to produce relaxation of the skeletal muscles during certain types of surgeries, such as those involving the chest or abdomen. They may also be used to facilitate the insertion of an endotracheal tube. Their onset of action is usually rapid (45 seconds to a few minutes) and the duration of action is 30 minutes or more.

Table 27-3. Muscle Relaxants Used During General Anesthesia

Generic Name	Trade Name*
atracurium besylate	Tracrium
doxacurium chloride	Nuromax
gallamine triethiodide	Flaxedil
metocurine iodide	Metubine, *generic*
mivacurium chloride	Mivacron
pancuronium bromide	Pavulon
pipecuronium bromide	Arduan
rocuronium bromide	Zemuron
succinylcholine chloride	Anectine, *generic*
tubocurarine chloride	*generic*
vecuronium bromide	Norcuron

*The term, *generic,* indicates that the drug is available in generic form.

THE STAGES OF GENERAL ANESTHESIA

General surgical anesthesia is divided into the following stages:

Stage I—the stage of analgesia
Stage II—the stage of delirium
Stage III—the stage of surgical analgesia
Stage IV—the stage of respiratory paralysis

With newer drugs and techniques, the stages of anesthesia may not be as prominent as described above. In addition, movement through the first two stages is usually very rapid.

Stage I

Induction is a part of stage I anesthesia. It begins with the administration of an anesthetic agent and lasts until consciousness is lost. With some induction agents, such as the short-acting barbiturates, this stage may last only 5 to 10 seconds.

Stage II

Stage II is the stage of delirium and is also brief. During this stage, the patient may move about and mumble incoherently. The muscles are somewhat rigid and the patient is unconscious and cannot feel pain. If surgery were attempted at this stage, there would be a physical reaction to painful stimuli, yet the patient would not remember sensing pain.

Stage III

Stage III is the stage of surgical analgesia and is divided into four parts, planes, or substages. The anesthesiologist differentiates these planes by the character of the respirations, eye movements, certain reflexes, pupil size, and so on. At plane 2 or 3, the patient is usually ready for the surgical procedure.

Stage IV

Stage IV is the stage of respiratory paralysis and is a rare and dangerous stage of anesthesia. At this stage, respiratory arrest and cessation of all vital signs may occur.

Anesthesia begins with a loss of consciousness. This is part of the induction stage (stage I). The patient is now relaxed and can no longer see or hear what is going on around him or her. After consciousness is lost, additional anesthetic agents are administered. Some of these agents are also used as part of the induction phase, as well as for deepening anesthesia. Depending on the type of surgery, an endotracheal tube may also be inserted into the trachea to provide an adequate airway and to assist in the administration of oxygen and other anesthetic agents. The endotracheal tube is removed during the postanesthesia period once the gag and swallowing reflexes have returned. If an IV line was not inserted before the patient's arrival in surgery, it is inserted by the anesthesiologist before the administration of an induction agent.

NURSING MANAGEMENT

Preanesthesia

Before surgery, the nurse has the following responsibilities:

- To perform the required tasks and procedures as prescribed by the physician and hospital policy the day or evening before or the morning of surgery. Examples of these tasks include administration of a hypnotic the night before surgery, shaving the operative area, taking vital signs, seeing that the operative consent is signed, checking to see if all jewelry or metal objects are removed, administering enemas, inserting a catheter, inserting a nasogastric tube, preoperative teaching, and so on. All tasks are recorded on the patient's chart.
- To check the chart for any recent, abnormal laboratory tests. If a recent, abnormal laboratory test was attached to the patient's chart shortly before surgery, the surgeon and the anesthesiologist must be made aware of the abnormality. A note can be attached to the front of the chart and the surgeon or anesthesiologist contacted by telephone.
- To place a list of known or suspected drug allergies or idiosyncrasies on the front of the chart
- To administer the preanesthetic (preoperative) medication.
- To instruct the patient to remain in bed and place the side rails up once the preanesthetic medication is administered

Nursing Alert

Preanesthetic agents *must* be administered *on time* to produce their intended effects. Failure to give the preanesthetic agent on time may result in events such as increased respiratory secretions due to the irritating effect of anesthetic gases and the need for an increased dose of the induction agent because the preanesthetic agent has not had time to sedate the patient.

Postanesthesia Recovery Room

After surgery, the nurse has the following responsibilities, which vary according to where the nurse first sees the postoperative patient:

- To admit the patient to the unit according to hospital procedure or policy
- To check the airway for patency, assess the respiratory status, and give oxygen as needed
- To position the patient to prevent aspiration of vomitus and secretions
- To check the following: blood pressure, pulse, intravenous lines, catheters, drainage tubes, surgical dressings, casts, and so forth
- To review the patient's surgical and anesthesia records
- To monitor the blood pressure, pulse, and respiratory rate every 5 to 15 minutes until the patient is discharged from the area
- To check the patient every 5 to 15 minutes for emergence from anesthesia
- To provide suction as needed
- To exercise caution in administering narcotics. The respiratory rate, blood pressure, and pulse must be checked before these drugs are given and 20 to 30 minutes after administration (see Chap. 16). The physician should be contacted if the respiratory rate is below 10 before the drug is given, and if the respirations fall below 10 after the drug is given.
- To discharge the patient from the area to his or her room or other specified area. All drugs administered and nursing tasks performed must be recorded before the patient leaves the postanesthesia recovery room.

Chapter Summary

- There are two types of anesthesia: local anesthesia and general anesthesia. Local anesthesia is the provision of a pain-free state in a specific area (or region). The patient is fully awake but does not feel pain in the area that has been anesthetized. When a general anesthetic is given, the patient loses consciousness and feels no pain. Reflexes, such as the swallowing and gag reflexes, are lost during deep general anesthesia.

- The various methods of administering a local anesthetic include topical application, local infiltration, or regional anesthesia. Topical anesthesia involves the application of the anesthetic agent to the surface of the skin, open area, or mucous membrane. Local infiltration anesthesia is the injection of a local anesthetic agent into tissues. Regional anesthesia is the injection of a local anesthetic agent around nerves so that the area supplied by these nerves will not send pain signals to the brain. Spinal anesthesia and a conduction block are types of regional anesthesia.

- Depending on the procedure performed, preparation for local anesthesia may or may not be similar to preparing the patient for general anesthesia. A local injectable anesthetic is administered by a physician or dentist.

- A preanesthetic agent is a drug given prior to the administration of anesthesia. A preanesthetic agent is most commonly given prior to the administration of general anesthesia but on occasion it may be given prior to injection of the local anesthetic to sedate the patient. The preanesthetic agent may consist of one drug or a combination of drugs whose purpose is to prepare the patient for anesthesia.

- The administration of general anesthesia requires the use of one or more agents. The choice of anesthetic agents depends on many factors, such as the general physical condition of the patient, the area, organ, or system being operated on, and the anticipated length of the surgical procedure.

- General surgical anesthesia is divided into Stage I—the stage of analgesia; Stage II—the stage of delirium, Stage III—the stage of surgical analgesia, and Stage IV—the stage of respiratory paralysis.

Critical Thinking Exercises

1. Mr. Brooks' family asks you why a drug is being given prior to his going to surgery for a bowel resection. When checking the chart you note that Mr. Brooks has an order for Demerol 50 mg IM and glycopyrrolate 0.35 mg IM 30 minutes before surgery. How would you explain to the family the purpose of the preanesthetic agents that are to be given to Mr. Brooks?

2. A nurse you are working with complains that she was reprimanded and asked to fill out an incident report for not giving a preanesthetic agent on time. She states that she feels she is being unfairly accused of a medication error since the medication was given 10 minutes before the patient was taken to surgery. What justification could you give for this being a potentially serious error?

Drugs That Affect the Respiratory System

V

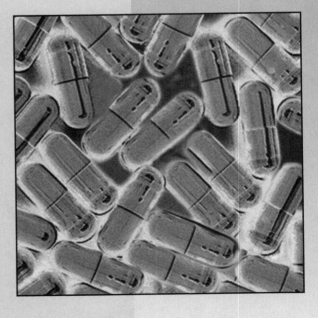

28

Antihistamines, Bronchodilators, and Decongestants

Key Terms

Antihistamine
Bronchodilator
Decongestant
Histamine
Sympathomimetic
Xanthine derivatives

Chapter Outline

Chapter Objectives

On completion of this chapter the student will:

- *Describe the uses and actions of the antihistamines, bronchodilators, or decongestants*
- *List some of the adverse reactions associated with the antihistamines, bronchodilators, or decongestants*
- *Discuss nursing management when administering an antihistamine, a bronchodilator, or a decongestant*
- *Use the nursing process when administering an antihistamine, a bronchodilator, or a decongestant*

The respiratory system consists of the upper and lower airways, the lungs, and the thoracic cavity. The function of the respiratory system is to provide a mechanism for the exchange of oxygen and carbon dioxide in the lungs. Any change in the respiratory status has the potential to affect every other body system since all cells need an adequate supply of oxygen for optimal functioning. This chapter will focus on drugs used to treat some of the more common disorders affecting the respiratory system, particularly allergies, bronchial asthma, and the congestion associated with certain respiratory disorders. Drugs used to treat these disorders include antihistamines, brochodilators and decongestants.

Antihistamines

Histamine is a substance present in various tissues of the body, such as the liver, lungs, intestines, and skin. The highest concentration of histamine is found in basophils (a type of white blood cell) and the mast cells that are found near capillaries. Histamine is produced in response to injury. Histamine acts on areas such as the vascular system and smooth muscle, producing dilatation of arterioles and an increased permeability of capillaries and venules. Dilatation of the arterioles results in localized redness. An increase in the permeability of small blood vessels produces an escape of fluid from these blood vessels into the surrounding tissues, which produces localized swelling. The release of histamine produces an inflammatory response. Histamine is also released in allergic reactions or hypersensitivity reactions, such as anaphylactic shock.

Antihistamines are drugs used to counteract the effects of histamine on body organs and structures. Examples of antihistamines include diphenhydramine (Benadryl), terfenadine (Seldane), brompheniramine (Dimetane), and astemizole (Hismanal).

ACTIONS OF THE ANTIHISTAMINES

Antihistamines block most, but not all, of the effects of histamine. They do this by competing for histamine at histamine receptor sites, thereby preventing histamine from entering these receptor sites and producing an effect on body tissues. Some antihistamines have additional effects, such as an antipruritic effect, an antiemetic effect, and a sedative effect.

USES OF THE ANTIHISTAMINES

The general uses of the antihistamines are the following:

- Relief of the symptoms of seasonal and perennial allergies
- Allergic and vasomotor rhinitis
- Allergic conjunctivitis
- Mild and uncomplicated angioneurotic edema and urticaria
- Relief of allergic reactions to drugs, blood, or plasma
- Relief of coughs due to colds or allergy
- Adjunctive therapy in anaphylactic shock
- Treatment of parkinsonism
- Relief of nausea and vomiting
- Relief of motion sickness
- Sedation
- As adjuncts to analgesics

Each antihistamine may be used for one or more of these reasons. The more specific uses of the various antihistamine preparations are given in Summary Drug Table 28-1.

ADVERSE REACTIONS ASSOCIATED WITH THE ADMINISTRATION OF THE ANTIHISTAMINES

Drowsiness and sedation are common adverse reactions seen with the use of many of the antihistamines. Some antihistamines appear to cause more drowsiness and sedation than others. Several newer preparations, for example, astemizole and terfenadine cause little, if any, drowsiness in most individuals.

Some antihistamines may cause dizziness, disturbed coordination, fatigue, hypotension, headache, epigastric distress, and photosensitivity (exaggerated response to brief exposure to the sun, resulting in moderately severe to severe sunburn.) Even though these drugs are sometimes used in the treatment of allergies, a drug allergy can occur with the use of an antihistamine. Symptoms that may indicate an allergy to these drugs include skin rash, urticaria, and anaphylactic shock. These drugs may also have anticholinergic (cholinergic blocking) effects, which may result in dryness of the mouth, nose, and throat and a thickening of bronchial secretions.

Serious cardiovascular adverse reactions, including cardiac arrest and death, have been reported in patients receiving astemizole and terfenadine. Severe arrhythmias may follow episodes of fainting (syncope).

Summary Drug Table 28-1. Antihistamines

Generic Name	Trade Name*	Uses	Adverse Reactions	Dose Ranges
astemizole	Hismanal	Allergic symptoms	Drowsiness, dry mouth, headache, increased appetite, weight gain, nausea, nervousness, dizziness, diarrhea	10 mg/d PO
brompheniramine maleate	Bromphen, Dimetane, *generic*	Allergic symptoms; allergic reactions to blood or plasma; adjunctive therapy in anaphylactic reactions	Drowsiness, sedation, dizziness, disturbed coordination, hypertension, headache, blurred vision, thickening of bronchial secretions	4 mg PO q4–6h; 8–12 mg PO of sustained release form q12h; up to 40 mg/d IM, SC, IV in divided doses
carbinoxamine maleate	Rondec (C)	Allergic rhinitis and vasomotor rhinitis	Sedation, dizziness, diplopia, vomiting, diarrhea, dry mouth, headache	PO 4–8 mg tid or qid
chlorpheniramine maleate	Chlor-Trimeton, *generic*	Allergic symptoms, hypersensitivity reactions, including anaphylaxis and transfusion reactions	Drowsiness, sedation, hypertension, palpitations, blurred vision, dry mouth, urinary hesitancy	4 mg PO q4–6h; sustained release form: 8–12 mg PO q8–12h; 5–20 mg IM, SC, IV
clemastine fumarate	Tavist	Allergic symptoms	Drowsiness, sedation, hypertension, palpitations, blurred vision, dry mouth, urinary hesitancy	1.34 mg PO bid to 2.68 mg PO tid
diphenhydramine hydrochloride	Benadryl *generic*	Allergic symptoms, hypersensitivity reactions, including anaphylaxis and transfusion reactions, motion sickness, antitussive, parkinsonism	Drowsiness, dry mouth, anorexia, blurred vision, urinary frequency	25–50 mg PO tid, qid; 10–100 mg IM, IV
loratadine	Claritin	Allergic symptoms	Dizziness, migraine headache, tremors, conjunctivitis, blurred vision, altered salivation	PO 10 mg/d
promethazine hydrochloride	Phenergan, Anergan, *generic*	Allergic symptoms, motion sickness, nausea and vomiting associated with anesthesia and surgery, adjunct to analgesics, sedation and apprehension, preoperative and postoperative sedation	Excessive sedation, confusion, disorientation, dizziness, fatigue, blurred vision, dry mouth	Allergy: 12.5–25 mg PO, 25 mg IM, IV; motion sickness, nausea, vomiting: 12.5–25 mg PO, IM, IV; 25–50 mg PO, IM, IV; preoperative: 25–50 mg IM or PO the night before surgery
terfenadine	Seldane	Allergic symptoms	Drowsiness, sedation, headache, visual disturbances, itching, urticaria, rash, nausea, vomiting, abdominal pain, dry mouth	60 mg PO bid
tripelennamine HCl	PZB, PZB-SR	Seasonal allergic rhinitis	Moderate sedation, mild GI distress, paradoxical excitation	PO 25–50 mg q4–6h; SR: 1(100 mg) tablet in AM and 1 tablet in PM

*The term, *generic,* indicates that the drug is available in generic form.

NURSING MANAGEMENT

Most antihistamines are given orally. Give these drugs with food to prevent gastrointestinal upset. Astemizole and loratadine are given on an empty stomach, at least 2 hours after meals or 1 hour before meals. The onset of action is within 15 to 30 minutes after oral administration with a duration of 3 to 4 hours. For parenteral administration, give deep intramuscularly, rather than subcutaneously because many of the antihistamines are irritating to subcutaneous tissue.

Observe the patient for the expected effects of the antihistamine and adverse reactions. Report adverse reactions to the physician. In some instances, for example, drowsiness or sedation may be present. When given to relieve preoperative anxiety, these adverse reactions are expected and are allowed to occur. Dryness of the mouth, nose, and throat may occur. Offer the patient frequent sips of water to relieve these symptoms. If the patient experiences dizziness or drowsiness provide assistance with ambulation.

If the antihistamine is given for a serious situation, such as a blood transfusion reaction or a severe drug allergy, assess the patient at frequent intervals until the symptoms appear relieved and for about 24 hours after the incident.

Nursing Alert

Do not administer antihistamines to patients with lower respiratory tract diseases. If these drugs are administered in disorders such as asthma, the drying effect on the respiratory tract may cause thickening of the respiratory secretions and make expectoration more difficult.

Immediately report any episodes of syncope (fainting) in patients receiving astemizole or terfenadine. This may be an indication of a potential cardiac arrhythmia. The physician may discontinue the medication to evaluate the patient's cardiac status.

Nursing Process
The Patient Receiving an Antihistamine

■ *Assessment*
Assessment of the patient receiving these drugs depends on the reason for use. Examples of assessments that may be performed include an assessment of the involved areas (eyes, nose, upper and lower respiratory tract) if the patient is receiving an anti-

histamine for the relief of symptoms of an allergy. If promethazine (Phenergan) is used with a narcotic to enhance the effects and reduce the dosage of the narcotic, take the blood pressure, pulse, and respiratory rate before the drug is given.

■ *Nursing Diagnoses*
Depending on the reason for administration, one or more of the following nursing diagnoses may apply to a person receiving an antihistamine:
- **Risk for Injury** related to adverse drug reactions (drowsiness, dizziness, disturbed coordination)
- **Risk for Ineffective Management of Therapeutic Regimen** related to lack of knowledge, adverse drug effects, other factors (specify)

■ *Planning and Implementation*
The major goals of the patient vary according to the reason the drug was administered and may include absence of injury and an understanding of and compliance to the prescribed therapeutic regimen. To make these goals measurable, more specific criteria must be added.

Risk for Injury. If drowsiness is severe or if other problems such as dizziness or a disturbance in muscle coordination occur, the patient may require assistance with ambulation and other activities. Place the call light within easy reach and instruct the patient to call before attempting to get out of bed or ambulate. Inform the patient that this adverse reaction may lessen with continued use of the drug.

■ *Patient and Family Teaching*
The dosage regimen and possible adverse drug reactions are reviewed with the patient. Include the following points in the patient teaching plan:
- Do not drive or perform other hazardous tasks if drowsiness occurs. This effect may diminish with continued use.
- Avoid the use of alcohol, as well as other drugs that cause sleepiness or drowsiness, while taking these drugs.
- These drugs may cause dryness of the mouth and throat. Frequent sips of water, hard candy, or chewing gum (preferably sugarless) may relieve this problem.
- Take this drug with food or meals because it may cause gastrointestinal upset.
- If the condition is not relieved, discuss this with the physician.
- Avoid ultraviolet light or sunlight because of the possibility of developing photosensitivity. Wear

sunglasses, protective clothing, and a sunscreen when exposed to sunlight.
- Take the drug 30 minutes prior to travel if used for motion sickness.

■ *Expected Outcomes for Evaluation*
- No evidence of injury
- Patient demonstrates understanding of drug regimen, adverse drug effects

Bronchodilators

A *bronchodilator* is a drug used to relieve bronchospasm associated with respiratory disorders such as bronchial asthma, chronic bronchitis, and emphysema. These conditions are progressive disorders characterized by a decrease in the inspiratory and expiratory capacity of the lung. Collectively, they are often referred to as chronic obstructive pulmonary disease. The patient with chronic obstructive pulmonary disease experiences dyspnea (difficulty breathing) with physical exertion, has difficulty inhaling and exhaling, and may exhibit a chronic cough.

ACTIONS OF THE BRONCHODILATORS

There are two types of bronchodilators: the *sympathomimetics* and the *xanthine derivatives*. Examples of sympathomimetic bronchodilators include terbutaline (Bricanyl) and albuterol (Ventolin). Examples of the xanthine derivatives are theophylline and aminophylline. Additional bronchodilators are listed in Summary Drug Table 28-2.

The *sympathomimetics* have beta-adrenergic activity (see Chap. 17), and therefore dilate the bronchi. The *xanthine derivatives*, although a different class of drugs, also have bronchodilating activity by means of their direct relaxation of the smooth muscles of the bronchi.

When bronchospasm occurs, there is a decrease in the lumen (or inside diameter) of the bronchi, which decreases the amount of air taken into the lungs with each breath. A decrease in the amount of air taken into the lungs results in respiratory distress. Use of a bronchodilating drug dilates the bronchi and allows more air to enter the lungs, which, in turn, completely or partially relieves respiratory distress.

USES OF THE BRONCHODILATORS

Bronchodilators are used primarily in the treatment of reversible airway obstruction due to bronchospasm associated with acute and chronic asthma, chronic bronchitis, emphysema or bronchiectasis (abnormal condition of the bronchial tree.) The more specific uses for the various bronchodilators are given in Summary Drug Table 28-2.

ADVERSE REACTIONS ASSOCIATED WITH THE ADMINISTRATION OF BRONCHODILATORS

Administration of a sympathomimetic bronchodilator may result in restlessness, anxiety, increase in blood pressure, palpitations, cardiac arrhythmias, and insomnia. Adverse reactions associated with administration of the xanthine derivatives include nausea, vomiting, restlessness, headache, palpitations, increased respirations, fever, hyperglycemia, and electrocardiographic changes.

NURSING MANAGEMENT

Nursing management of the patient receiving a bronchodilating drug requires careful monitoring of the patient and proper administration of the various drugs. These drugs may be given orally, parenterally or topically by inhalation or nebulization (see Chap. 2).

Oral preparations may be given with food or milk if gastric upset occurs. If a nebulizer or aerosol inhalator is used for administration, teach the patient how to use this method of delivering the drug to the lungs.

Some of these drugs, for example, aminophylline, may be given intravenously (IV)—either direct IV or as an IV infusion. Some of the sympathomimetics are extremely potent drugs. Exercise great care in reading the physician's order when preparing these drugs for administration. Note that the dose of drugs such as epinephrine and ethylnorepinephrine (Bronkephrine) are measured in *tenths* of a milliliter. Use a tuberculin syringe for measuring and administering these drugs by the parenteral route.

After administration of the drug, observe the patient for the effectiveness of drug therapy. Breathing should improve and the patient will appear less anxious. If relief does not occur, notify the physician because a different drug or an increase in dosage may be necessary.

Summary Drug Table 28-2. Systemic and Topical Bronchodilators

Generic Name	Trade Name*	Uses	Adverse Reactions	Dose Ranges
albuterol sulfate	Proventil, Ventolin	Bronchospasm, asthma	Restlessness, anxiety, fear, hypertension, palpitations, tachycardia, insomnia, tremors	2–4 mg PO tid, qid; 1–2 inhalations q4–6h or 2 inhalations prior to exercise; may also be given by nebulization
ephedrine sulfate	*generic*	Allergic disorders such as bronchial asthma	Tremors, anxiety, anorexia, nausea, vomiting, dizziness	25–50 mg PO, IM, SC, slow IV not to exceed 150 mg/24h
epinephrine	Adrenalin, Sus-Phrine, *generic*	Bronchial asthma, bronchospasm, hypersensitivity, reactions to drugs, sera, insect stings, or other allergens	Tremors, anxiety, arrhythmias, anorexia, nausea, vomiting, dyspnea	1:1000 solution: 0.3–0.5 mL (0.3–0.5 mg) SC, IM; 1:200 suspension: 0.1–0.3 mL SC; may also be given by inhalation or nebulization
ethylnorepinephrine hydrochloride	Bronkephrine	Bronchospasm	Anxiety, tremors, palpitations, headache, dizziness, anorexia, nausea, vomiting	0.5–1 mL SC, IM
isoproterenol hydrochloride	Isuprel	Bronchodilator in bronchopulmonary disease, bronchospasm	Nervousness, restlessness, tremors, insomnia, headache, hypertension, arrhythmias, nausea	10–20 mg sublingual q6–8h; bronchospasm under anesthesia: 0.01–0.02 mg IV; 1–2 inhalations 4–6 times/d; may also be given by nebulization
metaproterenol hydrochloride	Alupent, Metaprel	Bronchial asthma, bronchospasm	Tremors, anxiety, insomnia, dizziness, headache, palpitations, tachycardia	20 mg PO tid, qid; 2–3 inhalations q4–6h
terbutaline sulfate	Brethine, Bricanyl, Brethaire	Bronchospasm, bronchial asthma, emphysema	Tremors, anxiety, insomnia, dizziness, headache, palpitations, tachycardia	2.5–5 mg PO tid, 0.25 mg SC; 2 inhalations q3–4h
XANTHINE DERIVATIVES				
aminophylline	Amoline, Truphylline, *generic*	Bronchial asthma, bronchospasm	Nausea, vomiting, nervousness, anxiety, tachycardia, restlessness, headache, palpitations, insomnia	250–500 mg PO q6–8h; dosage may also be based on serum levels or body weight; IV infusion requires dilution and is given at a rate not exceeding 25 mg/min
dyphylline	Dilor, *generic*	Bronchial asthma, bronchospasm, COPD	Anxiety, restlessness, insomnia, dizziness, headache, palpitations, tachycardia, nausea, vomiting, anorexia	200–800 mg PO q6h; 250–500 mg IM
oxtriphylline	Choledyl, *generic*	Bronchial asthma, bronchospasm, COPD	Anxiety, restlessness, insomnia, dizziness, headache, palpitations, tachycardia, nausea, vomiting, anorexia	200 mg PO qid
theophylline	Slo-Phyllin, Elixophyllin, *generic*	Bronchial asthma, bronchospasm, COPD	Anxiety, restlessness, insomnia, dizziness, headache, palpitations, tachycardia, nausea, vomiting, anorexia	250–500 mg/q6h PO; dosage may also be based on serum levels

*The term, *generic*, indicates that the drug is available in generic form.

For patients receiving a xanthine derivative such as theophylline, the dosage is individualized and based on improvement of the patient's condition and serum theophylline drug levels. Therapeutic range of theophylline blood levels is 10 to 20 mcg/mL. Levels greater than 20 mcg/mL may cause toxicity.

> ### Nursing Alert
>
> Notify the physician immediately if any of the following signs of theophylline toxicity develop: anorexia, nausea, vomiting, restlessness, insomnia, tachycardia, arrhythmias, seizures.

If the patient has acute bronchospasm, check the blood pressure, pulse, respiratory rate, and response to the drug every 15 to 30 minutes until the patient's condition stabilizes and respiratory distress is relieved.

If a drug is given IV, administer through an infusion pump. Monitor the IV site closely for signs of extravasation. Check the IV infusion site at frequent intervals because these patients may be extremely restless. If aminophylline is given as a rectal suppository, check the patient every 15 to 30 minutes to be sure the suppository has been retained. If the patient is unable to retain the suppository, contact the physician because another route of administration may be necessary.

Adverse Drug Reactions

Observe the patient for adverse drug reactions. If adverse reactions occur, the next dose is withheld and the physician is contacted. Patients who have difficulty breathing and are receiving a sympathomimetic drug may experience extreme anxiety, nervousness, and restlessness, which may be due to their breathing difficulty, as well as the action of the sympathomimetic drug. In these patients, it may be difficult for the physician to determine if the patient is having an adverse drug reaction or if the problem is related to the respiratory disorder. Monitor blood pressure and pulse closely during therapy and report any significant changes.

Nursing Process
The Patient Receiving a Bronchodilator

■ Assessment
Assessment of the patient depends on the reason the drug is administered. Take the blood pressure, pulse, and respiratory rate before bronchodilator therapy is initiated and monitor throughout the course of therapy. Assess the lung fields and describe the sounds heard on the patient's chart both before and throughout therapy. If the patient is raising sputum, record a description of the sputum. Note and record the patient's general physical condition.

■ Nursing Diagnoses
Depending on the severity of bronchospasm, one or more of the following nursing diagnoses may apply to the patient receiving a bronchodilator:
- **Anxiety** related to difficulty breathing
- **Risk for Ineffective Management of Therapeutic Regimen** related to lack of knowledge of medication regimen, adverse drug effects, other (specify)

■ Planning and Implementation
The major goals of the patient may include a reduction in anxiety and an understanding of and compliance to the prescribed treatment regimen. To make these goals measurable, more specific criteria must be added.

Anxiety. The patient having difficulty breathing is bound to have anxiety, the extent of which depends on the degree of respiratory difficulty. Reassure the patient that the medication being administered will most likely relieve his or her respiratory distress in a short time. Observe patients who are extremely apprehensive more frequently until their respirations are near normal.

■ Patient and Family Teaching
If using an aerosol inhalator for administration of the bronchodilator, provide a thorough explanation of its use (see Chap. 2). Each brand is slightly different. Carefully review the instruction sheet that is provided with these products describing how the unit is assembled, used, and cleaned with the patient.

> ### Nursing Alert
>
> Do not assume that patient understands how to used an aerosol inhaler correctly. Many patients, even with repeated instruction, do not use the proper technique to administer the drug by inhalation. Along with verbal instructions, have the patient demonstrate to evaluate if he or she is using the proper technique. Repeat instructions at each follow-up visit.

Include the following points in the patient teaching plan:

- Take the drug exactly as prescribed by the physician.
- If symptoms become worse, do *not* increase the dose or frequency of use unless directed to do so by the physician.
- If gastrointestinal upset occurs, take this drug with food or milk (oral form).
- Drink six to eight glasses of water each day to decrease the thickness of secretions.
- Do not use nonprescription drugs (some may contain sympathomimetic drugs) unless use has been approved by the physician.
- Avoid smoking (when applicable). Smoking may make it difficult to adjust the dosage and may worsen breathing problems.
- These drugs may cause nervousness, insomnia, and restlessness (especially the sympathomimetics). Contact the physician if these symptoms become severe.
- When using an aerosol inhaler, if more than one inhalation is prescribed, wait at least 1 full minute between inhalations. When using isoproterenol and epinephrine, wait 3 to 5 minutes between inhalations. For metaprotererol, wait at least 10 minutes between inhalations.
- Stress the importance of frequent monitoring of theophylline serum levels.

■ *Expected Outcomes for Evaluation*
- Anxiety is reduced
- Patient demonstrates understanding of drug regimen, use of nebulizer, or aerosol inhalator

Decongestants

A *decongestant* is a drug that reduces swelling of the nasal passages, which, in turn, opens clogged nasal passages and enhances drainage of the sinuses.

ACTIONS OF THE DECONGESTANTS

The nasal decongestants are sympathomimetic agents, which produce localized vasoconstriction of the small blood vessels of the nasal membranes. Vasoconstriction reduces swelling in the nasal passages (decongestive activity). Nasal decongestants may be applied

topically and a few are available for oral use. Examples of nasal decongestants include phenylephrine (Neo-Synephrine) and oxymetazoline (Afrin), which are available as nasal sprays or drops and pseudoephedrine (Sudafed) which is taken orally. Additional nasal decongestants are listed in Summary Drug Table 28-3.

USES OF THE DECONGESTANTS

Decongestants are administered directly to the affected membranes by spray or drops or they can be administered systemically through the oral route. They are used to treat the congestion associated with rhinitis, hay fever, allergic rhinitis, sinusitis and the common cold.

ADVERSE REACTIONS ASSOCIATED WITH THE ADMINISTRATION OF THE DECONGESTANTS

When used topically in prescribed doses, there are usually minimal systemic effects in most individuals. On occasion, nasal burning, stinging, and dryness may be seen. *Overuse* of the topical form of these drugs can cause "rebound" nasal congestion, that is, the congestion becomes worse with the use of the drug. Although congestion may be relieved for a *brief* time after the drug is used, it recurs within a short time, which then prompts the patient to use the drug at more frequent intervals. When the topical form is used frequently or if the liquid is swallowed, the same adverse reactions seen with the oral decongestants may occur.

Use of oral decongestants may result in tachycardia and other cardiac arrhythmias, nervousness, restlessness, insomnia, blurred vision, nausea, and vomiting.

NURSING MANAGEMENT

Decongestants are used only occasionally in the clinical setting. Since some of these products are available without a prescription, the use of these products may be discovered during a patient history for other medical disorders. A history of the use of these products should be obtained including the name of the product used and frequency of use. Nonpre-

Summary Drug Table 28-3. Systemic and Topical Nasal Decongestants

Generic Name	Trade Name*	Uses	Adverse Reactions	Dose Ranges
ephedrine	Efedron	Nasal congestion	Nasal burning, stinging, dryness, rebound nasal congestion	2–3 drops or small amount of jelly in each nostril q4–6h
epinephrine hydrochloride	Adrenalin chloride	Nasal congestion	Nasal burning, stinging, dryness, rebound nasal congestion	1–2 drops in each nostril q4–6h
naphazoline hydrochloride	Privine	Nasal congestion	Nasal burning, stinging, dryness, rebound nasal congestion	2 drops in each nostril prn
oxymetazoline hydrochloride	Afrin, Dristan Long Lasting *generic*	Nasal congestion	Nasal burning, stinging, dryness, rebound nasal congestion	2–3 drops or sprays q12h
phenylephrine hydrochloride	Neo-Synephrine, Alconefrin	Nasal congestion	Nasal burning, stinging, dryness, rebound nasal congestion	1–2 drops or sprays in each nostril
phenyl-propanolamine hydrochloride	Propagest, *generic*	Nasal congestion	Anxiety, restlessness, anorexia, arrhythmias, nervousness, nausea, vomiting, blurred vision	25 mg PO q4h; 50 mg PO q8h
pseudoephedrine hydrochloride	Sudafed, *generic*	Nasal congestion	Anxiety, restlessness, anorexia, arrhythmias, nervousness, nausea, vomiting, blurred vision	60 mg PO q4–6h
tetrahydrozoline hydrochloride	Tyzine	Nasal congestion	Anxiety, restlessness, anorexia, arrhythmias, nervousness, nausea, vomiting, blurred vision	2–4 drops in each nostril
xylometazoline hydrochloride	Otrivin	Nasal congestion	Nasal burning, stinging, dryness, rebound nasal congestion	2–3 drops or sprays in each nostril q8–10h

*The term, *generic,* indicates that the drug is available in generic form.

scription nasal decongestants should not be used by those with hypertension or heart disease unless use is approved by the physician. The nurse should inform the physician if nasal congestion is not relieved.

Nursing Process
The Patient Using a Nasal Decongestant

■ *Assessment*
Assess the blood pressure, pulse, and congestion prior to and periodically throughout drug therapy when administering a decongestant. Assess and record lung sounds and bronchial secretions in the patient's record.

■ *Nursing Diagnosis*
● **Risk for Ineffective Management of Therapeutic Regimen** related to lack of knowledge of medication regimen, adverse drug effects, other (specify)

■ *Planning and Implementation*
The major goal of the patient may include an understanding of the use and adverse reactions associated with nasal decongestants. To make this goal measurable, more specific criteria must be added.

■ *Patient and Family Teaching*
Include the following points in the patient teaching plan:
● Use this product as directed by the physician or on the container label.

- Overuse of topical nasal decongestants can make the symptoms *worse*.
- Nasal burning and stinging may occur with the topical decongestants. If this becomes severe, discontinue use and discuss this problem with the physician, who may prescribe or recommend another drug.
- If using a spray, do not allow the tip of the container to touch the nasal mucosa and do not share the container with anyone.
- To administer the spray, sit upright and sniff hard for a few minutes after administration.
- To administer the drops, lie down on a bed with your head over the edge. Remain in this position several minutes after administering the drops.
- If symptoms do not improve within 7 days or if a high fever develops, contact the physician.

■ *Expected Outcomes for Evaluation*
- Patient verbalizes understanding of use of a decongestant and adverse reactions associated with use

Chapter Summary

- Histamine is a substance produced by the body in response to injury. Histamine acts on the vascular system and smooth muscle to produce vasodilation and increase the permeability of small vessels producing localized redness and edema. Antihistamines are drugs used to counteract the effects of histamine on the body organs and structures. Antihistamines block most of the effects of histamine by competing for histamine at the receptor sites. Antihistamines also have antipruritic, antiemetic, and sedative effects. Antihistamines are used primarily to relieve the symptoms associated with various types of allergies from seasonal allergic rhinitis to the life-threatening allergic response exhibited in anaphylactic shock. Drowsiness and sedation are the most common adverse reactions associated with administration of the antihistamines. The patient is warned to avoid any activity that requires mental alertness until the response of the drug in known.

- The bronchodilators are drugs used to relieve bronchospasms associated with bronchial asthma, chronic asthma, and emphysema. The two types of bronchodilators, the sympathomimetics and the xanthine derivatives, both have bronchodilating activity that acts to increase the lumen of the bronchi and allow more air to enter the respiratory tract. This either partially or completely relieves respiratory distress. Administration of a sympathomimetic bronchodilator may result in restlessness, anxiety, increase in blood pressure, and palpitations. Adverse reactions associated with the xanthine derivatives include nausea, vomiting, restlessness, and palpitations. Nursing management of the patient receiving a bronchodilating drug requires careful monitoring and proper administration of the various drugs.
- Decongestants are drugs used to reduce the swelling of the nasal passages, thereby opening clogged nasal passages and promoting sinus drainage. When used as prescribed, most individuals experience minimal adverse effects. However, overuse of the topical form of these drugs can cause rebound nasal congestion, that is, the congestion becomes worse with use. This is usually the result of not following the prescribed treatment regimen.

Critical Thinking Exercises

1. Mr. Potter, aged 57, is admitted to the pulmonary unit in acute respiratory distress. The physician orders IV aminophylline. In developing a care plan for Mr. Potter, you select the nursing diagnosis **Ineffective Airway Clearance**. What five nursing interventions would be most important in managing this problem?
2. Ms. Smith, aged 68, returned to the clinic for a follow-up visit after being diagnosed with chronic obstructive pulmonary disease. She is taking theophylline daily and using a metered-dose inhaler four times a day. What assessments would be most important for you to make at this time? What information is critical for you to be certain that Ms. Smith understands?

29

Antitussives, Mucolytics, and Expectorants

Key Terms

Chapter Outline

Chapter Objectives

On completion of this chapter the student will:

- *Define the terms antitussive, mucolytic, and expectorant*
- *Describe the uses and actions of antitussive, mucolytic, and expectorant drugs*
- *Discuss the nursing management of the patient receiving an antitussive, mucolytic, or expectorant*
- *Use the nursing process when administering an antitussive, mucolytic, or expectorant*

Upper respiratory infections are one of the most common afflictions of man. Many of the drugs used to treat the discomfort associated with an upper respiratory infection are available as nonprescription (over-the-counter) drugs, whereas others are only available by prescription.

Antitussives

An *antitussive* is a drug used to relieve coughing. Many antitussive drugs are combined with another drug, such as an antihistamine or expectorant, and sold as nonprescription cough medicine. Other antitussives, either alone or in combination with other drugs, are available by prescription only.

ACTIONS OF THE ANTITUSSIVES

Some antitussives depress the cough center located in the medulla and are called centrally-acting agents. Codeine and dextromethorphan are examples of centrally-acting antitussives. Other antitussives are peripherally-acting agents and act by anesthetizing stretch receptors in the respiratory passages, thereby decreasing coughing. An example of this type of antitussive is benzonatate (Tessalon Perles).

USES OF THE ANTITUSSIVES

Antitussives are used for the relief of a nonproductive cough. When the cough is productive of sputum, it should be treated by a physician who, based on a physical examination, may or may not prescribe or recommend an antitussive.

ADVERSE REACTIONS ASSOCIATED WITH THE ADMINISTRATION OF ANTITUSSIVES

Use of codeine may result in respiratory depression, euphoria, lightheadedness, sedation, nausea, vomiting, and hypersensitivity reactions. The more common adverse reactions associated with the antitussives are listed in Summary Drug Table 29-1. When used as directed, nonprescription cough medicines containing two or more ingredients have few adverse reactions, however, those that contain an antihistamine may cause drowsiness.

One problem associated with the use of an antitussive is related to its drug action. Although not an adverse reaction, depression of the cough reflex can cause a pooling of secretions in the lungs. A pooling of the secretions that are normally removed by coughing may result in more serious problems, such as pneumonia and atelectasis. For this reason, using an antitussive for a productive cough is often contraindicated.

Another problem can arise from the use of nonprescription cough medicine for self-treatment of a chronic cough. Indiscriminate use of antitussives by the general public may prevent early diagnosis and treatment of serious disorders, such as lung cancer and emphysema.

NURSING MANAGEMENT

When a patient has a cough, describe the type of cough (productive or nonproductive of sputum) and the frequency of coughing in the patient's chart. Also note and record whether the cough interrupts sleep or causes pain in the chest or other parts of the body.

Nursing Process
The Patient Receiving an Antitussive Drug

■ *Assessment*
A hospitalized patient may occasionally have an antitussive preparation prescribed, especially when a nonproductive cough causes discomfort, or threatens to cause more serious problems, such as raising pressure in the eye (increased intraocular pressure) following eye surgery or increasing intracranial pressure in those with disorders of the central nervous system. To assess, document the type of cough (productive, nonproductive) and, when present, describe the color and amount of the sputum. Take vital signs because some patients with a productive cough may have an infection.

■ *Nursing Diagnoses*
Depending on the reason for administration, one or more of the following nursing diagnoses may apply to a person receiving an antitussive drug:
● **Anxiety** related to need to cough frequently, pain or discomfort associated with coughing

Summary Drug Table 29-1. The Antitussives, Mucolytics, and Expectorants

Generic Name	Trade Name*	Uses	Adverse Reactions	Dose Ranges
ANTITUSSIVES				
Narcotics				
codeine sulfate	generic	Suppression of nonproductive cough	Respiratory depression, euphoria, lightheadedness, sedation, nausea, vomiting	10–20 mg PO q4–6h
Nonnarcotics				
benzonatate	Tessalon Perles	Same as codeine sulfate	Sedation, headache, mild dizziness, constipation, nausea, GI upset	100 mg PO tid
dextromethorphan hydrobromide	Hold DM, Suppress, Robitussin ES, generic	Same as codeine sulfate	Rare	10–30 mg PO q4–8h
diphenhydramine hydrochloride	Benylin Cough, generic	Same as codeine sulfate	Drowsiness, postural hypotension, epigastric distress, thickening of bronchial secretions, sedation	25 mg PO q4h
MUCOLYTICS				
acetylcysteine	Mucomyst, generic	Reduce viscosity of mucus in acute and chronic bronchopulmonary disease, tracheostomy care, atelectasis due to mucus obstruction	Stomatitis, nausea, vomiting, fever, drowsiness, bronchospasm, irritation of trachea and bronchi	1–10 mL of 20% solution or 2–20 mL of 10% solution by nebulization q2–6h; direct instillation; 1–2 mL of 10% or 20% solution as often as every hour
EXPECTORANTS				
guaifenesin (glyceryl guaiacolate)	Hytuss, Fenesin, generic	Relief of respiratory conditions characterized by dry, nonproductive cough and in the presence of mucus in the respiratory tract	Nausea, vomiting, dizziness, headache, rash	100–400 mg PO q4h; sustained release tablets 600 mg PO q12h
potassium iodide	SSKI, Pima, generic	Same as guaifenesin	Iodine sensitivity or iodinism (sore mouth, metallic taste, increased salivation, nausea, vomiting, epigastric pain, parotid swelling and pain)	300–1000 mg PO after meals 2–3 times daily and up to 1.5 g PO tid

*The term, *generic,* indicates that the drug is available in generic form.

- **Sleep Pattern Disturbance** related to coughing at night
- **Risk for Ineffective Management of Therapeutic Regimen** related to lack of knowledge of medication regimen, adverse drug effects

■ *Planning and Implementation*

The major goals of the patient may include a reduction in anxiety and an understanding of the prescribed treatment regimen. To make these goals measurable, more specific criteria must be added.

Anxiety. If the patient appears anxious over the need to cough at frequent intervals, reassure the patient that the medication will most likely relieve this problem. If the cough is not relieved, notify the physician.

Sleep Pattern Disturbance. Note whether coughing keeps the patient awake at night or if the patient has difficulty falling asleep after being awakened by coughing. If sleep is frequently interrupted by coughing, discuss the problem with the physician.

■ *Patient and Family Teaching*

Discourage the indiscriminate use of nonprescription cough medicines, especially when coughing produces sputum. Advise the patient to read the label carefully, follow the dosage recommendations, and consult a physician if the cough persists for more than 10 days or if fever or chest pain occurs. If an antitussive is prescribed for use at home, include the following in a teaching plan:

• Do not exceed the recommended dose.
• If chills, fever, chest pain, or sputum production occurs, contact the physician as soon as possible.
• Drink plenty of fluids.
• Oral capsules—Do not chew or break the capsules open; swallow them whole.
• If the cough is not relieved or becomes worse, contact the physician.

■ *Expected Outcomes for Evaluation*

• Reduces anxiety
• Relieves coughing
• Sleeps through night
• Patient and family demonstrate understanding of drug regimen

Mucolytics and Expectorants

A *mucolytic* is a drug that loosens respiratory secretions. An *expectorant* is a drug that aids in raising thick, tenacious mucus from the respiratory passages.

ACTIONS OF THE MUCOLYTICS AND EXPECTORANTS

A drug with mucolytic activity appears to reduce the viscosity (thickness) of respiratory secretions by direct action on the mucus. The only mucolytic presently in use is acetylcysteine (Mucomyst).

Expectorants increase the production of respiratory secretions, which, in turn, appears to decrease the viscosity of the mucus, which helps to raise secretions from the respiratory passages. An example of an expectorant is guaifenesin (Hytuss).

USES OF THE MUCOLYTICS AND EXPECTORANTS

The mucolytic acetylcysteine may be used as part of the treatment of bronchopulmonary diseases such as emphysema. It is primarily given by nebulization but also may be directly instilled into a tracheostomy to liquefy (thin) secretions.

Expectorants are used to help raise respiratory secretions. An expectorant may also be included along with one or more additional drugs, such as an antihistamine, decongestant, or antitussive, in some prescription and nonprescription cough medicines.

ADVERSE REACTIONS ASSOCIATED WITH THE ADMINISTRATION OF MUCOLYTICS AND EXPECTORANTS

The more common adverse reactions associated with mucolytic and expectorant drugs are listed in Summary Drug Table 29-1.

NURSING MANAGEMENT

On the patient's chart, record a description of the sputum raised. Patients with thick, tenacious mucus may have difficulty breathing. Notify the physician if the patient has difficulty breathing because of an inability to raise sputum and clear the respiratory passages.

Nursing Process
The Patient Receiving a Mucolytic or an Expectorant

■ *Assessment*

Determine the patient's degree of respiratory congestion by auscultating the lungs.

■ *Nursing Diagnoses*

• **Anxiety** related to respiratory difficulty, inability to raise sputum
• **Risk for Ineffective Management of Therapeutic Regimen** related to lack of knowledge of medication regimen, adverse drug effects, treatment modalities

■ *Planning and Implementation*

The major goals of the patient may include a reduction in anxiety and an understanding of the medication regimen. To make these goals measurable, more specific criteria must be added.

When the mucolytic acetylcysteine is administered by nebulization, explain the treatment to the patient and demonstrate how the nebulizer will be used. Remain with the patient during the first few treatments, especially when the patient is elderly or exhibits anxiety. Supply the patient with tissues and a paper bag for disposal of the tissues and place them within the patient's reach. Immediately before and after treatment, auscultate the lungs and record the findings of both assessments on the patient's chart. Between treatments, evaluate the patient's respiratory status and record these findings on the patient's chart. These evaluations aid the physician in determining the effectiveness of therapy. If any problem occurs during or after treatment, or if the patient is uncooperative, discuss the problem with the physician.

If acetylcysteine is ordered to be inserted into a tracheostomy, make sure suction equipment is at the bedside to be immediately available for aspiration of secretions. Record the effectiveness of therapy with acetylcysteine in the patient's chart.

When expectorants are given to those with chronic pulmonary disease, evaluate the effectiveness of drug therapy (ie, the patient's ability to raise sputum) and record this finding in the patient's chart.

Anxiety. Reassure the patient that the prescribed therapy will most likely help in raising secretions. Report any difficulty in breathing or severe anxiety over inability to breathe or to raise secretions to the physician.

■ *Patient and Family Teaching*
Acetylcysteine usually is administered in the hospital but may be prescribed for the patient being discharged and renting or buying respiratory therapy equipment for use at home. Give the patient or a family member full instruction in the use and maintenance of the equipment, as well as the technique of administration of acetylcysteine.

When an expectorant is prescribed, instruct the patient to take the drug as directed and to contact the physician if any unusual symptoms or other problems occur during use of the drug or if the drug appears to be ineffective.

■ *Expected Outcomes for Evaluation*
- Anxiety is reduced
- Patient and family demonstrate understanding of drug regimen, use of equipment to administer the drug (mucolytic)

Chapter Summary

- An antitussive is a drug used to relieve coughing. Many antitussive drugs are combined with another drug, such as an antihistamine or expectorant, and sold as nonprescription cough medicine. Other antitussives, either alone or in combination with other drugs, are available by prescription only.
- Some antitussives depress the cough center located in the medulla and are called centrally-acting agents. Codeine and dextromethorphan are examples of centrally-acting antitussives. Other antitussives are peripherally-acting agents and act by anesthetizing stretch receptors in the respiratory passages, thereby decreasing coughing. An example of this type of antitussive is benzonatate (Tessalon Perles). Antitussives are used for the relief of a nonproductive cough. When the cough is productive of sputum, it should be treated by a physician.
- A mucolytic is a drug that loosens respiratory secretions. An expectorant is a drug that aids in raising thick, tenacious mucus from the respiratory passages.
- A drug with mucolytic activity appears to reduce the thickness (viscosity) of respiratory secretions by direct action on the mucus. The only mucolytic presently in use is acetylcysteine (Mucomyst).
- Expectorants increase the production of respiratory secretions, which, in turn, appears to decrease the thickness of the mucus. An example of an expectorant is guaifenesin (Hytuss).
- When a patient has a cough, the type of cough (productive or nonproductive of sputum) and the frequency of coughing is described in the patient's chart. The nurse also notes and records whether the cough interrupts sleep or causes pain in the chest or other parts of the body.
- A description of the sputum raised is noted and recorded on the patient's chart. Patients with thick, tenacious mucus may have difficulty breathing. If the patient has difficulty breathing because of an inability to raise sputum and clear the respiratory passages, the physician is notified.

Critical Thinking Exercises

1. Your neighbor, Mr. Peterson, tells you that he has had a chronic cough for the past several months and asks you what is the best "cough medicine" to buy. What advice would you give to Mr. Peterson?
2. Ms. Moore, a patient in a nursing home, has had a cough for the past 3 weeks. Ms. Moore's physician is aware of her problem and has ordered an expectorant but told her that he wants her to cough and raise sputum. Ms. Moore's family asks you if something can be given to their mother to stop her from coughing. How would you discuss this problem and explain the prescribed therapy with Ms. Moore's family?

Drugs That Affect the Cardiovascular System

VI

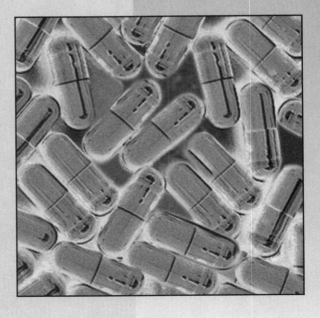

30

The Cardiotonics

Key Terms

Cardiac glycosides
Cardiac output
Digitalis glycosides
Digitalis toxicity
Digitalization
Positive inotropic action

Chapter Outline

Chapter Objectives

On completion of this chapter the student will:

- *Discuss the uses and general drug actions of the cardiotonics*
- *List the general adverse reactions seen with the administration of a cardiotonic*
- *Define and list the symptoms of digitalis toxicity*
- *Discuss nursing management when administering a cardiotonic*
- *Use the nursing process when administering a cardiotonic*

The cardiotonics are drugs used to increase the efficiency of the contraction of the heart muscle. The cardiotonics are the oldest and most effective drugs used to treat congestive heart failure (CHF), a condition in which the heart cannot pump enough blood to meet the tissue needs of the body. The cardiotonics improve the contraction of the heart muscle, which leads to improved blood flow to all tissues of the body.

The Cardiotonics

The cardiotonics include deslanoside (Cedilanid-D), digitoxin, and digoxin (Lanoxin). Other terms used to identify the cardiotonics are *cardiac glycosides* or *digitalis glycosides*. The digitalis or cardiac glycosides are obtained from the leaves of the purple foxglove or the *Digitalis purpurea* and the *Digitalis lanate*.

Miscellaneous drugs such as amrinone lactate (Inocor) and milrinone lactate (Primacor) are nonglycosides used in the short-term management of CHF. See Summary Drug Table 30-1 for information concerning the miscellaneous drugs.

ACTIONS OF THE CARDIOTONICS

The cardiotonics all have the same basic drug action; the only difference is in the speed and duration of action of each drug.

A heart weakened by disease or age sometimes cannot pump a sufficient amount of blood to meet the demands of the body leaving the patient in danger of developing CHF. In CHF, the heart is weakened causing a decrease in the amount of oxygenated blood leaving the left ventricle during each myocardial contraction. The amount of blood leaving the left ventricle at the time of each contraction is called the *cardiac output*. A marked decrease in cardiac output deprives the kidneys, brain, and other vital organs of an adequate blood supply. When the kidneys are deprived of an adequate blood supply, they are unable to effectively remove water, electrolytes, and waste products from the bloodstream. Excess fluid (edema) may occur in the lungs or tissues. The body then attempts to make up for this deficit by increasing the heart rate, which, in turn, circulates more blood through the kidneys, brain, and other vital organs. In many instances, an increase in the heart rate ultimately fails to deliver an adequate amount of blood to the kidneys, as well as to other vital organs. An increased heart rate also places added strain on the heart's muscle, which may further weaken the heart.

Cardiotonic drugs increase the force of contraction of the muscle (myocardium) of the heart. This is called a *positive inotropic action*. When the force of contraction of the myocardium is increased, cardiac output is increased. When cardiac output is increased, the blood supply to the kidneys and other vital organs is then increased. Water, electrolytes, and waste products are removed in adequate amounts and the symptoms of inadequate heart action or CHF are relieved. In most instances, the heart rate also decreases since vital organs are now receiving an adequate blood supply because of the increased force of myocardial contraction.

The cardiotonics also affect the transmission of electrical impulses along the pathway of the conduction system of the heart. The conduction system of the heart is a group of specialized nerve fibers consisting of the sinoatrial (SA) node, the atrioventricular node, the bundle of His, and the branches of Purkinje (Fig. 30-1). Each heartbeat (or contraction of the ventricles), which is the pulse felt at the wrist and other areas of the body where an artery is close to the surface or lies near a bone, is the result of an electrical impulse that normally starts in the SA node, is then received by the atrioventricular node, and travels down the bundle of His and through the Purkinje fibers (see Fig. 30-1). When the electrical impulse reaches the Purkinje fibers, the ventricles contract. Normally, once the ventricles contract, another electrical impulse is generated by the SA node and the cycle begins again. Cardiotonic drugs depress the SA node and slow conduction of the electrical impulse to the atrioventricular node. Slowing this part of the transmission of nerve impulses decreases the number of impulses and the number of ventricular contractions per minute.

USES OF THE CARDIOTONICS

The cardiotonics are used in the treatment of CHF, atrial fibrillation, atrial flutter, and paroxysmal atrial tachycardia.

ADVERSE REACTIONS ASSOCIATED WITH THE ADMINISTRATION OF THE CARDIOTONICS

There is a narrow margin of safety between the full therapeutic effects and the toxic effects of cardiotonic drugs. After a time, even normal doses of a car-

Summary Drug Table 30-1. Cardiotonics

Generic Name	Trade Name*	Uses	Adverse Reactions	Dose Ranges
deslanoside	Cedilanid-D	Congestive heart failure, atrial fibrillation and flutter, paroxysmal atrial tachycardia	Anorexia, nausea, vomiting, abdominal pain, blurred vision, yellow or green vision, halo effect around dark objects, arrhythmias	Loading dose: 1.6 mg IV, IM given as 1 injection or in portions of 0.8 mg each
digitoxin	Crystodigin, *generic*	Congestive heart failure, atrial fibrillation and flutter, paroxysmal atrial tachycardia	Anorexia, nausea, vomiting, abdominal pain, blurred vision, yellow or green vision, halo effect around dark objects, arrhythmias	Loading dose: rapid digitalization—0.6 mg followed by 0.4 mg PO, then 0.2 mg at 4–6 h intervals; slow digitalization: 0.2 mg PO bid for 4 d; maintenance dose: 0.05–0.3 mg/d PO
digoxin	Lanoxin, Lanoxicaps, *generic*	Congestive heart failure, atrial fibrillation and flutter, paroxysmal atrial tachycardia	Anorexia, nausea, vomiting, abdominal pain, blurred vision, yellow or green vision, halo effect around dark objects, arrhythmias	Loading dose: 0.4–0.6 mg IV or 0.5–0.75 mg PO but dosage for both routes varies, maintenance: based on serum digoxin levels
MISCELLANEOUS AGENTS				
amrinone lactate	Inocor	Short-term management of CHF patients who have not responded to digitalis, diuretics or vasodilators	Thrombocytopenia, nausea, abdominal pain, vomiting, hypotension	IV: 0.75 mg/kg bolus, may repeat in 30 min; maintenance: IV 5–10 mcg/kg/ min not to exceed 10 mg/ kg per day
milrinone lactate	Primacor	Congestive heart failure	Ventricular arrhythmias, headaches, hypokalemia, tremor, thrombocytopenia	IV: up to 1.13 mg/kg/d
ANTIDOTE-DIGOXIN SPECIFIC				
digoxin immune Fab (ovine)	Digibind	Digoxin toxicity	Rare; hypokalemia, reemergence of atrial fibrillation or CHF	IV: dosage depends on total dose or body load in mg. Normal dosage: up to 800 mg

*The term, *generic*, indicates that the drug is available in a generic form.

diotonic can cause toxic drug effects. The term *digitalis toxicity* (digitalis intoxication) is used when toxic drug effects occur when *any* cardiotonic is administered. The signs of digitalis toxicity include the following:

Gastrointestinal—anorexia, nausea, vomiting, diarrhea

Muscular—weakness (asthenia)

Central nervous system—headache, apathy, drowsiness, visual disturbances (blurred vision, disturbance in yellow/green vision, halo effect around dark objects), mental depression, confusion, disorientation, delirium.

Cardiac—changes in pulse rate or rhythm

Digitalis toxicity often results in electrocardiographic changes such as bradycardia, tachycardia, premature ventricular contractions, and a bigeminy (two beats followed by a pause) or trigeminy (three beats followed by a pause) pulse. Other arrhythmias (abnormal heart rhythm) may also be seen. Any change in the pulse rate or rhythm *may* indicate digitalis toxicity.

The physician may treat digitalis toxicity by temporarily discontinuing the drug until signs of toxicity disappear. The physician may also order a potassium salt to be given orally or intravenously. If severe bradycardia occurs, atropine (see Chap. 20) may be ordered. If digoxin or digitoxin has been

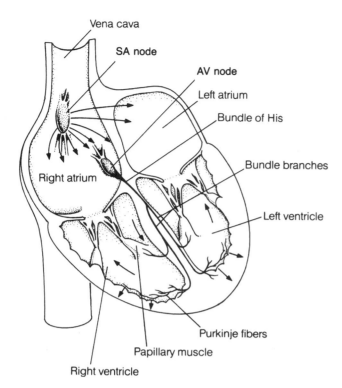

Figure 30-1

The conducting system of the heart. Impulses originating in the SA node are transmitted through the atria to the AV node down the bundle of His and the bundle branches through the Purkinje fibers to the ventricles.

given, the physician may order blood tests to determine drug serum levels. The therapeutic serum level of digoxin is 0.5 to 2 ng/mL (nanogram/milliliter) and the toxic serum level is more than 2.5 ng/mL. The therapeutic serum level of digitoxin is 20 to 35 ng/mL and the toxic serum level is more than 35 ng/mL.

Digoxin has a rapid onset and a short duration of action, whereas digitoxin has a slower onset and longer duration of action. Once the drug is withheld, the toxic effects of digoxin will disappear more rapidly than those of digitoxin. Digitalis has a slow onset and long duration of action. Deslanoside, which is only given parenterally, has an onset and duration of action similar to, but slightly longer than, parenteral digoxin.

NURSING MANAGEMENT

Digitalization

Patients started on therapy with a cardiotonic are being **digitalized**. Digitalizing doses are also referred to as **loading doses. Digitalization** is a

series of doses given until the drug begins to exert a **full therapeutic effect.** Once a full therapeutic effect is achieved, the patient is usually placed on a **maintenance dose** schedule. The ranges for digitalizing (loading) and maintenance doses are given in Summary Drug Table 30-1. There are variations in digitalizing doses, and the physician may decide to achieve full digitalization rapidly or slowly, depending on the patient's diagnosis, age, present condition, and other factors.

Administration

Before administering *each dose* of a cardiotonic, take the apical pulse rate for 60 seconds. Record the apical pulse in the designated area on the chart or the medication administration record and administer the medication. Withhold the drug and notify the physician if the pulse rate is 60 or below unless there is a written order giving different guidelines for withholding the drug.

Nursing Alert

The drug should also be withheld and the physician contacted if there are any signs of digitalis toxicity; if there is any change in the pulse rhythm; if there is a marked increase or decrease in the pulse rate since the last time it was taken; or if the patient's general condition appears to have worsened.

When a cardiotonic is given intravenously, administer slowly. When given intramuscularly, rotate the injection sites. To rotate injection sites correctly, a chart showing the order of rotation is inserted in the Kardex or the medication administration record. Each time the drug is given, record the injection site in the patient's chart.

During digitalization, the blood pressure, pulse, and respiratory rate are taken every 2 to 4 hours or as ordered by the physician. This time interval may be increased or decreased, depending on the patient's condition and the route used for administration.

Serum levels (digoxin or digitoxin) may be ordered daily during the period of digitalization and periodically during maintenance therapy. Periodic electrocardiograms, serum electrolytes, hepatic, and renal function tests, as well as other laboratory studies, may also be ordered.

Digitalis Toxicity and Adverse Drug Effects

Observe for signs of digitalis toxicity every 2 to 4 hours during digitalization and one to two times a day when a maintenance dose is being given. *Digitalis toxicity can occur even when normal doses are being administered or when the patient has been receiving a maintenance dose.*

Nursing Alert

Withhold the drug and report any of the following signs of digitalis toxicity to the physician immediately: loss of appetite (anorexia), nausea, vomiting, abdominal pain, visual disturbances (blurred, yellow or green vision and white halos, borders around dark objects) and arrhythmias (any type). Serum digoxin levels greater than 2.0 ng/mL and serum digitoxin levels greater than 35 ng/mL are also immediately reported.

When digitalis toxicity develops, the physician may discontinue digitalis until all signs of toxicity are gone.

Digoxin immune Fab (Digibind) is digoxin specific antigen binding fragments (fab) used as antidote in the treatment of digoxin overdosage. The dosage varies with the amount of digoxin ingested and is administered by the intravenous route over a 30-minute period. Most life-threatening states can be adequately treated with 800 mg of digoxin immune Fab. Few adverse reactions have been observed. However, worsening of CHF, low cardiac output, hypokalemia, or atrial fibrillation may occur (see Summary Drug Table 30-1).

Weigh patients receiving a cardiotonic drug daily or as ordered. Measure intake and output especially if the patient has edema, CHF, or is also receiving a diuretic. Diuretics (see Chap. 34) may be ordered for some patients receiving a cardiotonic drug. Diuretics, as well as other conditions or factors such as gastrointestinal suction, diarrhea, and old age, may produce low serum potassium levels (hypokalemia).

Nursing Alert

Hypokalemia makes the heart muscle more sensitive to digitalis, thereby increasing the possibility of developing digitalis toxicity. Patients with hypokalemia are observed closely and at frequent intervals for signs of digitalis toxicity.

The patient must also be closely observed for any adverse drug effects (see Adverse Reactions Associated With the Administration of the Cardiotonics), such as anorexia, nausea, vomiting, and diarrhea. Some adverse drug effects are also signs of digitalis toxicity, which can be serious. Any patient complaint or comment should be carefully considered, recorded on the patient's chart, and brought to the attention of the physician.

Great care must be taken in the administration of a cardiotonic drug. References should be consulted for average digitalizing and maintenance doses. The physician's order and the drug container must be checked carefully. If there is any doubt about the dosage or calculation of the dosage, check with the physician or pharmacist before giving the drug.

Nursing Process
The Patient Receiving a Cardiotonic

■ *Assessment*

The cardiotonics are potentially toxic drugs, therefore, observe the patient closely, especially during initial therapy. Before therapy is started, the physical assessment should include information that will establish a data base for comparison during therapy. Include the following in the physical assessment: (1) blood pressure, apical–radial pulse rate, respiratory rate; (2) auscultation of the lungs, noting any unusual sounds during inspiration and expiration; (3) examination of the extremities for edema; (4) checking the jugular veins for distention; (5) weight; (6) inspecting sputum raised (if any), and noting the appearance (eg, frothy, pink-tinged, clear, yellow, and so on); and (7) looking for evidence of other problems, such as cyanosis, shortness of breath on exertion (if the patient is allowed out of bed) or when lying flat, mental changes, and so on.

The physician may also order laboratory and diagnostic tests, such as an electrocardiogram, renal and hepatic function tests, complete blood count, serum enzymes, and serum electrolytes. These tests should be reviewed before the first dose is given. When subsequent laboratory tests are ordered, they also should be reviewed when the results are recorded on the patient's record.

■ *Nursing Diagnoses*

Depending on the drug, dose, reason for administration, and possible adverse drug reactions, one or more of the following nursing diagnoses may apply to a person receiving a cardiotonic drug:

- **Anxiety** related to diagnosis, possible lifetime drug therapy, other factors (specify)
- **Risk for Ineffective Management of Therapeutic Regimen**, related to lack of knowledge, indifference, other factors

■ *Planning and Implementation*

The major goals of the patient may include a reduction in anxiety, an absence of adverse drug effects, and an understanding of and compliance with the postdischarge medication regimen. To make these goals measurable, more specific criteria must be added.

Anxiety. Some patients may have varying degrees of anxiety related to their diagnosis or the fact that drug therapy may need to be continued for a long time. Allow time for the patient to express his or her concerns, as well as to identify any problems that may require a referral to individuals such as the physician, dietitian, or social worker.

■ *Patient and Family Teaching*

In some instances, a cardiotonic may be prescribed for a prolonged period. Some patients may discontinue their medication, especially if they feel better and their original symptoms have been relieved. The patient and family must understand that the prescribed medication must be taken *exactly* as directed by the physician.

The physician may want the patient to monitor his or her pulse rate daily while taking a cardiotonic. Show the patient or a family member the correct technique for taking the pulse. The physician may also want the patient to omit the next dose of the drug and call him or her if the pulse rate falls below a certain level (usually 60 beats/min). Emphasize these instructions at the time of patient teaching.

The following points are included in a teaching plan for the patient prescribed a cardiac glycoside:

- Do not discontinue this drug without first checking with the physician (unless instructed to do otherwise).
- Take this drug at the *same time* each day.
- Take pulse prior to taking the drug and withhold the drug and notify the physician if pulse rate is less than 60 or greater than 100 beats/min.
- Avoid antacids and nonprescription cough, cold, allergy, antidiarrheal, and diet (weight-reducing) drugs unless their use has been approved by the physician. Some of these drugs interfere with the action of the (cardiotonic) drug or cause other, potentially serious, problems.

- Contact the physician if nausea, vomiting, diarrhea, unusual fatigue, weakness, vision changes (such as blurred vision, changes in colors of objects, or halos around dark objects), or mental depression occurs.
- Keep drug in original container and do not mix in pill boxes.
- Follow the dietary recommendations made by the physician (if any).
- The physician will closely monitor therapy. Keep all appointments for physician visits or laboratory or diagnostic tests.

■ *Expected Outcomes for Evaluation*

- Anxiety is reduced
- Adverse reactions are identified and reported to the physician
- Patient and family demonstrate understanding of drug regimen
- Patient verbalizes importance of continued follow-up care
- Patient verbalizes importance of complying with the prescribed therapeutic regimen
- Patient complies to the prescribed drug regimen

Chapter Summary

- The cardiotonics include deslanoside (Cedilanid-D), digitoxin, and digoxin (Lanoxin) and are sometimes called cardiac glycosides or digitalis glycosides. The cardiac glycosides are the oldest and most effective drugs used to treat CHF, a condition in which the heart cannot pump enough blood to meet the tissue needs of the body. The cardiac glycosides improve the contraction of the heart muscle, which leads to improved blood flow to all tissues of the body.
- The heart that is weakened by disease, age, or both is often in need of drug therapy. Cardiotonic drugs increase the force of contraction of the myocardium (positive inotropic action) and increase cardiac output. The cardiotonics also depress the SA node and slow conduction of the electrical impulse to the atrioventricular node. Slowing this part of the transmission of nerve impulses decreases the number of ventricular contractions per minute.
- The cardiotonics are used in the treatment of CHF, atrial fibrillation, atrial flutter and atrial fibrillation. There is a very narrow range of safety between full therapeutic effects and the toxic effects. The signs of digitalis toxicity include: anorexia, nausea, vomiting, weakness, visual disturbances

(blurred vision, disturbance in yellow/green vision and halo effect around dark objects). Arrhythmias such as bradycardia, tachycardia, and premature ventricular contractions, are also observed with digitalis toxicity. The physician may treat digitalis toxicity by temporarily discontinuing the drug until signs of toxicity disappear.

- The cardiotonics are potentially toxic drugs and the patient must be observed closely during therapy. Before administering each dose of a cardiotonic, the apical pulse rate is taken for 60 seconds. The drug is withheld and the physician is notified if the pulse rate is 60 or below. The drug is also withheld if there are any signs of digitalis toxicity.

Critical Thinking Exercises

1. Mr. Taylor has been on digoxin for 3 weeks and has come to the clinic for a follow-up visit. When interviewing Mr. Taylor, what questions would you ask to evaluate his knowledge of the medication regimen and if he is experiencing any adverse reactions?

2. You are to participate in a team conference on the cardiac glycosides. Your topic to discuss is discharge teaching for the patient receiving a cardiac glycoside. Develop a teaching plan using the nursing process as a framework. What points would be most important for you to include?

31

Antiarrhythmic Drugs

Chapter Outline

Chapter Objectives

On completion of this chapter the student will:

- *Discuss the uses and general drug actions of the antiarrhythmic drugs*
- *List the general adverse reactions seen with the administration of an antiarrhythmic drug*
- *Discuss nursing management when administering an antiarrhythmic drug*
- *Use the nursing process when administering an antiarrhythmic drug*

Scherer JC, Roach S: INTRODUCTORY CLINICAL PHARMACOLOGY,
FIFTH EDITION © 1996 Lippincott-Raven Publishers

The antiarrhythmic drugs are primarily used to treat cardiac arrhythmias. A cardiac *arrhythmia* is a disturbance or irregularity in the heart rate, rhythm, or both and requires administration of one of the antiarrhythmic drugs. Some examples of cardiac arrhythmias are listed in Table 31-1.

Antiarrhythmic Drugs

An arrhythmia may occur as a result of heart disease or from a disorder that affects cardiovascular function. Conditions such as emotional stress, hypoxia, and electrolyte imbalance may also trigger an arrhythmia. An electrocardiogram (ECG) provides a record of the electrical activity of the heart. Careful interpretation of the ECG along with a thorough physical assessment is necessary to determine the cause and type of arrhythmia. The goal of antiarrhythmic drug therapy is to restore normal cardiac function and to prevent life-threatening arrhythmias.

ACTIONS OF THE ANTIARRHYTHMIC DRUGS

The cardiac muscle (myocardium) has attributes of both nerve and muscle and therefore has the proper-

Table 31-1. Types of Arrhythmias

Arrhythmia	Description
Atrial flutter	Rapid contraction of the atria (up to 300 beats/min) at a rate too rapid for the ventricles to pump efficiently
Atrial fibrillation	Irregular and rapid atrial contraction, resulting in a quivering of the atria and causing an irregular and inefficient ventricular contraction
Premature ventricular contractions	Beats originating in the ventricles instead of the SA node in the atria, causing the ventricles to contract before the atria and resulting in a decrease in the amount of blood pumped to the body
Ventricular tachycardia	A rapid heartbeat with a rate of more than 100 beats/min, usually originating in the ventricles
Ventricular fibrillation	Rapid disorganized contractions of the ventricles resulting in the inability of the heart to pump any blood to the body. This condition will result in death unless treated immediately.

Table 31-2. Antiarrhythmic Drug Classifications

Classification	Drug
Class I	Moricizine
Class I-A	Quinidine
	Procainamide
	Disopyramide
Class I-B	Lidocaine
	Phenytoin
	Tocainide
	Mexiletine
Class I-C	Flecainide
	Encainide
	Propafenone
Class II	Propanolol
	Esmolol
	Acebutolol
Class III	Bretylium
	Amiodarone
	Sotalol
Class IV	Verapamil

ties of both. Some cardiac arrhythmias are caused by the generation of an abnormal number of electrical impulses (stimuli). These abnormal impulses may come from the sinoatrial node or may be generated in other areas of the myocardium. The antiarrhythmic drugs are classified according to their effects on the myocardium and their presumed mechanism of action. As understanding of the pathophysiology of cardiac arrhythmias and the drugs used to treat these arrhythmias has increased, a method of classification has been developed that includes four basic classifications and several subclasses. Drugs in each class have certain similarities, yet each drug has subtle differences that make it unique. Table 31-2 identifies the classifications of the antiarrhythmic drugs.

Class I Antiarrhythmic Drugs

Class I antiarrhythmic drugs, such as moricizine, have a membrane-stabilizing or anesthetic effect on the cells of the myocardium, making them valuable in treating cardiac arrhythmias. Class I antiarrhythmic drugs contain the largest number of drugs of the four classifications. Because the actions differ slightly, they are subdivided into Class I-A, I-B, and I-C (see Table 31-2).

The drugs quinidine and procainamide (Procan SR and Pronestyl) are unrelated chemically but have similar drug actions. Quinidine and procainamide depress myocardial excitability or the ability of the myocardium to respond to an electrical stimulus. By depressing the myocardium and its ability to respond to some, but not all, electrical stimuli, the pulse rate decreases and the arrhythmia is corrected.

These drugs also prolong or lengthen the refractory (resting) period of the impulses traveling through the myocardium. Only one impulse can pass along a nerve fiber at any given time. Following the passage of an impulse, there is a brief pause or interval before the next impulse can pass along the nerve fiber. This pause is called the *refractory period,* which is the period between the transmission of nerve impulses along a nerve fiber. By lengthening the refractory period, the number of impulses traveling along a nerve fiber within a given time is decreased.

To illustrate this phenomenon, a patient has a pulse rate of 120 beats/min. By lengthening the refractory period between each impulse, fewer impulses would be generated each minute and the pulse rate would decrease.

Disopyramide (Norpace) decreases the rate of depolarization of myocardial fibers during the diastolic phase of the cardiac cycle. Nerve cells have positive ions on the outside and negative ions on the inside of the cell membrane when they are at rest. This is called *polarization.* When a stimulus passes along the nerve, the positive ions move from outside the cell into the cell, and the negative ions move from inside the cell to outside the cell. This movement of ions is called *depolarization.* Unless positive ions move into and negative ions move out of a nerve cell, a stimulus (or impulse) cannot pass along the nerve fiber. Once the stimulus has passed along the nerve fiber, the positive and negative ions move back to their original place, that is, the positive ions on the outside and the negative ions on the inside of the nerve cell. This movement back to the original place is called *repolarization.* Disopyramide decreases the rate (or speed) of depolarization and the stimulus must literally wait for this process before it can pass along the nerve fiber. Decreasing the rate of depolarization then decreases the number of impulses that can pass along a nerve fiber during a specific time period.

Lidocaine (Xylocaine) raises the threshold of the ventricular myocardium. *Threshold* is a term applied to any stimulus of the lowest intensity that will give rise to a response in a nerve fiber. A stimulus must be of a specific intensity (strength, amplitude) to pass along a given nerve fiber. To illustrate this phenomenon using plain figures instead of precise electrical values, a certain nerve fiber has a threshold of 10. If a stimulus rated as nine reaches the fiber, it will not pass along the fiber because its intensity is lower than the fiber's threshold of 10. If another

stimulus reaches the fiber and is rated at 14, it will pass along the fiber because its intensity is greater than the fiber's threshold of 10. By raising the threshold of a fiber that was originally 10 to 15, only those stimuli greater than 15 can pass along the nerve fiber.

Some cardiac arrhythmias result from many stimuli present in the myocardium. Some of these are weak or of low intensity but are still able to excite myocardial tissue. Lidocaine, by raising the threshold of myocardial fibers, reduces the number of stimuli that will pass along these fibers and therefore decreases the pulse rate and corrects the arrhythmia. Tocainide (Tonocard) and mexiletine (Mexitil) are also antiarrhythmic agents with actions similar to lidocaine.

The action of encainide (Enkaid) is unknown but is believed to be due to its ability to slow the rate of conduction of an electrical impulse along cardiac nerve fibers, as well as to reduce the response of the myocardium to electrical stimulation. This drug has been voluntary withdrawn from the market by the manufacturer because of uncertainty of its safety. However, it is available on a limited basis for patients with life-threatening arrhythmias who were stabilized on the drug prior to its withdrawal from the market.

Propafenone (Rythmol) and flecainide (Tambocor) have a direct stabilizing action on the myocardium, thus reducing the response of these fibers to electrical stimulation.

Class II Antiarrhythmic Drugs

Class II antiarrhythmic drugs include beta adrenergic blocking drugs, such as propranolol (Inderal), acebutolol (Sectral) and esmolol (Brevibloc). Propranolol has quinidine-like action (see earlier discussion of quinidine). It also decreases myocardial response to epinephrine and norepinephrine (adrenergic neurohormones) because of its ability to block stimulation of beta receptors of the heart (see Chap. 18). Adrenergic neurohormones stimulate the beta receptors of the myocardium and therefore increase the heart rate. Blocking the effect of these neurohormones decreases the heart rate. This is called a *blockade effect.*

Class III Antiarrhythmic Drugs

Bretylium (Bretylol) is the most important Class III antiarrhythmic drug. This drug acts to inhibit the release of norepinephrine by depressing adrenergic nerve excitability, thus producing an adrenergic blocking effect (see Chapter 18). The manner in which this drug corrects ventricular arrhythmias is not well-understood.

Amiodarone (Cordarone) appears to prolong the refractory period, as well as to exhibit alpha-adrenergic and beta-adrenergic blocking activity.

Class IV Antiarrhythmic Drugs

Class IV antiarrhythmic drugs include verapamil (Calan, Isoptin) and the other calcium channel blockers. Calcium channel blockers produce their antiarrhythmic action by inhibiting the movement of calcium through channels across the myocardial cell membranes and vascular smooth muscle. Contraction of cardiac and vascular smooth muscle depends on the movement of calcium ions into these cells through specific ion channels. By reducing the calcium flow, conduction through the SA and AV node is slowed and the refractory period is prolonged, resulting in suppression of the arrhythmia. The calcium channel blockers are also called slow channel blockers or calcium antagonists.

Dosage ranges for the antiarrhythmic drugs are given in Summary Drug Table 31-1.

USES OF THE ANTIARRHYTHMIC DRUGS

The uses of the antiarrhythmic drugs are given in Summary Drug Table 31-1.

In addition to its use as an antiarrhythmic, propranolol may also be used for patients with myocardial infarction. This drug has been shown to reduce the risk of death and repeated myocardial infarctions in those surviving the acute phase of a myocardial infarction. Additional uses include control of tachycardia in those with pheochromocytoma (a tumor of the adrenal gland that secretes excessive amounts of norepinephrine), migraine headaches, angina pectoris caused by atherosclerosis, and hypertrophic subaortic stenosis.

ADVERSE REACTIONS ASSOCIATED WITH THE ADMINISTRATION OF ANTIARRHYTHMIC DRUGS

The more common adverse reactions associated with the administration of antiarrhythmic agents are given in Summary Drug Table 31-1. Some of the

drugs discussed in this chapter are also used to treat hypertension (see Chap. 34).

The administration of quinidine may result in *cinchonism* (quinidine toxicity), the signs of which include ringing in the ears, headache, nausea, dizziness, fever, vertigo, and lightheadedness.

Procainamide administration may result in transient, but sometimes severe, hypotension and disturbances of cardiac rhythm such as ventricular asystole or fibrillation (when given intravenously), anorexia, urticaria or pruritus, nausea, and agranulocytosis following repeated use.

NURSING MANAGEMENT

Administration

During therapy with these drugs, take the patient's blood pressure, apical and radial pulse, and respiratory rate at periodic intervals, usually every 1 to 4 hours. Specific intervals are dependent on the physician's order or on nursing judgment and are based on the patient's general condition. Report significant changes in the blood pressure, the pulse rate or rhythm, respiratory difficulty, change in respiratory rate or rhythm, or a change in the patient's general condition to the physician immediately. Withhold the drug and notify the physician immediately when the pulse rate is above 120 or below 60. In some instances, the physician may establish additional or different guidelines for withholding the drug.

If the patient is acutely ill or is receiving one of these drugs parenterally, measure and record the intake and output. Additional points of nursing management for these drugs are given below.

Quinidine. If the patient is on a cardiac monitor, take an electrocardiogram (ECG) strip before treatment with quinidine is initiated. If the patient is not on a cardiac monitor, the physician may order an ECG to establish a baseline for comparison during therapy. When the patient is on a cardiac monitor, report any changes in the ECG pattern to the physician immediately. If the patient is not being monitored, report any changes in the pulse rate or rhythm to the physician. Monitor serum quinidine levels during administration of the drug. Therapeutic levels are 2 to 6 mcg/mL. Toxic effects usually occur at levels *greater* than 8 mcg/mL.

Summary Drug Table 31-1. Antiarrhythmic Drugs

Generic Name	Trade Name*	Uses	Adverse Reactions	Dose Ranges
CLASS I				
disopyramide	Norpace, Norpace CR *generic*	Suppression and treatment of ectopic ventricular contractions, ventricular tachycardia, paired ventricular contractions	Dry mouth, constipation, urinary hesitancy, blurred vision, nausea, dizziness, headache, hypotension, CHF	Ventricular arrhythmias, dosage individualized 200–300 mg initially followed by 400–800 mg/d in divided doses
encainide hydrochloride	Enkaid	Sustained ventricular tachycardia	Aggravation of ventricular arrhythmias, dizziness, headache, CHF, blurred or abnormal vision	Initial dose: 25 mg PO q8h; maintenance dose: up to 50 mg PO tid
flecainide acetate	Tambocor	Paroxysmal atrial fibrillation/flutter and atrioventricular tachycardia, ventricular arrhythmias	Dizziness, faintness, unsteadiness, blurred vision, headache, nausea, dyspnea, CHF, fatigue, palpitations, chest pain	Initial dose: 100 mg PO q 12h; maintenance dose up to 200 mg PO q12 h
lidocaine hydrochloride	Xylocaine, *generic*	Life-threatening arrhythmias (particularly those ventricular in origin)	Lightheadedness, nervousness, bradycardia, hypotension, drowsiness; apprehension	50–100 mg IV bolus; 1–4 mg/min IV infusion; 300 mg IM
mexiletine hydrochloride	Mexitil	Symptomatic ventricular arrhythmia	Palpitations, nausea, vomiting, chest pain, heartburn, dizziness, lightheadedness, rash	Initial dose: 200–300 mg PO q8h; maintenance dose: up to 450 mg PO q 12h
moricizine	Ethmozine	Ventricular arrhythmias	Cardiac rhythm disturbances, existing arrhythmia worsened, palpitations, dizziness, headache, nausea	600–900 mg/d q 8h in three equally divided doses
procainamide hydrochloride	Pronestyl, Pronestyl SR, Procan SR, *generic*	Premature ventricular contractions, ventricular tachycardia, atrial fibrillation, paroxysmal atrial tachycardia, cardiac arrhythmias associated with anesthesia and surgery	Hypotension, disturbances of cardiac rhythm, urticaria, fever, chills, nausea, vomiting, rash, confusion	PO, IM 50 mg/kg/d in divided doses q 3–6 h; IV 100 mg bolus q 5 min until arrhythmia is controlled up to 1000 mg loading infusion 500–600 mg over 30 mins; maintenance infusion 2–6 mg/min
propafenone	Rythmol	Life-threatening ventricular arrhythmias	Dizziness, nausea, vomiting, constipation, unusual taste, first degree AV block	Initial dose of 150 mg PO q8h; may be increased to 300 mg PO q8h
quinidine gluconate, quinidine sulfate, quinidine polyglacturonate	Quinaglute Dura-Tabs, *generic* Cardioquin, Quinidex Extend-Tabs	Premature atrial and ventricular contractions, atrial tachycardia and flutter, paroxysmal atrial fibrillation	Ringing in the ears, hearing loss, nausea, dizziness, vomiting, headache, disturbed vision	200–300 mg PO 3–4 times/d; sustained release forms 300–600 mg q 8–12 hr
tocainide hydrochloride	Tonocard	Life-threatening ventricular arrhythmia	Lightheadedness, nausea, vomiting, tremor, paresthesia/numbness, dizziness, hallucinations, restlessness, sedation, blurred vision, cardiac arrhythmias	Initial dose: 400 mg PO q8h; may be increased up to 1800 mg/d PO in divided doses

(continued)

Summary Drug Table 31-1 (Continued)

Generic Name	Trade Name*	Uses	Adverse Reactions	Dose Ranges
CLASS II				
acebutol	Sectral	Ventricular tachy-arrhythmias	Fatigue, weakness, brady-cardia, CHF, dizziness, impotence	400–1200 mg/d in single dose or two times/d
esmolol	Brevibloc	Short-term management of supra-ventricular tachyarrhythmias	Dizziness, headache, hypo-tension, nausea, phlebitis at IV site, visual distur-bances	Loading dose: 500 mcg/kg over 1 min followed by 50–200 mcg/min until therapeutic response; maintenance dose: 25 mcg/kg/min
propranolol hydrochloride	Inderal, Inderal-LA, *generic*	Cardiac arrhythmias	Fatigue, weakness, depres-sion, bradycardia, dizzi-ness, vertigo, rash, hyper-glycemia, bronchospasm, hypotension, agranulo-cytosis	Arrhythmias: 10–30 mg PO tid, qid: life-threaten-ing arrhythmias: up to 1 mg/min IV
CLASS III				
amiodarone	Cordarone	Life-threatening ven-tricular arrhythmias	Malaise, fatigue, tremor, nausea, vomiting, con-stipation, ataxia, anorexia, photosen--sitivity	Loading dose: 800–1600 mg/d PO in divided doses; maintenance dose: 400–600 mg/d PO
bretylium tosylate	Bretylol	Prophylaxis and ventric-ular fibrillation, life-threatening ventricular arrhythmias	Hypotension, nausea, vomit-ing, vertigo, dizziness	Immediate treatment: 5 mg/kg IV; mainte-nance: 5–10 mg/kg (diluted) q 6h or 1–2 mg/min by continuous IV infusion
CLASS IV				
verapamil hydrochloride	Calan, Calan SR, Isoptin, Isoptin SR, Verelan	Angina, supraventricular tachyarrhythmias, rapid ventricular arrhythmia in atrial flutter or fibrillation	Dizziness, bradycardia, hypotension, edema, constipation, nausea	Angina: 80–120 mg PO tid; arrhythmias: 240–320 mg/d tid or qid; SR: 240–360 mg/d in AM or in AM and PM

*The term, *generic*, indicates that the drug is available in a generic form.

Nursing Alert

Report any of the following signs or symptoms of cinchonism (quinidine toxicity): ringing in the ears (tinnitus), headache, nausea, dizziness, fever, vertigo, and lightheadedness.

Procainamide. The physician may order an ECG to provide baseline data for comparison during therapy. If the drug is given intravenously (IV), maintain continuous and close cardiac monitoring. When administered IV, discontinue the drug imme-diately if changes in the ECG pattern occur. Intra-venous administration is by IV piggyback. Hypoten-sion may be seen with IV administration; therefore, monitor the blood pressure every 15 minutes while the drug is being infused. Keep the patient supine during IV administration to minimize hypotension. If hypotension should occur, discontinue the drug and run the primary IV line at a rate to keep the vein open until the physician sees the patient.

When the drug is given orally, the patient is in-structed not to chew the capsule or tablet but to swallow it whole. For faster absorption, give the drug with a full glass of water on an empty stomach either 1 hour before meals or 2 hours after meals. If gas-trointestinal upset occurs, administer with or imme-diately after meals.

When given intramuscularly, use the gluteus muscle and rotate the injection sites.

Propranolol. Cardiac monitoring is recommended when the drug is given IV because severe bradycardia and hypotension may be seen. Obtain written instructions from the physician for propranolol administration. For example, the physician may want the drug to be withheld for a systolic blood pressure less than 90 mm Hg or a pulse rate less than 50. When assessing pulse rate also note the rate and quality.

Bretylium. Bretylium is a drug used in the emergency treatment of life-threatening ventricular arrhythmias. Because of its adverse reactions, bretylium is used when the arrhythmia is unresponsive to the other antiarrhythmic drugs. Baseline data will come from routine assessments made before the emergency. This drug is administered intramuscularly or IV, with *continuous* cardiac monitoring. Place the patient in a supine position and make suction equipment readily available in case vomiting should occur. A transient increase in arrhythmias and hypertension may occur within 1 hour after initial therapy is begun. Take the blood pressure and respiratory rate every 5 to 15 minutes and obtain the pulse rate from the cardiac monitor. Hypotension and postural hypotension may occur in approximately one-half of patients receiving bretylium. If systolic pressure is less than 75 mm Hg, notify the physician. Continue these activities until the arrhythmia is corrected. To discontinue the drug, the dosage should be gradually reduced over 3 to 5 days. After administration of the drug, observe the patient closely. An oral antiarrhythmic drug may be prescribed to provide continued stability to the cardiac muscle.

Disopyramide. Because of the cholinergic blocking effects of disopyramide (see Chap. 20), urinary retention may occur. Monitor the urinary output closely, especially during the initial period of therapy. If the patient's intake is sufficient but the output is low, palpate the lower abdomen for bladder distention. If urinary retention does occur, catheterization may be necessary.

Dryness of the mouth and throat due to the cholinergic blocking action of this drug also may be seen. Relieve dryness by offering frequent sips of water. Provide an adequate amount of fluid and instruct the patient to take sips of water to relieve this problem.

Postural hypotension may occur during the first few weeks of therapy. Advise the patient to make position changes slowly. In some instances, the patient may require assistance in getting out of the bed or chair.

Lidocaine. Lidocaine is an emergency drug used in the treatment of life-threatening ventricular arrhythmias. Constant cardiac monitoring is essential when this drug is administered by the IV or intramuscular routes. Observe the patient closely for signs of respiratory depression, respiratory arrest, convulsions, and hypotension. Keep an oropharyngeal airway and suction equipment at the bedside in case convulsions should occur.

Monitor the blood pressure and respiratory rate every 2 to 5 minutes when the drug is given IV and every 5 to 10 minutes when the drug is given intramuscularly. Check the pulse rate continually by means of the cardiac monitor. Contact the physician immediately if there are any changes in the vital signs or the ECG pattern or if respiratory problems or convulsions occur.

If pronounced bradycardia does occur, the physician may order emergency measures, such as the administration of IV atropine (see Chap. 20) or isoproterenol (see Chap. 17). Any sudden change in mental state should be reported to the physician immediately because a decrease in the dosage may be necessary. The administration of lidocaine is titrated to the patient's response and within institutional protocols.

Tocainide and Mexiletine. The dosage of these drugs must be individualized; therefore, monitor the vital signs at frequent intervals during initial therapy. Report changes in the pulse rate or rhythm to the physician. Adverse effects related to the central nervous system or gastrointestinal tract may occur during initial therapy and must be reported to the physician.

Encainide, Indecainide, Flecainide, and Propafenone. Observe the patient closely for a response to drug therapy, signs of congestive heart failure, the development of a new cardiac arrhythmia, or worsening of the arrhythmia being treated.

Amiodarone. This drug is only used when the patient does not respond to other antiarrhythmic drugs. Monitor the patient *closely* for adverse effects, especially congestive heart failure. Monitor the intake and output to detect early signs of fluid retention. Give this drug with food to reduce gastrointestinal irritation. Note any changes in the pulse rate or rhythm and report to the physician.

Verapamil. This drug is used to manage supraventricular arrhythmias and rapid ventricular rates in atrial flutter or fibrillation. Continuous cardiac monitoring is necessary during IV administration. Notify the physician if bradycardia or hypotension occurs. Patients receiving a cardiac glycoside (eg, digoxin) concurrently with verapamil must be monitored for an increased risk of digitalis toxicity. Administer orally with food or meals to minimize gastric upset.

Adverse Drug Reactions

Observe the patient for adverse drug reactions.

> ### Nursing Alert
>
> Antiarrhythmic drugs are capable of causing new arrhythmias, as well as an exacerbation of existing arrhythmias. Any new arrhythmia or exacerbation of an existing arrhythmia must be reported to the physician immediately.

Nursing judgment is necessary in reporting other adverse reactions to the physician. For example, the patient with a dry mouth is in no danger, even though the condition is uncomfortable. Although the occurrence of this is reported to the physician, it is not of an emergency nature. In some instances, minor adverse reactions must be tolerated by the patient. On the other hand, the patient with severe bradycardia or prolonged nausea and vomiting is in a potentially dangerous situation. Contact the physician immediately because additional treatment may be necessary.

Nursing Process
The Patient Receiving an Antiarrhythmic Drug

■ Assessment

Antiarrhythmic drugs are used in the treatment of various types of cardiac arrhythmias. There are initial assessments performed before starting therapy that are the same for all antiarrhythmic drugs and include the following:

* Take and record the blood pressure, an apical and radial pulse, and respiratory rate. This provides a database for comparison during therapy.
* Assess the patient's general condition and include observations such as skin color (pale, cyanotic, flushed, and so forth), orientation, level of con-

sciousness, and the patient's general status (appears acutely ill, appears somewhat ill, and so forth). Record all observations to provide a means of evaluating the response to drug therapy.
* Record any symptoms (subjective data) described by the patient.

The physician may also order laboratory and diagnostic tests, such as an ECG, renal and hepatic function tests, complete blood count, serum enzymes, and serum electrolytes. Review these test results before the first dose is given. When subsequent laboratory tests are ordered, review them as well.

■ Nursing Diagnoses

Depending on the drug, the dose, the patient's diagnosis, and other factors, one or more of the following may apply to the patient receiving an antiarrhythmic drug:

* **Anxiety** related to diagnosis, possible lifetime drug therapy, other factors (specify)
* **Risk for Injury** related to adverse drug reactions (dizziness, lightheadedness)
* **Risk for Ineffective Management of Therapeutic Regimen** related to lack of knowledge, indifference, other factors

■ Planning and Implementation

The major goals of the patient may include a reduction in anxiety, an absence of injury, an absence of adverse drug effects, and an understanding of and compliance with the postdischarge medication regimen. To make these goals measurable, more specific criteria must be added.

Anxiety. Varying degrees of anxiety may be seen in those with a cardiac disorder. Allow time for the patients to express their concerns, as well as to identify any problems that may require a referral to individuals, such as the physician, dietitian, or social worker.

Risk for Injury. Some of these drugs may cause dizziness and lightheadedness, especially during early therapy. Assist patients not on complete bed rest with ambulatory activities until these symptoms are no longer present.

■ Patient and Family Teaching

Explain the adverse drug effects that may occur to the patient and family. To ensure compliance to the prescribed drug regimen, emphasize the importance of taking these drugs as prescribed. It may be necessary to teach the patient or a family member how to take the pulse rate. Advise the patient to report any changes in the rate or rhythm to the physician.

The following points must be emphasized in teaching the patient and the family:

- Take the drug at the prescribed intervals. Do not omit a dose or increase or decrease the dose unless advised to do so by the physician. Do not stop the drug unless advised to do so by the physician.
- Do not take any nonprescription drug unless the use of a specific drug is approved by the physician.
- Avoid drinking alcoholic beverages or smoking unless these have been approved by the physician.
- Follow the directions on the label, such as taking the drug with food.
- Do not chew tablets or capsules; swallow them whole.
- Do not attempt to drive or perform hazardous tasks if lightheadedness or dizziness should occur.
- Notify the physician as soon as possible should any adverse effects occur.
- If a dry mouth should occur, take frequent sips of water, allow ice chips to dissolve in the mouth, or chew (sugar-free) gum.
- The wax matrix of sustained release tablets of procainamide (Procan SR only) is not absorbed by the body and may be found in the stool. This is normal.
- Keep all physician, clinic, or laboratory appointments because therapy will be closely monitored.
- Diabetic patients taking propranolol: adhere to the prescribed diet and check the blood glucose levels one to two times a day (or as recommended by the physician). Report elevated glucose levels to the physician as soon as possible because an adjustment in the dosage of insulin or oral hypoglycemic agents may be necessary.
- Keep all follow-up visits with the physician to monitor progress.

■ *Expected Outcomes for Evaluation*
- Anxiety is reduced
- Adverse reactions are identified and reported to the physician
- No evidence of injury
- Patient and family demonstrate understanding of drug regimen
- Patient verbalizes importance of continued follow-up care
- Patient verbalizes importance of complying with the prescribed treatment regimen
- Patient complies to the prescribed drug regimen

Chapter Summary

- Cardiac arrhythmias are irregularities in the rate and the rhythm of the heart. Drugs used to treat arrhythmias of the heart are called antiarrhythmic drugs. There are four classes of antiarrhythmic drugs.
- Class I antiarrhythmic drugs have a membrane stabilizing effect on the cells of the myocardium, making them valuable in treating cardiac arrhythmias. The major Class I antiarrhythmic drugs are quinidine, procainamide, and lidocaine. Quinidine and procainamide decrease the ability of the myocardium to respond to an electrical stimulus and prolong the refractory period. Lidocaine raises the threshold of the ventricular myocardium and reduces the number of stimuli that pass through the myocardium, resulting in a decrease in the pulse rate and a stabilization of the arrhythmia.
- Other Class I antiarrhythmic drugs include disopyramide, tocainide, and mexiletine.
- Class II antiarrhythmic drugs include beta adrenergic blocking drugs such as propranolol. The antiarrhythmic action results from a beta-adrenergic receptor blockade and a membrane stabilizing effect on the cells of the myocardium.
- The most significant Class III antiarrhythmic drug is bretylium. This drug acts to inhibit the release of norepinephrine by depressing adrenergic nerve excitability, thus producing an adrenergic blocking effect.
- Class IV antiarrhythmic drugs include verapamil (Calan, Isoptin) and the other calcium channel blockers. Calcium channel blockers produce their antiarrhythmic action by inhibiting the movement of calcium through channels across the myocardial cell membranes and vascular smooth muscle, thus slowing the influx of calcium into the myocardium. Reducing the calcium flow slows the AV conduction and prolongs the refractory period, resulting in a calming effect on the heart muscle.
- Initial assessments performed before starting therapy with any antiarrhythmic drug include the following: (1) take and record blood pressure, apical and radial pulse, and respiratory rate to provide data base for comparison during therapy; (2) assess the patient's general condition and include observations such as skin color, level of consciousness, and the patient's general status; record all observations to provide a means of evaluating the response to drug therapy; and (3) record any symptoms (subjective data) described by the patient.

• When these drugs are given IV, the patient must have continuous cardiac monitoring and close observation by the nurse. During therapy with these drugs, the patient's blood pressure, apical and radial pulse, and respiratory rate are taken at periodic intervals, usually every 1 to 4 hours. Specific intervals are dependent on the physicians's order or on nursing judgment and are based on the patient's general condition. Any significant change is reported to the physician immediately. The drug is withheld and the physician notified immediately when the pulse rate is above 120 or below 60. In some instances, the physician may establish additional guidelines for withholding the drug.

• The patient is observed for adverse drug reactions. Nursing judgment is necessary in reporting these to the physician. In some instances, minor adverse reactions must be tolerated by the patient. Other more serious reactions, such as severe bradycardia or prolonged nausea and vomiting, are potentially dangerous. Contact the physician immediately because additional treatment may be necessary.

Critical Thinking Exercises

1. Mr. Parker is at an outpatient clinic for a follow-up visit. He has been taking quinidine for several months for a cardiac arrhythmia. What assessments would you make on Mr. Parker to determine the effectiveness of quinidine therapy? What questions would you ask to determine the presence of any adverse reactions?

2. Ms. Grady, aged 48, will be dismissed in 2 days. The physician has prescribed propranolol to treat her arrhythmia. Develop a five point handout for Ms. Grady to take home with her explaining the most important points for her to know when taking propranolol.

32

Anticoagulant and Thrombolytic Drugs

Key Terms

Fibrolytic drugs
Prothrombin
Thrombolytic drugs
Thrombus

Chapter Outline

Chapter Objectives

On completion of this chapter the student will:

- *Discuss the uses and general drug actions of warfarin, heparin preparations, and the thrombolytic drugs*
- *List the adverse reactions associated with the administration of anticoagulants and the thrombolytic drugs*
- *Discuss the areas to be checked for evidence of bleeding when the patient is receiving an anticoagulant or thrombolytic drug*
- *Use the nursing process when administering an anticoagulant or thrombolytic drug*
- *Discuss nursing management when administering an anticoagulant or thrombolytic drug*

Scherer JC, Roach S: INTRODUCTORY CLINICAL PHARMACOLOGY,
FIFTH EDITION © 1996 Lippincott-Raven Publishers

Anticoagulants are used to prevent the formation and extension of a *thrombus* (blood clot). Although they do not thin the blood, they are sometimes called *blood thinners* by patients. The anticoagulants are a group of drugs that include oral warfarin (Coumadin) and parenteral heparin preparations. Initial therapy is usually begun with heparin because of its rapid onset of action. Warfarin is used for maintenance therapy and takes several days to reach a therapeutic effect.

Anticoagulants have *no* direct effect on an existing thrombus and *do not* reverse any damage from the thrombus. However, once the presence of a thrombus has been established, anticoagulant therapy can prevent additional clots from forming.

While the anticoagulants prevent thrombus formation, *thrombolytic drugs* are those used to dissolve blood clots that have already formed within the walls of a blood vessel. These drugs reopen blood vessels after they become occluded. Another term used to identify the thrombolytic drugs is *fibrolytic drugs*.

Warfarin

Warfarin is the oral anticoagulant currently in common use (see Summary Drug Table 32-1). Warfarin is given by the oral route although it is suitable for parenteral administration. Peak activity is reached 1.5 to 3 days after therapy is initiated.

ACTIONS OF WARFARIN

All anticoagulants interfere with the clotting mechanism of the blood; this is a complex chemical process. Warfarin interferes with the manufacture of vitamin K–dependent clotting factors by the liver. This results in the depletion of clotting factors II (prothrombin), VII, IX, and X. It is the depletion of *prothrombin* (Fig. 32-1), a substance that is essential for the clotting of blood, that accounts for most of the action of warfarin.

USES OF WARFARIN

Warfarin is used for the following:

- Prevention (prophylaxis) and treatment of venous thrombosis

- Treatment of atrial fibrillation with thrombus formation
- Prevention and treatment of pulmonary embolus
- As part of the treatment of coronary occlusion

ADVERSE REACTIONS ASSOCIATED WITH THE ADMINISTRATION OF WARFARIN

The principal adverse reaction associated with warfarin is bleeding, which may range from very mild to severe. Bleeding may be seen in many areas of the body, such as the bladder, bowel, stomach, uterus, and mucous membranes. Other adverse reactions are rare but may include nausea, vomiting, alopecia (loss of hair), urticaria (severe skin rash), abdominal cramping, diarrhea, rash, hepatitis (inflammation of the liver), jaundice (yellowish discoloration of the skin and mucous membranes), and blood dyscrasias (disorders).

NURSING MANAGEMENT

Laboratory Tests

A prothrombin time (PT) is ordered before and during warfarin therapy. The first dose of warfarin is *not* given until blood for a baseline PT is drawn.

Patients receiving warfarin for the first time often require daily adjustment of the dose, which is based on the *daily* PT results. The results of the PT are recorded on a flow sheet and reported as two figures. One figure is the patient's PT in seconds and the other is the control value in seconds. The control value is a method of laboratory standardization of the materials used to determine the PT. The daily dose of the oral anticoagulant is based on the patient's daily PT. Optimal therapeutic results are obtained when the patient's PT is 1.5 to 2.5 times the control value.

Most laboratories also report results for International Normalized Ratio (INR) along with the patient's prothrombin and the control value. The INR was devised as a way to standardize PT values and represents a way to "correct" the routine PT results from various laboratories. The test to determine PT is performed by adding a thromboplastin mixture to citrated (mixed with citric acid) plasma. However, thromboplastins vary greatly depending on their source and method of preparation, causing PT results to vary among laboratories using different thrombo-

Summary Drug Table 32-1. Anticoagulant and Thrombolytic Drugs

Generic Name	Trade Name*	Uses	Adverse Reactions	Dose Ranges
ANTICOAGULANTS				
heparin sodium	Liquaemin, *generic*	Prophylaxis of venous thrombosis, pulmonary embolus, peripheral arterial embolism, atrial fibrillation with embolization; disseminated intravascular coagulation	Hemorrhage, pain at injection site, thrombocytopenia	Dosage adjusted to individual patient according to coagulation test results
heparin sodium lock flush solution	Hep-Lock, *generic*	As IV flush to maintain patency of indwelling IV catheters used in intermittent IV therapy	Rare	1–2.5 mL as directed by the physician
warfarin sodium	Coumadin, Panwarfin, *generic*	Prophylaxis and treatment of venous thrombosis, pulmonary embolism, atrial fibrillation with embolism, adjunct in prophylaxis of embolism after MI	Hemorrhage	Initial dose: 10 mg/d for 2–4 days PO, maintenance: 2–10 mg/d depending on prothrombin time
ANTICOAGULANT ANTAGONISTS				
phytonadione (vitamin K₁)	Aquamephyton, Konakion, Mephyton	Anticoagulant-induced prothrombin deficiency (oral anticoagulants)	Hypersensitivity, anaphylaxis, nausea, vomiting (with oral use), rash	2.5–10 mg IM, SC, PO; dose may be repeated
protamine sulfate	*generic*	Heparin overdosage	Sudden fall in blood pressure, bradycardia, dyspnea, feeling of warmth, anaphylaxis	1 mg neutralizes 90–115 U heparin; dosage is individualized
THROMBOLYTIC				
alteplase, recombinant	Activase	Acute myocardial infarction, acute pulmonary embolism	Bleeding, urticaria, nausea, epistaxis	60 mg IV the first hr, 20 mg IV the second and third hr
anistreplase	Eminase	Acute myocardial infarction	Bleeding, hypotension, cardiac arrhythmias, nausea, vomiting, thrombocytopenia	30 U IV
streptokinase	Streptase	Acute transmural myocardial infarction, deep vein thrombosis, arterial thrombosis or embolism, occluded fever, arteriovenous cannula	Major or minor bleeding episodes, allergic reactions, bronchospasm	20,000–1,500,000 IU by IV infusion
urokinase	Abbokinase	Pulmonary emboli, coronary artery thrombosis; as IV	Bleeding, fever, skin rashes, bronchospasm	IV infusion: 4,400 IU/kg/h; coronary artery thrombi: 6000 IU/min for up to 2 hr
HEMOSTATIC				
aminocarproic acid	Amicar	Excessive bleeding associated with systemic hyperfibrinolysis	Nausea, cramping, dizziness, headache, tinnitus	PO: priming dose 5 g the first hr, 1–1.25 g h for 8h or until bleeding is controlled up to 30 g; IV; priming dose 4–5 g in first hr, then 1 g every 8h

*The term, *generic*, indicates that the drug is available in a generic form.

Blood coagulation

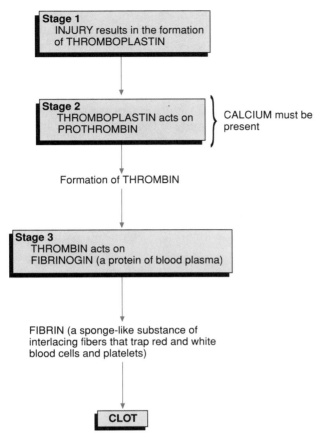

Figure 32-1

Blood coagulation.

plastins. These variations result in the possibility of the administration of inappropriate dosages of the anticoagulant. To prevent this, most laboratories now use a standard thromboplastin for the test and report an INR result. The INR is valuable in the management of patients maintained on long-term warfarin therapy. For patients on long-term warfarin therapy, the INR is maintained between 2 and 3. Levels *greater* than 4.5 are considered critical and should be reported to the physician immediately.

Administration

Before giving *each dose* of warfarin, check the prothrombin flow sheet or the laboratory report to determine the current PT results. Check the patient for any evidence of bleeding as well.

Nursing Alert

Withhold the drug and contact the physician immediately if any of the following occurs:

1. The PT exceeds 2.5 times (30% of normal) the control value.
2. There is evidence of bleeding.
3. The INR is greater than 3 (in patients on long-term warfarin therapy)

To hasten the onset of the therapeutic effect, a higher dosage (loading dose) may be prescribed for 2 to 4 days, followed by a maintenance dosage adjusted according to the daily PT.

Adverse Drug Reactions

Bleeding can occur any time during therapy with warfarin, even when the PT appears to be within a safe limit (eg, 1.5 to 2.5 times the control value). All nursing personnel and medical team members should be made aware of any patient receiving warfarin and the observations necessary with administration. Check the following for signs of bleeding:

Urinal, bedpan, catheter drainage unit—inspect the urine for a pink to red color; inspect the stool for signs of gastrointestinal bleeding (bright red to black stools); visually check the catheter drainage every 2 to 4 hours and when the unit is emptied. Oral anticoagulants may impart a red-orange color to alkaline urine, making hematuria difficult to detect visually. A urinalysis may be necessary to determine if blood is in the urine.
Emesis basin, nasogastric suction units—visually check the nasogastric suction unit every 2 to 4 hours and whenever the unit is emptied. Check the emesis basin each time it is emptied.
Skin, mucous membranes—inspect the patient's skin daily for evidence of easy bruising or bleeding. Be alert for bleeding from minor cuts and scratches, nosebleeds, or excessive bleeding following intramuscular (IM), subcutaneous (SC), or intravenous (IV) injections or following a venipuncture. After oral care, check the toothbrush and gums for signs of bleeding.

Apply prolonged pressure to the needle or catheter site after venipuncture, removal of central or peripheral IV lines, and IM and SC injections. Make laboratory personnel or those responsible for drawing blood for laboratory tests aware of anticoagulant therapy because prolonged pressure on the venipuncture site is necessary. All laboratory requests require a notation stating the patient is receiving anticoagulant therapy.

Overdosage

Symptoms of overdosage include blood in the stool (melena); petechiae (pinpoint sized red hemorrhagic spots on the skin); oozing from superficial injuries, such as cuts from shaving or bleeding from the gums after brushing the teeth; or excessive menstrual bleeding. Report any of these adverse reactions or evidence of bleeding to the physician immediately.

If bleeding occurs or if the PT exceeds 2.5 times the control value, the physician may either discontinue the anticoagulant for a few days or order vitamin K_1 (phytonadione), an oral anticoagulant antagonist, which must always be readily available when a patient is receiving warfarin. Since the warfarin interferes with the synthesis of vitamin K_1-dependent clotting factors, the administration of vitamin K_1 reverses the effects of warfarin by providing the necessary ingredient to enhance clot formation and stop bleeding.

Observe the patient for further evidence of bleeding until the PT is below 2.5 times the control value or until the bleeding episodes cease. PTs generally return to safe levels within 6 hours of administration of vitamin K_1. Administration of whole blood or plasma may be needed if severe bleeding occurs due to the delayed onset of vitamin K_1.

Nursing Process
The Patient Receiving Warfarin

■ *Assessment*

Before administering the first dose of warfarin, question the patient about *all* drugs taken during the previous 2 to 3 weeks (if the patient was recently admitted to the hospital). The activity of warfarin is influenced by many prescription and nonprescription drugs. If any drugs have been taken before admission, contact the physician before the first dose is administered.

During the course of therapy, continually assess for any signs of bleeding and hemorrhage. Areas of assessment include: gums, nose, stools, urine, or nasogastric drainage. See the section on Nursing Management for specific guidelines in these areas.

If the patient has a thrombus in an extremity, examine the area for color and skin temperature. Note any areas of redness or tenderness and ask the patient to describe any present symptoms. Take and record vital signs every 4 hours or more frequently.

■ *Nursing Diagnoses*

Depending on the patient's diagnosis, one or more of the following may apply to the patient receiving warfarin

- **Anxiety** related to diagnosis, therapeutic regimen, other factors (specify)
- **Risk for Ineffective Management of Therapeutic Regimen** related to indifference, lack of knowledge, other factors

■ *Planning and Implementation*

The major goals of the patient may include a reduction in anxiety and an understanding of the postdischarge medication regimen. To make these goals measurable, more specific criteria must be added.

Anxiety. Patients may be concerned over the need for an anticoagulant or the possibility that bleeding may occur. Reassure the patient that therapy will be closely monitored by members of the health team. Because use of an anticoagulant signifies a potentially serious problem, allow patients time to discuss their concerns.

■ *Patient and Family Teaching*

Provide a full explanation of their drug regimen to patients taking warfarin, including an explanation of the problems that can occur during therapy. A thorough review of the dose regimen, possible adverse drug reactions, and early signs of bleeding tendencies helps the patient cooperate with the prescribed therapy.

Include the following points in a patient and family teaching plan:
- Follow the dosage schedule prescribed by the physician.
- The PT will be monitored periodically. Keep all physician and laboratory appointments because dosage changes may be necessary during therapy.
- Do not take or discontinue other medications except on the advice of the physician. This includes nonprescription drugs, as well as those prescribed by a physician or dentist.
- Inform the dentist or other physicians of therapy with this drug *before* any treatment or procedure is started or medications are prescribed.

- Take the drug at the same time each day.
- Avoid alcohol unless use has been approved by the physician. Avoid eating excessive amounts of leafy green vegetables because they may contain large amounts of vitamin K that can interfere with the anticoagulant's effect.
- If evidence of bleeding should occur, for example, unusual bleeding or bruising, bleeding gums, blood in the urine or stool, black stool, or diarrhea, *omit* the next dose of the drug and contact the physician immediately.
- Use a soft toothbrush and consult a dentist regarding routine oral hygiene including the use of dental floss. Use an electric razor whenever possible to *avoid* small skin cuts.
- Wear or carry identification, such as Medic-Alert, to inform medical personnel and others of therapy with this drug.

■ *Expected Outcomes for Evaluation*
- Anxiety is reduced
- Patient and family demonstrate understanding of the drug regimen
- Patient verbalizes importance of complying with the prescribed therapeutic regimen
- Lists or describes early signs of bleeding

Heparin Preparations

Heparin preparations are available as heparin calcium and heparin sodium (see Summary Drug Table 32-1). Heparin preparations, unlike warfarin, *must* be given by the parenteral route, preferably SC or IV. The onset of anticoagulation is almost immediate after a single dose with maximum effects within 10 minutes of administration. Clotting time will return to normal within 4 hours unless subsequent doses are given.

ACTIONS OF HEPARIN

Heparin inhibits the formation of fibrin clots, inhibits the conversion of fibrinogen to fibrin, and inactivates several of the factors necessary for the clotting of blood. Heparin *cannot* be taken orally because it is inactivated by gastric acid in the stomach; therefore, it must be given by injection. Heparin has no effect on clots that have already formed and aids only in preventing the formation of new blood clots (thrombi).

USES OF HEPARIN

Heparin is used for the following:

- Prevention and treatment of venous thrombosis
- Atrial fibrillation with embolus formation
- Prevention of postoperative venous thrombosis and pulmonary embolism in certain patients undergoing surgical procedures, such as major abdominal surgery
- Prevention of clotting in arterial and heart surgery, in blood transfusions and dialysis procedures, and in blood samples for laboratory purposes
- Prevention of a repeat cerebral thrombosis in some stroke patients
- Treatment of coronary occlusion, acute myocardial infarction, and peripheral arterial embolism
- Diagnosis and treatment of disseminated intravascular coagulation, a severe hemorrhagic disorder

ADVERSE REACTIONS ASSOCIATED WITH THE ADMINISTRATION OF HEPARIN

Hemorrhage is the chief complication of heparin administration. Hemorrhage can range from minor local bruising to major hemorrhaging from any organ. Thrombocytopenia (low levels of platelets in the blood) may occur, causing bleeding from the small capillaries and resulting in easy bruising, petechiae (pinpoint hemorrhagic spots on the skin), and hemorrhage into the tissues. Other adverse reactions include local irritation when heparin is given by the SC route. Hypersensitivity reactions may also occur with any route of administration and include fever, chills, and urticaria. More serious hypersensitivity reactions include an asthmalike reaction and an anaphylactoid reaction.

NURSING MANAGEMENT

Nursing management of a patient receiving heparin requires close observation and careful monitoring. When heparin is given to prevent the formation of a thrombus, observe the patient for signs of thrombus formation every 2 to 4 hours. Because the signs and symptoms of thrombus formation vary and depend on the area or organ involved, carefully evaluate and report to the physician any complaint the patient may have or any change in the patient's condition.

Monitor for any indication of hypersensitivity reaction and report reactions such as chills, fever, or hives to the physician.

Laboratory Tests

Blood coagulation tests are usually ordered before and during heparin therapy, and the dose of heparin is adjusted to the test results. The partial thromboplastin time (PTT) and the activated partial thromboplastin time (aPTT) are used to monitor the administration of heparin. Both the PTT and the aPTT coagulation tests are essentially the same but the aPTT is faster and provides a narrow normal range. Optimal results of therapy are obtained when the PTT or the aPTT is 1.5 to 2.5 times the control value.

Whole blood clotting time, also known as Lee-White coagulation time, is the oldest and the least accurate of the coagulation tests. Whole blood clotting time is two and one-half to three times the control value.

Administration

The dosage of heparin is measured in *units* and is available in various dosage strengths as units per milliliter (U/mL), for example, 10,000 U/mL. When selecting the strength used for administration, choose the strength closest to the prescribed dose. For example, if 5000 U are ordered and the available strengths are 1000, 5000, 20,000, and 40,000 U/mL, use 1 mL of the 5000 U/mL for administration.

Heparin may be given by intermittent IV administration, continuous IV infusion, and the SC route. Intramuscular administration is avoided because of the possibility of the development of local irritation, pain, or hematoma (a collection of blood in the tissue). A solution of dilute heparin may be used to maintain patency of an IV site used for intermittent administration of any drug given by the IV route.

Heparin Lock

Intermittent IV administration requires the use of an adapter or heparin lock to provide ready access to a vein without having to maintain a continuous infusion. A solution of dilute heparin consisting of 10 to 100 units/1 mL may be ordered for injection into the heparin lock before and after the administration of the intermittent dose of heparin or any other drug administered by the intermittent IV route. This is called a heparin lock flush. The lock flush solution aids in preventing small clots from obstructing the needle of the intermittent administration set. To prevent incompatibility of heparin with other drugs, the heparin lock set is flushed with sterile water or sterile normal saline before and after any medication is given through the IV line. The physician or institutional policy dictates the use and type of lock flush solution.

Intermittent IV Infusion

Each time heparin is given, inspect the needle site for signs of inflammation, pain, and tenderness along the pathway of the vein. If these should occur, discontinue the use of this site and insert a new intermittent set at a different site. Coagulation tests are usually performed 30 minutes prior to the scheduled dose and from the extremity opposite the infusion site.

Continuous IV Infusion

An infusion pump must be used for the safe administration of heparin by continuous IV infusion. Check the infusion pump every 1 to 2 hours to ensure that it is working properly. Inspect the needle site for signs of inflammation, pain, and tenderness along the pathway of the vein. If these should occur, discontinue the infusion and restart it in another vein.

Blood coagulation tests for those receiving heparin by continuous IV infusion are taken at periodic intervals determined by the physician. If the patient is on prolonged heparin therapy, blood coagulation tests may be performed at less frequent intervals.

Subcutaneous Administration

Subcutaneous (SC) administration sites are rotated and the site used is recorded on the patient's chart. The recommended sites of administration are those on the abdomen. Avoid areas within 2 inches of the umbilicus because of the increased vascularity of that area. Give the injection at a 90 degree angle and do not aspirate or massage the site after the injection is given. Apply firm pressure to the injection site until all oozing of blood has stopped.

The "bunch" technique may be used when administering heparin SC. When using the "bunch" method, grasp the tissue around the site selected to form a tissue roll that is approximately 1/2 inch in diameter. Insert the needle into the tissue roll at a 90 degree angle and inject the medication. Release the tissue roll. Do not aspirate and apply pressure after the injection to prevent hematoma formation.

Ice may be applied to the injection site for 10 to 15 minutes before administration to reduce the possibility of bleeding or oozing at the injection site. The application of ice requires a physician's order or a written hospital policy. Each time heparin is given by this route, all recent injection sites are inspected for signs of inflammation (redness, swelling, tenderness) and hematoma formation.

Adverse Drug Reactions

Bleeding can occur during therapy with heparin. Vital signs are monitored every 2 to 4 hours or as ordered by the physician.

Nursing Alert

If a decided drop in blood pressure or rise in the pulse rate occurs, notify the physician because this may indicate internal bleeding.

Because hemorrhage may begin as a slight bleeding or bruising tendency, the patient is observed frequently for these occurrences (see earlier discussion of warfarin). At times, hemorrhage can occur without warning. If bleeding should occur, the physician may either decrease the dose, discontinue the heparin for a time, or order the administration of protamine sulfate.

Overdosage

In most instances, discontinuation of the drug is sufficient to correct overdosage because the duration of action of heparin is short. However, if hemorrhaging is severe, the physician may order protamine sulfate, the specific heparin antagonist. Protamine sulfate has an immediate onset of action and a duration of 2 hours. Protamine sulfate counteracts the effects of heparin, bringing blood coagulation tests within normal limits.

If administration of this drug is necessary, monitor the blood pressure and pulse rate every 15 to 30 minutes for 2 or more hours after administration of the heparin antagonist. Report any sudden decrease in blood pressure or increase in the pulse rate to the physician immediately. Observe the patient for new evidence of bleeding until blood coagulation tests are within normal limits.

To replace blood loss, the physician may order blood transfusions or fresh frozen plasma.

Nursing Process
The Patient Receiving Heparin

■ *Assessment*

Before administering the first dose of heparin, obtain vital signs. Laboratory studies related to heparin therapy include a PTT or an aPTT. Draw blood for laboratory studies *before* giving the first dose of heparin. Assess vital signs every 2 to 4 hours or more frequently during administration. Report any evidence of bleeding immediately.

■ *Nursing Diagnoses*

Depending on the reason for administration, one or more of the following nursing diagnoses may apply to a person receiving heparin:

● **Anxiety** related to diagnosis, drug therapy, other factors (specify)
● **Risk for Ineffective Management of Therapeutic Regimen** related to lack of knowledge, indifference, other (specify)

■ *Planning and Implementation*

The major goals of the patient may include a reduction in anxiety and an understanding of the therapeutic regimen. To make these goals measurable, more specific criteria must be added.

Anxiety. The diagnosis, as well as the insertion of an IV line or SC injection at scheduled intervals, may result in varying degrees of anxiety. Thoroughly explain the therapeutic regimen to the patient to ease the anxiety associated with knowledge deficit. Although the physician may explain the reason for heparin administration, an explanation by the nurse of the procedure is also important, and should include information about the injection schedule. After the explanation, allow the patient time to ask questions or discuss concerns.

■ *Patient and Family Teaching*

Include the following in a patient and family teaching plan:

- Report any signs of active bleeding immediately.
- Regular coagulation blood tests are critical for safe monitoring of the drug.
- Avoid IM injections while on anticoagulant therapy.
- Use a soft toothbrush when cleaning the teeth and an electric razor for shaving.
- Do not take *any* prescription or nonprescription drugs without consulting the physician. Drugs containing alcohol, aspirin, or ibuprofen may alter the effects of heparin.
- Alopecia, if observed, is temporary and reversible.
- Advise dentist or physician of anticoagulant therapy prior to any procedure or surgery.
- Carry appropriate identification with information concerning drug therapy or wear a Medic-Alert bracelet at all times.

■ *Expected Outcomes for Evaluation*

- Anxiety is reduced
- Patient verbalizes an understanding of treatment modalities

Thrombolytic Drugs

Alteplase, recombinant[1] (Activase), anistreplase (Eminase), streptokinase (Streptase, Kabikinase) and urokinase (Abbokinase) are a group of drugs used to dissolve certain types of blood clots and reopen blood vessels after they have been occluded. The potential benefits of these drugs must be carefully weighed against the potential dangers of bleeding.

---

[1]Alteplase is a tissue plasminogen activator (tPA) that is produced by recombinant DNA. Recombinant DNA is obtained by using gene splicing. Specific DNA segments of one organism are placed in the DNA of another organism. The genetic material of the recipient organism then reproduces itself and contains genetic material of its own plus the genetic material from the donor organism.

ACTIONS OF THROMBOLYTIC DRUGS

Although their exact action is slightly different, these drugs break down fibrin clots by converting plasminogen to plasmin (fibrolysin). Plasmin is an enzyme that breaks down the fibrin (see Fig. 32-1) of a blood clot. This reopens blood vessels after their occlusion and prevents tissue necrosis.

USES OF THROMBOLYTIC DRUGS

These drugs are used in the treatment of acute myocardial infarction to lyse (dissolve) a blood clot in a coronary artery. Urokinase is also used in the treatment of pulmonary emboli and for clearance of IV catheters obstructed by a blood clot. Streptokinase is also used in the treatment of deep vein thrombosis and obstructed arteriovenous cannulae.

ADVERSE REACTIONS ASSOCIATED WITH THE ADMINISTRATION OF THROMBOLYTIC DRUGS

Bleeding is the most frequent adverse reaction seen with the use of these drugs. Bleeding may be internal and involve areas such as the gastrointestinal tract, genitourinary tract, and the brain. Bleeding may also be external (superficial) and may be seen at areas of broken skin, such as venipuncture sites and recent surgical wounds. Allergic reactions may also be seen.

NURSING MANAGEMENT

These drugs are used as soon as possible after the formation of a thrombus, preferably within 6 hours. Initial patient assessments include vital signs and a review of the diagnostic tests performed to establish a diagnosis. Most of these patients are admitted or transferred to an intensive care unit because close monitoring for 48 or more hours after therapy is necessary.

Administration

Follow the physician's orders precisely regarding dosage and time of administration. These drugs are available in powder form and must be reconstituted according to the directions in the package insert.

Adverse Drug Reactions

Bleeding is the most common adverse reaction. Throughout administration of the thrombolytic drug, assess for signs of bleeding and hemorrhage (see earlier discussion on warfarin). If any bleeding is noted, contact the physician immediately because whole blood, packed red cells, or fresh, frozen plasma may be required.

Monitor vital signs every hour or more frequently during administration and for 48 hours after the drug is discontinued. Contact the physician if there is a marked change in one or more of the vital signs.

Monitor and report to the physician any signs of an allergic (hypersensitivity) reaction, namely difficulty breathing, wheezing, hives, skin rash, and hypotension.

Overdosage

Aminocaproic acid (Amicar) is used to control serious bleeding associated with hemorrhage caused by the thrombolytics. This drug is classified as a hemostatic and inhibits the activation of plasminogen. Aminocaproic acid is administered orally or by slow IV drip. Rapid intravenous infusion can cause hypotension, bradycardia, and arrhythmias. During IV infusion, vital signs must be monitored every 15 minutes until bleeding is controlled. Report adverse reactions, such as nausea, cramping or diarrhea to the physician. Notify physician immediately of positive Homans' sign (pain in the calf with dorsiflexion of the foot), leg pain, dyspnea, or chest pain.

Nursing Process
The Patient Receiving a Thrombolytic Drug

■ *Assessment*
Obtain a nursing history noting any history of prior conditions that might contraindicate the use of a thrombolytic drug (eg, recent surgery, ulcerative disease, tuberculosis). Identify any history of bleeding tendencies, heart disease, or allergic reactions to any drugs. Obtain a drug history of any drugs currently being taken. Report any relevant information to the physician prior to administration of the drug.

■ *Nursing Diagnoses*
Depending on the patient's diagnosis, one or more of the following may apply to the patient receiving a thrombolytic drug:

- **Anxiety** related to pain (acute myocardial infarction, pulmonary embolus, deep vein thrombosis), seriousness of disorder, other factors (specify)
- **Pain** related to obstruction of blood vessel
- **Risk for Ineffective Management of Therapeutic Regimen** related to lack of knowledge, indifference, other (specify)

■ *Planning and Implementation*
The major goals of the patient may include a reduction in anxiety, relief of pain, and an understanding of the therapeutic regimen. To make these goals measurable, more specific criteria must be added.

Pain. If pain is present, the physician may order a narcotic analgesic. Once the clot is dissolved and blood flows freely through the obstructed blood vessel, severe pain usually decreases.

Anxiety. If the patient is conscious, the procedure is explained to the patient and family. The patient also should be told that frequent monitoring techniques are necessary during and after therapy with the drug.

■ *Patient and Family Teaching*
Include the following in the patient and family teaching plan:
- An explanation of the purpose of the drug and the method of administration
- The need for continuous monitoring before and after administration of the thrombolytic drug
- The importance of reporting any evidence of hypersensitivity reaction (rash, difficulty breathing) or evidence of bleeding or bruising
- The need for bedrest and minimal handling during therapy to avoid injury

■ *Expected Outcomes for Evaluation*
- Anxiety is reduced
- Pain is relieved
- Patient and family demonstrate understanding of treatment and techniques necessary to monitor therapy

Chapter Summary

- The anticoagulants are a group of drugs that includes the oral anticoagulant warfarin (Coumadin) and the parenteral heparin preparations.

Anticoagulants are used to prevent the formation of a thrombus. The anticoagulants have no direct effect on an existing thrombus and do not reverse the damage from the thrombus. However, once the presence of a thrombus has been established, anticoagulant therapy can prevent additional clots from forming.

- The principal adverse reaction associated with all anticoagulants is bleeding, which may range from very mild to severe. Bleeding may be seen in many areas of the body, such as the bladder, bowel, stomach, uterus, and mucous membranes. Any evidence of bleeding (bleeding gums, epistaxis, easy bruising, black, tarry stools, oozing from wounds, or decrease in blood pressure) must be reported to the physician immediately.

- Warfarin, an oral anticoagulant, interferes with the clotting mechanism of the blood by interfering with the manufacture of vitamin K–dependent clotting factors by the liver.

- The coagulation test used to monitor warfarin therapy is prothrombin time (PT). Optimal therapeutic results are obtained when the patient's PT is 1.5 to 2.5 times the control value. If the PT exceeds 2.5 times the control value, the physician may discontinue the anticoagulant or order vitamin K_1. The administration of vitamin K_1 reverses the effects of warfarin and is considered a warfarin antagonist.

- Most laboratories also report results for International Normalized Ratio (INR) along with the patient's PT and the control value. The INR is used in the management of patients on long-term anticoagulant therapy. The INR should be between 2 and 3. Levels greater than 4.5 are considered critical and should be reported to the physician immediately.

- Warfarin should be withheld and the physician notified if the PT exceeds 2.5 times the control value, if there is evidence of bleeding, or if the INR is greater than 3.

- Heparin is an anticoagulant that is available as heparin calcium and heparin sodium. Heparin cannot be given orally because it is inactivated by the gastric acids in the stomach. Heparin is given only by injection (IV or SC).

- Heparin acts by inhibiting the formation of fibrin clots, by preventing the conversion of fibrinogen to fibrin. Heparin is used for the prevention and treatment of venous thrombosis, pulmonary emboli, atrial fibrillation with embolism, and during cardiac surgery and dialysis procedures.

- Blood coagulation tests used to monitor heparin therapy include the PTT and the aPTT. Optimal results of therapy are obtained when the PTT or the aPTT is 1.5 to 2.5 times the control value.

- Heparin may be given by intermittent IV administration, continuous IV infusion, and the SC route. Intramuscular administration is avoided because of the possibility of developing local irritation, pain, or hematoma. A solution of dilute heparin may be instilled into a heparin lock to maintain patency of an IV site used for intermittent administration of any drug given by the IV route.

- Because hemorrhage may begin as a slight bleeding or bruising tendency, the patient is observed frequently for any evidence of bleeding. At times, hemorrhage can occur without warning. If hemorrhage develops, the physician may either decrease the dose, discontinue the heparin, or order the administration of protamine sulfate, a heparin antagonist.

- The thrombolytics are a group of drugs used to dissolve certain types of blood clots and reopen blood vessels after they have been occluded. The thrombolytic drugs include alteplase, anistreplase, urokinase, and streptokinase.

- Although their mechanism of action is slightly different, these drugs break down fibrin clots by converting plasminogen to plasmin, an enzyme that breaks down the fibrin of a blood clot.

- These drugs are used in the treatment of acute myocardial infarction, to lyse a blood clot in a coronary artery, to treat pulmonary emboli, and to treat deep vein thrombosis.

- Bleeding is the most frequent adverse reaction seen with the use of these drugs. Bleeding may be internal and involve areas such as the gastrointestinal tract, genitourinary tract, and the brain. External bleeding may also be present and is observed at areas of broken skin, such as venipuncture sites and recent surgical wounds.

- These drugs are used as soon as possible, preferably within 6 hours, after the formation of a thrombus. Throughout administration of the thrombolytic drug, assess for signs of bleeding and hemorrhage. If any bleeding is noted, contact the physician immediately because whole blood, packed red cells, or fresh, frozen plasma may be required. Aminocaproic acid may be ordered to control serious bleeding associated with hemorrhage caused by the thrombolytics.

Critical Thinking Exercises

1. Ms. Jackson, aged 56, is hospitalized with a venous thrombosis. The physician orders SC heparin. In developing a care plan for Ms. Jackson, what four

nursing interventions would be most important to prevent complications while administering heparin? Give a rationale for each intervention.

2. Mr. Harris, aged 72, is a widower who has lived alone since his wife died 5 years ago. He has been prescribed warfarin to take at home after his dismissal from the hospital. What questions about his home environment would be important to ask Mr. Harris to best prepare him to care for himself and prevent any complications from the warfarin?

33

Antianginal, Peripheral Vasodilating, and Antihyperlipidemic Drugs

Key Terms

Atherosclerosis
Bile acid sequestrants
Catalyst
Cholesterol
Chylomicrons
High density
  lipoproteins
HMG-CoA reductase
  inhibitors
Hyperlipidemia
Lipids
Lipoproteins
Low density
  lipoproteins
Lumen
Prophylaxis
Sublingual
Transdermal systems
Transmucosal
Triglycerides
Vasodilatation
Very low density
  lipoproteins

Chapter Outline

Chapter Objectives

On completion of this chapter the student will:

- List the general actions, uses, and adverse reactions of antianginal drugs
- Discuss the nursing implications to be considered when administering an antianginal drug
- Use the nursing process when administering an anti-anginal drug
- List the general actions, uses, and adverse reactions of peripheral vasodilating drugs
- Discuss the nursing implications to be considered when administering a peripheral vasodilating drug

(continued)

Scherer JC, Roach S: INTRODUCTORY CLINICAL PHARMACOLOGY,
FIFTH EDITION © 1996 Lippincott-Raven Publishers

Chapter Objectives *(continued)*

- *Use the nursing process when administering a peripheral vasodilating drug*
- *List the general actions, uses, and adverse reactions of antihyperlipidemic drugs*
- *Discuss the nursing implications to be considered when administering an antihyperlipidemic drug*
- *Use the nursing process when administering an antihyperlipidemic drug*

Diseases of the arteries can cause serious problems, namely coronary artery disease, cerebral vascular disease, and peripheral vascular disease. Drug therapy for vascular diseases may include agents that dilate blood vessels and thereby increase blood supply to an area and drugs that lower serum lipid (fat or fatlike substances) levels. An increase in serum lipids is believed to contribute to or cause *atherosclerosis*, a disease characterized by deposits of fatty plaques on the inner wall of arteries. These deposits result in a narrowing of the *lumen* (inside diameter) of the artery and a decrease in blood supply to the area served by the artery.

This chapter discusses three different types of drugs whose primary purpose is to increase blood supply to an area: those that dilate blood vessels, namely the antianginal and peripheral vasodilating drugs, and those that prevent atherosclerosis by reducing serum lipoproteins and serum lipids (cholesterol and triglycerides), namely the antihyperlipidemic drugs. Vasodilating drugs sometimes relieve the symptoms of vascular disease, but in some cases drug therapy only gives minimal and temporary relief.

Antianginal Drugs

The antianginal drugs consist of the nitrates and a newer group of drugs called calcium channel blockers. See also Chapter 18 and Summary Drug Table 18-1 for the adrenergic blocking agents that are also used in the treatment of angina and other disorders.

ACTIONS OF THE ANTIANGINAL DRUGS

A vasodilating drug relaxes the smooth muscle layer of arterial blood vessels, which results in *vasodilatation,* an increase in the size of blood vessels, primar-

ily small arteries and arterioles. Because peripheral, cerebral, or coronary artery disease usually results in decreased blood flow to an area, drugs that *dilate* narrowed arterial blood vessels will carry more blood, followed by an increase in blood flow to the affected area. Increasing the blood flow to an area may result in complete or partial relief of symptoms.

Nitrates

The nitrates, for example, nitroglycerin and isosorbide (Isordil), have a direct relaxing effect on the smooth muscle layer of blood vessels. The end result of this effect is an increase in the lumen of the artery or arteriole and an increase in the amount of blood flowing through these structures. An increased blood flow then results in an increase in the oxygen supply to surrounding tissues.

Calcium Channel Blockers

Calcium is necessary for the transmission of nerve impulses. Calcium channel blockers, for example, nifedipine (Procardia), nicardipine (Cardene), diltiazem (Cardizem), and verapamil (Calan), inhibit the movement of calcium ions across cell membranes; therefore, less calcium is available for the transmission of nerve impulses. This drug action of the calcium channel blockers (also known as slow channel blockers) has several effects on the heart, including an effect on the smooth muscle of arteries and arterioles. These drugs dilate coronary arteries and arterioles, which, in turn, deliver more oxygen to cardiac muscle. The end effect of these drugs is the same as that of the nitrates.

USES OF THE ANTIANGINAL DRUGS

Nitrates

The nitrates are used in the treatment of angina pectoris. Some of these drugs, for example, erythrityl tetranitrate (Cardilate), are used for *prophylaxis* (prevention) and long-term treatment of angina, whereas others, such as sublingual nitroglycerin (Nitrostat), are used to relieve the pain of acute anginal attacks when they occur.

Calcium Channel Blockers

Calcium channel blockers are primarily used in the *prevention* of anginal pain associated with certain forms of angina, such as vasospastic (Prinzmetal's variant) angina and chronic stable angina. They are not used to abort (stop) anginal pain once it has occurred. When angina is due to coronary artery spasm, these drugs are recommended when the patient cannot tolerate therapy with the beta-adrenergic blocking agents (see Chap. 18) or the nitrates.

Some calcium channel blocking agents have additional uses. Verapamil affects the conduction system of the heart and may also be used in the treatment of cardiac arrhythmias. Nifedipine, verapamil, nicardipine, and diltiazem also are used in the treatment of essential hypertension (see Chap. 34).

The more specific uses of the nitrates and calcium channel blockers are given in Summary Drug Table 33-1.

ADVERSE REACTIONS ASSOCIATED WITH THE ADMINISTRATION OF ANTIANGINAL DRUGS

Nitrates

The nitrate antianginal drugs all have the same adverse reactions, although the intensity of some reactions may vary with the drug and the dose. A common adverse reaction seen with these drugs is headache, especially early in therapy. There may also be hypotension, dizziness, vertigo, and weakness associated with headache. Flushing due to dilatation of small capillaries near the surface of the skin may also be seen. In many instances, the adverse reactions associated with the nitrates lessen and often disappear with prolonged use of the drug. For some patients, these adverse reactions become severe, and the physician may lower the dose until symptoms subside. The dose may then be slowly increased if the lower dosage does not provide relief from the symptoms of angina.

Calcium Channel Blockers

Adverse reactions to these drugs usually are not serious and rarely require discontinuation of the drug. The more common adverse reactions seen include peripheral edema, dizziness, lightheadedness, nausea, dermatitis, skin rash, fever, and chills.

NURSING MANAGEMENT

Place *sublingual* (under the tongue) nitroglycerin under the tongue or between the cheek and the gum (buccal area). If this form of nitroglycerin has been prescribed, show the patient how and where to place the tablet in the mouth.

Translingual (under the tongue) nitroglycerin is a metered spray canister that is used to abort an acute anginal attack. Direct the spray from the canister onto or under the tongue. Each dose is metered so that when the canister top is depressed, the same dose is delivered each time. For some individuals, this is more convenient than the small tablets placed under the tongue.

> ### Nursing Alert
>
> The dose of sublingual nitroglycerin may usually be repeated every 5 minutes until pain is relieved. One to two sprays of translingual nitroglycerin may be used to relieve angina but no more than three metered doses are recommended within a 15-minute period.
>
> Instruct the patient to call the nurse if the pain is not relieved after three doses. Notify the physician if the patient has frequent anginal pain, if the pain worsens, or if the pain is not relieved after three doses within a 15-minute period because a change in the dose or the drug or other treatment may be necessary.

If the *transmucosal* (through or across the mucosa) form of nitroglycerin has been prescribed, instruct the patient to place the buccal tablet between the cheek and gum or between the upper lip and gum above the incisors and allow it to dissolve.

The dose of *topical* (ointment) nitroglycerin is measured in inches or millimeters (mm); about 25 mm equals 1 inch. Before the drug is measured and applied and after the ambulatory patient has rested for 10 to 15 minutes, obtain the blood pressure and pulse rate and compare with the baseline and previous vital signs. If the blood pressure is appreciably lower or the pulse rate higher than the resting baseline, contact the physician before the drug is applied. Applicator paper is supplied with the drug; use one paper for each application. While holding the paper, express the prescribed amount of ointment from the tube onto the paper. Remove the plastic wrap and paper from the previous application and cleanse the area as needed. Use the applicator paper to apply the ointment to the skin and *gently* spread the ointment over a 6 × 6-inch area in a thin, uniform layer. Ro-

Summary Drug Table 33-1. Antianginal Drugs

Generic Name	Trade Name*	Uses	Adverse Reactions	Dose Ranges
THE NITRATES				
amyl nitrite	*generic*	Relief of pain of angina pectoris	Headache, hypotension, dizziness, vertigo, weakness, flushing	Crush capsule and wave under nose taking 1–6 inhalations; may repeat in 3–5 min
erythrityl tetranitrate	Cardilate (tablets, sublingual)	Prophylaxis and long-term treatment of angina pectoris	Same as amyl nitrite	5–10 mg PO or sublingually
isosorbide dinitrate	Isordil, *generic* (sublingual, oral tablets or sustained release tablets or capsules), Sorbitrate (sublingual, chewable tablets, or oral tablets	Treatment and prevention of angina pectoris	Same as amyl nitrite	2.5–10 mg sublingual, 5 mg chewable tablets, 5–40 mg PO q6h, sustained release tablets or capsules 40–80 mg q8–12h
isosorbide mononitrate	Imdur, Monoket	Prevention of angina pectoris	Same as amyl nitrite	20 mg PO bid, extended release tablets 30–240 mg PO once daily
nitroglycerin, sublingual	Nitrostat	Prophylaxis and treatment of angina pectoris	Same as amyl nitrite	1 tablet sublingual or in buccal area as needed; may repeat every 5 min times 3
nitroglycerin, sustained release	Nitrong, *generic*	Prevention of angina pectoris	Same as amyl nitrite	2.5–26 mg PO tid, qid
nitroglycerin, topical	Nitro-Bid, *generic*	Prevention and treatment of angina pectoris	Same as amyl nitrite	1–2 inches q8h and up to 4–5 in q4h
nitroglycerin, translingual	Nitrolingual	Acute relief of an attack or prophylaxis of angina pectoris	Same as amyl nitrite	1–2 metered doses onto or under the tongue; may repeat in 5 min with no more than 3 metered doses in 15 min
nitroglycerin, transdermal system	Nitro-Dur, Nitrodisc, *generic*	Prevention of angina pectoris	Same as amyl nitrite	Apply 1 pad daily in the AM for 8–12 h, then remove
nitroglycerin, transmucosal	Nitrogard	Treatment and prevention of angina pectoris	Same as amyl nitrite	1 mg q3–5h while awake
CALCIUM CHANNEL BLOCKING AGENTS				
amlodipine	Norvasc	Chronic stable or vasospastic angina, hypertension	Dizziness, peripheral edema, lightheadedness, nausea, dermatitis, skin rash, fever, chills	2.5–10 mg/d PO
bepridil hydrochloride	Vascor	Chronic stable angina	Same as amlodipine	200–400 mg/d PO
diltiazem hydrochloride	Cardene, Cardene SR, Cardizem, Cardizem CD, *generic*	Chronic stable angina, hypertension	Same as amlodipine	Up to 480 mg/d PO in divided doses
nicardipine hydrochloride	Cardene, Cardene SR	Chronic stable angina, hypertension	Same as amlodipine	Up to 40 mg PO tid; sustained release: 30–60 mg PO bid
nifedipine	Procardia, Adalat, *generic*	Chronic stable or vasospastic angina, hypertension	Same as amlodipine	Up to 120 mg/d PO in divided doses; sustained release: up to 120 mg/d PO in divided doses

(continued)

Summary Drug Table 33-1 (Continued)

Generic Name	Trade Name*	Uses	Adverse Reactions	Dose Ranges
verapamil hydrochloride	Calan, Calan SR, Isoptin, Isoptin SR, *generic*	Chronic stable or vaso-spastic angina, hypertension, arrhythmias	Same as amlodipine	Angina: 40–120 mg PO tid; hypertension: up to 480 mg/d PO in divided doses; sustained release: up to 240 mg/d PO; arrhythmias: 5–10 mg IV bolus

*The term, *generic*, indicates the drug is available in generic form.

tate application sites to prevent inflammation of the skin. Areas that may be used for application include the chest (front and back), abdomen, and upper or lower arms and legs.

Nursing Alert

Do *not* rub the nitroglycerin ointment into the patient's skin because this will immediately deliver a large amount of the drug through the skin. Exercise care in applying topical nitroglycerin and do not allow the ointment to come in contact with the fingers or hands while measuring or applying the ointment because the drug will be absorbed through the skin of the person applying the drug. Wear disposable plastic gloves if drug contact is a problem. Following application of the ointment, cover the area with plastic wrap and secure the wrap with nonallergenic tape.

For most people, nitroglycerin *transdermal systems* are more convenient and easier to use. Transdermal systems have the drug, which is absorbed through the skin, impregnated in a pad. The pad is applied to the skin once a day for 10 to 12 hours. Research has shown that applying the patch in the morning and leaving it in place for 10 to 12 hours, followed by leaving the patch off for 10 to 12 hours yields better results and delays resistance to the drug.

When applying the transdermal system, inspect the skin site to be sure it is dry, free of hair, and not subject to excessive rubbing or movement. If needed, shave the application site. Apply the transdermal system at the same time each day and rotate the placement sites. The best time to apply the transdermal system is after morning care (bed bath, shower, tub bath) because it is important that the skin be thoroughly dry before applying the system. When removing the pad, cleanse the area as needed.

To avoid errors in applying and removing the patch, the person applying the patch can use a fiber-tipped pen to write his or her name (or initials), date, and time of application on the top side of the patch.

Nitroglycerin is also available as *oral tablets* that are swallowed. Give this form of nitroglycerin on an empty stomach unless the physician orders otherwise. If nausea occurs following administration, notify the physician. Taking the tablet or capsule with food may be ordered to relieve nausea.

If anginal attacks occur while the patient is receiving a calcium channel blocking agent, inform the physician of this problem, because a different approach to therapy for angina may be necessary.

Nursing Process
The Patient Receiving an Antianginal Agent

■ *Assessment*

Before administration of an antianginal drug, obtain and record a thorough description of the patient's anginal pain. Include the following information regarding the anginal pain: a description of the type of pain (eg, sharp, dull, squeezing); whether the pain radiates and to where; events that appear to cause anginal pain (eg, exercise, emotion); and events that appear to relieve the pain (eg, resting). Physical assessments include the blood pressure, an apical/radial pulse rate, and respiratory rate, after the patient has been at rest for about 10 minutes. Depending on the type of heart disease, additional physical assessments such as weight, inspection of the extremities for edema, and auscultation of the lungs may be appropriate.

■ *Nursing Diagnoses*

Depending on whether the antianginal drug is used each time anginal pain occurs or for prophylaxis

of angina, one or more of the following nursing diagnoses may apply to a person receiving an antianginal drug:
- **Pain** related to myocardial ischemia secondary to narrowing of the coronary arteries
- **Anxiety** related to diagnosis, pain, anticipation of pain, other factors (specify)
- **Fear** related to diagnosis, chest pain
- **Risk for Ineffective Management of Therapeutic Regimen** related to lack of knowledge of medication regimen, adverse drug effects

■ Planning and Implementation

The major goals of the patient may include a reduction in anxiety and fear, relief of pain, and an understanding of the postdischarge medication regimen. To make these goals measurable, more specific criteria must be added.

Relief of Pain. When a patient is receiving an antianginal agent, monitor the blood pressure and pulse rate every 3 to 4 hours or as ordered by the physician. If the patient has frequent chest pain or complains of dizziness or lightheadedness, monitor the blood pressure more frequently. In addition, evaluate the patient's response to therapy by questioning the patient about his or her anginal pain. In some patients, the pain may be entirely relieved, whereas in others it may be less intense or less frequent or may only occur with prolonged exercise. Record all information in the patient's chart because this helps the physician plan future therapy, as well as dose adjustment if required.

> **Nursing Alert**
>
> If the administration of sublingual or transmucosal nitrate fails to abort an anginal attack, notify the physician *immediately* because additional therapy or tests may be necessary. If an antianginal agent is used to prevent angina but the angina continues to occur, notify the physician immediately.

Adverse Drug Reactions. Observe patients receiving these drugs for adverse reactions. During initial therapy, headache and postural hypotension may be seen. If these reactions occur, notify the physician because a dose change may be necessary. Assist patients having episodes of postural hypotension with all ambulatory activities. Instruct those with episodes of postural hypotension to take the drug in a sitting or lying down position and to remain in that position until symptoms disappear. In many instances, headache, flushing, and postural hypotension that are seen with the administration of the nitrates become less severe or even disappear after a time.

Anxiety and Fear. Reassure the patient that the medication will relieve pain and if pain is not relieved, the physician will be contacted immediately. Allow patients time to discuss their concerns about their diagnosis, the occurrence of adverse reactions (if any), and treatment of the disorder.

■ Patient and Family Teaching

The patient and family must have a thorough understanding of the treatment of chest pain with an antianginal agent. These drugs are used either to prevent angina from occurring or to relieve the pain of angina. Explain the therapeutic regimen (dose, time of day the drug is taken, how often to take the drug, how to take or apply the drug) to the patient.

Adapt a teaching plan to the type of prescribed antianginal agent. The following are general areas included in a teaching plan, as well as those points relevant to specific forms of the drug.

Nitrates
- Avoid the use of alcohol unless use has been permitted by the physician.
- This drug may cause headache, flushing of the face and neck, and dizziness. Notify the physician if these or other reactions become severe.
- Notify the physician if the drug does not relieve pain or if pain becomes more intense despite use of this drug.
- Follow the recommendations of the physician regarding frequency of use.
- Take oral capsules or tablets (except sublingual) on an empty stomach unless the physician directs otherwise.
- Keep an adequate supply of the drug on hand for events, such as vacations, bad weather conditions, holidays, and so on.
- When taking nitroglycerin for an acute attack of angina, sit or lie down. To relieve severe lightheadedness or dizziness, lie down, elevate the extremities, move the extremities, and breathe deeply.
- Keep capsules and tablets in their original containers because nitroglycerin must be kept in a light-proof container and protected from exposure to light. *Never* mix this drug with any other drug in a container.
- Always replace the cover or cap of the container as soon as the oral drug or ointment is removed from

the container or tube. Replace caps or covers tightly because the drug deteriorates on contact with air.

- Keep a record of the frequency of acute anginal attacks (date, time of the attack, drug and dose used to relieve the acute pain); bring this record to each physician or clinic visit.
- Do not handle the tablets labeled as sublingual any more than necessary.
- Check the expiration date on the container of sublingual tablets. If it is past the expiration date, do not use the tablets. Instead, purchase a new supply.
- Do not swallow or chew sublingual or transmucosal tablets; allow them to dissolve slowly.
- The directions for use of translingual nitroglycerin are supplied with the product. Follow the instructions regarding using and cleaning the canister.
- Instructions for application of the topical ointment or transdermal system are available with the product. Read these instructions carefully.
- Apply the topical ointment or transdermal system at approximately the same time each day.
- Be sure the area is clean and *thoroughly dry* before applying the topical ointment or transdermal system and rotate application sites. Apply the transdermal system to the chest (front and back), abdomen, and upper or lower arms and legs. Apply the topical ointment to the front or the back of the chest. If applying to the back, have another person apply the ointment.
- When using the topical ointment form or transdermal system, cleanse old application sites with soap and warm water, as soon as the ointment or transdermal system is removed.
- To use the topical ointment, apply a thin layer on the skin using the paper applicator (the patient or family member may need instructions regarding this technique). Avoid finger contact with the ointment.
- Wash the hands before and after applying the ointment.

Calcium Channel Blockers
- Notify the physician if any of the following occurs: increased severity of chest pain or discomfort, irregular heartbeat, palpitations, nausea, shortness of breath, swelling of the hands or feet, or severe and prolonged episodes of lightheadedness and dizziness.
- If the physician prescribes one of these drugs plus a nitrate, take both exactly as directed to obtain the best results of the combined drug therapy.

■ Expected Outcomes for Evaluation
- Pain is relieved
- Anxiety is reduced
- Fear is reduced
- Patient verbalizes an understanding of treatment modalities
- Adverse reactions are identified and reported to the physician
- Patient and family demonstrate understanding of drug regimen

Peripheral Vasodilating Drugs

In contrast to the antianginal drugs, which are used primarily for angina, the peripheral vasodilating drugs are given for disorders affecting blood vessels of the extremities. Unfortunately, most of these drugs are labeled as "possibly effective" in the treatment of peripheral vascular disorders.

ACTIONS OF THE PERIPHERAL VASODILATING DRUGS

Peripheral vasodilating drugs, such as cyclandelate (Cyclan) and isoxsuprine (Vasodilan) act on the smooth muscle layers of peripheral blood vessels, primarily by blocking alpha-adrenergic nerves and stimulating beta-adrenergic nerves. For a review of the effect of stimulation and blocking (or blockade) effects on adrenergic nerve fibers, see Chapters 17 and 18.

USES OF THE PERIPHERAL VASODILATING DRUGS

Peripheral vasodilating drugs are chiefly used in the treatment of peripheral vascular diseases, such as arteriosclerosis obliterans, Raynaud's phenomenon, and spastic peripheral vascular disorders. These drugs also have other uses, such as the relief of symptoms associated with cerebral vascular insufficiency and circulatory disturbances of the inner ear. More specific uses of individual peripheral vasodilating drugs are given in Summary Drug Table 33-2.

Summary Drug Table 33-2. Peripheral Vasodilating Drugs

Generic Name	Trade Name*	Uses	Adverse Reactions	Dose Ranges
cyclandelate	Cyclan, *generic*	Intermittent claudication, arteriosclerosis obliterans, Raynaud's phenomena, nocturnal leg cramps, ischemic cerebral vascular disease	Heartburn, mild flushing, headache, weakness, tachycardia	Up to 800 mg/d PO in divided doses
isoxsuprine hydrochloride	Vasodilan, *generic*	Cerebral vascular insufficiency, arteriosclerosis obliterans, Raynaud's phenomena, thromboangiitis obliterans	Hypotension, tachycardia, chest pain, nausea, vomiting, dizziness, weakness	10–20 mg PO tid, qid
nylidrin hydrochloride	Adrin, Arlidin, *generic*	Arteriosclerosis obliterans, diabetic vascular disease, ischemic ulcer, frostbite, nocturnal leg cramps, thromboangiitis obliterans	Trembling, nervousness, nausea, vomiting, postural hypotension, palpitations	3–12 mg PO tid, qid
papaverine hydrochloride	Pavased, Cerespan, *generic*	Relief of cerebral and peripheral ischemia associated with arterial spasm, myocardial ischemia complicated by arrhythmias; may be given IV for vascular spasm associated with acute MI, angina, peripheral vascular disease	Nausea, abdominal distress, vertigo, drowsiness, sweating, flushing, rash	100–300 mg PO 3–5 times/day; timed release capsules: 150–300 mg PO q12h; 30–120 mg IM, IV q3h as needed

*The term *generic* indicates the drug is available in generic form.

ADVERSE REACTIONS ASSOCIATED WITH THE ADMINISTRATION OF PERIPHERAL VASODILATING DRUGS

Adverse reactions associated with these drugs are variable. Some of the more common adverse reactions are listed in Summary Drug Table 33-2. Because these drugs dilate peripheral arteries, some degree of hypotension may be associated with their administration. Along with hypotension, there is a physiologic increase in the pulse rate (tachycardia). Some of these drugs also cause flushing of the skin, which can range from mild to moderately severe. Nausea and vomiting may also be seen with these drugs.

NURSING MANAGEMENT

These drugs may be prescribed for outpatient use. Patients taking these drugs for relief of symptoms associated with peripheral vascular disorders often become discouraged over the lack of effectiveness of drug therapy. Encourage the patient to continue with the prescribed medication regimen, as well as to follow the physician's recommendations regarding additional methods of treating the disorder. The affected areas are examined at the time of each visit to a physician's office or outpatient clinic and findings are recorded in the patient's record.

Nursing Process
The Patient Receiving a Peripheral Vasodilating Drug

■ *Assessment*

Before the first dose of a peripheral vasodilating drug, obtain a thorough history of the patient's symptoms. Base the physical assessment on the patient's diagnosis. If cerebral vascular disease is present, evaluate the patient's mental status. If the diagnosis is a peripheral vascular disorder, examine the involved areas for general appearance, such as the color of the skin and evidence of drying or scaling. Note the skin temperature (warm, cool, cold) of the involved area and compare to other areas of the body and to the extremities not affected by peripheral vascular disease. Record these findings in the patient's record. Palpate the peripheral pulses in the affected extremities and record the strength and amplitude of each peripheral pulse. Obtain and record vital signs.

■ *Nursing Diagnoses*

Depending on the reason for administration, one or more of the following nursing diagnoses may apply to a person receiving a peripheral vasodilating drug:

- **Pain** related to narrowing of peripheral arteries, decreased blood supply to the extremities
- **Risk for Injury** related to hypotension, dizziness, lightheadedness secondary to drug action
- **Anxiety** related to pain or discomfort, diagnosis, other factors (specify)
- **Noncompliance** related to indifference, lack of knowledge, other factors
- **Risk for Ineffective Management of Therapeutic Regimen** related to lack of knowledge of medication regimen, adverse drug effects

■ *Planning and Implementation*

The major goals of the patient may include relief of pain, absence of injury, a reduction in anxiety, and an understanding of and compliance to the prescribed therapeutic regimen. To make these goals measurable, more specific criteria must be added.

Therapeutic results obtained from the administration of a peripheral vasodilating drug may not occur immediately. In some instances, results are minimal. Assess the involved extremities daily for changes in color and temperature and record the patient's comments regarding relief from pain or discomfort. The anticipated result of therapy for cerebral vascular disease is an improvement in the mental status.

Pain. Positive results of therapy for a peripheral vascular disorder may include a decrease in pain, discomfort, and cramping, increased warmth in the extremities, and an increase in amplitude of the peripheral pulses. Assess and record the patient's response to therapy. Monitor the blood pressure and pulse one to two times per day because these drugs can may cause a decrease in blood pressure.

Anxiety. Evaluation of the patient's response to the drug is important. To reduce anxiety associated with a slow response to therapy, remind the patient that while signs of improvement may be rapid, improvement usually occurs slowly over many weeks.

Adverse Drug Reactions. If adverse reactions occur, notify the physician. It is important to note the severity of the adverse reactions on the patient's record. In some instances, adverse reactions are mild and may need to be tolerated.

Risk for Injury. Some patients may experience dizziness and lightheadedness, especially during early therapy. If these effects should occur, assist the patient with all ambulatory activities and instruct the patient to ask for help when getting out of bed or ambulating.

Noncompliance. To ensure compliance to the drug regimen, tell the patient and family that improvement will most likely be gradual, although some improvement may be noted in a few days. Encourage the patient to continue with drug therapy and follow the physician's recommendations regarding care of the affected extremities, even though improvement may be slow.

■ *Patient and Family Teaching*

Develop a teaching plan to include the following:

- If nausea, vomiting, or diarrhea occurs, contact the physician.
- Dizziness may occur. Avoid driving and other potentially dangerous tasks, as well as sudden changes in position. Dangle the legs over the side of the bed for a few minutes when getting up in the morning or after lying down. If dizziness persists, contact the physician.
- Use caution when walking up or down stairs or when walking on ice, snow, a slick pavement, or slippery floors.
- Stop smoking (if applicable).
- Peripheral vascular disease: follow the physician's recommendations regarding exercise, avoiding exposure to cold, keeping the extremities warm, and avoiding injury to the extremities.

■ *Expected Outcomes for Evaluation*

- Pain is relieved
- No evidence of injury
- Anxiety is reduced
- Patient and family demonstrate understanding of drug regimen
- Patient verbalizes importance of complying with the prescribed therapeutic regimen

Antihyperlipidemic Drugs

Hyperlipidemia is an increase (hyper) in the *lipids* (lipi), which are a group of fats or fatlike substances in the blood (demia). *Cholesterol* and the *triglycerides* are the two lipids in the blood. Elevation of one or both of these lipids is seen in hyperlipidemia.

The term hyperlipidemia also includes changes (increase or decrease) in *lipoproteins* in the blood. The lipoproteins include *chylomicrons* (small particles of fat in the blood); *very low density lipoproteins* (VLDL); *low density lipoproteins* (LDL); and *high density lipoproteins* (HDL). In hyperlipidemia, chylomicrons may or may not be increased; VLDL and LDL may be normal, increased, or decreased; and the HDL may be normal or decreased. It is desirable to see an increase in the HDL (the "good" lipoprotein, which protects against the development of atherosclerosis). An elevation of the lipids and changes in the lipoproteins are believed to contribute to atherosclerosis.

ACTIONS OF THE ANTIHYPERLIPIDEMIC DRUGS

Antihyperlipidemic drugs decrease cholesterol and triglyceride levels in several ways. Cholestyramine (Questran) and colestipol (Colestid) are *bile acid sequestrants*. Bile, which is manufactured and secreted by the liver and stored in the gall bladder, emulsifies fat and lipids as these products pass through the intestine. Once emulsified, fats and lipids are readily absorbed in the intestine. These drugs bind to bile acids to form an insoluble substance that cannot be absorbed by the intestine and therefore is secreted in the feces. With increased loss of bile acids, the liver uses cholesterol to manufacture more bile. This is followed by a decrease in cholesterol levels.

Another group of drugs are called *HMG-CoA reductase inhibitors*. HMG-CoA reductase is an enzyme that is a *catalyst* (a substance that accelerates a chemical reaction without itself undergoing a change) in the manufacture of cholesterol. These drugs appear to have one of two activities, namely inhibiting the manufacture of cholesterol or promoting the breakdown of cholesterol. This drug activity lowers blood levels of cholesterol and serum triglycerides and increases blood levels of HDLs. Examples of these drugs are fluvastatin (Lescol), lovastatin (Mevacor), and simvastatin (Zocor).

The third group of antihyperlipidemic drugs work in a variety of ways. Probucol (Lorelco) appears to increase the excretion of bile acids, making the liver use cholesterol to manufacture more bile, and thus lower cholesterol levels. Dextrothyroxine (Choloxin) stimulates the liver to break down and excrete cholesterol through the biliary route into the feces. This drug activity thus lowers serum cholesterol. Gemfibrozil (Lopid) increases the excretion of cholesterol in the feces and reduces the production of triglycerides by the liver, thus lowering serum lipid levels. The ability of clofibrate (Atromid-S) and nicotinic acid (niacin) to lower cholesterol levels is not clearly understood.

USES OF THE ANTIHYPERLIPIDEMIC DRUGS

Antihyperlipidemic drug therapy plus control of the dietary intake of fat, particularly saturated fatty acids, are used to lower serum levels of cholesterol and triglycerides. The physician may use one drug or, in some instances, more than one antihyperlipidemic drug for those responding poorly to therapy with a single agent.

ADVERSE REACTIONS ASSOCIATED WITH THE ADMINISTRATION OF ANTIHYPERLIPIDEMIC DRUGS

Bile Acid Sequestrants

A common problem associated with the administration of this group of drugs is constipation. Additional adverse reactions include vitamin A and D deficiencies, bleeding tendencies (including gastrointestinal bleeding) due to a depletion of vitamin K, and abdominal pain and distention.

HMG-CoA Reductase Inhibitors

These drugs are often well tolerated. Adverse reactions, when they do occur, are often mild, transient, and do not require discontinuing therapy. The more common adverse reactions include nausea, vomiting, diarrhea, abdominal pain or cramps, and headache. A photosensitivity reaction also may be seen.

Miscellaneous Preparations

Clofibrate has been reported to pose a risk of cholecystitis (inflammation of the gall bladder) and cholelithiasis (stones in the gall bladder). Nicotinic acid may cause nausea, vomiting, abdominal pain, diarrhea, severe generalized flushing of the skin, a sensation of warmth, and severe itching or tingling.

Summary Drug Table 33-3 lists the adverse reactions for the miscellaneous preparations, as well as other antihyperlipidemic drugs.

NURSING MANAGEMENT

Hyperlipidemia is often treated on an outpatient basis. The drug regimen and possible adverse reac-

Summary Drug Table 33-3. Antihyperlipidemic Drugs

Generic Name	Trade Name*	Uses	Adverse Reactions	Dose Ranges
BILE ACID SEQUESTRANTS				
cholestyramine	Questran, Cholybar	Hyperlipidemia, relief of pruritus associated with partial biliary obstruction	Constipation, vitamin A, D, and K deficiencies, bleeding tendencies, abdominal pain and distention, hypersensitivity reactions, headache, backache	4 g PO 1–6 times/d
colestipol hydrochloride	Colestid	Same as cholestyramine	Same as cholestyramine	5–30 g/d PO as a single dose or in divided doses
HMG-CoA REDUCTASE INHIBITORS				
fluvastatin	Lescol	Reduction of elevated total and LDL cholesterol levels	Nausea, vomiting, diarrhea, abdominal pain or cramps, headache	20–40 mg/d PO hs
lovastatin	Mevacor	Same as fluvastatin	Same as fluvastatin	20–80 mg/d PO in single or divided doses
pravastatin	Pravachol	Same as fluvastatin	Same as fluvastatin	10–40 mg PO hs
simvastatin	Zocor	Same as fluvastatin	Same as fluvastatin	5–40 mg/ PO hs
MISCELLANEOUS PREPARATIONS				
clofibrate	Atromid-S, *generic*	Primary hyperlipidemia	Nausea, skin rash, muscle cramps and pain, fatigue, weight gain, cholecystitis, cholelithiasis	2 g/d PO in divided doses
dextrothyroxine sodium	Choloxin	Reduction of elevated cholesterol	Insomnia, angina, hair loss, skin rash, visual disturbances, nausea, vomiting, sweating, flushing	1–8 mg/d PO
gemfibrozil	Lopid	Hypertriglyceridemia	Abdominal discomfort, heartburn, nausea, vomiting, vertigo, headache	1200 mg/d PO in 2 divided doses 30 min before morning and evening meal
nicotinic acid (niacin)	*generic*	Reduction of elevated cholesterol or triglycerides	Nausea, vomiting, abdominal pain, diarrhea, severe generalized flushing, sensation of warmth, severe itching and tingling	1–2 g PO bid, tid with or after meals
probucol	Lorelco	Reduction of elevated cholesterol	Headache, dizziness, diarrhea, ECG changes, rash, itching, diminished sense of taste and smell	500 mg PO once or twice daily with morning and/or evening meals

*The term, *generic*, indicates the drug is available in generic form.

tions are explained to the patient. If a printed diet is given to the patient, the importance of following the recommended diet is emphasized.

Nursing Alert

Some patients experience moderate to severe generalized flushing of the skin, a sensation of warmth, and severe itching or tingling. Although these reactions are most often seen at higher dose levels, some patients may experience them even when small doses of nicotinic acid are administered. The sudden appearance of these reactions may frighten the patient. When giving nicotinic acid for the first time or when the drug is prescribed for outpatient use, explain to the patient that a feeling of warmth may occur and that this is not unusual. Advise the patient to put the call light on if discomfort is experienced. Contact the physician before the next dose is due should this adverse reaction occur. If the patient is in severe discomfort, contact the physician immediately. Outpatients can be advised to contact their physician if these reactions are severe or cause extreme discomfort.

Nursing Process
The Patient Receiving an Antihyperlipidemic Drug

■ *Assessment*

In many instances, there are no symptoms of hyperlipidemia and the disorder is not discovered until laboratory tests reveal elevated cholesterol and triglyceride levels, elevated low density lipoproteins, and decreased HDL levels. Often, these drugs are initially prescribed on an outpatient basis but initial administration may occur in the hospitalized patient.

Take a dietary history, focusing on the types of foods normally included in the diet. Take vital signs and weight, and inspect the skin and eyelids for evidence of xanthomas (flat or elevated yellowish deposits) that may be seen in the more severe forms of hyperlipidemia.

■ *Nursing Diagnoses*

● **Anxiety** related to identification of a risk factor in coronary artery disease (elevated lipids and lipoproteins)
● **Noncompliance** related to difficulty changing eating habits
● **Risk for Ineffective Management of Therapeutic Regimen** related to knowledge deficit of

diet control, lack of understanding of the required dietary regimen

■ *Planning and Implementation*

The major goals of the patient may include a reduction in anxiety, compliance to the dietary and drug treatment regimen proposed by the physician, and an understanding of the dietary measures necessary to reduce lipid and lipoprotein levels. To make these goals measurable, more specific criteria must be added.

Anxiety. Some patients may express concern over their diagnosis of hyperlipidemia and its link to atherosclerotic heart disease, as well as the need to change their dietary habits. Allow the patient time to ask questions about drug therapy or dietary changes. If available, refer the patient to a teaching dietitian to further explore ways to reduce the dietary intake of fat.

Noncompliance. Some patients may feel that it is difficult to change their dietary habits or that a low-fat diet is difficult to follow. Attempt to ensure compliance to the drug and diet regimen by answering questions as they arise. A referral to a dietitian or a thorough explanation of printed material explaining a low-fat diet may help ensure compliance to the therapeutic regimen.

■ *Patient and Family Teaching*

Stress the importance of following the diet recommended by the physician because drug therapy alone will not significantly lower cholesterol and triglyceride levels. Provide a copy of the recommended diet and review the contents of the diet with the patient and family. If necessary, refer the patient or family member to a teaching dietitian or a dietary teaching session or lecture provided by a hospital or community agency.

Develop a teaching plan to include the following:

Bile Acid Sequestrants
• Take the medication before meals unless the physician directs otherwise.
• Cholestyramine bar: chew each bar thoroughly and drink plenty of fluids. Cholestyramine powder: the prescribed dose *must* be mixed in 2 to 6 fluid ounces of water or *noncarbonated* beverage. The powder can also be mixed with highly fluid soups or pulpy fruits (applesauce, crushed pineapple).
• Colestipol granules: The prescribed dose *must* be mixed in liquids, soup, cereals, carbonated beverage, or pulpy fruits. The granules will not dissolve;

when mixing with a liquid, slowly stir the preparation until drinking. To be sure all the medication is taken, rinse the glass with a small amount of water and drink.

HMG-CoA Inhibitors
- Lovastatin is taken with meals. Fluvastatin, pravastatin, and simvastatin is taken without regard to meals.
- Avoid prolonged exposure to sunlight or ultraviolet light because a severe sunburn may occur. When exposure is unavoidable, wear a sunscreen and protective clothing.
- Contact the physician as soon as possible if nausea; vomiting; muscle pain, tenderness, or weakness; fever; upper respiratory infection; rash; itching; or extreme fatigue occurs.

Miscellaneous Preparations
- Clofibrate: if gastrointestinal upset occurs, take the drug with food. Notify the physician if chest pain, shortness of breath, palpitations, nausea, vomiting, fever, chills, or sore throat occurs.
- Dextrothyroxine: Notify the physician if chest pain, palpitations, sweating, diarrhea, headache, or skin rash occurs.
- Gemfibrozil: Dizziness or blurred vision may occur. Observe caution when driving or performing hazardous tasks. Notify the physician if epigastric pain, diarrhea, nausea, or vomiting occurs.
- Nicotinic acid: Take with meals. May cause mild to severe facial flushing, feeling of warmth, severe itching, or headache. These symptoms usually subside with continued therapy but contact the physician as soon as possible if symptoms are severe. If dizziness occurs, avoid sudden changes in posture.
- Probucol: Take the drug with meals. Notify the physician if diarrhea, abdominal pain, nausea, or vomiting occurs.

■ Expected Outcomes for Evaluation
- Anxiety is reduced
- Patient states willingness to comply to the prescribed treatment regimen
- Patient and family demonstrate understanding of treatment regimen

Chapter Summary

- Diseases of the arteries can cause serious problems, namely coronary artery disease, cerebral vascular disease, and peripheral vascular disease.

Drug therapy for vascular diseases may include agents that dilate blood vessels and thereby increase blood supply to an area and drugs that lower serum lipid (fat or fatlike substances) levels.
- The antianginal drugs consist of the nitrates, adrenergic blocking agents (discussed in Chap. 18), and a newer group of drugs called calcium channel blockers.
- The nitrates have a direct relaxing effect on the smooth muscle layer of blood vessels, thereby producing vasodilation. Calcium channel blockers inhibit the movement of calcium ions across cell membranes; therefore, less calcium is available for the transmission of nerve impulses. These drugs dilate coronary arteries and arterioles, which, in turn, deliver more oxygen to cardiac muscle. The end effect of these drugs is the same as the nitrates.
- The nitrates are used in the treatment of angina pectoris. Calcium channel blockers are primarily used in the *prevention* of anginal pain associated with certain forms of angina.
- A common adverse reaction seen with the nitrates is headache. Dizziness, hypotension, vertigo, weakness, and flushing may also be seen. Hypotension also may be seen. Adverse reactions of the calcium channel blockers may include peripheral edema, dizziness, lightheadedness, nausea, dermatitis, skin rash, fever, and chills.
- Peripheral vasodilating drugs act on the smooth muscle layers of peripheral blood vessels primarily by blocking alpha-adrenergic nerves and stimulating beta-adrenergic nerves. These drugs are chiefly used in the treatment of peripheral vascular diseases. Adverse reactions associated with these drugs are variable.
- Antihyperlipidemic drugs decrease cholesterol and triglyceride levels. Bile acid sequestrants bind to bile acids to form an insoluble substance that cannot be absorbed by the intestine and therefore are secreted in the feces. With increased loss of bile acids, the liver uses cholesterol to manufacture more bile. This is followed by a decrease in cholesterol levels.
- HMG-CoA reductase inhibitors appear to inhibit the manufacture of cholesterol or promote the breakdown of cholesterol which, in turn, lowers blood levels of cholesterol and serum triglycerides and increases blood levels of high density lipoproteins. The third group of antihyperlipidemic drugs work in a variety of ways.
- Antihyperlipidemic drug therapy plus control of the dietary intake of fat, particularly saturated fatty acids, are used to lower serum levels of cholesterol and triglycerides.

- Bile acid sequestrants may cause constipation, bleeding tendencies, vitamin A and D deficiencies, abdominal pain and distention, and gastrointestinal bleeding. HMG-CoA reductase inhibitors often are well tolerated, with only mild and transient adverse reactions. The miscellaneous antihyperlipidemics have a variety of adverse reactions, depending on the drug used. Nicotinic acid often produces the most notable adverse reactions, which include facial flushing and a feeling of warmth accompanied by severe itching or tingling.

Critical Thinking Exercises

1. Ms. Moore is admitted with severe chest pain and a possible myocardial infarction. Following tests, her physician prescribes transdermal nitroglycerin for her angina. Develop a teaching plan that will show Ms. Moore how and when to apply the transdermal form of nitroglycerin.

2. Mr. Lang, a patient in the medical clinic, is prescribed probucol (Lorelco) for hyperlipidemia and is given a copy of a low-fat diet. Mr. Lang tells you that he is a widower, that he often eats in a fast-food restaurant, and that he doesn't understand the diet he is to follow or the reason he is to take the prescribed medication. How would you explain the purpose of the medication to Mr. Lang? How could you help him understand his diet?

3. Mr. Billings is prescribed sublingual nitroglycerin for his angina. Develop a teaching plan that incorporates when and how to take the drug and what precautions he should take regarding handling and storage of the drug.

34

Antihypertensive Drugs

Key Terms

Aldosterone
Angiotensin-converting enzyme
Endogenous
Hypertension
Hypokalemia
Hyponatremia
Lumen
Orthostatic hypotension
Postural hypotension
Vasodilatation

Chapter Outline

Chapter Objectives

On completion of this chapter the student will:

- *List the general types, actions, and uses of the antihypertensive drugs*
- *Explain why blood pressure determinations are important during therapy with an antihypertensive drug*
- *Discuss the nursing implications to be considered when an antihypertensive drug is given*
- *Use the nursing process when administering an antihypertensive drug*

Scherer JC, Roach S: INTRODUCTORY CLINICAL PHARMACOLOGY,
FIFTH EDITION © 1996 Lippincott-Raven Publishers

Most cases of *hypertension* (high blood pressure) have no known cause. As in many other diseases and conditions, there is no one best drug, drug combination, or medical regimen for treatment of hypertension. Following examination and evaluation of the patient, the physician selects the antihypertensive drug and therapeutic regimen that will probably be most effective. In some instances, it may be necessary to change to another antihypertensive drug or add a second antihypertensive drug when the patient does not respond to therapy. In addition to drug therapy, the physician also may recommend additional measures, such as weight loss (if the patient is overweight), reduction of stress, and dietary changes, such as a decrease in the sodium (salt) intake. Once hypertension develops, management of this disorder becomes a lifetime task.

Antihypertensive Drugs

The types of drugs used for the treatment of hypertension include the following:

Alpha/beta-adrenergic blocking drugs—for example, labetalol (Normodyne)

Angiotensin-converting enzyme inhibitors—for example, captopril (Capoten), enalapril (Vasotec I.V.), lisinopril (Prinivil)

Antiadrenergic drugs (centrally acting)—for example, guanabenz (Wytensin), guanfacine (Tenex)

Antiadrenergic drugs (peripherally acting)—for example, guanadrel (Hylorel), guanethidine (Ismelin)

Beta-adrenergic blocking drugs—for example, atenolol (Tenormin), metoprolol (Lopressor), propranolol (Inderal)

Diuretics—for example, furosemide (Lasix), hydrochlorothiazide (HydroDIURIL)

Vasodilating drugs—for example, hydralazine (Apresoline), minoxidil (Loniten)

Calcium channel blocking drugs—for example, amlodipine (Norvasc), diltiazem (Cardizem CD)

ACTIONS OF ANTIHYPERTENSIVE DRUGS

Many antihypertensive drugs lower the blood pressure by dilating or increasing the size of arterial blood vessels (*vasodilatation*). Vasodilatation creates an increase in the *lumen* (the space or opening within an artery) of the arterial blood vessels, which,

in turn, increases the amount of space available for the blood to circulate. Because blood volume (the amount of blood) remains relatively constant, an increase in the space in which the blood circulates (ie, the blood vessels) lowers the pressure of the fluid (measured as blood pressure) in the blood vessels. Although the method by which antihypertensive drugs dilate blood vessels varies, the result remains basically the same. Antihypertensive drugs that have vasodilating activity include the **alpha/beta-adrenergic blocking drugs, antiadrenergic drugs, beta-adrenergic blocking drugs, calcium channel blocking drugs,** and **vasodilating drugs.** See Chapter 18 for additional discussion of adrenergic blocking drugs and antiadrenergic drugs.

The mechanism by which diuretics reduce elevated blood pressure is unknown, but is thought to be based, in part, on their ability to increase the excretion of sodium from the body. The actions and uses of diuretics are discussed in Chapter 35.

The mechanism of action of the angiotensin-converting enzyme inhibitors is not fully understood. It is believed that these drugs may prevent (or inhibit) the activity of *angiotensin-converting enzyme*, which converts angiotensin I to angiotensin II, a powerful vasoconstrictor. Both angiotensin I and angiotensin-converting enzyme normally are manufactured by the body and are called *endogenous* substances. The vasoconstricting activity of angiotensin II stimulates the secretion of the endogenous hormone *aldosterone* by the adrenal cortex. Aldosterone promotes the retention of sodium and water, which may contribute to a rise in blood pressure. By preventing the conversion of angiotensin I to angiotensin II, this chain of events is interrupted, sodium and water are not retained, and the blood pressure decreases.

USES OF ANTIHYPERTENSIVE DRUGS

These drugs are used in the treatment of hypertension. Although there are many antihypertensive drugs available, not all drugs may work equally well in a given patient. In some instances, the physician may find it necessary to prescribe a different antihypertensive drug when the patient fails to respond to therapy. Some antihypertensive drugs are used only in severe cases of hypertension and when other less potent drugs have failed to lower the blood pressure. At times, two antihypertensive drugs may be given together to achieve a better response.

Diazoxide (Hyperstat IV) and nitroprusside (Nipride) may be used to treat hypertensive emergencies, which are cases of extremely high blood pressure that do not respond to conventional antihypertensive drug therapy. These drugs are administered by the intravenous route.

ADVERSE REACTIONS ASSOCIATED WITH THE ADMINISTRATION OF ANTIHYPERTENSIVE DRUGS

The adverse reactions that may be seen when an antihypertensive drug is administered are listed in Summary Drug Table 34-1. For the adverse reactions

that may be seen when a diuretic is used as an antihypertensive agent, see Summary Drug Table 35-1.

When any antihypertensive drug is given, postural or orthostatic hypotension may be seen in some patients, especially early in therapy. *Postural hypotension* is the occurrence of dizziness and lightheadedness when the individual rises suddenly from a lying or sitting position. *Orthostatic hypotension* occurs when the individual has been standing in one place for a long time. These reactions can be avoided or minimized by having the patient rise slowly from a lying or sitting position and by avoiding standing in one place for a prolonged period.

Summary Drug Table 34-1. Antihypertensive Drugs

Generic Name	Trade Name*	Uses	Adverse Reactions	Dose Ranges
ANTIADRENERGIC DRUGS				
Centrally Acting				
clonidine hydrochloride	Catapres-TTS-1, -2, -3, Catapres	Hypertension	Dry mouth, drowsiness, dizziness, sedation, constipation, anorexia, malaise, weight gain, CHF, nightmares, rash, impotence, weakness	0.1–0.8 mg PO bid; transdermal: apply patch once every 7 d
guanfacine hydrochloride	Tenex	Hypertension	Dry mouth, weakness, dizziness, headache, impotence, constipation, fatigue	1–3 mg PO at hs
methyldopa and methyldopate hydrochloride	Aldomet, *generic*	Hypertension	Sedation, headache, weakness, bradycardia, nausea, vomiting, rash, fever, impotence, nasal congestion	Up to 3 g/d PO in divided doses; 250–500 mg IV q6h
Peripherally Acting				
doxazosin mesylate	Cardura	Hypertension	Palpitations, postural hypotension, nausea, vomiting, dry mouth, dyspnea, depression, headache	1–16 mg/d PO
guanadrel sulfate	Hylorel	Hypertension	Palpitations, chest pain, dyspnea, coughing, fatigue, headache, drowsiness, increased bowel movements, indigestion, nocturia, weight gain	10–75 mg/d PO in divided doses
guanethidine monosulfate	Ismelin	Hypertension	Bradycardia, fluid retention, dizziness, weakness, nausea, vomiting, dyspnea, diarrhea	10–50 mg/d PO
prazosin	Minipress, *generic*	Hypertension	Palpitations, nausea, dizziness, drowsiness, headache	2–15 mg/d PO in divided doses
terazosin	Hytrin	Hypertension	Same as prazosin	1–20 mg PO at hs

(continued)

Summary Drug Table 34-1 (Continued)

Generic Name	Trade Name*	Uses	Adverse Reactions	Dose Ranges
BETA-ADRENERGIC BLOCKING AGENTS				
acebutolol hydrochloride	Sectral	Hypertension, ventricular arrhythmias	Bradycardia, dizziness, vertigo, fatigue, gastric pain, sexual dysfunction, rash, pruritus, eye irritation, bronchospasm, joint pain	Hypertension: 200–800 mg PO bid; arrhythmias: up to 1200 mg/d PO
atenolol	Tenormin, *generic*	Hypertension, angina, acute MI	Same as acebutolol hydrochloride	Hypertension: 50–100 mg/d PO; angina: 50–200 mg/d PO; acute MI: 50–100 mg/d PO, 5 mg IV
betaxolol hydrochloride	Kerlone	Hypertension	Same as acebutolol hydrochloride	10–20 mg/d PO
bisoprolol fumarate	Zebeta	Hypertension	Same as acebutolol hydrochloride	2.5–20 mg/d PO
carteolol hydrochloride	Cartrol	Hypertension	Same as acebutolol hydrochloride	2.5–10 mg/d PO
metoprolol	Lopressor, Toprol XL	Hypertension, angina, acute MI	Same as acebutolol hydrochloride	100–450 mg/d PO in single or divided doses
nadolol	Corgard	Hypertension, angina	Same as acebutolol hydrochloride	Hypertension: 40–320 mg/d PO; angina: 40–240 mg/d PO
penbutolol sulfate	Levatol	Hypertension	Same as acebutolol hydrochloride	20–80 mg/d PO
pindolol	Visken, *generic*	Hypertension	Same as acebutolol hydrochloride	Up to 60 mg/d PO in single or divided doses
propranolol hydrochloride	Inderal, *generic*	Hypertension, cardiac arrhythmias, MI, angina, hypertrophic subaortic stenosis, migraine	Same as acebutolol hydrochloride	30–240 mg/d PO in single or divided doses depending on reason for use
timolol maleate	Blocadren, *generic*	Hypertension, migraine, MI	Same as acebutolol hydrochloride	Hypertension: 20–40 mg/d PO
ALPHA/BETA ADRENERGIC BLOCKERS				
labetalol hydrochloride	Normodyne, Trandate	Hypertension, control of blood pressure in severe hypertension	Fatigue, headache, drowsiness, dyspnea, bronchospasm, dizziness, nausea, vomiting, postural hypotension	100–400 mg PO bid; severe hypertension: up to 2.4 g/d PO, 20–80 mg IV injection, 50–300 mg IV infusion
VASODILATING DRUGS				
hydralazine hydrochloride	Apresoline, *generic*	Hypertension	Headache, anorexia, rash, urticaria, constipation, nasal congestion, dizziness	10–50 mg/d PO; 20–40 mg IV, IM
minoxidil	Loniten, *generic*	Severe hypertension	Hypersensitivity reactions, nausea, vomiting, increased body hair growth	Up to 100 mg/d PO in single or divided doses
ANGIOTENSIN-CONVERTING ENZYME (ACE) INHIBITORS				
benazepril hydrochloride	Lotensin	Hypertension	Hypotension, headache, abdominal pain, vomiting, nausea, cough, angioedema, constipation, dizziness, fatigue	10–40 mg/d PO in single or divided doses
captopril	Capoten	Hypertension, heart failure	Same as benazepril hydrochloride	Up to 450 mg/d PO in divided doses

(continued)

Summary Drug Table 34-1 (Continued)

Generic Name	Trade Name*	Uses	Adverse Reactions	Dose Ranges
enalapril maleate	Vasotec, Vasotec I.V.	Hypertension, heart failure	Same as benazepril hydrochloride	Up to 40 mg/d PO in single or divided doses; 0.625–1.25 mg IV q6h
fosinopril sodium	Monopril	Hypertension	Same as benazepril hydrochloride	10–80 mg/d PO
lisinopril	Prinivil, Zestril	Hypertension, CHF	Same as benazepril hydrochloride	Hypertension: 10–40 mg/d PO; CHF: 5–20 mg/d PO
quinapril hydrochloride	Accupril	Hypertension, CHF	Same as benazepril hydrochloride	Hypertension: 10–80 mg/d PO; CHF: 5–20 mg PO bid
ramipril	Altace	Hypertension	Same as benazepril hydrochloride	2.5–20 mg/d PO
CALCIUM CHANNEL BLOCKING DRUGS				
amlodipine	Norvasc	Hypertension, angina, vasospastic angina	Dizziness, lightheadedness, headache, nausea, diarrhea, peripheral edema, hypotension, rash, flushing, hypotension	Hypertension: 2.5–10 mg/d PO; angina: 5–10 mg/d PO
diltiazem hydrochloride	Cardizem, Cardizem CD, Cardizem SR, *generic*	Hypertension, angina, atrial fibrillation or flutter, paroxysmal supraventricular tachycardia	Same as amlodipine	Hypertension: 30–360 mg PO tid, qid; Cardizem CD: 180–360 mg/d PO; Cardizem SR: 60–360 mg/d PO; angina: Cardizem CD 120–480 mg/d PO; arrhythmias: 0.15–0.35 mg/kg IV bolus, 5–10 mg/hr IV infusion
felodipine	Plendil	Hypertension	Same as amlodipine	5–20 mg/d PO
isradipine	DynaCirc	Hypertension	Same as amlodipine	Up to 20 mg/d PO
nicardipine hydrochloride	Cardene, Cardene SR	Hypertension, angina	Same as amlodipine	Hypertension: 20–40 mg PO tid, sustained release 30 mg PO bid; angina: 20–40 mg PO tid
nifedipine	Procardia, Adalat, *generic*	Hypertension, angina	Same as amlodipine	Hypertension: 30–60 mg/d PO sustained release only; angina: up to 120 mg/d PO in divided doses
verapamil hydrochloride	Calan, Calan SR, Isoptin, Isoptin SR, *generic*	Hypertension, angina, atrial flutter or fibrillation, supraventricular tachyarrhythmias	Same as amlodipine	Hypertension: up to 480 mg/d PO in divided doses; sustained release up to 240 mg/d PO; angina: 40–120 mg PO tid; arrhythmias: 5–10 mg IV bolus
DRUGS FOR HYPERTENSIVE EMERGENCIES				
diazoxide, parenteral	Hyperstat IV, *generic*	Emergency reduction of blood pressure	Sodium and water retention, hypotension, myocardial ischemia, cerebral ischemia	1–3 mg/kg IV bolus
nitroprusside sodium	Nipride, Nitropress, *generic*	Emergency reduction of blood pressure	Abdominal pain, apprehension, bradycardia, diaphoresis, dizziness, headache	0.3–10 mcg/kg/ min IV infusion

*The term *generic* indicates the drug is available in generic form.

NURSING MANAGEMENT

Nurses can do much to educate others on the importance of having their blood pressure checked at periodic intervals. This includes people of all ages, since hypertension is not a disease seen only in older individuals. Once hypertension is detected, patient teaching is an important factor in successfully returning the blood pressure to normal or near normal levels.

Nursing Alert

Obtain the blood pressure and pulse rate immediately before each administration of an antihypertensive drug and compare to previous readings. If the blood pressure is significantly decreased from baseline values, do not give the drug and notify the physician. Also notify the physician if there is a significant increase in the blood pressure.

Monitoring and recording the blood pressure is important, especially early in therapy. The physician may need to adjust the dose of the drug upward or downward, try a different drug, or add another drug to the therapeutic regimen if the patient does not respond adequately to drug therapy. Each time the blood pressure is obtained, the same arm is used and the patient is placed in the same position (eg, standing, sitting, or lying down). In some instances, the physician may order the blood pressure taken in one or more positions, for example, standing and lying down. The blood pressure and pulse are monitored every 1 to 4 hours if the patient has severe hypertension, does not respond as expected to drug therapy, or is critically ill.

Nursing Alert

When diazoxide, nitroprusside, or trimethaphan are used for a hypertensive emergency, place the patient in a supine position immediately prior to, as well as after, administration of the drug. Monitor the rate of infusion (nitroprusside, trimethaphan) or rate of direct intravenous administration (diazoxide) and the patient's blood pressure closely during and after administration of the drug because severe hypotension can occur. The blood pressure and pulse rate may need to be monitored every 15 to 30 minutes until the blood pressure is reduced to safe levels.

Obtain daily to weekly weights when first starting drug therapy. Weigh the patient at regular intervals if a weight-reduction diet is used to lower the blood pressure, or if the patient is receiving a thiazide or related diuretic as part of antihypertensive therapy.

Clonidine is available as an oral tablet (Catapres) and transdermal patch (Catapres-TTS-1, -2, or -3). The transdermal patch is applied and kept in place for 7 days. Apply the adhesive overlay directly over the system to ensure the patch remains in place for the required period of time. If the patch loosens, the edges can be reinforced with nonallergenic tape. The date the patch was placed on and the date the patch is to be removed can be written on the surface of the patch with a fiber-tipped pen.

Nursing Process
The Patient Receiving an Antihypertensive Drug

■ *Assessment*
Before starting therapy with an antihypertensive drug, obtain the blood pressure and pulse rate on both arms with the patient in a standing, sitting, and lying position. Properly identify all readings (eg, the readings on each arm and the three positions used to obtain the readings) and record on the patient's chart. Obtain the patient's weight also, especially if a diuretic is part of therapy or the physician prescribes a weight-loss regimen.

■ *Nursing Diagnoses*
Depending on the drug, dose, and the type and severity of hypertension, one or more of the following nursing diagnoses may apply to a person receiving an antihypertensive drug:
- **Risk for Fluid Volume Deficit** related to administration of a diuretic as an antihypertensive drug (when appropriate)
- **Risk for Injury** related to dizziness or lightheadedness secondary to postural or orthostatic hypotensive episodes
- **Anxiety** related to diagnosis, other factors (specify)
- **Noncompliance** related to indifference, lack of knowledge, other factors
- **Risk for Ineffective Management of Therapeutic Regimen** related to lack of knowledge of medication regimen, adverse drug effects, treatment modalities

■ *Planning and Implementation*
The major goals of the patient may include a reduction in anxiety and an understanding of and compliance to the prescribed therapeutic regimen. To make

these goals measurable, more specific criteria must be added.

Adverse Drug Reactions. Observe the patient for adverse drug reactions because their occurrence may require a change in the dose or the drug. Notify the physician if any adverse reactions occur. In some instances, the patient may have to tolerate mild adverse reactions, such as dry mouth or mild anorexia.

Fluid Volume Deficit. Observe patients receiving a diuretic for hypertension for dehydration and electrolyte imbalances. A fluid volume deficit is most likely to occur if the patient fails to drink a sufficient amount of fluid. This is especially true in the elderly or confused patient. To prevent a fluid volume deficit in these patients, encourage oral fluids.

Electrolyte imbalances that may be seen during therapy with a diuretic include *hyponatremia* (low blood sodium) and *hypokalemia* (low blood potassium), although other imbalances may also be seen. See Chapter 48 and Table 48-1 for the signs and symptoms of electrolyte imbalances. Notify the physician if any signs or symptoms of an electrolyte imbalance occur.

Risk for Injury. If postural hypotension should occur, advise the patient to rise slowly from a sitting or lying position. Explain that when rising from a lying position, sitting on the edge of the bed for 1 or 2 minutes often minimizes these symptoms. Inform the patient that rising slowly from a chair and then standing for 1 to 2 minutes also minimizes the symptoms of postural hypotension. When symptoms of postural hypotension occur, assist the patient in getting out of bed or a chair and with ambulatory activities.

Anxiety. Some patients may exhibit anxiety related to their diagnosis or the fact that lifetime therapy for the control of hypertension is necessary. Allow the patient time to ask questions about the therapeutic and drug regimen prescribed by the physician. Tell the patient that most cases of hypertension can be controlled with drug therapy, thereby eliminating the dangers (stroke, heart attack) associated with hypertension.

Noncompliance. To ensure lifetime compliance to the prescribed therapeutic regimen, emphasize the importance of drug therapy, as well as other treatment modalities recommended by the physician, in the treatment of hypertension.

■ *Patient and Family Teaching*

Explain or describe the adverse reactions that may be seen with a particular antihypertensive agent and advise the patient to contact the physician if any should occur.

The physician may wish the patient or family to monitor blood pressure during therapy. Teach the technique of taking a blood pressure and pulse rate to the patient or family and allow sufficient time for supervised practice. Instruct the patient to keep a record of the blood pressure and bring this to each physician's office or clinic visit.

The following points are included in a teaching plan for the patient receiving an antihypertensive agent:

- Never discontinue this medication except on the advice of a physician.
- Avoid the use of any nonprescription drugs (some may contain drugs that are capable of raising the blood pressure) unless approved by the physician.
- Avoid alcohol unless use has been approved by the physician.
- This drug may produce dizziness or lightheadedness when rising suddenly from a sitting or lying position. To avoid these effects, rise slowly from a sitting or lying position.
- If the medication causes drowsiness, avoid hazardous tasks such as driving or performing tasks that require alertness. Drowsiness may disappear after a period of time.
- If unexplained weakness or fatigue occurs, contact the physician.
- Contact the physician if adverse drug effects occur.
- Follow the diet restrictions recommended by the physician. Do not use salt substitutes unless a particular brand of salt substitute is approved by the physician.

■ *Expected Outcomes for Evaluation*

- Fluid volume deficit is corrected (when appropriate)
- No evidence of injury
- Anxiety is reduced
- Patient complies to the prescribed drug regimen
- Patient and family demonstrate understanding of drug regimen
- Patient verbalizes importance of complying with the prescribed therapeutic regimen

Chapter Summary

- Most cases of hypertension have no known cause. As in many other diseases and conditions, there is no one best drug, drug combination, or medical regimen for treatment of hypertension. Following examination and evaluation of the patient, the physician selects the antihypertensive drug and therapeutic regimen that will probably be most effective.

- The types of drugs used for the treatment of hypertension include: alpha/beta-adrenergic blocking drugs, angiotensin-converting enzyme inhibitors, antiadrenergic drugs, beta-adrenergic blocking drugs, diuretics, vasodilating drugs, and calcium channel blocking drugs.
- Many antihypertensive drugs lower the blood pressure by dilating arterial blood vessels. Although the method by which antihypertensive drugs dilate blood vessels varies, the result remains basically the same. The mechanism by which diuretics reduce an elevated blood pressure is unknown but is thought to be based, in part, on their ability to increase the excretion of sodium from the body. The mechanism of action of the angiotensin-converting enzyme inhibitors is not fully understood. It is believed these drugs may prevent the activity of angiotensin-converting enzyme that converts angiotensin I to angiotensin II, which is a powerful vasoconstrictor. This activity of angiotensin II stimulates the secretion of the endogenous hormone aldosterone by the adrenal cortex.
- Although there are a variety of antihypertensive drugs available, not all drugs may work equally well in a given patient. In some instances, it may be necessary to prescribe a different antihypertensive drug when the patient fails to respond to therapy.

- When any antihypertensive drug is given, postural or orthostatic hypotension may be seen in some patients, especially early in therapy.
- Monitoring and recording the blood pressure is important, especially early in therapy. The dose of the drug may need to be adjusted upward or downward, or a different drug prescribed or added to the therapeutic regimen if the patient does not respond adequately to drug therapy. Each time the blood pressure is obtained, the same arm is used and the patient is placed in the same position (eg, standing, sitting, or lying down).

Critical Thinking Exercises

1. While working in the medical clinic of a hospital-associated healthcare satellite, a physician asks you to explain to a patient what can be done to avoid dizziness and lightheadedness when rising from a sitting or lying down position. When talking to the patient, you discover that he understands little English. How might you communicate to this patient what he can do to decrease the symptoms of postural and orthostatic hypotension?

2. Mr. Bates, who has been treated for hypertension, is admitted for treatment of a kidney stone. On admission, he had severe pain and his blood pressure was 160/96. For the past 2 days, his blood pressure has been between 140/92 and 148/92. When taking his blood pressure prior to giving him an oral antihypertensive drug you find that it now is 118/82. Would you give the drug? What further assessments would you perform?

Drugs That Affect the Urinary System

VII

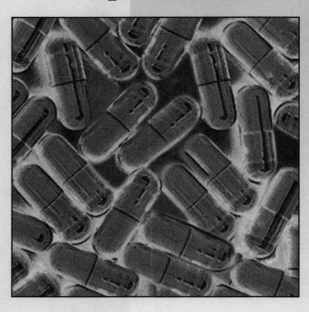

35

The Diuretics

Key Terms

Dehydration
Diuretic
Edema
Filtrate
Glaucoma
Hyperkalemia
Hypokalemia
Hyponatremia
Orthostatic
  hypotension
Postural hypotension

Chapter Outline

Chapter Objectives

On completion of this chapter the student will:

* ***List the general types, actions, and uses of the diuretics***
* ***Discuss the major adverse reactions associated with the administration of a diuretic***
* ***Discuss the nursing implications to be considered when a diuretic is given***
* ***Use the nursing process when administering a diuretic***

A *diuretic* is a drug that increases the secretion of urine by the kidneys. Many conditions or diseases, such as heart failure, endocrine disturbances, and kidney and liver diseases can cause retention of excess fluid (*edema*). When the retention of excess fluid occurs, the physician may order a diuretic, an agent that promotes the excretion of water and electrolytes. There are various types of diuretic agents, and the physician selects the agent that best suits the patient's needs and effectively reduces the amount of excess fluid in body tissues.

The Diuretics

The types of diuretic agents are **carbonic anhydrase inhibitors, loop diuretics, osmotic diuretics, potassium-sparing diuretics,** and **thiazides** and **related diuretics.** Summary Drug Table 35-1 lists examples of the different types of diuretic agents.

ACTIONS OF THE DIURETICS

Most diuretics act on the tubules of the kidney nephron. There are approximately one million nephrons in each kidney, filtering the bloodstream to remove waste products. During this process, water and electrolytes are also selectively removed.

The *filtrate* (ie, the fluid removed from the blood) normally contains ions (potassium, sodium, chloride); waste products (ammonia, urea); water; and, at times, other substances that are being excreted from the body, such as drugs. The filtrate then passes through the proximal tubule, the loop of Henle, and the distal tubules. At these points, selective reabsorption of amino acids, glucose, some electrolytes, and water takes place. Ions and water that are required by the body to maintain fluid and electrolyte balance are returned to the bloodstream by means of the minute capillaries that surround the distal and proximal tubules and the loop of Henle. Ions and water that are not needed by the body are then excreted in the urine.

Carbonic Anhydrase Inhibitors

Carbonic anhydrase is an enzyme that produces free hydrogen ions, which are then exchanged for sodium ions in the kidney tubules. Carbonic anhydrase in-

hibitors inhibit the action of the enzyme carbonic anhydrase. This effect results in the excretion of sodium, potassium, bicarbonate, and water. Carbonic anhydrase inhibitors also decrease the production of aqueous humor in the eye which, in turn, decreases intraocular pressure (IOP), that is, the pressure within the eye.

Loop Diuretics

The loop diuretics furosemide (Lasix) and ethacrynic acid (Edecrin) increase the excretion of sodium and chloride by inhibiting reabsorption of these ions in the distal and proximal tubules and in the loop of Henle. This mechanism of action at these three sites appears to increase their effectiveness as diuretics. Torsemide (Demadex) also increases urinary excretion of sodium, chloride, and water but acts primarily in the ascending portion of the loop of Henle. Bumetanide (Bumex) primarily increases the excretion of chloride but also has some sodium excreting ability, and has additional action on the proximal tubule of the nephron.

Osmotic Diuretics

Osmotic diuretics increase the density of the filtrate in the glomerulus. This prevents selective reabsorption of water, and water is excreted. Sodium and chloride excretion is also increased.

Potassium-Sparing Diuretics

Potassium-sparing diuretics may work in two ways. Triamterene (Dyrenium) and amiloride (Midamor) depress the reabsorption of sodium in the kidney tubules, and therefore increase sodium and water excretion. Both drugs additionally depress the excretion of potassium, and therefore are called potassium-sparing (or potassium-saving) diuretics. Spironolactone (Aldactone), also a potassium-sparing diuretic, antagonizes the action of aldosterone. Aldosterone, a hormone produced by the adrenal cortex, enhances the reabsorption of sodium in the distal convoluted tubules of the kidney. When this activity of aldosterone is blocked, sodium (but not potassium) and water are excreted.

Summary Drug Table 35-1. The Diuretics

Generic Name	Trade Name*	Uses	Adverse Reactions	Dose Ranges
CARBONIC ANHYDRASE INHIBITORS				
acetazolamide	Diamox, *generic*	Open-angle glaucoma, secondary glaucoma, preoperatively to lower IOP, edema due to CHF, drug-induced edema, control of petit mal and unlocalized seizures	Fever, rash, paresthesias, photosensitivity reactions, anorexia, crystalluria, acidosis, urticaria, pruritus	Glaucoma: up to 1 g/d PO in divided doses; acute glaucoma: 500 mg initially then 125–250 mg PO q4h; epilepsy: up to 1000 mg/d PO in divided doses; CHF: 250–375 mg/d PO
methazolamide	Neptazane	Glaucoma	Same as acetazolamide	50–100 mg PO bid, tid
LOOP DIURETICS				
bumetanide	Bumex	Edema due to CHF, cirrhosis of the liver, renal disease	Anorexia, nausea, vomiting, dizziness, rash, photosensitivity reactions, postural or orthostatic hypotension, glycosuria	0.5–10 mg/d PO, IV
ethacrynic acid	Edecrin, Edecrin Sodium	Same as bumetanide plus ascites due to malignancy, idiopathic edema, lymphedema	Same as bumetanide	50–400 mg/d PO in divided doses; 0.5–1 mg/kg IV
furosemide	Lasix, *generic*	Same as bumetanide plus hypertension	Same as bumetanide	Edema: up to 600 mg/d PO in single or two divided doses, 20–40 mg IM, IV; hypertension: up to 40 mg PO bid; CHF and chronic renal failure: up to 2–2.5 g/d IV
torsemide	Demadex	Same as bumetanide plus hypertension	Same as bumetanide	CHF:10–20 mg/d PO, IV; Renal failure: 20 mg/d PO, IV; cirrhosis, hypertension: 5–10 mg/d PO, IV
OSMOTIC DIURETICS				
glycerin (glycerol)	Osmoglyn	Glaucoma, prior to and after eye surgery	Fluid and electrolye imbalance	1–2 g/kg/ PO
isosorbide	Ismotic	Same as glycerin	Same as glycerin	1–3 g/kg PO
mannitol	Osmitrol, *generic*	To promote diuresis in acute renal failure, reduction of IOP, treatment of cerebral edema	Edema, fluid and electrolyte imbalance, headache, blurred vision, nausea, vomiting, diarrhea, urinary retention	20–200 g/24 hr IV
urea	Ureaphil	Reduction of IOP, reduction of intracranial pressure	Headache, nausea, vomiting, fluid and electrolyte imbalance, syncope	Up to 120 g/d IV
POTASSIUM-SPARING DIURETICS				
amiloride hydrochloride	Midamor	CHF, hypertension, hypokalemia from other diuretics, prevention of hypokalemia in at-risk patients	Headache, nausea, anorexia, diarrhea, vomiting, weakness, hyperkalemia	5–20 mg/d PO

(continued)

Summary Drug Table 35-1 (Continued)

Generic Name	Trade Name*	Uses	Adverse Reactions	Dose Ranges
spironolactone	Aldactone, *generic*	Hypertension; edema due to CHF, cirrhosis, renal disease; hypokalemia, prophylaxis of hypokalemia in those taking digitalis, hyperaldosteronism	Cramping, diarrhea, drowsiness, lethargy, rash, drug fever, hyperkalemia	Up to 400 mg/d PO in single dose or divided doses
triamterene	Dyrenium	Prevention of hypokalemia, edema due to CHF, cirrhosis, renal disease	Diarrhea, nausea, vomiting, hyperkalemia, photosensitivity reactions	Up to 300 mg/d PO in divided doses
THIAZIDES AND RELATED DIURETICS				
chlorothiazide	Diuril, *generic*	Hypertension; edema due to CHF, cirrhosis, corticosteroid and estrogen therapy	Hypotension, dizziness, vertigo, lightheadedness, anorexia, gastric distress, impotence, hematologic changes, photosensitivity reactions, hyperglycemia, fluid and electrolyte imbalances, weakness	Hypertension: up to 2 g/d PO in divided doses; edema: 0.5–1 g PO, IV daily or bid
chlorthalidone	Hygroton, *generic*	Same as chlorothiazide	Same as chlorothiazide	Hypertension: 25–100 mg/d PO; edema: 50–200 mg/d PO
hydrochlorothiazide	HydroDIURIL, Esidrix, *generic*	Same as chlorothiazide	Same as chlorothiazide	Hypertension: 25–50 mg/d PO; edema: 25–200 mg/d PO
hydroflumethiazide	Diucardin, Saluron	Same as chlorothiazide	Same as chlorothiazide	Hypertension: 50–100 mg/d PO; edema: 25–200 mg/d PO
indapamide	Lozol	Hypertension, edema due to CHF	Same as chlorothiazide	Hypertension: 1.25–5 mg/d PO; edema: 2.5–5 mg/d PO
methychlothiazide	Enduron, *generic*	Same as chlorothiazide	Same as chlorothiazide	Hypertension: 2.5–5 mg/d PO; edema: 2.5–10 mg/d PO
polythiazide	Renese	Same as chlorothiazide	Same as chlorothiazide	Hypertension: 2–4 mg/d PO; edema: 1–4 mg/d PO

*The term *generic* indicates the drug is available in generic form.

Thiazides and Related Diuretics

Thiazides and related diuretics inhibit the reabsorption of sodium and chloride ions in the ascending portion of the loop of Henle and distal tubule of the nephron. This action results in the excretion of sodium, chloride, and water.

USES OF THE DIURETICS

Diuretics are used in a variety of medical disorders. The physician selects the type of diuretic that will most likely be effective for treatment of a specific disorder. In some instances, hypertension may be treated with the administration of an antihypertensive drug and a diuretic. The diuretics used for this combination therapy include loop diuretics and the thiazides and related diuretics. The specific uses of each type of diuretic agent are discussed below.

Carbonic Anhydrase Inhibitors

Glaucoma is an increase in the IOP that, if left untreated, can result in blindness. Acetazolamide (Diamox) is used in the treatment of simple (open-angle) glaucoma, secondary glaucoma, and preoperatively in acute angle-closure glaucoma when delay of surgery is desired to lower IOP. These drugs are also used in the treatment of edema due to congestive heart failure (CHF), drug-induced edema, and control of epilepsy (petit mal and unlocalized seizures). Methazolamide (Neptazane) is used in the treatment of glaucoma.

Loop Diuretics

Loop diuretics are used in the treatment of edema associated with CHF, cirrhosis of the liver, and renal disease, including the nephrotic syndrome. These drugs are particularly useful when a greater diuretic effect is desired. Furosemide and torsemide are also used to treat hypertension. Ethacrynic acid is also used for the short-term management of ascites due to a malignancy, idiopathic edema, and lymphedema.

Osmotic Diuretics

Mannitol (Osmitrol) is used for the promotion of diuresis in the prevention and treatment of the oliguric phase of acute renal failure, as well as the reduction of IOP and the treatment of cerebral edema. Urea is useful in reducing cerebral edema and in the reduction of IOP. Glycerin (Osmoglyn) and isosorbide (Ismotic) are used in the treatment of acute glaucoma and to reduce IOP before and after eye surgery.

Potassium-Sparing Diuretics

Potassium-sparing diuretics may be used in the treatment of some disorders because of their ability to conserve potassium. Amiloride (Midamor) is used in the treatment of CHF and hypertension and is often used with a thiazide diuretic. Spironolactone and triamterene are also used in the treatment of hypertension and edema due to CHF, cirrhosis, and the nephrotic syndrome. Amiloride, spironolactone and triamterene are also available with hydrochlorothiazide, a thiazide diuretic that enhances the antihypertensive and diuretic effects of the drug combination while still conserving potassium.

Thiazides and Related Diuretics

Thiazides and related diuretics are used in the treatment of hypertension, edema caused by CHF, hepatic cirrhosis, corticosteroid and estrogen therapy, and renal dysfunction.

ADVERSE REACTIONS ASSOCIATED WITH THE ADMINISTRATION OF DIURETICS

The administration of any diuretic may result in a fluid and electrolyte imbalance. The most common imbalances are a loss of potassium and water. When too much potassium is lost, *hypokalemia* (low blood potassium) occurs. In certain patients, such as those also receiving a digitalis glycoside or who currently have a cardiac arrhythmia, hypokalemia has the potential to create a serious problem. If too much water is lost, dehydration occurs, which also can be serious, especially in elderly patients.

Other electrolytes, namely magnesium, sodium, and chlorides, are also lost. Whether a fluid or electrolyte imbalance occurs depends on the amount of fluid and electrolytes lost and the ability of the individual to replace them. For example, if a patient receiving a diuretic eats poorly and does not drink extra fluids, an electrolyte and water imbalance is likely to occur, especially during initial therapy with the drug. However, even when a patient drinks adequate amounts of fluid and eats a well-balanced diet, an electrolyte imbalance may still occur and require electrolyte replacement (see Chap. 48).

Carbonic Anhydrase Inhibitors

Adverse reactions associated with short-term therapy with carbonic anhydrase inhibitors are rare. Long-term use of these drugs may result in fever, rash, paresthesia (numbness, tingling), photosensitivity reactions (exaggerated sunburn reaction when the skin is exposed to sunlight or ultraviolet light), anorexia, and crystalluria (crystals in the urine). On occasion, acidosis may occur and oral sodium bicarbonate may be used to correct this imbalance.

Loop Diuretics

Adverse reactions seen with the loop diuretics may include anorexia, nausea, vomiting, dizziness, rash, *postural hypotension* (dizziness and lightheadedness when rising suddenly from a sitting or lying position) or *orthostatic hypotension* (hypotension after standing in one place for a long time), photosensitivity reactions, and glycosuria (glucose in the urine). Diabetics taking these drugs may experience an elevation of their blood glucose.

Osmotic Diuretics

The osmotic diuretics, urea and mannitol, are administered intravenously (IV), whereas glycerin and isosorbide are administered orally. Administration by the IV route may result in a rapid fluid and electrolyte imbalance, especially when these drugs are administered prior to surgery with the patient in a fasting state.

Potassium-Sparing Diuretics

Hyperkalemia (increase in potassium in the blood), a serious event, may be seen with the administration of potassium-sparing diuretics. Hyperkalemia is most likely to occur in those with an inadequate fluid intake and urine output, those with diabetes or renal disease, the elderly, and those who are severely ill.

Additional adverse reactions of these drugs are listed in Summary Drug Table 35-1. When a potassium-sparing and thiazide diuretic are given together, the adverse reactions associated with both agents may be seen.

Thiazides and Related Diuretics

Administration of thiazides and related diuretics may be associated with numerous adverse reactions. However, many patients take these drugs without experiencing adverse reactions other than excessive fluid and electrolyte loss, which often can be corrected with an adequate fluid intake, a well-balanced diet, supplemental oral electrolytes, or the eating of foods or fluids high in the electrolytes that are being lost. Some of the adverse reactions that may be seen, in addition to those listed in Summary Drug Table 35-1, include gastric irritation, abdominal bloating, reduced libido, dizziness, vertigo, headache, photosensitivity, and weakness. The ad-

ministration of a thiazide diuretic *and* a digitalis glycoside may result in cardiac arrhythmias.

NURSING MANAGEMENT

Fluid and electrolyte imbalances are most likely to occur early in therapy or in those who fail to drink adequate fluids or eat a well-balanced diet. Some of the signs and symptoms of an excessive loss of sodium (*hyponatremia*) include cold, clammy skin, decreased skin turgor, confusion, hypotension, irritability, and tachycardia. Examples of signs and symptoms of excessive water loss (*dehydration*) include thirst, poor skin turgor, dry mucous membranes, weakness, dizziness, fever, and a low urine output. Signs and symptoms of hypokalemia may include anorexia, nausea, vomiting, depression, confusion, cardiac arrhythmias, impaired thought processes, and drowsiness. Signs and symptoms of hyperkalemia may include irritability, anxiety, confusion, nausea, diarrhea, cardiac arrhythmias, and abdominal distress. See Chapter 48 and Table 48-3 for additional discussion of fluid and electrolyte imbalances.

> ### *Nursing Alert*
>
> The most common adverse reaction associated with the administration of a diuretic is the loss of fluid and electrolytes, especially during initial therapy with the drug. In some patients, the diuretic effect is moderate, whereas in others a large volume of fluid is lost. Regardless of the amount of fluid lost, there is always the possibility of excessive electrolyte loss, which is potentially serious. Closely observe patients receiving a potassium-sparing diuretic for signs of hyperkalemia, a serious and potentially fatal electrolyte imbalance. Patients receiving a thiazide diuretic and a digitalis glycoside concurrently require frequent monitoring of the pulse rate and rhythm. Immediately report any significant changes in the pulse rate and rhythm to the physician.

During initial therapy, observe patients for the effects of drug therapy. The type of assessment will depend on factors such as the reason for the administration of the diuretic, the type of diuretic administered, the route of administration, and the condition of the patient. Measure intake and output and record any marked decrease to the physician. During initial therapy, weigh patients at the same time daily. Be sure they are wearing the same amount or type of clothing.

The Patient with Edema

Weigh patients with edema due to congestive heart failure or other causes daily or as ordered by the physician. Measure and record the intake and output every 8 hours. The critically ill patient or the patient with renal disease may require more frequent measurements of urinary output. Obtain the blood pressure, pulse, and respiratory rate every 4 hours or as ordered by the physician. An acutely ill patient may require more frequent monitoring of the vital signs.

Examine areas of edema daily to evaluate the effectiveness of drug therapy, and record the findings in the patient's chart. Evaluate the patient's general appearance and condition daily or more often if the patient is acutely ill.

The Patient with Glaucoma

If a diuretic is given for glaucoma, evaluate the patient's response to drug therapy (relief of eye pain) every 2 hours.

Nursing Alert

Notify the physician immediately if eye pain increases or if it has not begun to decrease 3 to 4 hours after the first dose. If the patient has acute closed-angle glaucoma, check the pupil of the affected eye every two hours for dilation and response to light.

If the patient is ambulatory and has reduced vision because of glaucoma, assistance may be needed with ambulatory and self-care activities.

The Patient with Hypertension

Monitor the blood pressure, pulse, and respiratory rate of patients with hypertension receiving a diuretic, or a diuretic along with an antihypertensive drug, prior to the administration of the drug. More frequent monitoring may be necessary if the patient is critically ill or the blood pressure excessively high.

The Patient with Epilepsy

If a carbonic anhydrase inhibitor is being given for petit mal or unlocalized epileptic seizures, assess the patient at frequent intervals for the occurrence of seizures, especially early in therapy and in those known to have seizures at frequent intervals. If a seizure does occur, record a description of the seizure in the patient's chart, including time of onset, and duration. Accurate descriptions of the pattern and the number of seizures occurring each day helps the physician plan future therapy and adjust drug dosages as needed.

The Patient With Increased Intracranial Pressure

If a patient is receiving the osmotic diuretic mannitol or urea for treatment of increased intracranial pressure due to cerebral edema, monitor the blood pressure, pulse, and respiratory rate every 30 to 60 minutes or as ordered by the physician. Immediately report any increase in blood pressure or decrease in the pulse or respiratory rate or any changes in the neurological status to the physician. Perform neurologic assessments (vital signs, response of the pupils to light, level of consciousness, response to a painful stimulus, and so on) at the time intervals ordered by the physician. Evaluate and record the patient's response to the drug, that is, the signs and symptoms that may indicate a *decrease* in intracranial pressure.

Nursing Process
The Patient Receiving a Diuretic

■ *Assessment*

Before administering a diuretic, take the vital signs and weigh the patient. Review current laboratory tests, especially the levels of serum electrolytes. If the patient has peripheral edema, inspect the involved areas and record in the patient's chart the degree and extent of edema. If the patient is receiving a carbonic anhydrase inhibitor for increased IOP, record the patient's description of pain and obtain vital signs. The physical assessment of the patient receiving a diuretic for epilepsy includes vital signs and weight. Review the patient's chart for a description of the seizures and the frequency of their occurrence.

If the patient is to receive an osmotic diuretic, focus the assessment on the patient's disease or disorder and the symptoms being treated. For example, if the patient has a low urinary output and the osmotic diuretic is given to increase urinary output, review the intake and output ratio and symptoms the patient is experiencing, weigh the patient, and take the vital signs as part of the physical assessment before starting drug therapy.

■ *Nursing Diagnoses*

Depending on the drug, dose, and reason for administration, one or more of the following nursing diagnoses may apply to a person receiving a diuretic:

- **Risk for Fluid Volume Deficit** related to excessive diuresis secondary to administration of a diuretic
- **Risk for Injury** related to adverse drug effects (lightheadedness, dizziness)
- **Anxiety** related to diagnosis, frequent urination, other factors (specify)
- **Noncompliance** related to indifference, lack of knowledge, other factors
- **Risk for Ineffective Management of Therapeutic Regimen** related to knowledge deficit of medication regimen, adverse drug effects

■ *Planning and Implementation*

The major goals of the patient may include correction of a fluid volume deficit, absence of injury, a reduction in anxiety, and an understanding of and compliance with the postdischarge medication regimen. To make these goals measurable, more specific criteria must be added.

Fluid Volume Deficit and Electrolyte Imbalance. On occasion, a fluid volume deficit may occur if the patient experiences diuresis but fails to take a sufficient amount of fluid orally to correct the deficit. This is especially true in the elderly or confused patient. To prevent a fluid volume deficit in these patients, encourage oral fluids at frequent intervals during waking hours.

A well-balanced diet may prevent electrolyte imbalances. Encourage patients to eat and drink all food and fluids served at mealtime. Encourage patients, especially the elderly, to eat or drink between meals and in the evening (when allowed). Monitor the intake and output and notify the physician if the patient fails to drink an adequate amount of fluid, if the urinary output is low, if the urine appears concentrated, if the patient appears dehydrated, or if signs and symptoms of an electrolyte imbalance are apparent.

Risk for Injury. Some patients experience dizziness or lightheadedness, especially during the first few days of therapy or when a rapid diuresis has occurred. Assist patients allowed out of bed with ambulatory activities until these adverse drug effects disappear.

Anxiety. Some patients may exhibit anxiety related to their diagnosis or the fact that it will be necessary to urinate at frequent intervals. To reduce anxiety, explain the purpose and effects of the drug. Tell the patient that the need to urinate frequently will probably decrease. For some patients, the need to urinate frequently decreases after a few weeks of therapy. Provide the patient on bed rest with a call light and, when necessary, place a bedpan or urinal within easy reach.

Inform the patient that the drug will be given early in the day so nighttime sleep will not be interrupted. Although the duration of activity of most diuretics is around 8 hours or less, some diuretics have a longer activity, which may result in a need to urinate during nighttime hours. This is especially true early in therapy.

Noncompliance. Before the first dose of a diuretic is given, the purpose of the drug (ie, to rid the body of excess fluid), when diuresis may be expected to occur, and how long diuresis will last (Table 35-1) is explained to the patient. To ensure compliance to the prescribed drug regimen, stress the importance of diuretic therapy in treating the patient's disorder.

Table 35-1. Examples of Onset and Duration of Activity of Diuretic Agents

Drug	Onset	Duration of Activity
acetazolamide		
tablets	1–1.5 hr	8–12 hr
sustained-release capsules	2 hr	18–24 hr
IV	2 min	4–5 hr
amiloride	2 hr	24 hr
bumetanide	30–60 min	4–6 hr
ethacrynic acid		
PO	Within 30 min	6–8 hr
IV	Within 5 min	2 hr
furosemide		
PO	Within 1 hr	6–8 hr
IV	Within 5 min	2 hr
Mannitol (IV)	30–60 min	6–8 hr
spironolactone	24–48 hr	48–72 hr
thiazides and related diuretics	1–2 hr	Varies*
triamterene	2–4 hr	12–16 hr
urea (V)	30–45 min	5–6 hr

*Duration varies with drug used. Average duration is 12–24/hr with polythiazide, chlorthalidone, and indapamide having a duration of more than 24 hr.

If the patient states that taking a diuretic at a specific time will be a problem, question the patient in an attempt to identify the difficulty associated with drug therapy. Once a problem is identified, solutions or suggestions can be made.

■ *Patient and Family Teaching*

The patient and the family require a full explanation of the prescribed drug therapy, including when to take the drug (diuretics taken once a day are best taken early in the morning); if the drug is to be taken with food; and the importance of following the dosage schedule printed on the container label. The onset and duration of the drug's diuretic effect are also explained. The patient and family must also be made aware of the signs and symptoms of fluid and electrolyte imbalances and adverse reactions that may occur when using a diuretic.

Additional teaching points should include the following:
- Do not stop the drug or omit doses except on the advice of a physician.
- Take the drug early in the morning (once a day dosage, only) unless directed otherwise.
- Avoid alcohol and nonprescription drugs unless their use has been approved by the physician.
- Notify the physician if any of the following should occur: muscle cramps or weakness, dizziness, nausea, vomiting, diarrhea, dry mouth, thirst, general weakness, rapid pulse, or gastrointestinal distress.
- If dizziness or weakness occurs, observe caution while driving or performing hazardous tasks, rise slowly from a sitting or lying position, and avoid standing in one place for an extended time.
- Weigh self weekly or as recommended by the physician. Keep a record of these weekly weights and contact the physician if weight loss exceeds three to five pounds per week.
- If foods or fluids high in potassium are recommended by the physician, eat the amount recommended. Do not exceed this amount or eliminate these foods from the diet for more than 1 day except when told to do so by the physician.
- After a time, the diuretic effect of the drug may be minimal because most of the body's excess fluid has been removed. Continue therapy to prevent further accumulation of fluid.
- Thiazide and related diuretics, loop diuretics, carbonic anhydrase inhibitors, triamterene: avoid exposure to sunlight or ultraviolet light (sun lamps, tanning beds) because exposure may cause an exaggerated sunburn (photosensitivity reaction).

- Loop diuretics and patients with diabetes mellitus: blood glucometer tests for glucose may be elevated (blood) or the urine positive for glucose. Contact the physician if home testing of blood glucose levels are higher than previously or if urine tests positive for glucose.
- Potassium-sparing diuretics: avoid eating foods high in potassium and avoid the use of salt substitutes containing potassium. Read food labels carefully. Do not use a salt substitute unless a particular brand has been approved by the physician.
- The patient with glaucoma: contact the physician immediately if eye pain is not relieved or if it increases.
- A family member of the patient with epilepsy should keep a record of all seizures witnessed and bring this to the physician at the time of the next visit. Contact the physician immediately if the seizures increase in number.

■ *Expected Outcomes for Evaluation*
- Fluid volume deficit (if present) is corrected
- No evidence of injury
- Anxiety is reduced
- Patient verbalizes importance of complying with the prescribed treatment regimen
- Patient and family demonstrate understanding of drug regimen

Chapter Summary

- A *diuretic* is a drug that increases the secretion of urine by the kidneys. Many conditions or diseases, such as heart failure, endocrine disturbances, and kidney and liver diseases can cause retention of excess fluid.
- The types of diuretic agents are **carbonic anhydrase inhibitors, loop diuretics, osmotic diuretics, potassium-sparing diuretics,** and **thiazides and related diuretics.**
- Most diuretics act on the tubules of the kidney nephron. The filtrate normally contains ions, waste products, water, and, at times, other substances that are being excreted from the body. The filtrate passes through the proximal tubule, the loop of Henle, and the distal tubules. At these points, selective reabsorption of amino acids, glucose, some electrolytes, and water takes place.

Ions and water that are required by the body to maintain fluid and electrolyte balance are returned to the bloodstream by means of the minute capillaries that surround the distal and proximal tubules and the loop of Henle. Ions and water that are not needed by the body are then excreted in the urine.

- Diuretics are used in a variety of medical disorders. The physician selects the type of diuretic that will most likely be effective for treatment of a specific disorder. In some instances, hypertension may be treated with the administration of an antihypertensive drug and a diuretic.

- The administration of any diuretic may result in a fluid and electrolyte imbalance. The most common imbalances are a loss of potassium and water. When too much potassium is lost, hypokalemia occurs. Fluid and electrolyte imbalances are most likely to occur early in therapy or in those who fail to drink adequate fluids or eat a well-balanced diet.

Critical Thinking Exercises

1. Mr. Walsh, aged 46, sees his physician and is prescribed a thiazide diuretic for hypertension. He tells you that it will be very inconvenient for him to take his medication in the morning and he would prefer to take it at night. Other than asking him why taking the drug in the evening is more convenient, what other questions would you ask Mr. Walsh? What explanation regarding present and future actions of this diuretic could you tell this patient?

2. A nurse asks you why it is important to give a diuretic early in the morning. What explanation could you give this person?

3. Ms. Palmer, aged 88, is a patient in a nursing home. Her physician prescribes a thiazide diuretic for CHF and hypertension. The nurse in charge advises you to evaluate Ms. Palmer for signs and symptoms of dehydration and hyponatremia. What would you look for? Which of these signs and symptoms might be difficult to evaluate considering her age?

36

Urinary Antiinfectives

Key Terms

Antiinfectives
Bactericidal
Bacteriostatic

Chapter Outline

Chapter Objectives

On completion of this chapter the student will:

- *List the general actions and use of the urinary anti-infectives*
- *Discuss the nursing implications to be considered when a urinary antiinfective is given*
- *Use the nursing process when administering urinary anti-infective drugs*

Some drugs used in the treatment of urinary tract infections (UTIs) do not belong to antibiotic or sulfonamide groups of drugs. The drugs discussed in this chapter are *antiinfectives* (against infection) used in the treatment of UTIs and have an effect on bacteria in the urinary tract. Although administered systemically, that is, by the oral or parenteral route, they do not achieve significant levels in the bloodstream and are of no value in the treatment of systemic infections. They are primarily excreted by the kidneys and exert their major antibacterial effects in the urine.

Urinary Antiinfectives

Examples of urinary antiinfectives include nalidixic acid (NegGram), cinoxacin (Cinobac), nitrofurantoin (Furadantin), and methenamine mandelate (Mandelamine).

There are additional drugs used in the treatment of UTIs. Examples of these drugs include ampicillin (see Chap. 6), the cephalosporins (see Chap. 7), sulfonamides (see Chap. 11), and norfloxacin (see Chap. 9). There also are drugs available in combination, for example oxytetracycline (an antibiotic) combined with sulfamethizole (a sulfonamide), and phenazopyridine (a urinary tract analgesic). Summary Drug Table 36-1 gives examples of the combination drugs used for UTIs.

ACTIONS OF THE URINARY ANTIINFECTIVES

As a result of their high concentration in the urine, nalidixic acid and cinoxacin appear to interfere with bacterial multiplication by interfering with the manufacture (replication) of DNA. Nitrofurantoin may be *bacteriostatic* (slows or retards the multiplication of bacteria) or *bactericidal* (destroys bacteria), depending on the concentration of the drug in the urine. Methenamine and methenamine salts break down and form ammonia and formaldehyde, which is bactericidal. Trimethoprim (Trimpex) interferes with the bacteria's ability to metabolize folinic acid, thereby exerting bacteriostatic activity. Phenazopyridine (Pyridium) is a dye that exerts a topical analgesic effect on the lining of the urinary tract. It has no antiinfective activity.

The actions of other urinary antiinfectives, such as the cephalosporins and sulfonamides, are discussed in their appropriate chapters.

USES OF THE URINARY ANTIINFECTIVES

Like the sulfonamides and other antiinfectives, the systemic antiinfectives are used for UTIs that are caused by susceptible microorganisms. Phenazopyridine is available as a separate drug but is also included in some urinary antiinfective combination drugs. This drug is used for the relief of symptoms associated with UTIs.

ADVERSE REACTIONS ASSOCIATED WITH THE ADMINISTRATION OF THE URINARY ANTIINFECTIVES

Cinoxacin. Nausea, abdominal pain, vomiting, anorexia, diarrhea, perineal burning, headache, photophobia, and dizziness may be seen with the administration of cinoxacin.

Methenamine and Methenamine Salts. Administration may result in gastrointestinal disturbances, such as anorexia, nausea, vomiting, stomatitis, and cramps. Large doses may result in burning on urination and bladder irritation.

Nalidixic Acid. Abdominal pain, nausea, vomiting, anorexia, diarrhea, rash, drowsiness, dizziness, photosensitivity reactions, blurred vision, weakness, and headache may occur with the administration of nalidixic acid. Visual disturbances, when they do occur, are noted after each dose and often disappear after a few days of therapy.

Nitrofurantoin. Nitrofurantoin administration may result in nausea, vomiting, anorexia, rash, peripheral neuropathy, headache, brown discoloration of the urine, and hypersensitivity reactions, which may range from mild to severe. Acute and chronic pulmonary reactions also have been seen.

Trimethoprim. Trimethoprim administration may result in rash, pruritus, epigastric distress, nausea,

Summary Drug Table 36-1. Urinary Antiinfectives

Generic Name	Trade Name*	Uses	Adverse Reactions	Dose Ranges
cinoxacin	Cinobac Pulvules	Initial or recurrent UTIs	Nausea, abdominal pain, vomiting, anorexia, diarrhea, perineal burning, headache, photophobia, dizziness	1 g/d PO in 2–4 divided doses for 7–14 d
methenamine hippurate	Hiprex, Urex	Suppression or elimination of bacteriuria associated with pyelonephritis, cystitis, other chronic urinary tract infections, infected residual urine	Anorexia, nausea, vomiting, stomatitis, cramps	1 g PO bid
methenamine mandelate	Mandelamine, *generic*	Same as methenamine hippurate	Same as methenamine hippurate	1 g PO qid
nalidixic acid	NegGram	UTIs caused by susceptible microorganisms	Abdominal pain, nausea, vomiting, anorexia, diarrhea, rash, drowsiness, dizziness, photosensitivity reactions, blurred vision, weakness, headache	1 g PO qid for 1–2 wk
nitrofurantoin	Furan, Furadantin, *generic*	UTIs caused by susceptible microorganisms	Nausea, vomiting, anorexia, rash, peripheral neuropathy, headache, brown discoloration of urine, hypersensitivity reactions	50–100 mg PO qid
nitrofurantoin macrocrystals	Macrodantin	Same as nitrofurantoin	Same as nitrofurantoin	50–100 mg PO qid
phenazopyridine	Pyridium, Urogesic, *generic*	Relief of symptoms associated with irritation of the lower genitourinary tract	Headache, rash, pruritus	200 mg PO tid
trimethoprim (TMP)	Trimpex, *generic*	UTIs caused by susceptible microorganisms	Rash, pruritus, epigastric distress, nausea, vomiting	100 mg PO q12h or 200 mg PO q24h for 10 d
URINARY ANTIINFECTIVE COMBINATIONS				
sulfamethizole and phenazopyridine	Thiosulfil-A	UTIs caused by susceptible microorganisms	Same as phenazopyridine and sulfamethizole (Chap. 11)	2–4 tablets PO tid, qid
sulfamethizole, oxytetracycline, and phenazopyridine	Urobiotic–250	UTIs caused by susceptible microorganisms	Same as phenazopyridine-sulfamethizole (Chap. 11), and oxytetracycline (Chap. 8)	1 capsule PO qid
trimethoprim and sulfamethoxazole (TMP--SMZ)	Bactrim, Septra, *generic*	UTIs caused by susceptible microorganisms	GI disturbances, allergic skin reactions, headache, anorexia, glossitis	160 mg, TMP/800 mg SMZ PO q12h; 8–10 mg/kg/d (based on TMP) IV in 2–3 divided doses

*The term *generic* indicates that the drug is available in generic form.

and vomiting. When trimethoprim is combined with sulfamethoxazole (Septra), the adverse effects associated with a sulfonamide may also occur.

The adverse reactions seen with other antiinfectives, such as ampicillin, the sulfonamides, and cephalosporins are given in their appropriate chapters.

NURSING MANAGEMENT

Many UTIs are treated on an outpatient basis since in many cases hospitalization is not required. UTIs may be seen in the hospitalized or nursing home patient with an indwelling urethral catheter or a disorder, such as a stone in the urinary tract.

Monitor vital signs every 4 hours or as ordered by the physician. Report any significant rise in temperature to the physician because methods of reducing the fever or repeat culture and sensitivity tests may be necessary.

Measure the intake and output especially when the physician orders an increase in fluid intake or a kidney infection is being treated. The physician may also order daily urinary pH levels when methenamine or nitrofurantoin is administered. These drugs work best in acid urine; failure of the urine to remain acidic may require administration of a urinary acidifier, such as ascorbic acid.

Monitor the patient's response to therapy daily. If after several days the symptoms of the UTI have not improved or if they become worse, notify the physician as soon as possible. Periodic urinalysis and urine culture and sensitivity tests may be ordered to monitor the effects of drug therapy.

Nursing Alert

Pulmonary reactions have been reported with the use of nitrofurantoin and may be seen within hours and up to 3 weeks after therapy with this drug is initiated. Signs and symptoms of an acute pulmonary reaction include dyspnea, chest pain, cough, fever, and chills. If these reactions occur, the physician is notified immediately and the next dose of the drug withheld until the patient is seen by a physician. Signs and symptoms of chronic pulmonary reactions, which may be seen during prolonged therapy, include dyspnea, nonproductive cough, and malaise.

Nursing Process
The Patient Receiving a Urinary Antiinfective

■ Assessment

When a UTI has been diagnosed, sensitivity tests are performed to determine bacterial sensitivity to the drugs (antibiotics and urinary antiinfectives) that will control the infection. Question the patient regarding symptoms of the infection before instituting therapy. Note in the patient's chart the color and appearance of the urine. Take vital signs. Obtain a urine sample for culture and sensitivity before giving the first dose of the drug.

■ Nursing Diagnoses

Depending on the patient and the severity of the UTI, one or more of the following may apply to a person receiving a urinary antiinfective:

- **Anxiety** related to symptoms
- **Noncompliance** related to indifference, lack of knowledge, other factors
- **Risk for Ineffective Management of Therapeutic Regimen** related to knowledge deficit of medication regimen, adverse drug effects

■ Planning and Implementation

The major goals of the patient may include a reduction in anxiety and an understanding of and compliance to the prescribed therapeutic regimen. To make these goals measurable, more specific criteria must be added.

Administration. Give these drugs with food to prevent gastrointestinal upset. Give nitrofurantoin with food, meals, or milk because this drug is irritating to the stomach.

Fluids. Advise the patient to drink at least 2000 mL or more of fluids each day unless the physician orders otherwise. Drinking extra fluids aids in the physical removal of bacteria from the genitourinary tract and is an important part of the treatment of UTIs.

Offer fluids at regular intervals to elderly patients or those that seem unable to increase their fluid intake without supervision. Notify the physician if the patient fails to drink extra fluids, if the urine output is low, or if the urine appears concentrated during daytime hours. The urine of those drinking 2000 mL or more per day will appear dilute and light in color.

Adverse Drug Reactions. Observe the patient for adverse drug reactions. If an adverse reaction occurs, contact the physician before the next dose of the drug is due. Report serious drug reactions immediately. Observe patients receiving nitrofurantoin for signs of a pulmonary reaction, which can be serious. Notify the physician immediately of any symptoms believed to be related to the respiratory system.

Anxiety. The symptoms of a UTI, for example, burning and pain on urination and frequent urination, often are distressing to the patient. Reassure the patient that symptoms most likely will decrease or disappear in a few days.

Noncompliance. In many cases, symptoms are relieved after several days of drug therapy. To ensure compliance to the prescribed drug regimen, stress the importance of completing the full course of drug therapy even though symptoms have been relieved. A full course of therapy is necessary to be sure all bacteria have been eliminated from the urinary tract.

■ *Patient and Family Teaching*

Include the following points in a patient and family teaching plan:

- Take the drug with food or meals (nitrofurantoin *must* be taken with food or milk). If gastrointestinal upset occurs despite taking the drug with food, contact the physician.
- Take the drug at the prescribed intervals. Complete the full course of therapy. Do not discontinue taking the medication even though the symptoms have disappeared, unless directed to do so by the physician.
- If drowsiness or dizziness occurs, avoid driving and performing tasks that require alertness.
- During therapy with this drug, avoid alcoholic beverages and do not take any nonprescription drug unless use has been approved by the physician.
- Notify the physician immediately if symptoms do not improve after 3 or 4 days.
- Nitrofurantoin: notify the physician immediately if any of the following occur: fever, chills, cough, shortness of breath, chest pain, or difficulty breathing. Do not take the next dose of the drug until the physician has been contacted. The urine may appear brown during therapy with this drug; this is not abnormal.
- Nalidixic acid: avoid prolonged exposure to sunlight or ultraviolet light (tanning beds or lamps) because an exaggerated sunburn may occur.
- Methenamine, methenamine salts: avoid excessive intake of citrus products, milk and milk products.
- Phenazopyridine: may cause a reddish-orange discoloration of the urine and may stain fabrics. This is not abnormal.

■ *Expected Outcomes for Evaluation*

- Anxiety is reduced
- Patient verbalizes an understanding of treatment modalities
- Patient and family demonstrate understanding of drug regimen
- Patient verbalizes importance of complying with the prescribed therapeutic regimen

Chapter Summary

- Some drugs used in the treatment of urinary tract infections (UTIs) do not belong to antibiotic or sulfonamide groups of drugs. The drugs discussed in this chapter are antiinfectives used in the treatment of UTIs and have an effect on bacteria in the urinary tract. Although administered systemically, they do not achieve significant levels in the bloodstream, are of no value in the treatment of systemic infections, are primarily excreted by the kidneys, and exert their major antibacterial effects in the urine.
- Additional drugs used in the treatment of UTIs include ampicillin, the cephalosporins, sulfonamides, and norfloxacin. There also are drugs available in combination.
- As a result of their high concentration in the urine, nalidixic acid and cinoxacin appear to interfere with bacterial multiplication by interfering with the manufacture of DNA. Nitrofurantoin may be bacteriostatic or bactericidal, depending on the concentration of the drug in the urine. Methenamine and methenamine salts break down and form ammonia and formaldehyde, which is bactericidal. Trimethoprim interferes with the bacteria's ability to metabolize folinic acid, thereby exerting bacteriostatic activity. Phenazopyridine is a dye that exerts a topical analgesic effect on the lining of the urinary tract. It has no antiinfective activity.
- Like the sulfonamides and other antiinfectives, the systemic antiinfectives are used for UTIs that are caused by susceptible microorganisms. Phenazopyridine is available as a separate drug but is also included in some urinary antiinfective combination drugs. This drug is used for the relief of symptoms associated with UTIs.
- Many UTIs are treated on an outpatient basis since in many cases hospitalization is not required. UTIs may be seen in the hospitalized or nursing home patient with an indwelling urethral catheter or a disorder, such as a stone in the urinary tract.

Critical Thinking Exercises

1. Mr. Elliott, aged 42, sees his physician because his symptoms of a UTI have recurred. His last UTI was 8 weeks ago and he failed to see his physician for a follow-up urine sample 2 weeks after completing his course of drug therapy. The physician suspects that Mr. Elliott may not have followed instructions regarding treatment for his UTI. What points would you stress in a teaching plan for this patient?
2. Ms. Howard, aged 86, has Alzheimer's disease and is a patient in a nursing home. She has developed a UTI and is prescribed cinoxacin (Cinobac Pulvules). What specific nursing tasks would you include in a nursing care plan for this patient?

Drugs That Affect the Endocrine System

VIII

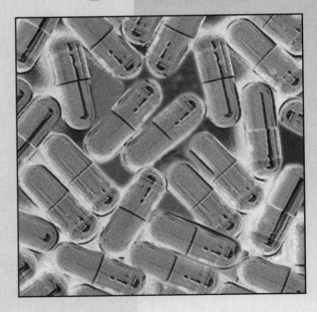

37

Insulin and Oral Hypoglycemic Agents

Key Terms

Diabetes mellitus

Diabetic ketoacidosis

Escherichia coli

Glucagon

Glucometer

Hyperglycemia

Hyperinsulinism

Hyperosmolar Hyperglycemic nonketotic syndrome

Hypoglycemia

Hypoinsulinism

Insulin

Lipodystrophy

Sulfonylurea

Chapter Outline

Chapter Objectives

On completion of this chapter the student will:

- *List the types and uses of insulins*
- *Discuss the adverse reactions associated with the administration of insulin*
- *Discuss nursing management when administering insulin*
- *Use the nursing process when administering insulin*
- *List the types and uses of oral hypoglycemic agents*
- *Discuss the adverse reactions associated with the administration of oral hypoglycemic agents*
- *Discuss nursing management when administering the oral hypoglycemic agents*
- *Use the nursing process when administering an oral hypoglycemic agent*

Diabetes mellitus is a metabolic disorder of the pancreas in which glucose intolerance results from varying degrees of insulin insufficiency. Although no age group is exempt, diabetes is most frequently seen in people between ages 40 and 60.

As a result of the disease, diabetics are at greater risk for a number of disorders including myocardial infarction, cerebrovascular accident (stroke), and peripheral vascular disease. In addition, diabetes is a leading cause of blindness in the United States.

Insulin and the oral hypoglycemic drugs, along with diet and exercise, are the cornerstone of treatment and are used to prevent episodes of hypoglycemia and to normalize carbohydrate metabolism.

The two major types of diabetes mellitus are:

Type I—Insulin-dependent diabetes mellitus (IDDM). Former names of this type of diabetes mellitus include juvenile diabetes, juvenile-onset diabetes, and brittle diabetes.

Type II—Non–insulin-dependent diabetes mellitus (NIDDM). Former names of this type of diabetes mellitus include maturity-onset diabetes, adult-onset diabetes, and stable diabetes.

Those with type I diabetes produce insulin in insufficient amounts and therefore must have insulin supplementation to survive. Those with type II diabetes have a decreased production of insulin or a decrease in the sensitivity of the tissues to insulin. Many type II diabetics are able to control their diabetes with diet, exercise, and oral hypoglycemics.

Insulin

Insulin is a hormone manufactured by the beta cells of the pancreas. It is the principal hormone required for the proper use of glucose (carbohydrate) by the body.

ACTIONS OF INSULIN

Insulin appears to activate a process that helps glucose molecules enter the cells of striated muscle and adipose tissue. Insulin also stimulates the synthesis of glycogen by the liver. In addition, insulin promotes protein synthesis and helps the body store fat by preventing its breakdown for energy. When the production of insulin by the pancreas is insufficient, the patient has diabetes mellitus.

Duration of Action

Onset, peak, and duration are three properties of insulin that are of clinical importance. **Onset** is when insulin first begins to act in the body; **peak** is when the insulin is exerting maximum action; and **duration** is the length of time the insulin remains in effect. To meet the needs of those with diabetes mellitus, various insulin preparations have been developed to delay the onset and prolong the duration of action of insulin. When insulin is combined with protamine (a protein), the absorption of insulin from the injection site is slowed and the duration of action is prolonged. The addition of zinc also modifies the onset and duration of action of insulin.

Insulin preparations are classified as rapid-acting, intermediate-acting, or long-acting. Table 37-1 lists the types of insulin preparations and compares their onset, peak, and duration of action.

Availability of Insulin

Insulin is available as purified extracts from beef and pork pancreas and is biologically similar to human insulin. These animal source insulins are used less frequently today than in years past. They are being replaced by synthetic insulin called human insulin.

Human insulin is derived by two methods. One method is by genetic engineering using strains of Escherichia coli, a microorganism found in the gastrointestinal tract. The other method is by chemical modification of pork insulin. Human insulin appears to cause fewer allergic reactions than insulin obtained from animal sources.

USES OF INSULIN

Insulin is necessary for controlling type I diabetes mellitus where there is an marked decrease in the amount of insulin produced by the pancreas. Insulin may be necessary for controlling the more severe and complicated forms of type II diabetes mellitus, although many patients with type II diabetes can be controlled on diet alone or diet and an oral hypoglycemic agent (see section on oral hypoglycemic drugs). Insulin may also be used in the treatment of severe diabetic ketoacidosis (DKA) or diabetic coma.

Table 37-1. Onset, Peak, and Duration of Action of Various Insulin Preparations*

Preparation	Onset (Hrs)	Peak (Hrs)	Duration (Hrs)
RAPID-ACTING INSULINS			
Insulin injection (regular)	½–1	5–10	6–8
Prompt insulin zinc suspension (semi-lente)	1–1½	5–10	12–16
INTERMEDIATE-ACTING INSULIN			
Isophane insulin suspension (NPH)	1–1½	4–12	24
Insulin zinc suspension (lente)	1–2½	7–15	24
LONG-ACTING INSULINS			
Protamine zinc insulin (PZI)	4–8	14–24	36
Extended insulin zinc suspension	4–8	10–30	>36

*References may vary slightly on these figures.

ADVERSE REACTIONS ASSOCIATED WITH THE ADMINISTRATION OF INSULIN

The two major adverse reactions seen with insulin administration are hypoglycemia (low blood glucose or sugar) and hyperglycemia (elevated blood glucose or sugar). The signs and symptoms of hypoglycemia and hyperglycemia are listed in Table 37-2.

Hypoglycemia occurs when there is too much insulin in the bloodstream in relation to the available glucose (hyperinsulinism). Hypoglycemia may occur when the patient eats too little food; when the insulin dose is incorrectly measured and is greater than that prescribed; or when the patient drastically increases physical activity. Hyperglycemia may occur if there is too little insulin in the bloodstream in relation to the available glucose (hypoinsulinism). Hyperglycemia also may occur when the patient eats too much food; when too little or no insulin is given; or when the patient experiences emotional stress, infection, surgery, pregnancy, or an acute illness.

The patient may develop an allergy to the animal (pig or cow) from which insulin is obtained, or an allergy may develop to the protein or zinc added to insulin. To minimize the possibility of an allergic reaction, some physicians prescribe human insulin or purified insulin. However, on rare occasions, some individuals become allergic to the human and purified insulins as well.

Table 37-2. Hypoglycemia versus Hyperglycemia

Symptoms	Hypoglycemia	Hyperglycemia
Blood glucose	Less than 60 mg/dl	Greater than 200 mg/dl
Central nervous system	Fatigue, weakness, nervousness, confusion, headache, diplopia, convulsions, psychosis, dizziness, unconsciousness	Drowsiness, dim vision
Respirations	Rapid, slow	Deep, rapid (air hunger)
Gastrointestinal	Hunger, nausea, pain, loss of appetite	Thirst, nausea, vomiting, abdominal pain
Skin	Pale, moist, or dry	Dry, flushed
Urine	Negative for glucose and acetone	Positive for glucose and acetone
Pulse	Normal	Rapid
Miscellaneous	Numbness, tingling	Acetone breath

An individual can also become insulin-resistant (or resistant to insulin) because of the development of antibodies against insulin. These patients have impaired receptor function and become so unresponsive to insulin that the daily dose requirement may be in excess of 500 units per day rather than the usual 40 to 60 units per day. High potency insulin in a concentrated form (U500; see Concentration of Insulin) is used to manage patients requiring greater than 200 units per day.

NURSING MANAGEMENT

Nursing management of a patient with diabetes requires diligent, skillful, and comprehensive nursing care.

Insulin Administration

Insulin must be administered by the parenteral route, usually the subcutaneous route (SC). Regular insulin is the only insulin preparation given intravenously (IV). Insulin cannot be administered orally because it is a protein and readily destroyed in the gastrointestinal tract.

There are several methods used to administered insulin. One method is the use of a needle and syringe. Use of the microfine needles has reduced the discomfort associated with an injection. Another method is the jet injection system, which uses pressure to deliver a fine stream of insulin below the skin. Another method uses a disposable needle and special syringe. The syringe uses a cartridge that is prefilled with a specific type of insulin (regular human insulin, isophane [NPH] insulin, or a mixture of isophane and regular insulin). The number of desired units are then selected by turning a dial and then the locking ring.

Another method of insulin delivery is the insulin pump, which is intended for a select group of individuals, such as the pregnant diabetic with early long-term complications and those with, or candidates for, renal transplantation. This system attempts to mimic the body's normal pancreatic function, uses only regular insulin, is battery-powered, and requires insertion of a needle into SC tissue. The needle is changed every 1 to 3 days. The amount of insulin injected can be adjusted according to blood glucose monitoring, which is usually done four to eight times per day.

Many patients are maintained on a single dose of intermediate-acting insulin in the morning or at bedtime. However, the insulin dosage pattern that most closely follows normal insulin production is a multiple dose plan sometimes called **intensive insulin therapy**. In this regimen, a single dose of intermediate or long-acting insulin is taken at bedtime. Small doses of regular insulin are taken before meals based on the patient's blood glucose levels. This allows for greater flexibility in the patient's lifestyle, but can also inconvenience the patient as well (eg, the need to always have supplies with them, the lack of privacy, inconvenient schedules).

Nursing Alert

Insulin requirements may change when the patient experiences any form of stress and with any illness, particularly illnesses resulting in nausea and vomiting.

Insulin is ordered by trade (brand) name or by the generic name, for example, Ultralente Iletin (trade name) or insulin zinc suspension, extended (generic name; Summary Drug Table 37-1). Do not substitute one brand of insulin for another unless substitution is approved by the physician because some patients may be sensitive to changes in brands of insulin. In addition, never substitute one type of insulin for another. For example, do not use insulin zinc suspension instead of the prescribed protamine zinc insulin.

Concentration of Insulin

Insulin is available in concentrations of U100 and U500. Most diabetics use U100. The U500 concentration is used for patients who are resistant to insulin and require large insulin doses. Read the label of the insulin bottle carefully for the name, source of insulin (eg, human, beef, pork, beef and pork, purified beef, and so forth), and the number of units per milliliter (U/mL). The dose of insulin is measured in units (U). U100 insulin has 100 units in each milliliter; U500 has 500 units is each milliliter.

Mixing Insulins

If the patient is to receive regular insulin and NPH, or regular and lente insulin, clarify with the physician whether two separate injections are to be given

Summary Drug Table 37-1. Insulin Preparations	
Types of Insulins	**Trade Name**
RAPID-ACTING INSULINS	
Insulin injection	Regular Iletin I
	Regular Iletin
	Pork Regular Iletin II
	Regular Purified Pork
	Humulin R
	Novolin R
	Velosulin Human
	Novolin R PenFill
INTERMEDIATE-ACTING INSULINS	
Isophane insulin suspension	NPH Iletin I
	NPH Insulin
	NPH-N
	Pork NPH Iletin II
	Humulin N
	Novolin N
	Novolin N PenFill
Insulin Zinc Suspension (Lente)	Lente Iletin I
	Lente Insulin
	Lente Iletin II
	Lente L
	Humulin L
	Novolin L
LONG-ACTING INSULINS	
Insulin Zinc Suspension (Ultralente)	Ultralente U
	Humulin U Ultralente
MIXED INSULINS	
Isophane insulin and insulin injection	Humulin 70/30
	Novolin 70/30
	Novolin 70/30 PenFill
	Humulin 50/50

or if the insulins may be mixed in the same syringe. If the two insulins are to be given in the same syringe, draw the regular, short-acting insulin into the syringe first. Even small amounts of intermediate or long-acting insulin, if mixed with the regular, can bind with the regular insulin and delay its onset.

An unexpected response may be obtained when changing from mixed injections to separate injections or vice versa. If the patient had been using insulin mixtures before admission, ask whether the insulins were given separately or together.

Several types of premixed insulins are currently available. These insulins combine regular insulin with the longer acting NPH insulin. The mixtures are available in ratios of 70/30 and 50/50 of NPH to regular. While these premixed insulins are helpful for patients who have difficulty drawing up their insulin or seeing the markings on the syringe, they prohibit individualizing the dosage. For patients

that have difficulty controlling their diabetes, these premixed insulins may not be effective.

Administering Insulin

The physician selects the dosage and type of insulin that will most likely meet the requirements of an individual patient. There is no standard dose range of insulin as there is for most other drugs. The dose prescribed for the patient may require changes until the dosage is found that best meets the patient's needs.

The expiration date printed on the label of the insulin bottle is always checked before withdrawing the insulin.

Always use an insulin syringe that matches the concentration of insulin to be given. For example, a syringe labeled as U100 is used only with insulin labeled U100. U500 insulin is only given SC or intramuscularly (IM), never IV, and may be administered using a tuberculin syringe. Close observation is necessary because secondary hypoglycemic reactions may occur up to 24 hours after the administration of U500 insulin. Accuracy is of the utmost importance when measuring any insulin preparation because of the potential danger of administering an incorrect dosage.

When insulin is in a suspension (this can be seen when looking at a vial that has been untouched for approximately 1 hour), gently rotate the vial between the palms of the hands and tilt gently end-to-end immediately before withdrawing the insulin. This ensures even distribution of the suspended particles. Do not shake insulin vigorously.

Carefully check the physician's order for the type and dosage of insulin immediately before withdrawing the insulin from the vial. All air bubbles must be eliminated from the syringe barrel and hub of the needle before the syringe is withdrawn from the insulin vial. When regular insulin and another insulin are mixed in the same syringe, administer the insulin within 5 minutes of withdrawing the two insulins from the two vials.

Give the insulin injection (regular insulin) 15 to 30 minutes before a meal because the onset of action is 30 to 60 minutes. Give the longer-acting insulins before breakfast or at bedtime (depending on the physician's instructions). Insulin is given SC. Only regular insulin may be given IM or IV, as well as by the SC route.

Rotating Injection Sites

Insulin may be injected into the arms, thighs, abdomen, or buttocks. Rotate insulin injection sites to prevent lipodystrophy (atrophy of SC fat), a problem that can interfere with the absorption of insulin from the injection site. Because absorption rates vary at the different sites, with the abdomen having the most rapid rate of absorption followed by the upper arm, thigh, and buttocks, some physicians now recommend rotating the injection sites within one specific area rather than rotating areas. Carefully plan the pattern of rotation of the injection sites and then write it in the patient's chart. Before each dose of insulin is given, check the patient's chart for the site of the previous injection and use the next site (according to the rotation plan) for injection. Record the site used for injection.

Each time insulin is given, inspect previous injection sites for signs of inflammation, which may indicate a localized allergic reaction. Note any inflammation or other skin reactions. Report localized allergic reactions, signs of inflammation, or other skin changes to the physician as soon as possible because a different type of insulin may be necessary.

Adverse Reactions

Close observation of the diabetic patient is important, especially when the patient is a new diabetic, the insulin dosage is changed, the patient is pregnant, the patient has a medical illness or has had surgery, or the patient failed to adhere to the prescribed diet.

Nursing Alert

Check the patient at the expected time of onset and peak of action (see Table 37-1) of the insulin given and observed for signs of hypoglycemia. Hypoglycemia (see Table 37-2), which can develop suddenly, may indicate a need for an adjustment in the insulin dosage or other changes in treatment, such as a change in diet.

Signs of hyperglycemia may also occur but are more likely to be less prominent and develop slowly.

Correct episodes of hypoglycemia as soon as the symptoms are recognized. Methods of terminating a hypoglycemic reaction include the administration of one or more of the following:

Orange juice or other fruit juice
Hard candy or honey
Commercial glucose products
Glucagon by the SC, IM, or IV route
Glucose 10% or 50% IV

Selection of any one or more of the above methods for terminating a hypoglycemic reaction, as well as other procedures to be followed, such as drawing blood for glucose levels, depends on the written order of the physician or hospital policy. Never give an oral fluid or substance to terminate a hypoglycemic reaction unless swallowing and gag reflexes are present. Absence of these reflexes may result in aspiration of the oral fluid or substance into the lungs, which can result in extremely serious consequences and even death. If swallowing and gag reflexes are absent or if the patient is unconscious, give glucose or glucagon by the parenteral route.

Glucagon is a hormone produced by the alpha cells of the pancreas; it acts to increase blood sugar by stimulating the conversion of glycogen to glucose in the liver. A return of consciousness is observed within 5 to 20 minutes after parenteral administration of glucagon. Glucagon is effective in treating hypoglycemia only if liver glycogen is available.

Notify the physician of any hypoglycemic reaction, the substance and amount used to terminate the reaction, blood samples drawn (if any), the length of time required for the symptoms of hypoglycemia to disappear, and the present status of the patient. After termination of a hypoglycemic reaction, observe the patient closely for additional hypoglycemic reactions. The length of time close observation is required depends on the peak and duration of the insulin administered.

Nursing Alert

In patients taking human insulin symptoms of hypoglycemia are less pronounced than in patients taking animal-based products.

Diabetic Ketoacidosis

Diabetic ketoacidosis (DKA) is a potentially life-threatening deficiency of insulin (hypoinsulinism), resulting in severe hyperglycemia and requiring prompt diagnosis and treatment. Since insulin is unavailable to allow glucose to enter the cell, dangerously high levels of glucose builds up in the blood (hyperglycemia). The body, needing energy, begins to break down fat for energy. As fats are broken down, ketones are produced by the liver. As more and more fat is used for energy, higher levels of ketones accumulate in the blood. This increase in ketones disrupts the acid-base balance within the body leading to DKA. Insulin is essential to treat this potentially dangerous complication.

Immediately report any of the following symptoms: elevated blood glucose levels (greater than 200 mg/dL), headache, increased thirst, epigastric pain, nausea, vomiting, hot, dry, flushed skin, restlessness, diaphoresis (sweating) and fruity odor to the breath.

Hyperosmolar Hyperglycemic Nonketotic Syndrome

Another complication of diabetes is hyperosmolar hyperglycemic nonketotic syndrome. This syndrome occurs most often as a result of a stressor, such as acute illness and is manifested by hyperglycemia and hyperosmolarity, resulting in cellular dehydration and diuresis (excessive urination). A serious consequence is an electrolyte imbalance caused by a loss of sodium and potassium during diuresis. Ketosis and acidosis do not occur as in DKA. Treatment consists of administration of IV insulin and correction of fluid and electrolyte imbalance.

Blood and Urine Testing

Blood glucose levels are monitored often in the diabetic. The physician may order blood glucose levels to be tested before meals, after meals, and at bedtime. Less frequent monitoring may be performed if the patient's glucose levels are well-controlled. The glucometer is a device used by the diabetic or the nursing personnel to monitor blood glucose levels (Fig. 37-1). Since blood glucose monitoring devices vary greatly, the manufacturer's instructions should be followed carefully.

Most glucometers require a small sample of capillary blood that is obtained from the fingertip using a spring-loaded lancet. The blood sample is dropped on a reagent test strip and placed in the glucometer that automatically uses the sample to determine a numerical reading that represents the current blood glucose level. Blood glucose level should be maintained between 70 mg/dl and 100 mg/dl.

Perform the finger stick on the side of a finger where there are fewer nerve endings and more capillaries and milk the finger to produce a large, hanging drop of blood, which is distributed over the entire pad. Do not smear the blood or try to obtain an extra drop. Use of this technique to obtain a blood sample will help prevent inaccurate readings.

Urine testing has been widely used to monitor glucose levels in the past but this method has largely been replaced with blood glucose monitoring. Urine testing is less expensive than blood glucose monitoring and is noninvasive. Severely immunosuppressed patients may prefer urine testing to avoid the potential for infection with the finger stick required with blood glucose monitoring. However, it is essential that patients understand that urine testing for glucose is not as accurate as blood glucose monitoring. Urine testing can play a role in identifying ketone excretion in those patients prone to ketoacidosis.

Nursing Process
The Patient Receiving Insulin

■ *Assessment*

If the patient has been recently diagnosed as having diabetes mellitus and has not received insulin or if the patient is a known diabetic, the initial physical assessment before administering the first dose of insulin includes taking the blood pressure, pulse and respiratory rates, and weighing the patient. Make a general assessment of the skin, mucous membranes, and extremities with special attention to any sores or cuts that appear to be infected or healing poorly, as well as any ulcerations or other skin or mucous mem-

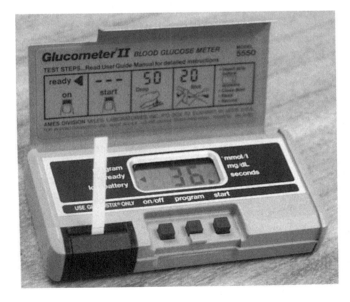

Figure 37-1

The Glucometer II is an example of a glucose testing device that can be used by the patient or by members of the healthcare team to monitor blood glucose levels.

brane changes. Include in the patient history dietary habits, a family history of diabetes (if any), and an inquiry into the type and duration of symptoms experienced. Review the patient's chart for recent laboratory and diagnostic tests.

If the patient has diabetes and has been receiving insulin, also include in the history the type and dosage of insulin used, the type of diabetic diet, and the average results of glucose testing. Evaluate the patient's past compliance to the prescribed therapeutic regimen, such as diet, weight control, and periodic evaluation by a physician.

■ *Nursing Diagnoses*

The nursing diagnoses depend on the patient's individual needs and are based on the information obtained during assessment.

The extent of the nursing diagnoses depends on factors such as whether the patient is a new diabetic, has had treatment for diabetes, or has not followed the prescribed medical regimen.

- **Anxiety** related to diagnosis, fear of giving own injections, dietary restrictions, other factors (specify)
- **Ineffective Individual Coping** related to inability to accept diagnosis, other factors (specify)
- **Fear** related to diagnosis, consequences of diabetes
- **Altered Health Maintenance** related to inability to comprehend drug regimen, lack of equipment to monitor drug effects, lack of knowledge
- **Risk for Ineffective Management of Therapeutic Regimen** related to lack of knowledge, misunderstanding, or complexity of prescribed treatment program, other factors (specify)

■ *Planning and Implementation*

The major goals of the patient may include a reduction in anxiety and fear, improved ability to cope with the diagnosis, and an understanding of and compliance to the prescribed therapeutic regimen. More specific criteria must be added to make these goals measurable.

Anxiety and Fear. The new diabetic often has many concerns regarding the diagnosis. For some, initially coping with diabetes and the methods required for controlling the disorder creates many problems. Some of the fears and concerns of new diabetics may include having to give themselves an injection, having to follow a diet, weight control, the complications associated with diabetes, and changes in eating times and habits. An effective teaching pro-

gram helps relieve some of the anxiety seen in the new diabetic. The newly diagnosed diabetic needs time to talk about the disorder, express concerns, and ask questions.

Impaired Adjustment, Coping, and Altered Health Maintenance. The new diabetic may have difficulty accepting the diagnosis, and the complexity of the therapeutic regimen can seem overwhelming. Before patients can be expected to carry out treatment, they must accept the fact that they have diabetes, and deal with their feelings about having the disorder. The nurse has an important role in helping these patients gradually accept the diagnosis and begin to understand their feelings. Understanding diabetes may help patients work with physicians and other medical personnel in managing their diabetes.

■ *Patient and Family Teaching*

Noncompliance is a problem with some diabetics, making patient and family teaching vital to proper management of diabetes. An occasional lapse in adherence to the prescribed diet occurs in most patients, for example, around holidays or other special occasions. This slip may not cause a problem if it is brief, not excessive, and there is an immediate return to the prescribed regimen. On the other hand, there are those who frequently stray from the prescribed regimen, take extra insulin to cover dietary indiscretions, fast for several days before follow-up blood glucose determinations, and engage in other dangerous behaviors.

Whereas some patients can be convinced that failure to adhere to the prescribed therapeutic regimen is detrimental to their health, others continue to deviate from the prescribed regimen until serious complications develop. Make every effort to stress the importance of adherence to the prescribed treatment during the initial teaching session and during follow-up office or clinic visits.

Establish a thorough teaching plan for all new diabetics, for those who have had any change in the management of their diabetes (eg, diet, insulin type, insulin dosage), and for those whose management has changed because of an illness or disability, for example, loss of sight or disabling arthritis. The newly diagnosed diabetic patient and family must have an explanation of the disease and methods of treatment as soon as the physician has revealed the diagnosis to the patient. Always individualize the teaching plan because the needs of each patient are different.

Self-monitoring of blood glucose is an important component in the management of diabetes. It is the preferred method for monitoring glucose by most physicians for all diabetics, with variations only in the suggested frequency of testing. If the patient is to use a blood glucose monitoring device, review the method of obtaining a small sample of blood from the finger and the use of the device with the patient. Printed instructions and illustrations are supplied with the device and must be reviewed with the patient. Encourage the patient to purchase the brand recommended by the physician. Allow time for supervised practice.

Include the following areas in a diabetic teaching plan:

- Blood glucose or urine testing—the testing material recommended by the physician; a review of the instructions included with the glucometer or the materials used for urine testing; the technique of collecting the specimen; interpreting test results; number of times a day or week the blood or urine is tested (as recommended by the physician); a record of test results
- Insulin—types; how dosage is expressed; calculating the insulin dosage; importance of using only the type, source, and brand name recommended by the physician; importance of not changing brands unless the physician approves; keeping a spare vial on hand; prescription for insulin purchase is not required
- Storage of insulin—insulin is kept at room temperature away from heat and direct sunlight if used within 1 month; vials not in use are stored in the refrigerator; prefilled insulin in glass or plastic syringes are stable for 1 week under refrigeration
- Needle and syringe—Purchase requires a prescription; purchase the same brand and needle size each time; parts of the syringe; reading the syringe scale
- Preparation for administration—principles of aseptic technique; how to hold the syringe; how to withdraw insulin from the vial; measurement of insulin in the syringe using the syringe scale; mixing insulin in the same syringe (when appropriate); elimination of air in the syringe and needle; what to do if the syringe or needle is contaminated
- Administration of insulin—sites to be used; rotation of injection sites; angle of injection; administration at the time of day prescribed by the physician; disposal of the needle and syringe
- Diet—importance of following the prescribed diet; calories allowed; food exchanges; planning daily menus; establishing meal schedules; selecting food from a restaurant menu; reading food labels; using of artificial sweeteners
- Traveling—importance of carrying an extra supply of insulin and a prescription for needles and syringes; storage of insulin when traveling; protecting needles and syringes from theft; importance of discussing travel plans (especially foreign travel) with the physician
- Hypoglycemia/hyperglycemia—signs and symptoms of hypoglycemia and hyperglycemia; food or fluid used to terminate a hypoglycemic reaction; importance of notifying the physician immediately if either reaction occurs
- Personal hygiene—importance of good skin and foot care, personal cleanliness, frequent dental checkups, and routine eye examinations
- Exercise—importance of following the physician's recommendations regarding physical activity
- When to notify the physician—increase in blood glucose levels; urine positive for ketones; if pregnancy occurs (female patient of childbearing age); occurrence of hypoglycemic or hyperglycemic episodes; occurrence of illness, infection, or diarrhea (insulin dosage may require adjustment); appearance of new problems (eg, leg ulcers, numbness of the extremities, significant weight gain or loss)
- Identification—wear identification, such as Medic-Alert, to inform medical personnel and others of the use of insulin to control the disease

■ *Expected Outcomes for Evaluation*

- Anxiety and fear is reduced
- Demonstrates beginning ability to cope with the disorder and its required treatment
- Patient demonstrates positive outlook and adjustment to diagnosis
- Patient verbalizes willingness to comply to the prescribed therapeutic regimen
- Patient and family demonstrate understanding of drug regimen
- Patient demonstrates understanding of the information presented in teaching sessions
- Patient is able to test blood glucose levels, give own insulin injections

Oral Hypoglycemics

The oral hypoglycemic drugs, also called sulfonylureas, are not oral insulins. They are oral agents used to treat type II diabetics who are not well-controlled on diet and exercise alone. These drugs are not effective in type I diabetes. The various oral hypoglycemic drugs are listed in Summary Drug Table 37-2.

to release a sufficient amount of insulin to meet the individual's needs.

ACTIONS OF THE ORAL HYPOGLYCEMICS

The oral hypoglycemic drugs appear to lower blood glucose by stimulating the beta cells of the pancreas to release insulin. Oral hypoglycemic drugs are not effective if the beta cells of the pancreas are unable

USES OF THE ORAL HYPOGLYCEMICS

The oral hypoglycemic drugs are of value only in the treatment of patients with type II (non–insulin-dependent or maturity-onset) diabetes mellitus whose condition cannot be controlled by diet alone. These drugs may also be used with insulin in the manage-

Summary Drug Table 37-2. Oral Hypoglycemic Agents

Generic Name	Trade Name*	Uses	Adverse Reactions	Dose Ranges
acetohexamide	Dymelor, generic	As adjunct to diet to lower the blood glucose in NIDDM	Hypoglycemia, nausea, epigastric fullness, heartburn, allergic skin reaction, leukopenia, thrombocytopenia, weakness, paresthesia, tinnitus, fatigue, dizziness	250 mg to 1.5 g/d in AM or before morning and evening meals
chlorpropamide	Diabinese generic	As adjunct to diet to lower the blood glucose in NIDDM	Same as acetohexamide; also dizziness	Initial dose: 100–250 mg/d; maintenance dose: 100–500 mg/d
glipizide	Glucotrol, generic	As adjunct to diet to lower the blood glucose in NIDDM	Same as acetohexamide; also diarrhea	5–40 mg/d either in AM or in divided doses
glyburide	Diabeta, Micronase, Glynase Press Tab	As adjunct to diet to lower the blood glucose in NIDDM	Same as acetohexamide	Diabeta/Micronase: Initial dose 2.5–5 mg/d; Maintenance: 1.25–20 mg/d single or divided doses; Glynase: initial 1.5–3 mg/d with breakfast; maintenance: 0.75–12 mg/d in single or divided doses
metformin	Glucophage	As adjunct to diet to lower blood glucose in NIDDM, in conjunction with a sulfonylurea when diet and sulfonylurea do not control hyperglycemia	Diarrhea, nausea, vomiting, abdominal bloating, flatulence, anorexia	500–2500 mg/d with meals in AM and PM or t.i.d. with meals
tolbutamide	Orinase, generic	As adjunct to diet to lower the blood glucose in NIDDM	Same as acetohexamide; also taste alteration	1–2 g/d with breakfast or in divided doses
tolazamide	Tolinase, generic	As adjunct to diet to lower the blood glucose in NIDDM	Same as acetohexamide	100–250 mg/d with breakfast. Adjust dosage to response. If dosage greater than 500 mg/d give in divided doses

*The term generic indicates that the drug is available in generic form.

ment of some patients with diabetes mellitus. Use of an oral hypoglycemic agent with insulin may decrease the insulin dosage in some individuals.

ADVERSE REACTIONS ASSOCIATED WITH THE ADMINISTRATION OF ORAL HYPOGLYCEMICS

All oral hypoglycemic drugs may produce severe hypoglycemia. The elderly, debilitated, or malnourished patient is more likely to experience hypoglycemia; however, this reaction may occur in any individual taking these drugs.

Other adverse reactions seen with these drugs are anorexia, nausea, vomiting, epigastric discomfort, heartburn, and various vague neurologic symptoms, such as weakness and numbness of the extremities. Often, these can be eliminated by reducing the dosage or giving the drug in divided doses. If these reactions become severe, the physician may try another oral hypoglycemic agent or discontinue the use of these drugs. If the drug is discontinued, it may be necessary to control the diabetes with insulin.

Additional adverse reactions include pruritus, urticaria, jaundice, leukopenia, mild anemia, thrombocytopenia, weakness, fatigue, dizziness, and skin rashes.

NURSING MANAGEMENT

Administration of Oral Hypoglycemic Agents

Give oral hypoglycemic agents as a single daily dose or in divided doses. Give acetohexamide (Dymelor), chlorpropamide (Diabinese), tolazamide (Tolinase), and tolbutamide (Orinase) with food to prevent gastrointestinal upset. Give glipizide (Glucotrol) 30 minutes before a meal, and glyburide (Micronase) with breakfast or with the first main meal of the day. The physician orders the meal with which glyburide is given.

Conduct ongoing assessments daily to include monitoring vital signs and observing for adverse drug reactions. The physician may also order daily to weekly weights. Notify the physician if an adverse reaction occurs or if there is a significant weight gain or loss.

> **Nursing Alert**
>
> Exposure to stress such as infection, fever, surgery, or trauma may cause a loss of control in patients stabilized on oral hypoglycemic drugs. Should this occur, the physician may discontinue the oral agent and administer insulin.

Hypoglycemia

Observe the patient every 2 to 4 hours for episodes of hypoglycemia during initial therapy or following a change in dosage. If both an oral hypoglycemic agent and insulin are given, observe the patient more frequently for hypoglycemic episodes during the initial period of combination therapy. If the patient is receiving only an oral hypoglycemic agent and a hypoglycemic reaction does occur, it is often (but not always) less intense than one seen with insulin administration.

As discussed earlier, terminate hypoglycemic reactions immediately. The method of terminating a hypoglycemic reaction is the same as for a hypoglycemic reaction occurring with insulin administration. Notify the physician as soon as possible if episodes of hypoglycemia occur because the dosage of the oral hypoglycemic agent (or insulin, when both insulin and an oral hypoglycemic agent are given) may need to be changed.

> **Nursing Alert**
>
> Although elderly patients taking the oral hypoglycemic drugs are particularly susceptible to hypoglycemic reactions, these reactions may be difficult to detect in the elderly. Notify the physician of any of the following symptoms: confusion, fatigue, excessive hunger, sweating, or numbness of the extremities.

Glucose/Ketone Testing

Capillary blood specimens are obtained and tested in the same manner as for insulin (see previous section). Notify the physician if blood sugar levels are elevated (consistently over 200 mg/dL) or if ketones are present in the urine.

Nursing Process
The Patient Receiving an Oral Hypoglycemic Agent

■ *Assessment*

If the patient has been recently diagnosed as having diabetes mellitus and has not received an oral hypoglycemic agent, or if the patient is a known diabetic and has been taking one of these drugs, include weight, blood pressure, pulse, and respiratory rate in the initial assessment. Make a general assessment of the skin, mucous membranes, and extremities with special attention to sores or cuts that appear to be healing poorly and ulcerations or other skin or mucous membrane changes. In the history include dietary habits, a family history of diabetes (if any), and an inquiry into the type and duration of symptoms experienced. Review the patient's chart for recent laboratory and diagnostic tests. If the patient has diabetes and has been receiving an oral hypoglycemic drug, include the name of the drug and the dosage, the type of diabetic diet, the average results of blood glucose testing, and an inquiry into adherence to the dietary and weight control regimen prescribed by the physician.

■ *Nursing Diagnoses*

The nursing diagnoses may depend on the patient's individual needs and are based on the information obtained during assessment.

The extent of the nursing diagnoses depends on factors such as whether the patient is a new diabetic, has had treatment for diabetes, or has not followed the prescribed medical regimen.

- **Anxiety** related to diagnosis, dietary restrictions, other factors (specify)
- **Ineffective Individual Coping** related to inability to accept diagnosis
- **Altered Health Maintenance** related to inability to comprehend drug regimen, lack of knowledge
- **Risk of Ineffective Management of Therapeutic Regimen** related to lack of knowledge, misunderstanding, or complexity of prescribed treatment program, other factors (specify)

■ *Planning and Implementation*

The major goals of the patient may include a reduction in anxiety, improved ability in coping with the diagnosis, and an understanding of and compliance to the prescribed therapeutic regimen. For these goals to be measurable, more specific criteria must be added.

Anxiety and Coping. As discussed in the section on insulin, the newly diagnosed diabetic often has many concerns about the management of the disease. Some patients, when learning that management of their diabetes can be achieved by diet and an oral drug, may have a tendency to discount the seriousness of their disorder. Without creating additional anxiety, emphasize the importance of following the prescribed treatment regimen.

Encourage the newly diagnosed diabetic to talk about the disorder, express concerns, and ask questions. Allowing these patients time to talk may also help them begin to cope with their diabetes.

Impaired Adjustment and Altered Health Maintenance. In addition to the material regarding impaired adjustment, noncompliance, and altered health maintenance discussed in the previous section on insulin, the patient receiving an oral hypoglycemic drug may also express concern about the possibility of having to take insulin in the future. Encourage the patient to discuss this and other concerns with the physician.

■ *Patient and Family Teaching*

Failing to comply with the prescribed treatment regimen may be a problem with patients taking an oral hypoglycemic drug because of the erroneous belief that not having to take insulin means that their disease is not serious and therefore does not require strict adherence to the recommended dietary plan. Inform these patients that control of their diabetes is just as important as for patients requiring insulin and that control is achieved only when they adhere to the treatment regimen prescribed by the physician.

If the patient is newly diagnosed as having diabetes mellitus, discuss the disease and methods of control with the patient and family after the physician has revealed the diagnosis to the patient. Although taking an oral hypoglycemic agent is less complicated than self-administration of insulin, the diabetic taking one of these agents needs a thorough explanation of the management of the disease. Individualize the teaching plan because the needs of each patient are different.

Include the following information in a teaching plan:
- Take the drug exactly as directed on the container (eg, with food, 30 minutes before a meal, and so forth).

- To control diabetes, follow the diet and drug regimen prescribed by the physician exactly.
- This drug is not oral insulin and cannot be substituted for insulin.
- Never stop taking this drug or increase or decrease the dose unless told to do so by the physician.
- Take the drug at the same time or times each day.
- Eat meals at approximately the same time each day. Erratic meal hours or skipped meals may result in difficulty in controlling diabetes with this drug.
- Avoid alcohol, dieting, commercial weight loss products, and strenuous exercise programs unless use or participation has been approved by the physician.
- Test blood for glucose and urine for ketones as directed by the physician. Keep a record of test results and bring this record to each physician or clinic visit.
- Maintain good foot and skin care and routine eye and dental examinations for the early detection of the complications that occur in some diabetics.
- Exercise should be moderate: avoid strenuous exercise and erratic periods of exercise.
- Wear identification, such as Medic-Alert, to inform medical personnel and others of diabetes and the drug or drugs currently being used to treat the disease.
- Notify the physician if any of the following occurs: episodes of hypoglycemia, apparent symptoms of hyperglycemia, elevated blood glucose levels, positive results of urine tests for glucose or ketone bodies, pregnancy (female patient of childbearing age), gastrointestinal upset, fever, sore throat, unusual bruising or bleeding, diarrhea, rash, yellowing of the skin. Notify the physician also if any serious illness not requiring hospitalization occurs.
- Give symptoms of hypoglycemia and hyperglycemia to the patient in printed form and then give full explanation. Explain the method recommended by the physician for terminating a hypoglycemic reaction.

■ *Expected Outcomes for Evaluation*

- Anxiety is reduced
- Patient demonstrates beginning ability to cope with the disorder and its required treatment
- Patient demonstrates positive outlook and adjustment to diagnosis
- Patient verbalizes willingness to comply to the prescribed treatment regimen
- Patient and family demonstrate understanding of drug regimen
- Patient and family demonstrate understanding of the information presented in teaching sessions
- Patient is able to use the glucometer to monitor blood sugar or test urine for glucose and ketones

Chapter Summary

- Diabetes mellitus is a metabolic disorder of the pancreas in which glucose intolerance results from varying degrees of insulin insufficiency. Insulin or the oral hypoglycemic drugs, along with diet and exercise, are used to treat diabetes.
- The two major types of diabetes mellitus are: Type I—insulin-dependent diabetes mellitus; and Type II—non–insulin-dependent diabetes mellitus. Those with type I diabetes produce no insulin and therefore need insulin to survive. Those with type II diabetes produce some insulin and many are able to control their diabetes with diet alone or diet and an oral hypoglycemic agent. Insulin may be necessary for the control of the more severe and complicated forms of type II diabetes mellitus.
- Insulin is a hormone manufactured by the beta cells of the pancreas and is the principal hormone required for the proper use of glucose by the body. In addition, insulin promotes protein synthesis and helps the body store fat by preventing its breakdown for energy.
- Onset, peak, and duration are three properties of insulin that are of clinical importance. To meet the needs of those with diabetes mellitus, various insulin preparations have been developed to delay the onset and prolong the duration of action of insulin. Insulin preparations are classified as rapid-acting, intermediate-acting, or long-acting.
- Insulin is available as purified extracts from beef and pork pancreas and is biologically similar to human insulin. These animal source insulins are used less frequently today than in years past and are being replaced by synthetic insulin called human insulin.
- The two major adverse reactions seen with insulin administration are hypoglycemia and hyperglycemia. Hypoglycemia occurs when there is too much insulin in the bloodstream in relation to the available glucose, such as occurs when the patient eats too little food, when the insulin dose is incorrectly measured and is greater than that prescribed, or when the patient drastically increases physical activity. Hyperglycemia may occur if there is too little insulin in the bloodstream in relation to the available glucose, such as when the patient eats too much food, when too little or no in-

sulin is given, or when the patient experiences emotional stress, infection, surgery, pregnancy, or an acute illness.

- Nursing management of a patient with diabetes requires diligent, skillful, and comprehensive nursing care. Insulin may be administered with the use of a needle and syringe, the jet injection system, a disposable needle and a special syringe that is prefilled with a specific type of insulin, or the insulin pump.

- Insulin is available in concentrations of U100 and U500. Most diabetics use U100. The U500 concentration is used for patients who are resistant to insulin and require large insulin doses.

- The physician selects the dosage and type of insulin that will most likely meet the individual's requirements. There is no standard dose range of insulin as there is for most other drugs. The dose prescribed for the patient may require changes until the dosage is found that best meets the patient's needs.

- Episodes of hypoglycemia should be corrected as soon as the symptoms are recognized by administering one or more of the following: orange juice or other fruit juice, hard candy or honey, commercial glucose products, glucagon by the SC, IM, or IV route, or glucose 10% or 50%. Notify the physician of any hypoglycemic reaction, the substance and amount used to terminate the reaction, blood samples drawn (if any), the length of time required for the symptoms of hypoglycemia to disappear, and the present status of the patient. After termination of a hypoglycemic reaction, observe the patient closely for additional hypoglycemic reactions.

- Diabetic ketoacidosis (DKA) is a potentially life-threatening deficiency of insulin resulting in severe hyperglycemia and requiring prompt diagnosis and treatment. Insulin is essential to treat this potentially dangerous complication. The symptoms of hyperglycemia (blood glucose levels greater than 200 mg/dL; headache; increased thirst; epigastric pain; nausea; vomiting; hot, dry, flushed skin; restlessness; diaphoresis (sweating); and fruity odor to the breath) are immediately reported to the physician.

- Another complication of diabetes, hyperosmolar hyperglycemic nonketotic syndrome, occurs most often as a result of a stressor, such as acute illness, and is manifested by hyperglycemia and hyperosmolarity, resulting in cellular dehydration and diuresis. Treatment consists of administration of IV insulin and correction of fluid and electrolyte imbalance.

- Blood glucose levels are monitored often in the diabetic. The physician may order blood glucose levels to be tested before meals, after meals, and at bedtime. Less frequent monitoring may be performed if the patient's glucose levels are well-controlled. The glucometer is a device used by the diabetic or the nursing personnel to monitor blood glucose levels. Urine testing may be ordered by the physician under certain circumstances.

- The oral hypoglycemic drugs or sulfonylureas are not oral insulins. They are oral agents used to treat type II diabetics who are not well-controlled on diet and exercise alone. These drugs are not effective in type I diabetes. The oral hypoglycemic drugs appear to lower blood glucose by stimulating the beta cells of the pancreas to release insulin. Oral hypoglycemic drugs are not effective if the beta cells of the pancreas are unable to release a sufficient amount of insulin to meet the individual's needs.

- All oral hypoglycemic drugs may produce severe hypoglycemia. The elderly, debilitated, or malnourished patient is more likely to experience hypoglycemia; however, this reaction may occur in any individual taking these drugs. Exposure to stress such as infection, fever, surgery, or trauma may cause a loss of control in patients stabilized on oral hypoglycemic drugs. Should this occur, the physician may discontinue the oral agent and administer insulin.

- As with insulin administration, hypoglycemic reactions are terminated immediately using the same method of terminating a hypoglycemic reaction as for a hypoglycemic reaction occurring with insulin administration. The physician is notified as soon as possible if episodes of hypoglycemia occur because the dosage of the oral hypoglycemic agent (or insulin, when both insulin and an oral hypoglycemic agent are given) may need to be changed.

- Capillary blood specimens are obtained and tested in the same manner as for insulin. The physician is notified if blood sugar levels are elevated (consistently over 200 mg/dL) or if ketones are present in the urine.

- Failing to comply with the prescribed treatment regimen may be a problem with patients taking either an oral hypoglycemic drug or insulin. If the patient is newly diagnosed as having diabetes mellitus, the disease and methods of control are discussed with the patient and family after the physician has revealed the diagnosis to the patient. Whether taking an oral hypoglycemic drug or insulin, the diabetic needs a thorough explanation of the disease and its management. Symptoms of hypoglycemia and hyperglycemia are given to the patient in printed form along with a full explanation. The method recommended by the physician for terminating a hypoglycemic reaction is explained. The teaching plan for each patient is individualized because the needs of each patient are different.

Critical Thinking Exercises

1. Ms. Baxter, aged 47, has been taking insulin for the past 6 years for IDDM. An assessment at the outpatient clinic reveals a blood sugar of 110 mg/dL. In examining Ms. Baxter's skin, the nurse notices several areas on the thighs that appear scarred and other areas that appear as dimples or-pitting in the skin. How would you investigate this problem with Ms. Baxter? What suggestions would you make for her care?

2. James, aged 16, has recently been diagnosed with diabetes mellitus and the physician has ordered insulin. He is having difficulty dealing with this diagnosis. What three areas of instruction would you make as your priority in preparing James for discharge?

38

Pituitary and Adrenocortical Hormones

Key Terms

Adenohypophysis
Adrenal insufficiency
Corticosteroids
Cushing's syndrome
Diabetes insipidus
Feedback mechanism
Glucocorticoids
Gonadotropins
Gonads
Mineralocorticoids
Neurohypophysis
Somatotropic hormone

Chapter Outline

Chapter Objectives

On completion of this chapter the student will:

- *List the hormones produced by the pituitary gland and the adrenal cortex*
- *State the functions of the pituitary and adrenocortical hormones*
- *List the actions, uses, and adverse reactions of pituitary and adrenocortical hormones*
- *Discuss the major adverse reactions of the pituitary and adrenocortical hormones*
- *Discuss nursing management when administering a pituitary or adrenocortical hormone*
- *Use the nursing process when administering pituitary and adrenocortical hormones.*

The pituitary gland lies deep within the cranial vault, connected to the brain by a stalk and protected by an indentation of the sphenoid bone called the sella turcica. There are two parts to the pituitary gland: the *anterior* pituitary or *adenohypophysis* and the *posterior* pituitary or *neurohypophysis*. The hormones of the pituitary and the organs or structures influenced by these hormones are shown in Figure 38-1.

Pituitary hormones regulate growth, metabolism, the reproductive cycle, electrolyte balance, and water retention or loss. Anterior and posterior pituitary hormones are summarized in Summary Drug Table 38-1.

Hormones of the anterior and posterior pituitary gland

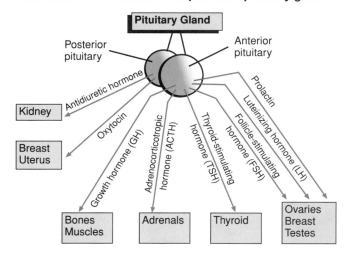

Figure 38-1

Hormones of the anterior and posterior pituitary gland.

Anterior Pituitary Hormones

The hormones of the anterior pituitary include growth hormone, adrenocorticotropic hormone (ACTH), thyroid-stimulating hormone, follicle-stimulating hormone (FSH), luteinizing hormone (LH), and prolactin. All but prolactin are used medically.

THE GONADOTROPINS

Follicle-stimulating hormone and *luteinizing hormone* are called *gonadotropins* because they influence the *gonads* (the organs of reproduction). In both sexes, FSH and LH influence the secretion of sex hormones, development of secondary sex characteristics, and the reproductive cycle.

Prolactin, which is also secreted by the anterior pituitary, stimulates the production of breast milk in the postpartum patient. Additional functions of prolactin are not well understood.

ACTIONS AND USES OF THE GONADOTROPINS

Menotropins and Urofollitropin

Menotropins (Pergonal) and urofollitropin (Metrodin) are purified preparations of the gonadotropins (FSH and LH) extracted from the urine of postmenopausal women. Menotropins is used to induce ovulation and pregnancy in the anovulatory (failure to produce an ovum or failure to ovulate) female. In the male, it is used to induce the production of sperm (spermatogenesis).

Urofollitropin is used to induce ovulation in women with polycystic ovarian disease.

Clomiphene and Chorionic Gonadotropin

Clomiphene (Clomid) is a synthetic nonsteroidal compound used to induce ovulation and pregnancy in the anovulatory female.

Chorionic gonadotropin (human chorionic gonadotropin) is extracted from human placentas and contains FSH and LH. It is used to induce ovulation and pregnancy in the anovulatory female. This drug is also

Summary Drug Table 38-1. Anterior and Posterior Pituitary Hormones

Generic Name	Trade Name*	Uses	Adverse Reactions	Dose Ranges
ANTERIOR PITUITARY HORMONES				
adrenocorticotropic hormone (cortico-tropin, ACTH)	Acthar, *generic*	Diagnostic testing of adrenocortical function, acute exacerbation of multiple sclerosis, nonsuppurative thyroiditis, hypercalcemia associated with malignancies	Same as glucocorticoids (see table 38-2)	Diagnostic: 10–25 U in 500 mL 5% dextrose IV infused over 8-h period; other uses: 20–120 U/d IM, SC
chorionic gonado-tropin (HCG)	Glukor, A.P.L., *generic*	Ovulatory failure, prepubertal cryptorchism	Headache, irritability, nervousness, edema, fatigue, restlessness, precocious puberty	Dosage, frequency, length of treatment is individualized; ranges are 500–10,000U/dose IM
clomiphene citrate	Clomid, Serophene	Ovulatory failure	Vasomotor flushes, abdominal discomfort, blurred vision, ovarian enlargement, nausea, vomiting, nervousness	First course: 50 mg/d PO for 5 d; second and third course (if necessary) 100 mg/d PO for 5 d
menotropins	Pergonal	Ovulatory failure, stimulation of spermatogenesis	Ovarian enlargement, hemoperitoneum, febrile reactions, hypersensitivity	75–150 IU IM
somatrem	Protropin	Growth failure due to deficiency of pituitary growth hormone in children	Failure to respond to therapy due to development of antibodies	Up to 0.1 mg/kg SC, IM 3 times/wk
somatropin	Humatrope	Growth failure due to deficiency of pituitary growth hormone in children	Failure to respond to therapy due to development of antibodies	Up to 0.06 mg/kg SC, IM 3 times/wk
urofollitropin	Metrodin	Induction of ovulation	Ovarian enlargement, nausea, vomiting, breast tenderness, ectopic pregnancy	75–100 IU IM
POSTERIOR PITUITARY HORMONES				
desmopressin acetate	DDAVP	Nocturnal enuresis, diabetes insipidus, hemophilia A, von Willebrand's disease	Headache, nausea, nasal congestion, abdominal cramps	0.1–0.4 mL/d as a nasal solution (dosage may be divided); 0.5–1 mL/d SC, IV
lypressin	Diapid	Nocturnal enuresis, diabetes insipidus, hemophilia A, von Willebrand's disease	Rhinorrhea, nasal congestion, irritation of nasal passages, headache	1–2 sprays in each nostril
oxytocin	Pitocin	Induction of labor, control of postpartum bleeding	Postpartum hemorrhage, cardiac arrhythmias, nausea, vomiting, fetal bradycardia	1–2 m U/min (maximum dose 20 m U/min) IV; 10 U after delivery of the placenta IM
vasopressin	Pitressin Synthetic	Diabetes insipidus, prevention and treatment of postoperative abdominal distention	Tremor, sweating, vertigo, nausea, vomiting, abdominal cramps, hypersensitivity reactions, headache	Diabetes insipidus: 5–10 U SC, IM; abdominal distention: 5–10 U IM

*The term, *generic*, indicates that the drug is available in generic form.

used for the treatment of prepubertal cryptorchism (failure of the testes to descend into the scrotum).

ADVERSE REACTIONS ASSOCIATED WITH THE ADMINISTRATION OF GONADOTROPINS

Menotropins and Urofollitropin

The adverse reactions associated with menotropins include ovarian enlargement, hemoperitoneum (blood in the peritoneal cavity), and febrile reactions. Multiple births and birth defects have been reported with the use of this drug.

Urofollitropin administration may result in mild to moderate ovarian enlargement, nausea, vomiting, breast tenderness, and ectopic pregnancy.

Clomiphene and Chorionic Gonadotropins

Administration of clomiphene may result in vasomotor flushes (which are like the hot flashes of menopause), abdominal discomfort, ovarian enlargement, blurred vision, nausea, vomiting, and nervousness. Chorionic gonadotropin administration may result in headache, irritability, restlessness, fatigue, edema, and precocious puberty (when given for cryptorchism).

NURSING MANAGEMENT

Menotropins and chorionic gonadotropin injections are given in the physician's office or clinic. Administer these drugs intramuscularly (IM) because they are destroyed in the gastrointestinal tract. Clomiphene is an oral tablet and is prescribed for self-administration. At the time of each office or clinic visit, question the patient regarding the occurrence of adverse reactions. Vital signs and weight may also be taken at this time.

Nursing Process
The Patient Receiving a Gonadotropin

■ *Assessment*
These drugs are almost always administered on an outpatient basis. Before prescribing any one of these drugs, the physician will take a thorough medical history and perform a physical examination. Additional laboratory and diagnostic tests for ovarian function and tubal patency may also be performed.

Take and record vital signs and weight before therapy is instituted.

■ *Nursing Diagnoses*
Depending on the individual, one or more of the following nursing diagnoses may apply to the patient receiving a gonadotropin:
● **Anxiety** related to inability to conceive, treatment outcome, other factors
● **Risk for Ineffective Management of Therapeutic Regimen**, related to lack of knowledge, adverse drug reactions, other (specify)

■ *Planning and Implementation*
The major goals of the patient may include a reduction in anxiety and an understanding of the therapeutic regimen. To make these goals measurable, more specific criteria must be added.

Anxiety. Patients wishing to become pregnant often experience a great deal of anxiety. The success rate of these drugs varies and depends on many factors. The physician usually discusses the value of this, as well as other approaches, with the patient and her sexual partner. Offer encouragement to relieve anxiety. Allow the patient time to talk about her problems or concerns about the proposed treatment program.

■ *Patient and Family Teaching*
Encourage the patient receiving menotropins, chorionic gonadotropin, or both of these drugs, to keep all physician appointments. The physician explains the possible risks associated with therapy for ovulatory failure. Explain to the patient any symptoms that require notifying the physician.

Include the following information when clomiphene is prescribed for ovulatory failure:
• Take the drug as prescribed (5 days); do not stop taking the drug before the course of therapy is finished unless told to do so by the physician.
• Notify the physician if bloating, stomach or pelvic pain, jaundice, blurred vision, hot flashes, breast discomfort, headache, nausea, or vomiting occurs.
• This drug may cause dizziness or lightheadedness. If these occur, do not drive or perform other tasks requiring alertness.

- If ovulation has not occurred after the first course, a second or third course (if the first and second are not successful) of therapy may be used.
- Prior to the beginning therapy, advise the patient of the possibility of multiple births.

■ Expected Outcomes for Evaluation
- Anxiety is reduced
- Patient demonstrates knowledge of treatment and dosage regimen, adverse drug reactions, involved risks of treatment, and importance of complying with the physician's recommendations

GROWTH HORMONE

Growth hormone, also called *somatotropic hormone*, is secreted by the anterior pituitary. This hormone regulates the growth of the individual until somewhere around early adulthood or the time when the person no longer gains height.

Growth hormone is available as the synthetic products somatrem (Protropin) and somatropin (Humatrope). Both are of recombinant DNA origin and are identical to human growth hormone. These drugs are administered to children who have failed to grow because of a deficiency of pituitary growth hormone.

These drugs must be used before closure of bone epiphyses (the ends of bones, separated from the main bone but joined to its cartilage, that allow for growth or lengthening of the bone) and are ineffective in those with closed epiphyses. When the epiphyses close, growth (in height) can no longer occur.

ADVERSE REACTIONS ASSOCIATED WITH ADMINISTRATION OF GROWTH HORMONE

Antibodies to somatropin and somatrem may develop in a small number of patients, resulting in a failure to respond to therapy, namely, failure of the drug to produce growth in the child.

NURSING MANAGEMENT

Children may increase their growth rate from 3.5 to 4 cm per year before treatment to 8 to 10 cm per year during the first year of treatment. Growth hormone is given either IM or subcutaneously (SC). The drug may be given at bedtime to most closely adhere to the body's natural release of the hormone. If the drug is to be given at bedtime, instruct parents on the proper technique to administer SC injections.

Each time the child visits the physician's office or clinic, record height and weight measurements to evaluate the response to therapy. Perform periodic laboratory tests and yearly bone surveys. The bone surveys check bone growth, as well as detect epiphyseal closure, at which time therapy must be stopped.

Nursing Process
The Patient Receiving a Growth Hormone

■ Assessment
Perform a thorough physical examination and laboratory and diagnostic tests before a child is accepted in a growth program. Before starting therapy, take and record vital signs and the height and weight.

■ Nursing Diagnoses
- **Anxiety** related to failure to grow (parents and child)
- **Knowledge Deficit** related to therapeutic regimen, adverse effects other (specify)

■ Planning and Implementation
The major goals of the patient and parents may include a reduction in anxiety and an understanding of the treatment program. To make these goals measurable, more specific criteria must be added.

Anxiety. The parents, and sometimes the children, may be concerned over a failure to grow, as well as the success or possible failure of treatment with a growth hormone. Allow time for the parents and children to ask questions not only before therapy is started but also during the months of growth hormone treatment.

Knowledge Deficit. When the patient is receiving growth hormone, the physician discusses in detail the therapeutic regimen for increasing growth (height) with the child's parents or guardians. Encourage the parents to keep all clinic or physician's office visits.

■ Expected Outcomes for Evaluation
- Anxiety is reduced
- Parents verbalize understanding of treatment program

ADRENOCORTICOTROPIC HORMONE

ACTH (corticotropin) is an anterior pituitary hormone that stimulates the adrenal cortex to produce and secrete adrenocortical hormones, primarily the glucocorticoids. ACTH is used for diagnostic testing of adrenocortical function. This drug may also be used for the management of acute exacerbations of multiple sclerosis, nonsuppurative thyroiditis, and hypercalcemia associated with cancer. It is also used as an antiinflammatory and immunosuppressant drug when conventional glucocorticoid therapy has not proven effective.

ADVERSE REACTIONS ASSOCIATED WITH THE ADMINISTRATION OF ADRENOCORTICOTROPIC HORMONE

Because ACTH stimulates the release of glucocorticoids from the adrenal gland, adverse reactions seen with the administration of this hormone are similar to the glucocorticoids (see Adrenocortical Hormones) and affect many body systems. The most common adverse reactions include:

Central nervous system—mental depression, psychosis, euphoria, nervousness
Cardiovascular system—hypertension, edema, congestive heart failure, thromboembolism
Gastrointestinal system—nausea, vomiting, increased appetite, weight gain, peptic ulcer
Integumentary system—petechiae, ecchymosis, decreased wound healing, hirsutism, acne
Musculoskeletal system—weakness, osteoporosis
Endocrine system—menstrual irregularities, hyperglycemia, decreased growth in children
Miscellaneous—hypersensitivity reactions, hypokalemia, hypernatremia, increased susceptibility to infection, cushingoid appearance (eg, moon face, buffalo hump, hirsutism), cataracts, increased intraocular pressure

NURSING MANAGEMENT

Nursing management depends on the patient's diagnosis, physical status, and the reason for use of the drug and may include vital signs every 4 hours, and observation for the adverse reactions seen with

glucocorticoid administration (see Adrenocortical Hormones).

Administration

This drug may be given by the intravenous (IV), SC, or IM route. During parenteral administration of ACTH, observe the patient for hypersensitivity reactions. Symptoms may include a rash, urticaria, hypotension, tachycardia, or difficulty in breathing. If the drug is given IM or SC, observe the patient for hypersensitivity reactions immediately and for about 2 hours after the drug is given. If a hypersensitivity reaction occurs, notify the physician immediately. Long-term use increases the risk of hypersensitivity.

> **Nursing Alert**
>
> ACTH may mask signs of infection including fungal or viral eye infection. There may be a decreased resistance and inability to localize infection. Report any complaints of sore throat, cough, fever, malaise, sores that do not heal, or redness or irritation of the eyes.

ACTH can cause alterations in the psyche. Observe and report any evidence of behavior change, such as mental depression, insomnia, euphoria, mood swings, or nervousness.

During therapy monitor intake and output and obtain a daily weight. Observe for and report any evidence of edema such as weight gain, rales, increased pulse or dyspnea. Monitor blood glucose levels for a rise in blood glucose.

Check stools for evidence of bleeding (dark or tarry in color, positive guaiac).

Nursing Process
The Patient Receiving an Adrenocorticotropic Hormone

■ *Assessment*

Review the patient's chart for the diagnosis, laboratory tests, and other pertinent information. Take and record vital signs. Additional assessments depend on the patient's condition and diagnosis.

■ *Nursing Diagnoses*

Depending on the patient's condition and reason for administration, one or more of the following may apply to the patient receiving ACTH:

- **Anxiety** related to diagnosis, treatment regimen, other factors
- **Risk for Ineffective Management of Therapeutic Regimen** related to lack of knowledge, adverse reactions, other (specify)

■ *Planning and Implementation*

The major goals of the patient may include a reduction in anxiety and an understanding of the therapeutic regimen. To make these goals measurable, more specific criteria must be added.

Anxiety. Anxiety is decreased with understanding of the therapeutic regimen. Allow time for a thorough explanation, as well as to answer any questions.

■ *Patient and Family Teaching*

Include the following in a teaching plan for the patient receiving ACTH:

- Explain the method of administration (IM, IV, SC) and possible adverse reactions to expect and to report.
- Instruct the patient to avoid contact with those who have an infection because resistance to infection may be decreased.
- Report any symptoms of infection immediately (eg, sore throat, fever, cough, or sores that do not heal).
- Advise the diabetic patient to monitor blood glucose (if self-monitoring is being done) or urine closely and notify the physician if glucose appears in the urine or the blood glucose shows a significant rise.
- Advise the patient to notify the physician of a marked weight gain, swelling in the extremities, muscle weakness, persistent headache, visual disturbances, or behavior change.

■ *Expected Outcomes for Evaluation*

- Anxiety is reduced
- Patient verbalizes understanding of therapeutic regimen, adverse effects requiring notification of the physician

Posterior Pituitary Hormones

The posterior pituitary gland produces two hormones: *vasopressin (antidiuretic hormone)* and *oxytocin* (see Chap. 41). Posterior pituitary hormones are summarized in Summary Drug Table 38-1.

VASOPRESSIN

Vasopressin (Pitressin Synthetic) and its derivatives, namely lypressin (Diapid) and desmopressin (DDAVP), regulate the reabsorption of water by the kidneys. Vasopressin is secreted by the pituitary when body fluids must be conserved. An example of this mechanism may be seen when an individual has severe vomiting and diarrhea with little or no fluid intake. When this and similar conditions are present, the posterior pituitary releases the hormone vasopressin; water in the kidneys is reabsorbed into the blood (ie, conserved); and the urine becomes concentrated. Vasopressin also has some vasopressor activity.

Vasopressin and its derivatives are used in the treatment of *diabetes insipidus,* a disease resulting from the failure of the pituitary to secrete vasopressin or from surgical removal of the pituitary. Vasopressin may also be used for the prevention and treatment of postoperative abdominal distention.

ADVERSE REACTIONS ASSOCIATED WITH ADMINISTRATION OF VASOPRESSIN

Local or systemic hypersensitivity reactions may occur in some patients receiving vasopressin. Tremor, sweating, vertigo, nausea, vomiting, and abdominal cramps may also be seen.

NURSING MANAGEMENT

Abdominal Distention

Only vasopressin is used for the management of abdominal distention. After administration of vasopressin for abdominal distention, a rectal tube may be ordered. Insert the lubricated end of the tube past the anal sphincter and tape in place. Leave the tube in place for 1 hour or as prescribed by the physician. Auscultate the abdomen every 15 to 30 minutes and measure the abdominal girth every hour or as ordered by the physician.

Diabetes Insipidus

Vasopressin may be given IM or SC to treat diabetes insipidus. Vasopressin tannate is given IM. Lypressin is given intranasally and desmopressin may be given intranasally, SC, or IV. The physician orders the method of administration.

Lypressin is administered intranasally by spraying 1 or 2 sprays to one or both nostrils usually 4 times per day. Dosages greater than 10 sprays in each nostril every 3 to 4 hours is not recommended. Patients learn to regulate their dosage based on the frequency of urination and increase of thirst. When administering, have the patient hold the bottle upright with the head in a vertical position.

Vasopressin tannate, which is given IM, is suspended in peanut oil. Because the fluid in the ampule is thick, warm the ampule to body temperature before withdrawing the drug.

Monitor the blood pressure, pulse, and respiratory rate every 4 hours or as ordered by the physician. Notify the physician if there are any significant changes in these vital signs because a dosage adjustment may be necessary.

The dosage of vasopressin or its derivatives may require periodic adjustments. After administration of the drug, observe the patient every 10 to 15 minutes for signs of an excessive dosage (eg, blanching of the skin, abdominal cramps, and nausea). If these occur, reassure the patient that recovery from these effects will occur in a few minutes. Adverse reactions, such as skin blanching, abdominal cramps, and nausea may be decreased if vasopressin is administered with one or two glasses of water.

Nursing Alert

Excessive dosage is manifested as water intoxication (fluid overload). Symptoms of water intoxication include: drowsiness, listlessness, confusion, headache (which may precede convulsions and coma). If signs of excessive dosage occur, notify the physician before the next dose of the drug is due because a change in the dosage, the restriction of oral or IV fluids, and the administration of a diuretic may be necessary.

Notify the physician immediately if a hypersensitivity reaction occurs (eg, difficulty breathing, pruritus, hives, or asthma-like symptoms).

Nursing Process
The Patient Receiving Vasopressin

■ Assessment
Before administering the first dose of vasopressin for the management of diabetes insipidus, take the blood pressure, pulse, and respiratory rate. Weigh

the patient to obtain a baseline weight for future comparison. Serum electrolyte levels and other laboratory tests may be ordered by the physician.

Before administering vasopressin to relieve abdominal distention, obtain the blood pressure, pulse, and respiratory rate. Auscultate the abdomen and record the findings. Measure and record the abdominal girth.

■ Nursing Diagnoses
Depending on the route of administration and the patient's diagnosis, one or more of the following nursing diagnoses may apply to a person receiving vasopressin:

* **Anxiety** related to symptoms of diabetes insipidus, methods of treatment, pain or discomfort due to abdominal distention, other factors
* **Fluid Volume Deficit** related to inadequate fluid intake, need to increase dose of drug, failure to recognize symptoms of dehydration (diabetes insipidus)
* **Risk for Ineffective Management of Therapeutic Regimen** related to noncompliance, lack of knowledge (diabetes insipidus), adverse drug reactions, dosage adjustment, use of nasal spray, other (specify)

■ Planning and Implementation
The major goals of the patient may include a reduction in anxiety, correction of a fluid volume deficit, and an understanding of and compliance to the prescribed therapeutic regimen. To make these goals measurable, more specific criteria must be added.

Anxiety. The symptoms of diabetes insipidus include the voiding of a large volume of urine at frequent intervals during the day and throughout the night. Accompanied by frequent urination is the need to drink large volumes of fluid because these patients are continually thirsty. Until controlled by medication, these symptoms cause a great deal of anxiety. Reassure the patient that with medication these symptoms will most likely be reduced or eliminated.

If the patient is receiving vasopressin for abdominal distention, explain in detail the method of treating this problem and the necessary monitoring of drug effectiveness (auscultation of the abdomen for bowel sounds, insertion of a rectal tube, measurement of the abdomen).

Fluid Volume Deficit. When the patient has diabetes insipidus, measure the intake and output accurately and observe the patient for signs of dehydration. This is especially important early in treatment and until such time as the optimum dosage is determined and symptoms have diminished. If the patient's output greatly exceeds his or her intake, notify the physician. In some instances, the physician may order specific gravity and volume measurements of each voiding or at hourly intervals. Record these results in the chart to aid the physician in adjusting the dosage to the patient's needs.

It is most important that these patients be supplied with large amounts of drinking water. Refill the water container at frequent intervals. This is especially important when the patient has limited ambulatory activities.

■ *Patient and Family Teaching*

If lypressin or desmopressin is to be used in the form of a nasal spray for the patient with diabetes insipidus, demonstrate the technique of instillation. Include illustrated patient instructions with the drug and review them with the patient. If possible, have the patient demonstrate the technique of administration. Discuss the need to take the medication only as directed by the physician. Do not increase the dosage (ie, the number or frequency of sprays) unless advised to do so by the physician.

On occasion, a patient may need to self-administer vasopressin by the parenteral route. If so, instruct the patient or a family member in the preparation and administration of the drug and measurement of the specific gravity of the urine.

Stress the importance of adhering to the prescribed treatment program to control symptoms. In addition to instruction in administration, include the following in a patient and family teaching plan:

* Drink one or two glasses of water immediately before taking the drug.
* Measure the amount of fluids taken each day.
* Measure the amount of urine passed at each voiding, and then total the amount for each 24-hour period.
* Rotate injection sites for parenteral administration.
* Contact the physician immediately if any of the following occur: a significant increase or decrease in urinary output, abdominal cramps, blanching of the skin, nausea, signs of inflammation or infection at the injection sites, confusion, headache, or drowsiness.

■ *Expected Outcomes for Evaluation*
* Anxiety is reduced
* Signs of a fluid volume deficit are absent (diabetes insipidus)

* Patient verbalizes an understanding of treatment modalities and importance of continued follow-up care (diabetes insipidus)
* Patient and family demonstrate understanding of drug regimen
* Adverse reactions are identified and reported to the physician (diabetes insipidus)
* Patient verbalizes importance of complying with the prescribed therapeutic regimen (diabetes insipidus)

The Adrenocortical Hormones

The adrenal gland lies on the superior surface of each kidney. It is a double organ composed of an outer cortex and an inner medulla. In response to ACTH secreted by the anterior pituitary, the adrenal cortex secretes several hormones (the glucocorticoids, the mineralocorticoids, and small amounts of sex hormones).

The *glucocorticoids* and *mineralocorticoids* are essential to life and influence many organs and structures of the body. The glucocorticoids and mineralocorticoids are collectively called *corticosteroids*. Their uses and dose ranges are given in Summary Drug Table 38-2.

THE GLUCOCORTICOIDS

Although there are several glucocorticoids produced by the adrenal cortex, the two most prominent are hydrocortisone and cortisone. The *glucocorticoids* influence or regulate functions, such as the immune response system, the regulation of glucose, fat and protein metabolism, and control of the antiinflammatory response. Examples of the glucocorticoids include cortisone, hydrocortisone, prednisone, prednisolone, and triamcinolone.

USES OF THE GLUCOCORTICOIDS

The glucocorticoids are used as antiinflammatory and as immunosupressants to suppress inflammation and modify the immune response. The specific uses of the glucocorticoids are given in Table 38-1.

Summary Drug Table 38-2. Glucocorticoids and Mineralocorticoids

Generic Name	Trade Name*	Uses	Adverse Reactions	Dose Ranges
GLUCOCORTICOIDS				
cortisone	Cortone Acetate, *generic*	See Table 38–1	See Table 38–2	25–300 mg/d PO
dexamethasone	Decadron, *generic*	See Table 38–1	See Table 38–2	Initial dosage: 0.75–9 mg/d PO; further doses depend on disease being treated
dexamethasone acetate	Decadron-LA, *generic*	See Table 38–1	See Table 38–2	8–16 mg IM; may be repeated in 1–3 wk
hydrocortisone (cortisol)	Cortef, *generic*	See Table 38–1	See Table 38–2	Initial dosage 20–240 mg/d PO; ⅓–½ oral dosage IM
methylprednisolone	Medrol, *generic*	See Table 38–1	See Table 38–2	Initial dosage: 4–48 mg/d PO; maintenance dose based on response to therapy
methylprednisolone acetate	Depo-Medrol, *generic*	See Table 38–1	See Table 38–2	40–120 mg IM
prednisolone	Delta-Cortef, *generic*	See Table 38–1	See Table 38–2	5–60 mg/d PO
prednisone	Metricorten, Deltasone, *generic*	See Table 38–1	See Table 38–2	Initial dosage: 5–60 mg/d PO
triamcinolone	Aristocort, *generic*	See Table 38–1	See Table 38–2	Initial dosage: 4–60 mg/d PO
triamcinolone diacetate	Aristocort L.A., *generic*	See Table 38–1	See Table 38–2	40 mg/wk IM (average dose)
MINERALOCORTICOIDS				
fludrocortisone acetate (has both glucocorticoid and mineralocorticoid activity)	Florinef Acetate	Partial replacement therapy for Addison's disease, salt-losing adrenogenital syndrome	See Table 38–2	Addison's disease: 0.05–0.2 mg/d PO; adrenogenital syndrome: 0.1–0.2 mg/d

*The term, *generic,* indicates that the drug is available in generic form.

ADVERSE REACTIONS ASSOCIATED WITH THE ADMINISTRATION OF THE GLUCOCORTICOIDS

The adverse reactions that may be seen with the administration of the glucocorticoids are given in Table 38-2. Long- or short-term high-dose therapy may also produce many of the signs and symptoms seen with *Cushing's syndrome,* a disease due to the overproduction of endogenous glucocorticoids. Some of the signs and symptoms of this Cushing's-like (or cushingoid) state include a "buffalo" hump (a hump on the back of the neck), moon face, oily skin and acne, osteoporosis, purple striae on the abdomen and hips, skin pigmentation, and weight gain. When a serious disease or disorder is being treated, it is often necessary to allow these effects to occur since therapy with these drugs is absolutely necessary.

NURSING MANAGEMENT

The glucocorticoids may be administered orally, IM, SC, IV, topically, or as an inhalant. The physician may also inject the drug into a joint (intraarticular), a lesion (intralesional), soft tissue, or bursa.

The dosage of the glucocorticoids is individualized and based on the severity of the condition and the patient's response. Daily oral doses are generally given prior to 9:00 AM to minimize adrenal suppression and

Table 38-1. Uses of Glucocorticoids

ENDOCRINE DISORDERS

Primary or secondary adrenal cortical insufficiency, congenital adrenal hyperplasia, nonsuppressive thyroiditis, hypercalcemia associated with cancer

RHEUMATIC DISORDERS

Short-term management of acute ankylosing spondylitis, acute and subacute bursitis, acute nonspecific tenosynovitis, acute gouty arthritis, psoriatic arthritis, rheumatoid arthritis, posttraumatic osteoarthritis, synovitis of osteoarthritis, epicondylitis

COLLAGEN DISEASES

Lupus erythematosus, acute rheumatic carditis, systemic dermatomyositis

DERMATOLOGIC DISEASES

Pemphigus, bullous dermatitis herpetiformis, severe erythema multiforme (Stevens-Johnson syndrome), exfoliative dermatitis, mycosis fungoides, severe psoriasis, severe seborrheic dermatitis, angioedema, urticaria, various skin disorders, such as lichen planus or keloids

ALLERGIC STATES

Control of severe or incapacitating allergic conditions not controlled by other methods, bronchial asthma (including status asthmaticus), contact dermatitis, atopic dermatitis, serum sickness, drug hypersensitivity reactions

OPHTHALMIC DISEASES

Severe acute and chronic allergic and inflammatory processes, keratitis, allergic corneal marginal ulcers, herpes zoster of the eye, iritis, iridocyclitis, chorioretinitis, diffuse posterior uveitis, optic neuritis, sympathetic ophthalmia, anterior segment inflammation

RESPIRATORY DISEASES

Sarcoidosis, berylliosis, fulminating or disseminated pulmonary tuberculosis, aspiration pneumonia

HEMATOLOGIC DISORDERS

Idiopathic or secondary thrombocytopenic purpura, hemolytic anemia, red blood cell anemia, congenital hypoplastic anemia

NEOPLASTIC DISEASES

Leukemias, lymphomas

EDEMATOUS STATES

To induce diuresis or remission of proteinuria in the nephrotic state

GASTROINTESTINAL DISEASES

During critical period of ulcerative colitis, regional enteritis, intractable sprue

NERVOUS SYSTEM

Acute exacerbations of multiple sclerosis

---

to coincide with normal adrenal function. However, alternate-day therapy may be prescribed for patients on long-term therapy.

Alternate-Day Therapy

The alternate-day therapy approach to glucocorticoid administration is used in the treatment of diseases and disorders requiring long-term therapy, especially the arthritic disorders. This regimen involves giving twice the daily dose of the glucocorticoid every other day. The drug is given only once on the alternate day and *before* 9 AM. The purpose of alternate-day administration is to provide the patient requiring long-term glucocorticoid therapy with the beneficial effects of the drug while minimizing certain undesirable reactions (see Table 38-2).

Plasma levels of the endogenous adrenocortical hormones vary throughout the day and nighttime hours. They are normally *higher* between 2 AM and about 8 AM, and *lower* between 4 PM and midnight. When plasma levels are lower, the anterior pituitary releases ACTH, which, in turn, stimulates the adrenal cortex to manufacture and release glucocorticoids. When plasma levels are high, the pituitary gland does not release ACTH. The response of the pituitary to high or low plasma levels of glucocorticoids and the resulting release or nonrelease of ACTH is

an example of the *feedback mechanism,* which may also be seen in other glands of the body, such as the thyroid gland.

Administration of glucocorticoids several times a day and over a short time (as little as 5 to 10 days) results in shutting off the pituitary release of ACTH because there are always high levels of the glucocorticoids in the plasma (which is due to the body's own glucocorticoid production plus the administration of a glucocorticoid drug). Ultimately, the pituitary atrophies and ceases to release ACTH. Without ACTH, the adrenals fail to manufacture and release (endogenous) glucocorticoids. When this happens, the patient has acute *adrenal insufficiency,* which is a life-threatening situation until corrected with the administration of an exogenous glucocorticoid.

Administration of a short-acting glucocorticoid on *alternate* days and before 9 AM, when glucocorticoid plasma levels are still relatively high, does *not* affect the release of ACTH later on in the day, yet gives the patient the benefit of exogenous glucocorticoid therapy.

Daily Assessments

Daily assessments of the patient receiving a glucocorticoid and the frequency of these assessments depend largely on the disease being treated. Areas to

Table 38-2. Adverse Effects of Glucocorticoids

FLUID AND ELECTROLYTE DISTURBANCES

Sodium and fluid retention, congestive heart failure in susceptible patients, potassium loss, hypokalemic alkalosis, hypertension, hypocalcemia, hypotension or shock-like reactions.

MUSCULOSKELETAL

Muscle weakness, loss of muscle mass, tendon rupture, osteoporosis, aseptic necrosis of femoral and humoral heads, spontaneous fractures.

CARDIOVASCULAR

Thromboembolism or fat embolism, thrombophlebitis, necrotizing angiitis, syncopal episodes, cardiac arrhythmias, aggravation of hypertension.

GASTROINTESTINAL

Pancreatitis, abdominal distention, ulcerative esophagitis, nausea, increased appetite and weight gain, possible peptic ulcer with perforation, hemorrhage.

DERMATOLOGIC

Impaired wound healing, thin fragile skin, petechiae, ecchymoses, erythema, increased sweating, supression of skin test reactions, subcutaneous fat atrophy, purpura, striae, hyperpigmentation, hirsutism, acneiform eruptions, urticaria, agioneurotic edema.

NEUROLOGIC

Convulsions, steroid-induced catatonia, increased intracranial pressure with papilledema (usually after treatment is discontinued), vertigo, headache, neuritis or paresthesias, steroid psychosis, insomnia.

ENDOCRINE

Amenorrhea, other menstrual irregularities, development of cushingoid state, suppression of growth in children, secondary adrenocortical and pituitary unresponsiveness (particularly in times of stress), decreased carbohydrate tolerance, manifestation of latent diabetes mellitus, increased requirements for insulin or oral hypoglycemic agents (in diabetics).

OPHTHALMIC

Posterior subcapsular cataracts, increased intraocular pressure, glaucoma, exophthalmos.

METABOLIC

Negative nitrogen balance (due to protein catabolism).

OTHER

Anaphylactoid or hypersensitivity reactions, aggravation of existing infections, malaise, increase or decrease in sperm motility and number.

---

be included in the patient care plan must be based on nursing judgment, as well as specific orders written by the physician.

- Monitor vital signs every 4 to 8 hours.
- Evaluate the patient's response to the drug daily; make evaluations more frequently if a glucocorticoid is used for emergency situations. Because these drugs are used to treat a great many diseases and conditions, base an evaluation of drug response on the patient's diagnosis and the signs and symptoms of his or her disease.
- Weigh the patient daily to weekly. Observe for signs of electrolyte imbalance, especially hypocalcemia, hypokalemia, and hypernatremia (see Chap. 48).
- Assess daily for signs of adverse effects of the mineralocorticoid or glucocorticoid.
- Monitor patients receiving a glucocorticoid for mental changes, especially if there is a history of depression or other psychiatric problems or if high doses of the drug are being given. Document mental changes accurately and inform the physician of their occurrence. Closely observe patients that appear extremely depressed.
- Observe the patient for signs of an infection, which may be masked by glucocorticoid therapy. Report any slight rise in temperature, sore throat, or other signs of infection to the physician as soon as possible.

- Because of a possible decreased resistance to infection during glucocorticoid therapy, nursing personnel and visitors with any type of infection or recent exposure to an infectious disease should avoid patient contact.
- Administration of the glucocorticoids poses the threat of adrenal gland insufficiency (particularly if the alternate-day therapy is *not* prescribed). Assess throughout therapy for hypotension, weight loss, weakness, nausea, anorexia, and lethargy, which indicate the possibility of adrenal insufficiency.
- Diabetic patients receiving a glucocorticoid may require frequent adjustment of their insulin or oral hypoglycemic drug dosage. If the blood glucose levels increase or urine is positive for glucose or ketones, notify the physician.
- Check the blood or urine of the nondiabetic patient weekly for glucose and ketone bodies because glucocorticoids may aggravate latent diabetes.
- Make dietary adjustment for the increased loss of potassium and the retention of sodium if necessary.
- Observe patients on long-term glucocorticoid therapy, especially those allowed limited activity, for signs of compression fractures of the vertebrae and pathological fractures of the long bones. If the patient complains of back or bone pain, notify the physician. Extra care is also necessary to prevent

falls and other injuries when the patient is confused or is allowed out of bed.

- Peptic ulcer has been associated with glucocorticoid therapy. Bring any complaints of epigastric burning or pain, or the passing of tarry stools to the physician's attention immediately.
- Always inform the physician if signs of electrolyte imbalance or glucocorticoid drug effects are noted.
- If the patient is receiving alternate-day therapy, give the drug *before* 9 AM.
- Never omit the dose of a glucocorticoid. If the patient cannot take the drug orally because of nausea or vomiting, notify the physician immediately because the drug needs to be ordered given by the parenteral route. Patients who are receiving nothing by mouth for any reason must have the glucocorticoid given by the parenteral route.

Nursing Alert

At no time must a glucocorticoid be discontinued suddenly. When administration of a glucocorticoid extends beyond 5 days and the drug is to be discontinued, *taper the dosage* over several days. In some instances, it may be necessary to taper the dose over 7 to 10 or more days. Abrupt discontinuation of a glucocorticoid usually results in acute adrenal insufficiency, which, if not recognized in time, can result in death.

Adrenal insufficiency is a critical deficiency of the mineralocorticoids and the glucocorticoids requiring immediate treatment. Symptoms of adrenal insufficiency as a result of too rapid withdrawal include: nausea, fatigue, anorexia, dyspnea, hypotension, hypoglycemia, fever, malaise, dizziness, and fainting. Death due to circulatory collapse will result unless the condition is treated promptly.

Situations producing stress (eg, trauma, surgery, severe illness) may precipitate the need for an increase in dosage of the corticosteroids until the crisis situation or stressful situation is resolved.

THE MINERALOCORTICOIDS

The *mineralocorticoids* consist of aldosterone and desoxycorticosterone, and play an important role in conserving sodium and increasing the excretion of potassium. Because of these activities, the mineralocorticoids play an important role in controlling salt and water balance. Of these two hormones, aldosterone is the more potent. Deficiencies of the miner-

alocorticoids result in a loss of sodium and water and a retention of potassium.

Fludrocortisone (Florinef) is a drug that has both glucocorticoid and mineralocorticoid activity and is the only presently available mineralocorticoid drug.

USES OF THE MINERALOCORTICOIDS

Fludrocortisone is used for replacement therapy for primary and secondary adrenocortical deficiency. Even though this drug has *both* mineralocorticoid and glucocorticoid activity, it is used only for its mineralocorticoid effects.

ADVERSE REACTIONS ASSOCIATED WITH ADMINISTRATION OF THE MINERALOCORTICOIDS

Adverse reactions may occur if dosage is too high or prolonged or if withdrawal is too rapid. Administration of fludrocortisone may cause edema, hypertension, congestive heart failure, enlargement of the heart, increased sweating, or allergic skin rash. Additional adverse reactions include hypokalemia, muscular weakness, headache, and hypersensitivity reactions. Because this drug has glucocorticoid and mineralocorticoid activity and is often given with the glucocorticoids, adverse reactions of the glucocorticoids must be closely monitored as well (see Table 38-2).

NURSING MANAGEMENT

Fludrocortisone is given orally and is well-tolerated in the gastrointestinal tract. Monitor the blood pressure at frequent intervals. Hypotension may indicate insufficient dosage. Weigh the patient daily. Assess for edema particularly swelling of the feet and hands. Auscultate lungs for adventitious sounds (eg, rales/crackles).

Nursing Process
The Patient Receiving a Glucocorticoid or Mineralocorticoid

■ *Assessment*

Before the administration of a glucocorticoid or mineralocorticoid, take the blood pressure, pulse, and respiratory rate. Additional physical assessments depend on the reason for use and the general condition of the patient. When feasible, perform an assessment of the area of disease involvement, such as the respiratory tract or skin, and record the findings in the patient's record. These findings provide baseline data for the evaluation of the patient's response to drug therapy. Weigh patients who are acutely ill or have a serious systemic disease before starting therapy.

■ Nursing Diagnoses
Depending on the drug, dose, and reason for administration, one or more of the following nursing diagnoses may apply to a person receiving a glucocorticoid or mineralocorticoid:
- **Anxiety** related to symptoms of disorder, diagnosis, other factors
- **Risk for Ineffective Management of Therapeutic Regimen** related to noncompliance, lack of knowledge, adverse drug effects, treatment modalities, other factors (specify)

■ Planning and Implementation
The major goals of the patient may include a reduction in anxiety and an understanding of and compliance to the prescribed treatment regimen. To make these goals measurable, more specific criteria must be added.

Anxiety. Depending on the situation, patients may experience anxiety because of the symptoms of their disorder, their diagnosis, or the required treatment regimen. Some of the anxiety in these patients may be lessened by assuring them that their symptoms will most likely be relieved. A thorough teaching plan may also help relieve anxiety due to prolonged therapy or alternate-day therapy.

■ Patient and Family Teaching
To prevent noncompliance, the patient and family must receive thorough instructions and warnings about the drug regimen.

Short-Term Glucocorticoid Therapy
- Take exactly as directed in the prescription container. Do not increase, decrease, or omit a dose unless advised to do so by the physician.
- Follow the instructions for tapering the dose because they are extremely important.
- If the problem does not improve, contact the physician.

Alternate-Day Glucocorticoid Therapy
- Take this drug *before* 9 AM once every other day. Use a calendar or some other method to identify the days of each week the drug is taken.
- Do not stop taking the drug unless advised to do so by the physician.
- If the problem becomes worse, especially on the days the drug is not taken, contact the physician.

Most of the teaching points given below may also apply to alternate-day therapy, especially when higher doses are used and therapy extends over many months.

Long-Term or High-Dose Glucocorticoid Therapy
- Do not omit this drug or increase or decrease the dosage except on the advice of the physician.
- Inform other physicians, dentists, and all medical personnel of therapy with this drug. Wear a Medic-Alert tag or other form of identification to alert medical personnel of long-term therapy with a glucocorticoid.
- Do not take any nonprescription drug unless its use has been approved by the physician.
- Whenever possible, avoid exposure to infections. Contact the physician if minor cuts or abrasions fail to heal, persistent joint swelling or tenderness is noted, or fever, sore throat, upper respiratory infection, or other signs of infection occur.
- If the drug cannot be taken orally for any reason or if diarrhea occurs, contact the physician immediately. If unable to contact the physician before the next dose is due, go to the nearest hospital emergency department (preferably where the original treatment was started or where the physician is on the hospital staff) because the drug has to be given by injection.
- Weigh weekly. If significant weight gain or swelling of the extremities is noted, contact the physician.
- If dietary recommendations are made by the physician, these are an important part of therapy and must be followed.
- Follow the physician's recommendations regarding periodic eye examinations and laboratory tests.

Include the following in a teaching plan for the patient taking the mineralocorticoid, fludrocortisone:
- Take as directed. Do not increase or decrease dosage except if instructed to do so by the physician.
- Do not discontinue the drug abruptly.
- Inform the physician if the following adverse reactions occur: edema, muscle weakness, weight gain, anorexia, swelling of the extremities, dizziness, severe headache, or shortness of breath.

- Carry patient identification such as Medic Alert so that drug therapy will be known to medical personnel during an emergency situation.
- Keep follow-up appointments to determine if a dosage adjustment is necessary.

■ *Expected Outcomes for Evaluation*
- Anxiety is reduced
- Patient verbalizes an understanding of dosage regimen
- Patient verbalizes importance of complying with the prescribed therapeutic regimen and importance of continued follow-up care
- Patient and family demonstrate understanding of drug regimen
- Patient demonstrates understanding of importance in not suddenly discontinuing therapy (long-term or high-dose therapy)

Chapter Summary

- Pituitary hormones regulate growth, metabolism, the reproductive cycle, electrolyte balance, and water retention or loss. The pituitary gland consists of the anterior pituitary or the adenohypophysis and the posterior pituitary or the neurohypophysis. The hormones of the anterior pituitary include growth hormone, adrenocorticotropic hormone, thyroid-stimulating hormone, follicle-stimulating hormone, luteinizing hormone, and prolactin. All but prolactin are use medically.
- The gonadotropins influence the gonads (the organs of reproduction) and include menotropins, urofollitropin, clomiphene, and chorionic gonadotropin. The drugs are used to induce ovulation and pregnancy in the anovulatory female. In addition, menotropins are used in the male to induce the production of sperm. Chorionic gonadotropin is used to treat prepubertal cryptorchism. These drugs are almost always administered on an outpatient basis. Any adverse reactions are reported to the physician.
- Growth hormone is called somatotropic hormone and is secreted by the anterior pituitary. This hormone regulates the growth of the individual until early adulthood or until closure of bone epiphyses. When the epiphyses closes, growth in height can no longer occur. Synthetic hormones somatrem or somatropin are administered to children who have failed to grow because of a deficiency of pituitary growth hormone. The drugs must be used before the epiphyses close.

- ACTH is an anterior pituitary hormone that stimulates the adrenal cortex to produce and secrete adrenocortical hormones. ACTH is used for diagnostic testing of adrenocortical function and for acute exacerbation of certain conditions, such as multiple sclerosis, nonsuppurative thyroiditis, and hypercalcemia associated with cancer. Adverse reactions are similar to the adverse reactions of the glucocorticoids. ACTH may mask signs of infection. The physician must be notified of sore throat, cough, fever, or malaise. Any behavior change such as mental depression, insomnia, mood swings, or nervousness must be reported as well.
- The posterior pituitary gland produces two hormones: vasopressin (antidiuretic hormone) and oxytocin. Vasopressin regulates the reabsorption of water by the kidneys and is secreted by the pituitary when body fluids must be conserved. Vasopressin and its derivatives are used in the treatment of diabetes insipidus (a disease caused by the failure of the pituitary to secrete vasopressin or to surgical removal of the pituitary gland). The dosage of vasopressin may require periodic adjustments. Adverse reactions such as a significant increase or decrease in urinary output, abdominal cramps, blanching of the skin, nausea, signs of inflammation, confusion, headache, or drowsiness are reported to the physician.
- The adrenal cortex manufactures the corticosteroids, which include the glucocorticoids and the mineralocorticoids. The glucocorticoids have multiple uses and act primarily as antiinflammatory and immunosuppressant drugs. The two most prominent glucocorticoids are hydrocortisone and cortisone. Many adverse reactions are associated with the administration of the glucocorticoids. The most prominent of the adverse reactions include symptoms of Cushing's syndrome, such as "buffalo" hump, moon face, oily skin, hypertension, and acne. Other adverse reactions include osteoporosis, purple striae on the abdomen, and weight gain. Sometimes the presence of these adverse reactions must be tolerated since therapy with these drugs is absolutely necessary. The drugs may be given parenterally, orally, or as an inhalant, or applied topically. The dosage is individualized and based on the severity of the condition and the patient's response.
- The alternate-day treatment regimen may be given to provide the patient requiring long-term glucocorticoid therapy with the beneficial effects of the drug while minimizing certain undesirable reactions. This regimen involves giving twice the

daily dose of the glucocorticoid every other day before 9 AM. Administration of glucocorticoids even for short-term therapy (5 to 10 days) may result in shutting off release of the glucocorticoids from the adrenal cortex. The adrenal cortex decreases production of the glucocorticoids because the administration of the drug maintains adequate plasma levels of the hormone. When the drug is discontinued, the patient may suffer acute adrenal insufficiency. To prevent the occurrence of this potentially fatal condition, the dosage of the glucocorticoids is tapered over several days until the medication is discontinued.

- The mineralocorticoids play an important role in conserving sodium and increasing the excretion of potassium. Because of this, they play an important role in maintaining water balance. Fludrocortisone (Florinef) is the only presently available mineralocorticoid drug. This drug is used for replacement therapy for primary and secondary adrenocortical deficiency.

Critical Thinking Exercises

1. Judy Cowan, aged 28, has been prescribed clomiphen to induce ovulation and pregnancy. Judy is very anxious and wants desperately to become pregnant. Her husband, Jim, has come to the clinic with her. What assessments would be important prior to initiating treatment with clomiphen? What information would the nurse include in a teaching plan for Jim and Judy?

2. Plan a team conference to discuss the administration of ACTH (corticotropin). Identify three critical points that would be essential to discuss. Explain your rationale for choosing each point.

3. Ms. Susan Talbot, aged 38, is taking prednisone for rheumatoid arthritis. Therapy will continue for several months in an effort to manage the inflammatory process. Her care plan includes the nursing diagnosis **Body Image Disturbance** related to the medication regimen. What five nursing interventions would be most appropriate for the nursing staff to include for this nursing diagnosis?

39

Thyroid and Antithyroid Drugs

Key Terms

Chapter Outline

Chapter Objectives

On completion of this chapter the student will:

- *Discuss the role of the thyroid gland in the regulation of physiologic processes*
- *Discuss the actions and uses of thyroid and antithyroid drugs*
- *List the signs and symptoms of iodism and iodine allergy*
- *List the general adverse reactions associated with the administration of thyroid and antithyroid drugs*
- *Discuss nursing management when administering a thyroid or antithyroid drug*
- *Use the nursing process when administering a thyroid or antithyroid drug*

Scherer JC, Roach S: INTRODUCTORY CLINICAL PHARMACOLOGY,
FIFTH EDITION © 1996 Lippincott-Raven Publishers

The *thyroid gland* is located in the neck in front of the trachea. This highly vascular gland manufactures and secretes two hormones: *thyroxine* (T$_4$) and *triiodothyronine* (T$_3$). *Iodine* is an essential element for the manufacture of both of these hormones.

The activity of the thyroid gland is regulated by thyroid-stimulating hormone, produced by the anterior pituitary gland (see Fig. 38-1). When the level of circulating thyroid hormones decreases, the anterior pituitary secretes thyroid-stimulating hormone, which then activates the cells of the thyroid to release stored thyroid hormones. This is another example of the feedback mechanism (see Chap. 38).

Two diseases are related to the hormone-producing activity of the thyroid gland: (1) *hypothyroidism*, which is a **decrease** in the amount of thyroid hormones manufactured and secreted, and (2) *hyperthyroidism*, which is an **increase** in the amount of thyroid hormones manufactured and secreted. The symptoms of hypothyroidism and hyperthyroidism are given in Table 39-1.

Thyroid Hormones

Thyroid hormones used in medicine include both the natural and synthetic hormones. The synthetic hormones are generally preferred because they are more uniform in potency than the natural hormones obtained from animals. Thyroid hormones are listed in Summary Drug Table 39-1.

ACTIONS OF THE THYROID HORMONES

The thyroid hormones have an influence on every organ and tissue of the body. These hormones are principally concerned with increasing the metabolic rate of tissues, which results in increases in the heart and respiratory rate, body temperature, cardiac output, oxygen consumption, and the metabolism of fats, proteins, and carbohydrates. The exact mechanisms by which the thyroid hormones exert their influence on body organs and tissues is not well understood.

USES OF THE THYROID HORMONES

Thyroid hormones are used as replacement therapy when the patient is hypothyroid. By supplementing the decreased endogenous thyroid production and secretion with exogenous thyroid hormones, an attempt is made to create a *euthyroid* (normal thyroid) state.

Thyroid hormones may also be used with antithyroid drugs in the treatment of *thyrotoxicosis* or *thyroid storm*. Thyrotoxicosis or thyroid storm is a form of severe hyperthyroidism that is characterized by symptoms such as high fever, extreme tachycardia, and altered mental status.

ADVERSE REACTIONS ASSOCIATED WITH THE ADMINISTRATION OF THYROID HORMONES

The dose of thyroid hormones must be carefully adjusted according to the patient's hormone requirements. At times, several upward or downward dosage

Table 39-1. Signs and Symptoms of Thyroid Dysfunction

Body system or function	Hypothyroidism	Hyperthyroidism
Metabolism	Decreased with anorexia, intolerance to cold, low body temperature, weight gain despite anorexia	Increased with increased appetite, intolerance to heat, elevated body temperature, weight loss despite increased appetite
Cardiovascular	Bradycardia, moderate hypotension	Tachycardia, moderate hypertension
Central nervous system	Lethargy, sleepiness	Nervousness, anxiety, insominia, tremors
Skin, skin structures	Pale, cool, dry skin, face appears puffy, hair coarse, nails thick and hard	Flushed, warm, moist skin
Ovarian function	Heavy menses, may be unable to conceive, loss of fetus possible	Irregular or scant menses
Testicular function	Low sperm count	

Summary Drug Table 39-1. Thyroid and Antithyroid Drugs

Generic Name	Trade Name*	Uses	Adverse Reactions	Dose Ranges
THYROID HORMONES				
levothyroxine sodium (T$_4$)	Levothroid, Levoxyl, Synthroid, *generic*	Hypothyroidism, thyrotoxicosis	Palpitations, tachycardia, tremors, headache, nervousness, insomnia, diarrhea, vomiting, weight loss, sweating, heat intolerance	0.025–0.3 mg/d PO; 0.1–0.5 mg IV
liothyronine sodium (T$_3$)	Cytomel, *generic*	Hypothyroidism, thyrotoxicosis	Same as levothyroxine	5–100 µg/d PO
liotrix (T$_3$, T$_4$)	Euthroid, Thyrolar	Hypothyroidism, thyrotoxicosis	Same as levothyroxine	15–120 mg/d PO and increased PRN
thyroid dessicated	Armour Thyroid, *generic*	Hypothyroidism	Same as levothyroxine	32–195 mg/d PO
ANTITHYROID PREPARATIONS				
methimazole	Tapazole	Hyperthyroidism, preparation for thyroidectomy or radioactive iodine therapy	Agranulocytosis, headache, exfoliative dermatitis, granulocytopenia, thrombocytopenia, hepatitis, hypoprothrombinemia, jaundice, loss of hair, nausea, vomiting	5–60 mg/d PO, usually in divided doses at about 8 h intervals
propylthiouracil (PTU)	*generic*	Same as methimazole	Same as methimazole	300–900 mg/d PO, usually in divided doses at about 8 h intervals
IODINE PRODUCTS				
strong iodine solution (Lugol's solution)	*generic*	To prepare hyperthyroid patients for thyroid surgery	Rash, swelling of salivary glands, "Iodism" (metallic taste, burning mouth and throat, sore teeth, and gums, symptoms of a head cold, diarrhea, nausea), allergic reactions (fever, joint pains, swelling of parts of face and body)	2–6 drops PO tid for 10 d before surgery
sodium iodide (^{131}I)	Iodotope, *generic*	Thyrotoxicosis, selected cases of thyroid cancer	Bone marrow depression, anemia, blood dyscrasias, nausea, vomiting, tachycardia, itching, rash, hives, tenderness and swelling of the neck, sore throat and cough	Measured by a radioactivity calibration system prior to administering PO 4–10 mCi; Thyroid cancer: 50–150 mCi
potassium iodide (oral)	*generic*	Preparation for thyroidectomy, radiation protectant following administration of radioactive isotopes	Same as strong iodine solution	300–1500 mg tid PO

*The term, *generic*, indicates that the drug is available in generic form.

adjustments must be made until the optimal therapeutic dosage is reached and the patient becomes euthyroid. During initial therapy, the most common adverse reactions seen are signs of overdose and hyperthyroidism (see Table 39-1). Adverse reactions other than symptoms of hyperthyroidism are rare.

NURSING MANAGEMENT

The full effects of thyroid hormone replacement therapy may not be apparent for several weeks or more but early effects may be apparent in as little as 48 hours. Monitor the vital signs daily or as ordered and observe the patient for signs of hyperthyroidism, which is a sign of excessive drug dosage.

Nursing Alert

If signs of hyperthyroidism (eg, nervousness, anxiety, increased appetite, elevated body temperature, tachycardia, moderate hypertension or flushed, warm, moist skin) are apparent, report these to the physician before the next dose is due because it may be necessary to decrease the daily dosage.

Signs of a therapeutic response include weight loss, mild diuresis, a sense of well-being, increased appetite, an increased pulse rate, an increase in mental activity, and decreased puffiness of the face, hands, and feet. If the dosage is inadequate, the patient will continue to experience signs of hypothyroidism.

Closely monitor patients with diabetes mellitus during therapy, especially during the initial stages of dosage adjustment. Observe the patient for signs of hyperglycemia (see Chap. 37) and notify the physician if this problem occurs.

Administer thyroid hormones once a day, early in the morning and preferably before breakfast. An empty stomach increases the absorption of the oral preparation. Levothyroxine (Synthroid) is also given intravenously and is prepared for administration immediately before use.

Nursing Process
The Patient Receiving a Thyroid Hormone

■ *Assessment*
After a diagnosis of hypothyroidism and before starting therapy, take vital signs and weigh the patient. Obtain a history of the patient's signs and symptoms and perform a general physical assessment to determine outward signs of hypothyroidism.

■ *Nursing Diagnoses*
Depending on the individual and his or her symptoms, one or more of the following nursing diagnoses may apply to a person receiving a thyroid hormone:
* **Anxiety** related to diagnosis, symptoms of disorder
* **Risk for Ineffective Management of Therapeutic Regimen** related to indifference, lack of

knowledge, adverse drug reactions, treatment modalities, other factors

■ *Planning and Implementation*
The major goals of the patient may include a reduction in anxiety and an understanding of and compliance to the prescribed therapeutic regimen. To make these goals measurable, more specific criteria must be added.

Anxiety. Some patients may exhibit anxiety due to the symptoms of their disorder, as well as concern about relief of their symptoms. The patient should be reassured that although relief may not be immediate, symptoms should begin to decrease or even disappear in a few weeks.

■ *Patient and Family Teaching*
Thyroid hormones are usually given on an outpatient basis. Emphasize the importance of taking the drug exactly as directed and not stopping the drug even though symptoms have improved.

Provide the following information to the patient and family when thyroid hormone replacement therapy is prescribed:
* Replacement therapy is for life (exception: transient hypothyroidism seen in those with thyroiditis).
* Do not increase, decrease, or skip a dose unless advised to do so by the physician.
* Take this drug in the morning, preferably before breakfast, unless advised by the physician to take it at a different time of day.
* Notify the physician if any of the following occur: headache, nervousness, palpitations, diarrhea, excessive sweating, heat intolerance, chest pain, increased pulse rate, or any unusual physical change or event.
* The dosage of this drug may require periodic adjustments; this is normal. Dosage changes are based on a response to therapy.
* Therapy needs to be evaluated at periodic intervals, which may vary from every 2 weeks during the beginning of therapy to every 6 to 12 months once symptoms are controlled.
* Weigh self weekly. Report any significant weight gain or loss to the physician.
* Do not change from one brand of this drug to another without consulting the physician.

■ *Expected Outcomes for Evaluation*
* Anxiety is reduced
* Patient verbalizes importance of complying with the prescribed treatment regimen

- Patient verbalizes an understanding of treatment modalities and importance of continued follow-up care
- Patient and family demonstrate understanding of drug regimen

Antithyroid Drugs

Antithyroid drugs or thyroid antagonists are used to treat hyperthyroidism. In addition to the antithyroid drugs, hyperthyroidism may be treated with surgical removal of some or almost all of the thyroid gland (subtotal thyroidectomy) or by the administration of radioactive iodine (^{131}I).

ACTIONS OF THE ANTITHYROID DRUGS

Antithyroid drugs inhibit the manufacture of thyroid hormones. They do not affect existing thyroid hormones that are circulating in the blood or stored in the thyroid gland. For this reason, therapeutic effects of the antithyroid drugs may not be observed for 3 to 4 weeks. Antithyroid drugs are listed in Summary Drug Table 39-1.

Radioactive iodine is also used to treat hyperthyroidism. After oral administration, the iodine is distributed within the cellular fluid and excreted. The radioactive isotope accumulates in the cells of the thyroid gland where destruction of thyroid cells occurs without damaging other cells throughout the body.

USES OF THE ANTITHYROID DRUGS

Methimazole (Tapazole) and propylthiouracil (PTU) are used for the medical management of hyperthyroidism. Not all patients respond adequately to antithyroid drugs; therefore, a thyroidectomy may be necessary. Antithyroid drugs may also be administered before surgery to temporarily return the patient to a euthyroid state. When used for this reason, the vascularity of the thyroid gland is reduced and the tendency to bleed excessively during and immediately after surgery is decreased.

Strong iodine solution, also known as Lugol's solution, may be given orally with methimazole or propylthiouracil to prepare for thyroid surgery. Io-dine solutions are also used for rapid treatment of hyperthyroidism because they can decrease symptoms in 2 to 7 days.

Radioactive iodine (^{131}I) may be used for treatment of hyperthyroidism and selected cases of cancer of the thyroid. The drug is given orally either as a solution or in a gelatin capsule.

ADVERSE REACTIONS ASSOCIATED WITH THE ADMINISTRATION OF ANTITHYROID DRUGS

Methimazole and Propylthiouracil. The most serious adverse reaction associated with these drugs is agranulocytosis (decrease in the number of white blood cells, eg, neutrophils, basophils, and eosinophils). Reactions observed with agranulocytosis include hay fever, sore throat, skin rash, fever, or headache. Other major reactions include exfoliative dermatitis, granulocytopenia, aplastic anemia, hypoprothrombinemia, and hepatitis. Minor reactions, such as nausea, vomiting and paresthesias, may be also be seen.

Iodine Solutions. Reactions that may be seen with strong iodine solution include symptoms of *iodism* (excessive amounts of iodine in the body), which are a metallic taste in the mouth, swelling and soreness of the parotid glands, burning of the mouth and throat, sore teeth and gums, symptoms of a head cold, and occasionally gastrointestinal upset. Allergy to iodine may also be seen and can be serious. Symptoms of iodine allergy include swelling of parts of the face and body, fever, joint pains, and sometimes difficulty in breathing. The last problem requires immediate medical attention.

Radioactive Iodine (^{131}I). Reactions after administration of radioactive iodine include sore throat, swelling in the neck, nausea, vomiting, cough, and pain on swallowing. Other reactions include bone marrow depression, anemia, leukopenia, thrombocytopenia, and tachycardia.

NURSING MANAGEMENT

Administration

The patient with an enlarged thyroid gland may have difficulty swallowing the tablet. If this occurs, discuss the problem with the physician.

Strong iodine solution is measured in drops, which are added to water or fruit juice. This drug has a strong, salty taste. Allow the patient to experiment with various types of fruit juices to determine which one best disguises the taste of the drug. Iodine solutions should be drunk through a straw since they may cause tooth discoloration.

Radioactive iodine is given by the physician, orally as a single dose. If the patient is hospitalized, radiation safety precautions identified by the hospital's department of nuclear medicine are followed.

Adverse Drug Reactions

Observe the patient for adverse drug effects. During short-term therapy before surgery, adverse drug reactions are usually minimal. Long-term therapy is usually on an outpatient basis. Question the patient regarding a relief of symptoms, as well as signs or symptoms indicating an adverse reaction related to the blood cells, such as fever, sore throat, easy bruising or bleeding, fever, cough, or any other signs of infection.

Nursing Alert

Agranulocytosis is potentially the most serious adverse reaction to methimazole and propylthiouracil. Notify the physician if fever, sore throat, rash, headache, hay fever, yellow discoloration of the skin or vomiting occurs.

Once a euthyroid state is achieved, the physician may add a thyroid hormone to the therapeutic regimen to prevent or treat hypothyroidism, which may develop slowly during long-term antithyroid drug therapy or after administration of radioactive iodine.

When iodine solutions are administered, observe the patient closely for symptoms of iodism and iodine allergy (see Adverse Reactions). If these occur, withhold the drug and notify the physician immediately. This is especially important if swelling around or in the mouth or difficulty in breathing occurs.

Nursing Process
The Patient Receiving an Antithyroid Drug

■ *Assessment*

Before starting therapy with an antithyroid drug, obtain a history of the symptoms of hyperthyroidism. Include in the physical assessment vital signs, weight, and a notation regarding the outward symptoms of the hyperthyroidism (see Table 39-1). If the patient is prescribed an iodine solution, take a careful allergy history, particularly to iodine or seafood (which contains iodine).

■ *Nursing Diagnoses*

Depending on the individual, one or more of the following nursing diagnoses may apply to a person receiving an antithyroid drug:

● **Anxiety** related to symptoms of the disorder
● **Risk for Ineffective Management of Therapeutic Regimen** related to indifference, lack of knowledge, adverse drug reactions, treatment modalities, other factors

■ *Planning and Implementation*

The major goals of the patient may include a reduction in anxiety and an understanding of and compliance to the prescribed therapeutic regimen.

Anxiety. The patient with hyperthyroidism may be concerned with the results of medical treatment and with the problem with taking the drug at regular intervals around the clock (usually every 8 hours). Whereas some patients may be awake early in the morning and retire late at night, others may experience difficulty in an every 8 hour dosage schedule. Another concern may be a tendency to forget the first dose early in the morning, thus, causing a problem with the two following doses.

If the patient expresses a concern about the dosage schedule, the nurse may be able to offer suggestions. For example, suggest for an 8-hour interval schedule: 7 AM, 3 PM, and 11 PM. The nurse may also suggest pasting a notice on a bathroom mirror to remind the individual that the first dose is due immediately after rising. After a week or more of therapy, most patients remember to take their morning dose on time. If the first or last dose interferes with sleep, the nurse should suggest the patient discuss this with the physician.

■ *Patient and Family Teaching*

Review the dosage and times the drug is to be taken with the patient and family. Include the following additional teaching points:

Methimazole and Propylthiouracil
● Take these drugs at regular intervals around the clock (eg, every 8 hours) unless directed otherwise by the physician.

- Do not take these drugs in larger doses or more frequently than as directed on the prescription container.
- Notify the physician promptly if any of the following occur: sore throat, fever, cough, easy bleeding or bruising, headache, or a general feeling of malaise.
- Record weight twice a week. Notify the physician if there is any sudden weight gain or loss. (*Note:* the physician may also want the patient to monitor pulse rate. If this is recommended, the patient needs instruction in the proper technique and a recommendation to record the pulse rate and bring the record to the physician's office or clinic).
- Avoid the use of nonprescription drugs unless the physician has approved the use of a specific drug.

Strong Iodine Solution

- Dilute the solution with water or fruit juice. Fruit juice often disguises the taste more than water does. Experiment with the types of fruit juice that best reduce the unpleasant taste of this drug.
- Discontinue the use of this drug and notify the physician if any of the following occur: skin rash, metallic taste in the mouth, swelling and soreness in front of the ears, sore teeth and gums, severe gastrointestinal distress, or head-cold symptoms.

Radioactive Iodine

- Follow the directions of the department of nuclear medicine regarding precautions to be taken. (*Note:* In some instances, the dosage is small and no special precautions may be necessary).
- Thyroid hormone replacement therapy may be necessary if hypothyroidism develops.
- Follow-up evaluations of the thyroid gland and the effectiveness of treatment with this drug are necessary.

■ Expected Outcomes for Evaluation

- Anxiety is reduced
- Patient verbalizes an understanding of dosage regimen
- Patient verbalizes importance of complying with the prescribed treatment regimen
- Patient and family demonstrate understanding of drug regimen

Chapter Summary

- The thyroid gland is a highly vascular gland located in the neck and functions to manufacture and secrete two hormones, thyroxine (T_4) and tri-

dothyronine (T_3). Two disorders related to the hormone-producing activity of the thyroid gland are hypothyroidism and hyperthyroidism.

- Hypothyroidism is a decrease in the production and secretion of the thyroid hormones. The symptoms of hypothyroidism include decreased metabolism, lethargy, bradycardia, intolerance to cold, low body temperature and weight gain. Thyroid hormones are used as replacement therapy when the patient is hypothyroid or they may be used with antithyroid drugs in the treatment of thyrotoxicosis. The dose of thyroid hormones must be carefully adjusted according to the patient's hormone requirements. During initial therapy, the most common adverse reactions seen are signs of overdose and symptoms of hyperthyroidism.
- The full effects of thyroid hormone replacement therapy may not be apparent for several weeks or more but early effects may be apparent in as little as 48 hours. If signs of hyperthyroidism develop during therapy, report these to the physician before the next dose is due because it may be necessary to decrease the daily dosage. If the dosage is inadequate, the patient will continue to experience signs of hypothyroidism.
- Hyperthyroidism is treated with the antithyroid drugs, surgical removal of some or almost all of the thyroid gland, or by the administration of radioactive iodine (^{131}I). The symptoms of hyperthyroidism include increased metabolism with increased weight, intolerance to heat, elevated body temperature, weight loss, nervousness, and tachycardia.
- The antithyroid drugs, methimazole (Tapazole) and propylthiouracil, inhibit the manufacture of thyroid hormones and are used for the medical management of hyperthyroidism. Not all patients respond adequately to antithyroid drugs; therefore, a thyroidectomy may be necessary. Antithyroid drugs may also be administered before surgery to try to temporarily return the patient to a euthyroid state. The use of these drugs prior to surgery reduces the vascularity of the thyroid gland so that the tendency to bleed excessively during and immediately after surgery is decreased. The most serious adverse reaction associated with methimazole and propylthiouracil is agranulocytosis.
- Strong iodine solution (Lugol's solution) may be given orally with methimazole or propylthiouracil to prepare the patient for thyroid surgery. Reactions that may be seen with strong iodine solution include symptoms of iodism, which include a metallic taste in the mouth, swelling and soreness of the parotid glands, and burning of the mouth

and throat. Allergy to iodine may also be seen and can be serious. Symptoms of iodine allergy in-clude swelling of parts of the face and body, fever, joint pains, and sometimes difficulty in breath-ing. Iodine allergy requires immediate medical attention.

- Radioactive iodine (^{131}I) may be used for treatment of hyperthyroidism and selected cases of cancer of the thyroid. The drug is given orally either as a solution or in a gelatin capsule. Reactions after administration of radioactive iodine include sore throat, swelling in the neck, nausea, vomiting, cough, and pain on swallowing. The patient is observed for adverse drug effects. During short-term therapy before surgery, adverse drug reactions are usually minimal. Long-term therapy is usually on an outpatient basis.
- Once a euthyroid state is achieved, the physician may add a thyroid hormone to the therapeutic regimen to prevent or treat hypothyroidism, which may develop slowly during long-term antithyroid drug therapy or after administration of radioactive iodine.

Critical Thinking Exercises

1. Ms. Hartman, aged 47, has been prescribed levothyroxine (Synthroid) for hypothyroidism. Develop a teaching plan for Ms. Hartman that would provide her with the knowledge she needs to maintain a therapeutic treatment regime.

2. Mr. Conrad will receive a dose of radioactive iodine from the physician. How would you prepare Mr. Conrad prior to his taking the drug? In preparation for dismissal, what would be the most important points to stress to Mr. Conrad about radioactive iodine?

40

Male and Female Hormones

Key Terms

5α-dihydrotestosterone
Anabolism
Androgens
Catabolism
Endogenous
Estradiol
Estriol
Estrogen
Estrone
Menarche
Progesterone
Progestins
Testosterone

Chapter Outline

Chapter Objectives

On completion of this chapter the student will:

- *Discuss the medical uses of male and female hormones*
- *List and discuss the major adverse reactions associated with the administration of male or female hormones*
- *Use the nursing process when administering male or female hormones*
- *Discuss the nursing implications associated with the administration of male and female hormones*

Scherer JC, Roach S: INTRODUCTORY CLINICAL PHARMACOLOGY, FIFTH EDITION © 1996 Lippincott-Raven Publishers

Male and female hormones play an vital role because they actuate the reproduction potential, aid in development and maintenance of secondary sex characteristics, and are necessary for human reproduction. Although hormones are naturally produced by the body, there are situations when administration of a male or female hormone is indicated in the treatment of certain disorders, such as inoperable breast cancer, male hypogonadism, male or female hormone deficiency, contraception, and the treatment of the symptoms of menopause.

The Male Hormones

Male hormones—*testosterone* and its derivatives—are collectively called *androgens*. Androgen secretion is under the influence of the anterior pituitary gland. Small amounts of male and female hormones are also produced by the adrenal cortex (see Chap. 38).

ACTIONS OF THE MALE HORMONES

Androgens

The male hormone testosterone and its derivatives actuate the reproductive potential in the adolescent male. From puberty onward, androgens continue to aid in the development and maintenance of secondary sex characteristics: facial hair, deep voice, body hair, body fat distribution, and muscle development. Testosterone also affects the accessory sex organs (penis, testes, vas deferens, prostate) at the time of puberty. Under the influence of testosterone, the accessory sex organs grow in size. The androgens also promote tissue-building processes (*anabolism*) and reverse tissue-depleting processes (*catabolism*). Examples of androgens are fluoxymesterone (Halotestin), methyltestosterone (Oreton Methyl), and testosterone. Examples of androgens are given in Summary Drug Table 40-1.

Anabolic Steroids

The anabolic steroids are synthetic drugs chemically related to the androgens. Like the androgens, they promote tissue-building processes. Given in normal doses, they have a minimal effect on the accessory sex organs and secondary sex characteristics. Examples of anabolic steroids are given in Summary Drug Table 40-1.

Androgen Hormone Inhibitor

The androgen hormone inhibitor finasteride (Proscar) is a synthetic compound drug that inhibits the conversion of testosterone into the potent androgen *5α-dihydrotestosterone* (*DHT*). The development of the prostate gland is dependent on DHT. The lowering of serum levels of DHT reduce the effect of this hormone on the prostate gland, resulting in a decrease in the size of the gland and the symptoms associated with prostatic gland enlargement.

USES OF THE MALE HORMONES

Androgens

In the male, androgen therapy may be given as replacement therapy for testosterone deficiency. Deficiency states in the male, such as hypogonadism (failure of the testes to develop); selected cases of delayed puberty; and the development of testosterone deficiency after puberty may be treated with androgens. The transdermal testosterone system is used as replacement therapy when endogenous testosterone is deficient or absent.

In the female, androgen therapy may be used as part of the treatment for inoperable metastatic breast carcinoma in patients who are 1 to 5 years *past* menopause. In addition, some breast carcinomas in women are "hormone-dependent" tumors, that is, their growth and spread are influenced by the female hormone estrogen. Administration of an androgen to patients with this type of malignant breast tumor counteracts the effect of estrogen on these tumors. Androgens may also be administered to premenopausal women with metastatic breast carcinoma that is believed to be hormone-dependent and whose tumor growth and spread have been slowed after an oophorectomy (removal of the ovaries). Androgen therapy may also be used to reduce postpartum breast pain and engorgement. The uses of the androgens are also given in Summary Drug Table 28-1.

Summary Drug Table 40-1. The Androgens, Anabolic Steroids, and Androgen Hormone Inhibitor

Generic Name	Trade Name*	Uses	Adverse Reactions	Dose Ranges
ANDROGENS				
fluoxymesterone	Halotestin, *generic*	Males: hypogonadism; Females inoperable breast cancer, prevention of postpartum breast pain and engorgement	Males: gynecomastia, testicular atrophy, inhibition of testicular function, impotence, enlargement of the penis, nausea, jaundice, headache, anxiety, male pattern baldness, acne, depression; Females: amenorrhea, virilization	Males: hypogonadism 5–20 mg/d PO; Females: breast cancer 10–40 mg/d PO in divided doses; postpartum: 2.5 mg immediately after delivery then 5–10 mg/d PO
methyltestosterone	Oreton Methyl, Android-25, *generic*	Males: hypogonadism, male climacteric, impotence, androgen deficiency, postpubertal cryptorchidism; Females: breast cancer, postpartum breast pain and engorgement	Same as fluoxymesterone	Males: 10–50 mg/d PO, 5–25 mg/d buccal tablets; Females: breast cancer: 50–200 mg/d PO, 25–100 mg/d buccal tablets; postpartum: 80 mg/d PO
testosterone, aqueous	Tesamone, *generic*	Males: delayed puberty, androgen replacement therapy, hypogonadism; Females: palliation of breast cancer, postpartum breast pain and engorgement	Same as fluoxymesterone	Males: androgen replacement 25–50 mg IM 2–3 times/wk; hypogonadism 50–400 mg/dose IM; Females: breast cancer: 50–100 mg IM 3 times/wk; postpartum: 25–50 mg IM
testosterone cypionate (in oil)	depAndro 100, *generic*	Males: hypogonadism, delayed puberty; Females: palliation of inoperable breast cancer	Same as fluoxymesterone	Males: 50–400 mg/dose IM; Females: 200–400 mg/dose IM
testosterone transdermal system	Testoderm	Males: androgen replacement therapy	Same as fluoxymesterone	One system applied daily
ANABOLIC STEROIDS				
nandrolone decanoate	Deca-Durabolin, *generic*	Management of anemia of renal insufficiency	Acne, nausea, vomiting, fluid and electrolyte imbalances, jaundice, anorexia, muscle cramps, malignant and benign liver tumors, increased risk of atherosclerosis, mental changes, testicular atrophy, virilization (females)	50–200 mg/wk IM
nandrolone phenpropionate	Durabolin, *generic*	Control of metastatic breast cancer in women	Same as nandrolone decanoate	50–100 mg/wk IM
oxandrolone	Oxandrin	Promote weight gain in those with weight loss after extensive surgery, severe trauma, severe infections	Same as nandrolone decanoate	2.5 mg PO bid to qid
ANDROGEN HORMONE INHIBITOR				
finasteride	Proscar	Benign prostatic hypertrophy	Impotence, decreased libido, decreased volume of ejaculate	5 mg/d PO

*The term, *generic*, indicates the drug is available in generic form.

Anabolic Steroids

The specific uses of the various anabolic steroids are listed in Summary Drug Table 40-1.

The use of anabolic steroids to promote an increase in muscle mass and strength has become a serious problem. Anabolic steroids are *not* intended for this use. Unfortunately, there have been deaths in young, healthy individuals directly attributed to the use of these drugs.

Androgen Hormone Inhibitor

Finasteride is used in the treatment of the symptoms associated with benign prostatic hypertrophy (BPH), such as difficulty starting the urinary stream, frequent passage of small amounts of urine, and having to urinate during the night (nocturia). Several months of therapy may be required before a significant improvement is noted and symptoms of BPH decrease.

ADVERSE REACTIONS ASSOCIATED WITH THE ADMINISTRATION OF MALE HORMONES

Androgens

In the male, administration of an androgen may result in breast enlargement (gynecomastia), testicular atrophy, inhibition of testicular function, impotence, enlargement of the penis, nausea, jaundice, headache, anxiety, male pattern baldness, acne, and depression. Fluid and electrolyte imbalances, which include sodium, water, chloride, potassium, calcium, and phosphate retention, may also be seen.

In the female receiving an androgen preparation for breast carcinoma, the most common adverse reactions are amenorrhea and other menstrual irregularities, and virilization. Virilization in the female produces facial hair, a deepening of the voice, and enlargement of the clitoris. Male pattern baldness and acne may also be seen.

Adverse reactions are minimal when an androgen is given to the postpartum female because the drug is only given for 3 to 5 days.

Anabolic Steroids

Virilization in the female is the most common reaction associated with anabolic steroids, especially when higher doses are used. Acne occurs frequently in all age groups and both sexes. Nausea, vomiting, diarrhea, fluid and electrolyte imbalances (the same as for the androgens, discussed previously), testicular atrophy in the male, jaundice, anorexia, and muscle cramps may also be seen. Blood-filled cysts of the liver and sometimes the spleen, malignant and benign liver tumors, an increased risk of atherosclerosis, and mental changes are the most serious adverse reactions that may occur during prolonged use.

Many serious adverse drug reactions are being reported in healthy individuals using anabolic steroids. There is some indication that prolonged high-dose use has resulted in psychologic and possibly physical addiction and some individuals have required treatment in drug abuse centers. Severe mental changes such as uncontrolled rage ("roid rage"), severe depression, suicidal tendencies, malignant and benign liver tumors, aggressive behavior, increased risk of atherosclerosis, inability to concentrate, and personality changes are not uncommon. In addition, the incidence of the severe adverse reactions cited earlier appears to be increased in those using anabolic steroids for this purpose.

Androgen Hormone Inhibitor

Usually, adverse reactions are mild and do not require discontinuing the drug. Adverse reactions, when they do occur, are related to the sexual drive and include impotence, decreased libido, and a decreased volume of ejaculate.

NURSING MANAGEMENT

Oral and parenteral androgens are often taken or given by injection on an outpatient basis. The male receiving an androgen or anabolic steroid is questioned by the physician or nurse regarding the effectiveness of drug therapy. Male patients in long-term care facilities may be given finasteride for BPH.

Nurses should discourage the illegal use of anabolic steroids to increase muscle mass. Serious, and sometimes fatal, consequences have occurred with the illegal use of these drugs.

Inoperable Breast Carcinoma

Weigh the patient daily or as ordered by the physician. If the patient is on complete bedrest, weights may be taken every 3 to 4 days (or as ordered) using a bed scale. Notify the physician if there is a significant increase or decrease in the weight. Check the lower extremities daily for signs of edema.

Nursing Alert

Observe the patient each day for adverse drug reactions, especially signs of fluid and electrolyte imbalance, jaundice (which may indicate hepatotoxicity), and virilization. Alert the physician to any signs of fluid and electrolyte imbalance or jaundice.

Monitor vital signs every 4 to 8 hours. Evaluate the patient's response to drug therapy based on original assessments. Responses that may be seen include a decrease in pain, an increase in the appetite, and a feeling of well-being.

Postpartum Breast Pain and Engorgement

Evaluate the patient for drug response. Inform the physician if breast pain or engorgement is not relieved.

Anabolic Steroids

When anabolic steroids are used for weight gain, weigh the patient at intervals ranging from daily to weekly. A good dietary regimen is necessary to promote weight gain. Consult the dietitian if the patient eats poorly.

Nursing Process
The Patient Receiving a Male Hormone

■ *Assessment*
Assessment of the patient receiving an androgen or anabolic steroid depends on the drug, the patient, and the reason for administration.

Androgens. In most instances, androgens are administered to the male on an outpatient basis. Before and during therapy, the physician may order electrolyte studies because use of these drugs can result in fluid and electrolyte imbalances.

When these drugs are given to the female patient with inoperable breast carcinoma, evaluate the patient's present status (physical, emotional, and nutritional) carefully and record the findings in the patient's chart. Carefully evaluate and record problem areas, such as pain, any limitation of motion, and the ability to participate in the activities of daily living. Take and record the vital signs and weight. Baseline laboratory tests may include a complete blood count, hepatic function tests, serum electrolytes, and serum and urinary calcium levels. Review these tests and note any abnormalities.

When given as short-term therapy to the female patient with postpartum breast pain and engorgement, record a summary of the symptoms in the patient's chart.

Anabolic Steroids. Evaluate and record the patient's physical and nutritional status before starting therapy with anabolic steroids. Take the weight, blood pressure, pulse, and respiratory rate. Baseline laboratory studies may include a complete blood count, hepatic function tests, and serum electrolytes and serum lipid levels. Review these studies and note any abnormal laboratory tests.

Androgen Hormone Inhibitor. Question the patient at length about symptoms of BPH, such as frequency of voiding during the day and night, difficulty starting the urinary stream, and so on. Record all symptoms in the patient's chart.

■ *Nursing Diagnoses*
Depending on the drug, dose, and reason for administration, one or more of the following nursing diagnoses may apply to a person receiving an androgen or anabolic steroid:
- **Anxiety** related to diagnosis, adverse effects of drug therapy (female patient), other factors
- **Risk for Ineffective Management of Therapeutic Regimen** related to lack of knowledge of medication regimen, adverse drug effects, treatment modalities

■ *Planning and Implementation*
The major goals of the patient may include a reduction in anxiety and an understanding of and compliance to the prescribed therapeutic regimen. To make these goals measurable, more specific criteria must be added.

Administration. If the androgen is to be administered as a buccal tablet, demonstrate the placement of the tablet and warn the patient not to swallow the tablet but to allow it to dissolve in the mouth. Remind the patient not to smoke or drink water until the tablet is dissolved. When the testosterone transdermal system is prescribed, place the system on clean, dry scrotal skin. Optimal skin contact of the transdermal system is achieved by dry shaving scrotal hair prior to placement of the system. The system is worn for 22 to 24 hours, removed, and a new system applied. Before application of a new system, wash and then dry the skin of the scrotum. Periodically check the scrotum for scrotal hair and dry shave as needed.

Adverse Reactions. Observe patients receiving an androgen or anabolic steroid for signs of adverse drug reactions. In the female, masculinization may been seen with long-term administration but must be tolerated to obtain the desired effect of the drug.

Anxiety. With long-term administration, the female patient may develop mild to moderate masculine changes (virilization), namely, facial hair, a deepening of the voice, and enlargement of the clitoris. Male pattern baldness, patchy hair loss, skin pigmentation, and acne may also be seen. Although these adverse effects are not life-threatening, they often are distressing and only add to the patient's discomfort and anxiety. These problems may be easy to identify but they are not always easy to solve. If hair loss occurs, suggest the wearing of a wig. Advise the patient that mild skin pigmentation may be covered with makeup but severe and widespread pigmented areas and acne are often difficult to conceal. Each patient is different, and the emotional responses to these outward changes may range from severe depression to a positive attitude and acceptance. Work with the patient as an individual, first identifying the problems, and then helping the patient, whenever possible, to deal with these changes.

■ Patient and Family Teaching
Explain the dosage regimen and possible adverse drug reactions to the patient and family.

Develop a teaching plan to include the following:

Androgens
- Notify the physician if any of the following occur: nausea, vomiting, swelling of the legs, jaundice. Female patients should report any signs of virilization to the physician.
- Oral Tablets—take with food or a snack to avoid gastrointestinal upset.
- Buccal tablets—place the tablet between the cheek and molars and allow it to dissolve in the mouth. Do not smoke or drink water until the tablet is dissolved.

- Testosterone transdermal system—apply according to the directions supplied with the product. Be sure the skin is clean and dry and the placement area is free of hair.

Anabolic Steroids
- These drugs may cause nausea and gastrointestinal upset. Take this drug with food or meals.
- Keep all physician or clinic visits because close monitoring of therapy is essential.
- Female patient—Notify the physician if signs of virilization occur.

Androgen Hormone Inhibitor
- May be taken without regard to meals.
- Inform the physician immediately if sexual partner is or may become pregnant because additional measures such as discontinuing the drug or use of a condom may be necessary.

■ Expected Outcomes for Evaluation
- Anxiety is reduced
- Adverse reactions are identified and reported to the physician
- Patient verbalizes importance of complying with the prescribed treatment regimen
- Patient and family demonstrate understanding of drug regimen
- Patient verbalizes an understanding of treatment modalities and importance of continued follow-up care

The Female Hormones

The two *endogenous* (produced by the body) female hormones are the *estrogens* and *progesterone*. Like the androgens, their production is under the influence of the anterior pituitary gland. The endogenous estrogens are *estradiol, estrone,* and *estriol.* The most potent of these three estrogens is estradiol. There are natural and synthetic progesterones, which are collectively called *progestins.* Examples of estrogens used as drugs include chlorotrianisene (Tace) and estradiol (Estrace). Examples of progestins used as drugs include medroxyprogesterone (Provera) and norethindrone (Norlutin). Examples of estrogens and progestins are given in Summary Drug Table 40-2.

Summary Drug Table 40-2. The Female Hormones

Generic Name	Trade Name*	Uses	Adverse Reactions	Dose Ranges
ESTROGENS				
chlorotrianisene	Tace	Postpartum breast engorgement, symptoms of menopause, female hypogonadism, inoperable prostatic carcinoma	Nausea, vomiting, breakthrough bleeding, abdominal cramps, headache, cholasma, melasma, migraine, weight gain or loss, bloating, change in menstrual flow, dizziness	Postpartum: 12 mg PO qid or 50 mg PO q6h; symptoms of menopause, hypogonadism: 12–25 mg/d PO; prostatic cancer: 12–25 mg/d PO
conjugated estrogens, oral	Premarin	Symptoms of menopause, female hypogonadism, female castration, primary ovarian failure, osteoporosis, palliation of breast and prostate cancer, prevention of postpartum breast engorgement	Same as chlorotrianisene	Menopause, female castration, primary ovarian failure: 1.25 mg/d PO; female hypogonadism: 2.5–7.5 mg/d PO; osteoporosis: 0.625 mg/d PO; prostate cancer: 1.25–2.5 mg PO tid; postpartum: 3.75 mg PO q4h
diethylstilbestrol (DES)	*generic*	Inoperable progressing prostatic and breast cancer (males, females past menopause)	Same as chlorotrianisene	Prostate cancer: 1–3 mg/d PO; breast cancer: 15 mg/d PO
esterified estrogens	Menest, Estratab	Symptoms of menopause, female hypogonadism, female castration, primary ovarian failure, prostatic cancer, breast cancer (males, females past menopause)	Same as chlorotrianisene	Menopause: 0.3–1.25 mg/d PO; female hypogonadism: 2.5–7.5 mg/d PO; female castration, primary ovarian failure: 1.25 mg/d PO; Prostatic cancer: 1.25–2.5 mg PO tid; breast cancer (male, female) 10 mg PO tid
estradiol transdermal system	Estraderm	Symptoms of menopause, female hypogonadism, female castration, primary ovarian failure, osteoporosis	Same as chlorotrianisene	Apply as directed by the physician
estradiol valerate in oil	Delestrogen, *generic*	Symptoms of menopause, postpartum breast engorgement, prostatic cancer, female hypogonadism	Same as chlorotrianisene	Menopause, female hypogonadism: 10–20 mg IM every 4 weeks; postpartum: 10–25 mg IM as single injection; prostatic cancer: 30 or more mg IM every 1–2 weeks
PROGESTINS				
medroxyprogesterone acetate	Provera, *generic*	Amenorrhea, abnormal uterine bleeding	Breakthrough bleeding, spotting, change in menstrual flow, amenorrhea, breast tenderness, edema, weight gain or loss, acne, cholasma, melasma, mental depression	5–10 mg/d PO
norethindrone acetate	Norlutate	Amenorrhea, abnormal uterine bleeding, endometriosis	Same as medroxyprogesterone acetate	Amenorrhea, abnormal uterine bleeding 2.5–5 mg/d PO; endometriosis: up to 15 mg/d PO
progesterone in oil	Gesterol 50, *generic*	Amenorrhea, functional uterine bleeding	Same as medroxyprogesterone acetate	5–10 mg/d IM

*The term, *generic*, indicates the drug is available in generic form.

ACTIONS OF THE FEMALE HORMONES

Estrogens

The estrogens are secreted by the ovarian follicle and in smaller amounts by the adrenal cortex. Estrogens are important in the development and maintenance of the female reproductive system and the primary and secondary sex characteristics. At puberty, they promote growth and development of the vagina, uterus, and Fallopian tubes, and enlargement of the breasts. They also affect the release of pituitary gonadotropins (see Chap. 38). Other actions of estrogen include fluid retention, protein anabolism, thinning of the cervical mucus, and the inhibition of ovulation. Estrogens contribute to the conservation of calcium and phosphorus; the growth of pubic and axillary hair; and pigmentation of the breast nipples and genitals. Estrogens also stimulate contraction of the Fallopian tubes (which promotes movement of the ovum); modify the physical and chemical properties of the cervical mucus; and restore the endometrium after menstruation.

Progestins

Progesterone is secreted by the corpus luteum, placenta, and, in small amounts, by the adrenal cortex. Progesterone and its derivatives (ie, the progestins) transform the proliferative endometrium into a secretory endometrium. Progestins are necessary for the development of the placenta and inhibit the secretion of pituitary gonadotropins, which, in turn, prevents maturation of the ovarian follicle and ovulation. The synthetic progestins are usually preferred for medical use because of the decreased effectiveness of progesterone when administered orally.

USES OF THE FEMALE HORMONES

Estrogens

The estrogens are used in the treatment of postpartum breast engorgement, inoperable prostatic carcinoma, relief of moderate to severe vasomotor symptoms of menopause (flushing, sweating), female hypogonadism, atrophic vaginitis, osteoporosis in females past menopause, and in selected cases of inoperable breast carcinoma. The estradiol transdermal system is used for moderate to severe vasomotor symptoms associated with menopause, female hypogonadism, following removal of the ovaries in premenopausal women (female castration), primary ovarian failure, atrophic vaginitis, and prevention of osteoporosis.

The estrogens, in combination with a progestin, are also used as oral contraceptives (Summary Drug Table 40-3). The uses of individual estrogens are given in Summary Drug Table 40-2. The use of estrogens in the treatment of carcinoma are discussed in Chapter 47.

Progestins

The progestins are used in the treatment of amenorrhea, endometriosis, and functional uterine bleeding. Progestins are also used as oral contraceptives, either alone or in combination with an estrogen (see Summary Drug Table 28-2).

Oral Contraceptives

Estrogens and progestins (combination oral contraceptives) or progestins only are used as oral contraceptives. There are three types of estrogen and progestin combination oral contraceptives: monophasic, biphasic, and triphasic. The monophasic oral contraceptives provide a fixed dose of estrogen and progestin. The biphasic and triphasic oral contraceptives deliver hormones similar to the levels naturally produced by the body.

Implant Contraceptive System
Levonorgestrel, a progestin, is available as an implant contraceptive system (Norplant System). Six capsules, each containing levonorgestrel, are implanted under local anesthesia in the subdermal (below the skin) tissues of the mid-portion of the upper arm. The capsules provide contraceptive protection for 5 years but may be removed at any time at the request of the patient.

Intrauterine Progesterone Contraceptive System
The progesterone intrauterine system (Progestasert) is a T-shaped unit containing progesterone and is inserted in the uterine cavity. This system exerts contraceptive effectiveness for 1 year at which time it is removed by the physician and a new system inserted.

Summary Drug Table 40-3. Oral and Implantable Contraceptives

Combination Products (Estrogen and Progestin)*

MONOPHASIC ORAL CONTRACEPTIVES

50 mcg mestranol 1/50 M, 1 mg norethindrone	Genora 1/50, Nelova 1/50 M, Norethin Norinyl 1 + 50, Ortho-novum 1/50
50 mcg ethinyl estradiol, 1 mg norethindrone	Ovcon-50
50 mcg ethinyl estradiol, 1 mg ethynodiol diacetate	Demulen 1/50
50 mcg ethinyl estradiol, 0.5 mg norgestrel	Ovral
35 mcg ethinyl estradiol, 1 mg norethindrone	Genora 1/35, N.E.E. 1/35, Norinyl 1 + 35, Nelova 1/35E, Norethin 1/35E, Ortho-Novum 1/35
35 mcg ethinyl estradiol, 0.5 mg norethindrone	Brevicon, Genora 0.5/35, Modicon, Nelova 0.5/35E
35 mcg ethinyl estradiol, 0.4 mg norethindrone	Ovcon-35
35 mcg ethinyl estradiol, 0.25 mg norgestimate	Ortho-Cyclen
35 mcg ethinyl estradiol, 1 mg ethynodiol diacetate	Demulen 1/35
30 mcg ethinyl estradiol, 1.5 mg norethindrone acetate	Loestrin 21 1.5/30, Loestrin Fe 1.5/30
30 mcg ethinyl estradiol, 0.3 mg norgestrel	Lo/Ovral
30 mcg ethinyl estradiol, 0.15 mg desogestrel	Desogen, Ortho-Cept
30 mcg ethinyl estradiol, 0.15 mg levonorgestrel	Levlen, Levora, Nordette
20 mcg ethinyl estradiol, 1 mg norethindrone acetate	Loestrin 21 1/20, Loestrin Fe 1/20

BIPHASIC ORAL CONTRACEPTIVES

Phase one: 35 mcg ethinyl estradiol, 10/11, 0.5 mg norethindrone; Phase two: 35 mcg ethinyl estradiol, 1 mg norethrindrone	Jenest–28, Nelova 10/11, Ortho–Novum

TRIPHASIC ORAL CONTRACEPTIVES

Phase one: 35 mcg ethinyl estradiol, 0.5 mg norethindrone; Phase two: 35 mcg ethinyl estradiol, 1 mg norethindrone; Phase three: 35 mcg ethinyl estradiol, 0.5 mg norethindrone	Tri-Norinyl
Phase one: 35 mcg ethinyl estradiol, 0.5 mg norethindrone; Phase two: 35 mcg ethinyl estradiol; 0.75 mg norethindrone; Phase three: 35 mcg ethinyl estradiol, 1 mg norethindrone	Ortho-Novum 7/7/7
Phase one: 30 mcg ethinyl estradiol, 0.05 mg levonorgestrel; Phase two: 40 mcg ethinyl estradiol, 0.075 mg levonorgestrel; Phase three: 30 mcg ethinyl estradiol, 0.125 mg levonorgestrel	Tri-Levlen, Triphasil
Phase one: 35 mcg ethinyl estradiol, 0.18 mg norgestimate; Phase two: 35 mcg ethinyl estradiol, 0.125 mg norgestimate; Phase three: 35 mcg ethinyl estradiol, 0.25 mg norgestimate	Ortho Tri-Cyclen

Progestin Only

0.35 mg norethindrone	Micronor, Nor-O.D.
0.075 mg norgestrol	Ovrette

Implant Contraceptive Systems (Progestins)

levonorgestrel—6 capsules each containing 35 mg levonorgestrel for subdermal implantation	Norplant System
progesterone—T-shaped unit containing 38 mg progesterone for insertion in the uterine cavity	Progestasert

*Estrogens are listed first and progestins second.

Medroxyprogesterone Acetate Contraceptive Injection

Medroxyprogesterone acetate (Depo-Provera), a synthetic progestin used in the treatment of abnormal uterine bleeding and secondary amenorrhea, is also used as a contraceptive. This drug is given intramuscularly every 3 months.

ADVERSE REACTIONS ASSOCIATED WITH THE ADMINISTRATION OF THE FEMALE HORMONES

Administration of estrogens or progestins by any route of administration may result in many adverse reactions although the incidence and intensity of these reactions varies. Some of the adverse reactions seen with the administration of estrogens include nausea, vomiting, breakthrough bleeding (bleeding or spotting between menstrual periods), abdominal cramps, headache, intolerance to contact lenses, pain at the injection site, chloasma (pigmentation of the skin) or melasma (discoloration of the skin), migraine, weight increase or decrease, change in menstrual flow, bloating, and dizziness. Warnings associated with the administration of estrogen include an increased risk of endometrial cancer, gallbladder disease, hypertension, hepatic adenoma (a benign tumor of the liver), photosensitivity reactions, increased risk of thromboembolic disease, and hypercalcemia in those with breast cancer and bone metastases.

Progestin administration may result in breakthrough bleeding, spotting, change in the menstrual flow, amenorrhea, breast tenderness, edema, weight increase or decrease, acne, chloasma or melasma, and mental depression.

When used as combination oral contraceptives, the adverse reactions associated with the estrogens and the progestins must be considered.

The warnings associated with the use of oral contraceptives include cigarette smoking, which increases the risk of cardiovascular side effects, such as venous and arterial thromboembolism, myocardial infarction, and thrombotic and hemorrhagic stroke. Also reported with oral contraceptive use are hepatic adenomas and tumors, visual disturbances, gallbladder disease, hypertension, and fetal abnormalities.

In addition to the adverse reactions seen with progestins, the use of a levonorgestrel implant system may result in bruising following insertion; scar tissue formation at the site of insertion; and hyperpigmentation at the implant site. In addition to the adverse reactions seen with progestins, the intrauterine progesterone contraceptive system may result in bleeding and cramps during the first few weeks after insertion, septicemia, pelvic infection, cervical erosion, vaginitis, spontaneous abortion, and the system being embedded into the wall of the uterus. The use of medroxyprogesterone acetate contraceptive injection may result in the same adverse reactions as those associated with administration of any progestin.

NURSING MANAGEMENT

Evaluation of drug therapy, as well as nursing management, is based on the reason for use of the female hormone.

The Outpatient

At the time of each office or clinic visit, obtain the blood pressure, pulse, respiratory rate, and weight. Question the patient regarding any adverse drug effects, as well as the result of drug therapy. For example, if the patient is receiving an estrogen for the symptoms of menopause, she is asked to compare her original symptoms with the symptoms she is currently experiencing, if any. A periodic (usually annual) physical examination is performed by the physician and may include a pelvic examination, breast examination, Pap smear, and laboratory tests. The patient with a prostatic or breast carcinoma usually requires more frequent evaluations of response to drug therapy.

The instructions for starting oral contraceptive therapy vary slightly with the product used. Each product has detailed patient instruction sheets regarding starting oral contraception therapy and are reviewed with the patient. The instructions for missed doses also are included in the package insert and are reviewed with the patient.

The Hospital Patient

The following are included in a nursing care plan for the hospitalized patient receiving a female hormone:

- Monitor the vital signs daily or more often, depending on the patient's physical condition and the reason for drug use.
- Diabetic patient—Notify the physician if blood glucose levels tested with a glucometer are elevated or the urine is positive for glucose or ketone bodies because a change in the dosage of insulin or the oral hypoglycemic agent may be required.
- Observe the patient for adverse drug reactions, especially those related to the liver (the development of jaundice) or the cardiovascular system (thromboembolism).
- Weigh the patient weekly or as ordered by the physician. Report any significant weight gain or loss to the physician.
- Patients with breast carcinoma or prostatic carcinoma should observe for and evaluate signs indicating a response to therapy, for example, a relief of pain, an increase in appetite, a feeling of well-being. In prostatic carcinoma, the response to therapy may be rapid, but in breast carcinoma the response is usually slow.
- Postpartum breast engorgement—A breast binder may be ordered for 3 days. Remove the breast binder and reapply every 4 hours or as needed and record the patient's response to therapy.

Nursing Process
The Patient Receiving a Female Hormone

■ *Assessment*

Before the administration of an estrogen or progestin, obtain a complete health history including a menstrual history, which includes the *menarche* (age of onset of first menstruation); menstrual pattern; and any changes in the menstrual pattern including a menopause history, when applicable. In those prescribed an estrogen (including oral contraceptives), obtain a history of thrombophlebitis or other vascular disorders, a smoking history, and a history of liver diseases. Take the blood pressure, pulse, and respiratory rate. The physician usually performs a breast and pelvic examination and obtains a Pap smear before starting therapy. He or she may also order hepatic function tests.

If the male or female patient is being treated for a malignancy, determine and enter in the patient's record a general evaluation of the patient's physical and mental status. The physician may also order laboratory tests, such as serum electrolytes and liver function tests.

■ *Nursing Diagnoses*

Depending on the patient and reason for administration, one or more of the following may apply to the patient receiving a female hormone:
- **Anxiety** related to diagnosis, other factors
- **Noncompliance** related to lack of knowledge, other factors
- **Risk for Ineffective Management of Therapeutic Regimen** related to lack of knowledge of medication regimen, adverse drug effects

■ *Planning and Implementation*

The major goals of the patient may include a reduction in anxiety and an understanding of and compliance to the prescribed therapeutic regimen. To make these goals measurable, more specific criteria must be added.

Anxiety. The female patient taking female hormones may have many concerns about therapy with these drugs. Some concerns may be based on inaccurate knowledge, for example, the woman who hears of incorrect facts about certain dangers associated with female hormones. Although there are dangers associated with long-term use of female hormones, many of these adverse reactions occur in a small number of patients. When the patient is closely followed by the physician, the dangers associated with long-term use are often minimized.

Encourage the patient and allow her time to ask questions about her therapy. Clarify information that is inaccurate before therapy is started. Refer to the physician questions that cannot or should not be answered by a nurse.

The male patient with inoperable prostatic carcinoma also may have concerns over taking a female hormone. Assure the patient that the dosage is carefully regulated and that feminizing effects, if they occur, are usually minimal.

Noncompliance. Give the patient a thorough explanation of the dose regimen and adverse reactions that may be seen with the prescribed drug. Advise those taking oral contraceptives that skipping a dose could result in pregnancy.

In most instances, the physician performs periodic examinations, for example, laboratory tests, a pelvic examination, or a Pap smear. Encourage the patient to keep all appointments for follow-up evaluation of therapy.

■ *Patient and Family Teaching*

Estrogens and Progestins

- A patient package insert is available with the drug. Read the information carefully. If there are any questions about this information, discuss them with the physician.
- If gastrointestinal upset occurs, take the drug with food.
- Notify the physician if any of the following occurs: pain in the legs or groin area; sharp chest pain or sudden shortness of breath; lumps in the breast; sudden severe headache; dizziness or fainting; vision or speech disturbances; weakness or numbness in the arms or legs, severe abdominal pain, depression, or yellowing of the skin or eyes.
- Female patient: If pregnancy is suspected or abnormal vaginal bleeding occurs, stop taking the drug and contact the physician immediately.
- Avoid exposure to sunlight or ultraviolet light because a severe skin reaction (similar to a severe sunburn) may occur. A sunscreen (sun protection factor of 12 or above) should be worn on exposed skin surfaces when exposure to the sun is necessary.
- Diabetic patient: Check the blood glucose or urine daily or more often. Contact the physician if the blood glucose is elevated or if the urine is positive for glucose or ketones. An elevated blood glucose or urine positive for glucose or ketones may require a change in diabetic medication (insulin,

oral hypoglycemic agent) or diet; these changes must be made by the physician.

Oral Contraceptives

- A patient package insert is available with the drug. Read the information carefully. Begin the first dose as directed in the package insert or as directed by the physician. If there are any questions about this information, discuss them with the physician.
- Avoid smoking or excessive exposure to second-hand smoke while taking these drugs.
- Avoid prolonged exposure to sunlight or ultraviolet light (tanning lamps and beds) and wear a sunscreen when outdoors.
- To obtain a maximum effect, take this drug as prescribed and at intervals not exceeding once every 24 hours. An oral contraceptive is best taken with the evening meal or at bedtime. The effectiveness of this drug depends on following the prescribed dosage schedule. Failure to comply with the dosage schedule may result in a pregnancy.
- Use an additional method of birth control (as recommended by the physician) until after the first week in the initial cycle.
- While taking these drugs, periodic examinations by the physician and laboratory tests are necessary.
- If there are any questions regarding what to do about a missed dose, discuss the procedure to follow with the physician.

Estradiol Transdermal System

- Apply the system immediately after opening the pouch, with the adhesive side down. Apply to clean, dry skin of the trunk preferably the abdomen below the waistline. Press the system firmly in place with the palm of the hand for about 10 seconds.
- The old system is removed each day and a new system applied unless the physician directs otherwise. Rotate application sites.
- Follow the directions of the physician regarding application of the system (eg, continuous, 3 weeks use followed by 1 week off).
- If the system falls off, it may be reapplied or a new system applied.

■ Expected Outcomes for Evaluation

- Anxiety is reduced
- Patient verbalizes an understanding of dosage regimen and importance of continued follow-up care
- Patient verbalizes importance of complying with the prescribed therapeutic regimen

Chapter Summary

- Male and female hormones play an vital role because they actuate the reproduction potential, aid in development and maintenance of secondary sex characteristics, and are necessary for human reproduction.
- Male hormones—*testosterone* and its derivatives—are collectively called *androgens*. Androgen secretion is under the influence of the anterior pituitary gland. Small amounts of male and female hormones are also produced by the adrenal cortex.
- The male hormone testosterone and its derivatives actuate the reproductive potential in the adolescent male. From puberty onward, androgens continue to aid in the development and maintenance of secondary sex characteristics. The androgens also promote anabolism and reverse catabolism.
- The anabolic steroids are synthetic drugs chemically related to the androgens. Like the androgens, they promote tissue-building processes. Given in normal doses, they have a minimal affect on the accessory sex organs and secondary sex characteristics.
- The androgen hormone inhibitor finasteride inhibits the conversion of testosterone into the potent androgen *5α-dihydrotestosterone* (*DHT*). The lowering of serum levels of DHT reduce the effect of this hormone on the prostate gland, resulting in a decrease in the size of the gland and the symptoms associated with prostatic gland enlargement.
- In the male, androgen therapy may be given as replacement therapy for testosterone deficiency. In the female, androgen therapy may be used as part of the treatment for inoperable metastatic breast carcinoma in patients who are 1 to 5 years *past* menopause and in those with "hormone-dependent" tumors. Anabolic steroids may be used to promote weight gain in those who are underweight; in the management of osteoporosis occurring past menopause and in reversing the profound catabolism; in the control of metastatic breast cancer; and in the treatment of certain types of anemia. Finasteride is used in the treatment of the symptoms associated with BPH.
- The two *endogenous* female hormones are the *estrogens* and *progesterone*; like the androgens, their production is under the influence of the anterior pituitary gland. The endogenous estrogens are *estradiol*, *estrone*, and *estriol*. The most potent of these three estrogens is estradiol. There are nat-

ural and synthetic progesterones, which are collectively called *progestins*.

- The estrogens are secreted by the ovarian follicle and in smaller amounts by the adrenal cortex and are important in the development and maintenance of the female reproductive system and the primary and secondary sex characteristics.
- Progesterone is secreted by the corpus luteum, placenta, and, in small amounts, by the adrenal cortex. Progesterone and its derivatives (ie, the progestins) transform the proliferative endometrium into a secretory endometrium. Progestins are necessary for the development of the placenta and inhibit the secretion of pituitary gonadotropins, which, in turn, prevents maturation of the ovarian follicle and ovulation.
- The estrogens are used in the treatment of postpartum breast engorgement; inoperable prostatic carcinoma; relief of moderate to severe vasomotor symptoms of menopause (flushing, sweating); female hypogonadism; atrophic vaginitis; osteoporosis in females past menopause; and in selected cases of inoperable breast carcinoma.
- The estrogens, in combination with a progestin, are also used as oral contraceptives. The progestins are used in the treatment of amenorrhea, endometriosis, and functional uterine bleeding.

Progestins are also used as oral contraceptives, either alone or in combination with an estrogen.

Critical Thinking Exercises

1. Ms. Burton is receiving methyltestosterone (Oreton Methyl) for treatment of metastatic breast cancer. The drug has caused changes in her appearance, namely deepening of her voice, some male pattern baldness, and facial hair. What suggestions could you give this patient who has a limited income and may be unable to afford extensive cosmetic and wardrobe changes?
2. John, a friend of your brother, has started to use anabolic steroids to increase his strength and muscle mass to improve his chances of getting a football scholarship. Your brother tells you that this is acceptable because his friend wants an education. What would you tell your brother?
3. You have been asked to give information to a 17-year-old single patient who has been prescribed an oral contraceptive. What information and explanations would you give to this patient? What might be the best way to give this information to this patient?

41

Drugs Acting on the Uterus

Key Terms

Abortifacients
Oxytocic
Oxytocin
Uterine atony
Water intoxication

Chapter Outline

Chapter Objectives

On completion of this chapter the student will:

- *Discuss the actions and uses of drugs acting on the uterus*
- *List some of the major adverse reactions associated with the administration of drugs acting on the uterus*
- *Discuss nursing management when administering an oxytocic drug, uterine relaxant, or abortifacient*
- *Use the nursing process when administering an oxytocic drug, uterine relaxant, or abortifacient*

Drug therapy is beneficial for use in labor and delivery to promote the well-being of the mother and fetus. Depending on the patient's need, drugs may be used to stimulate, intensify, or inhibit uterine contractions. The three principal types of drugs used for their effect on the uterus are the *oxytocics,* the *uterine relaxants,* and the *abortifacients.* Drugs acting on the uterus are listed in Summary Drug Table 41-1.

The Oxytocic Drugs

Oxytocic drugs are drugs that are used to induce uterine contractions similar to those of normal labor. These drugs are desirable when delivery is in the best interest of the mother and the fetus.

Summary Drug Table 41-1. Drugs Acting on the Uterus

Generic Name	Trade Name*	Uses	Adverse Reactions	Dose Ranges
OXYTOCICS				
ergonovine maleate	Ergotrate, *generic*	Uterine atony and hemorrhage	Nausea, vomiting, diarrhea, blood pressure elevation	0.2 mg IM, IV; 0.2–0.4 mg PO q6–12h
methylergonovine maleate	Methergine	Routine management after delivery of the placenta, uterine atony and hemorrhage	Nausea, vomiting, dizziness, hypertension, headache, palpitations	0.2 mg IM, IV after delivery of the placenta; 0.2 mg PO tid, qid
oxytocin (parenteral)	Pitocin, Syntocin, *generic*	Antepartum: to initiate or improve uterine contractions; postpartum: to produce uterine contractions in third stage of labor, control of postpartum bleeding and hemorrhage	Uterine rupture, fetal bradycardia, neonatal jaundice, anaphylactic reaction, nausea, vomiting, water intoxication, cardiac arrhythmias	Induction of labor: 1–2 mU/min IV infusion, gradually increase dosage by 1–2 mU/min with maximum dosage 20 mU/min; postpartum bleeding: IV infusion of 10–40 U in 1000 mL; 10 U Im
UTERINE RELAXANTS				
ritodrine hydrochloride	Yutopar	Preterm labor	Alterations in fetal and maternal heart rates and maternal blood pressure, palpitations, headache, nausea, vomiting	IV; 0.1 mg/min and increased depending on patient response; PO: 10–20 mg q2–6h
terbutaline	Brethine, Brethaire	Preterm labor	Nervousness, restlessness, nausea, vomiting, transient hyperglycemia, insomnia, tremor, headache, hypertension, tachycardia, palpitations, hypokalemia, pulmonary edema	Preterm labor: IV 10 mcg/min q10 min up to 80 mcg/min increased by 5 mcg/min; SQ: 250 mcg qh until contractions stop; PO: 2.5 mg q4–6h until delivery
ABORTIFACIENTS				
carboprost tromethamine	Hemabate	Termination of pregnancy	Nausea, vomiting, diarrhea, headache, paresthesia, perforated uterus or cervix	Initially: 250 mcg IM; subsequent doses of 250–500 mcg may be necessary
dinoprostone (prostaglandin E2)	Prostin E2	Termination of pregnancy	Vomiting, diarrhea, nausea, headache, hypotension, chills	1 suppository high into vagina; may be repeated
sodium chloride 20%	*generic*	Termination of pregnancy	Fever, flushing, fluid overload, pulmonary embolus, changes in the coagulation mechanism	Up to 250 mL by transabdominal intra-amniotic instillation

*The term, *generic,* indicates that the drug is available in generic form.

ACTIONS AND USES OF THE OXYTOCIC DRUGS

An *oxytocic* drug is one that stimulates the uterus. Included in this group of drugs are ergonovine (Ergotrate), methylergonovine (Methergine), and oxytocin (Pitocin).

Ergonovine and Methylergonovine. Ergonovine and methylergonovine both increase the strength, duration, and frequency of uterine contractions and decrease the incidence of uterine bleeding. They are given after the delivery of the placenta and are used to prevent postpartum and postabortal hemorrhage due to *uterine atony* (marked relaxation of the uterine muscle).

Oxytocin. *Oxytocin* is an endogenous hormone produced by the posterior pituitary gland (see Chap. 38). This hormone has uterine-stimulating properties, especially on the pregnant uterus. As pregnancy progresses, the sensitivity of the uterus to oxytocin increases, reaching peak sensitivity immediately prior to the birth of the infant. This sensitivity enables oxytocin drugs to exert their full therapeutic effect on the uterus and produce the desired results. Oxytocin also has antidiuretic and vasopressor effects. The exact role of oxytocin in normal labor and medically induced labor is not well understood.

Oxytocin is administered intravenously (IV) for starting or improving labor contractions to obtain an early vaginal delivery of the fetus. An early vaginal delivery may be indicated when there are fetal or maternal problems, for example, a diabetic mother with a large fetus, Rh problems, premature rupture of the membranes, uterine inertia, and eclampsia or preeclampsia (also called pregnancy-induced hypertension). Oxytocin may also be used in the management of inevitable or incomplete abortion.

Oxytocin may also be given intramuscularly (IM) during the third stage of labor (period from the time the baby is expelled until the placenta is expelled) to produce uterine contractions and control postpartum bleeding and hemorrhage. It may be used topically as a nasal spray to stimulate the milk ejection (milk letdown) reflex.

ADVERSE REACTIONS ASSOCIATED WITH THE ADMINISTRATION OF THE OXYTOCIC DRUGS

Ergonovine and Methylergonovine. The adverse reactions associated with ergonovine and methylergonovine include nausea, vomiting, diarrhea, elevated blood pressure, temporary chest pain, dizziness, and headache. Allergic reactions may also be seen.

Oxytocin. Administration of oxytocin may result in fetal bradycardia, uterine rupture, neonatal jaundice, nausea, vomiting, *water intoxication* (fluid overload, fluid volume excess), cardiac arrhythmias, and anaphylactic reactions. When used as a nasal spray, adverse reactions are rare. Occasionally, abdominal cramping may be noted.

NURSING MANAGEMENT

Ergonovine and Methylergonovine. Ergonovine and methylergonovine are administered at the direction of the physician. Ergonovine is usually given during the third stage of labor after the placenta has been delivered. Methylergonovine is usually given at the time of the delivery of the anterior shoulder or after the delivery of the placenta. Take and record the mother's blood pressure, pulse, and respiratory rate immediately before the drug is administered.

After injection of the drug, monitor the blood pressure, pulse, and respiratory rate at the intervals ordered by the physician. After leaving the delivery room, palpate the uterine fundus for firmness and position. Report any excess bleeding to the physician immediately.

Ergonovine and methylergonovine may also be given orally during the postpartum period to reduce the possibility of postpartum hemorrhage and to prevent relaxation of the uterus. Monitor the vital signs every 4 hours. The patient may complain of abdominal cramping with the administration of these drugs. If cramping is moderately severe to severe, notify the physician because it may be necessary to discontinue the medication.

Oxytocin. When oxytocin is prescribed, the physician orders the type and amount of IV fluid; the number of units of oxytocin added to the IV solution; and the IV infusion rate. Use an electronic infusion device to control the infusion rate. Place the patient on a fetal monitor to assess the fetal heart rate. Monitoring of the uterine contractions for strength and length of the contractions is also essential and can be done with the use of an external monitor or by an internal uterine catheter with an electronic monitor. Piggyback the IV or use a Y-tubing system so that the one bottle contains the diluent and the oxytocin and the other contains only the IV solution. This allows the solution containing the drug to be discontinued while the other line is available to keep to maintain the patency of the IV when it is necessary to interrupt the infusion of oxytocin.

The physician establishes guidelines for the administration of the oxytocin solution and for increasing or decreasing the flow rate or discontinuing administration of oxytocin based on standards established by the Association of Women's Health, Obstetrics and Neonatal Nurses. Usually, the flow rate is increased every 20 to 30 minutes but this may vary according to the patient's response.

Nursing Alert

All patients receiving IV oxytocin must be under constant observation to identify complications. A one-to-one nurse-patient ratio is recommended when monitoring a patient on a oxytocin infusion. In addition, a qualified physician should be immediately available at all times.

Assess the patient's blood pressure, pulse, and respiratory rate every 30 minutes. Assess the fetal heart rate (FHR) and uterine contractions every 15 minutes or as ordered by the physician. When monitoring uterine contractions, notify the physician immediately if any of the following occurs:

- Any significant change in the FHR or rhythm
- Any marked change in the frequency, rate, or rhythm of uterine contractions: uterine contractions lasting more than 60 seconds or contractions occurring more frequently than every 2 to 3 minutes
- A marked increase or decrease in the patient's blood pressure or pulse or any significant change in the patient's general condition

If any of the above are noted, immediately discontinue the oxytocin infusion and run the primary IV line at the rate prescribed by the physician until the physician examines the patient.

Report any signs of water intoxication or fluid overload (eg, drowsiness, confusion, headache, listlessness, and wheezing, coughing, rapid breathing) to the physician immediately.

Oxytocin may be given IM after delivery of the placenta. Obtain the blood pressure, pulse, and respiratory rate immediately before and every 5 to 10 minutes after the drug is administered. Palpate the fundus of the uterus for a response to the drug.

When administering oxytocin topically, place the patient in an upright position, and, with the squeeze

bottle held upright, deliver the prescribed number of sprays to one or both nostrils. Have the patient then wait 2 to 3 minutes before nursing the infant or pumping the breasts. If a breast pump is being used, record the amount of milk pumped from the breasts.

Notify the physician if milk drips from the breast before or after nursing, if milk drips from the breast not being nursed, or if abdominal cramps occur during nursing because the drug may need to be discontinued.

Nursing Process
The Patient Receiving an Oxytocic Drug

◼ *Assessment*

Before starting an IV infusion of oxytocin, obtain an obstetric history (parity, gravidity, previous obstetric problems, type of labor, stillbirths, abortions, live birth infant abnormalities, and so forth) and a general health history.

Assess the FHR and the mother's blood pressure, pulse, and respiratory rate immediately before starting an IV infusion of oxytocin for the induction of labor. In addition, assess and record the activity of the uterus (strength, duration, and frequency of contractions, if any).

When the patient is to receive ergonovine or methylergonovine, take the blood pressure, pulse, and respiratory rate before administration of either of these drugs.

◼ *Nursing Diagnoses*

Depending on the drug and reason for use, one or more of the following may apply to the patient receiving an oxytocic drug:
- **Anxiety** related to labor and delivery
- **Fluid Volume Excess** related to rapid administration of IV fluids containing oxytocin
- **Knowledge deficit** of therapeutic regimen

◼ *Planning and Implementation*

The major goals of the patient may include a reduction in anxiety, absence of a fluid volume excess (oxytocin administration), and an understanding of the treatment regimen.

Fluid Volume Excess. When oxytocin is administered IV, there is a danger of a fluid volume excess (water intoxication) because oxytocin has an antidiuretic effect. Measure the intake and output. In some instances, hourly measurements of the output are necessary. Observe the patient for signs of fluid overload (see Chap. 48). If these are apparent, notify the physician *immediately* because it may be necessary to change the rate of infusion or discontinue the use of oxytocin.

Anxiety and Knowledge Deficit. When ergonovine or methylergonovine are administered in the delivery room, briefly explain the purpose of the injection to the patient. If either of these drugs is given after delivery of the infant, explain the purpose of the drug (eg, to improve the tone of the uterus and help the uterus to return to its [near] normal size) to the patient.

The patient receiving oxytocin to induce labor may have concern over the use of the drug to produce contractions. Explain the purpose of the IV infusion and the results expected to the patient. Since the patient receiving oxytocin must be closely supervised, spending time with the patient and offering encouragement and reassurance may help reduce anxiety.

■ *Expected Outcomes for Evaluation*

- Anxiety is reduced
- No evidence of a fluid volume excess (oxytocin administration)
- Patient demonstrates understanding of treatment

Uterine Relaxants

Uterine relaxants are useful in the management of preterm labor. These drugs will decrease uterine activity and prolong the pregnancy to allow the fetus to develop more fully thereby increasing the chance of fetal survival. Ritodrine (Yutopar) and terbutaline (Brethine) are two drugs currently used as uterine relaxants in the management of preterm (or premature) labor.

ACTIONS AND USES OF UTERINE RELAXANTS

Ritodrine. Ritodrine has an effect on beta-adrenergic receptors, principally those that innervate the uterus. Stimulation of these beta-adrenergic receptors inhibits uterine smooth muscle contractions. Ritodrine administration initially requires hospital-

ization. If treatment is successful, the patient may continue to take the drug orally at home.

Terbutaline. Terbutaline (Brethine) is also classified as a beta-adrenergic agonist (see Chap. 17) and used primarily as a bronchodilator for patients with asthma and chronic obstructive pulmonary disease. Terbutaline is not approved by the Food and Drug Administration for treatment of preterm labor. Its use in the management of premature labor is investigational. However, many physicians prefer terbutaline to manage preterm labor and it has proven to be highly effective for this purpose. When prescribed, most agencies have the patient sign an informed consent prior to initiating therapy.

ADVERSE REACTIONS ASSOCIATED WITH THE ADMINISTRATION OF UTERINE RELAXANTS

Ritodrine. Alterations in fetal and maternal heart rates and maternal blood pressure frequently occur when ritodrine is administered IV. Additional frequent adverse reactions associated with IV administration include nausea, vomiting, headache, palpitations, and erythema. Oral administration frequently produces a slight increase in the maternal heart rate. Palpitations, tremors, nausea, and vomiting also are seen in a small number of patients.

Terbutaline. Adverse reactions observed with the administration of terbutaline include nervousness, restlessness, tremor, headache, anxiety, hypertension, hypokalemia (low serum potassium), arrhythmias and palpitations. A serious, but rare adverse reaction is pulmonary edema.

NURSING MANAGEMENT

Nursing management for ritodrine and terbutaline is similar. For IV administration, prepare the solution according to the physician's instructions. Use an infusion pump to control the rate of flow. Piggyback ritodrine or terbutaline to the primary line, keeping the primary line to maintain the patency of the IV should it be necessary to temporarily discontinue the infusion of the drug. Place the patient on a cardiac monitor. To minimize hypotension, place the patient in a left lateral position unless the physician orders a different position.

Nursing Alert

Perform the following tasks at 15- to 30-minute intervals:

- Obtain blood pressure, pulse, and respiratory rate
- Obtain FHR
- Check the IV infusion rate
- Examine the area around the IV needle insertion for signs of extravasation
- Monitor uterine contractions (frequency, intensity, length)

Keep the physician informed of the patient's response to the drug because a dosage change may be necessary. The physician establishes guidelines for the regulation of the IV infusion rate, as well as the blood pressure and pulse ranges that require stopping the IV infusion. After contractions cease, the dosage is tapered to the least effective dose by decreasing the infusion rate of the drug at regular intervals prescribed by the physician. Continue the IV infusion for at least 12 hours after uterine contractions have ceased.

Oral maintenance therapy, if ordered, usually begins approximately 30 minutes before the IV infusion is discontinued and continues after the patient is discharged from the hospital or until the delivery of a mature fetus is assured.

With terbutaline, monitor the patient for symptoms of hypokalemia (eg, weakness, fatigue, arrhythmias). Assess respiratory status for symptoms of pulmonary edema (eg, dyspnea, tachycardia, increased respiratory rate, rales, frothy sputum). The physician may prescribe terbutaline for administration by the oral or the subcutaneous route throughout the treatment rather than use the IV route.

Nursing Process

The Patient Receiving a Uterine Relaxant

■ Assessment

Before starting an IV infusion containing ritodrine or terbutaline, obtain the patient's vital signs and the FHR. Auscultate lung sounds to provide a baseline assessment. Assess uterine contractions and FHR prior to administration.

■ Nursing Diagnoses

- **Anxiety** related to preterm labor
- **Risk for Ineffective Management of Therapeutic Regimen** related to lack of knowledge, indifference, other (specify)

■ Planning and Implementation

The major goals of the patient may include a reduction in anxiety and an understanding of the treatment of preterm labor.

Anxiety. The patient in preterm labor may have many concerns about her pregnancy, as well as the effectiveness of drug therapy. Offer emotional support and encouragement during the time the drug is being administered.

■ Patient and Family Teaching

Explain the treatment regimen to the patient. The physician usually discusses the expected outcome of treatment with the patient.

Include the following instructions for patients taking oral ritodrine at home:

- Take the drug exactly as prescribed.
- Do not use any nonprescription drugs unless their use has been approved by the physician.
- Notify the physician immediately if any of the following occur: uterine contractions, nausea, vomiting, palpitations, or shortness of breath.
- Frequent examinations are necessary to monitor therapy.

■ Expected Outcomes for Evaluation

- Anxiety is reduced
- Patient demonstrates understanding of in-hospital treatment
- Patient demonstrates understanding of dosage regimen to be followed at home
- Patient verbalizes understanding of when to notify the physician if problems occur after discharge from the hospital

Abortifacients

Abortifacients are drugs that are used to abort or terminate a pregnancy. Administration of these drugs is one of several methods, such as a hysterotomy or dilation and curettage, that may be used to terminate a pregnancy. The method that is selected to terminate a pregnancy is individualized and is based on many factors, such as the health of the patient, the length of pregnancy, and the facilities available.

ACTIONS OF THE ABORTIFACIENTS

Carboprost (Hemabate) and dinoprostone (Prostin E2) are prostaglandins (fatty acid derivatives whose release is thought to increase the sensitivity of peripheral pain receptors), which stimulate the uterus to contract. By stimulating uterine contractions, the uterus is emptied of the products of pregnancy, that is, the fetus, the placenta, and the amniotic fluid. The manner in which each of these drugs stimulate the uterine muscle is not well understood.

Sodium chloride 20% is injected into the amniotic fluid and produces death of the fetus. The fetus is then expelled.

USES OF THE ABORTIFACIENTS

Carboprost. Carboprost is given IM and is used to abort the fetus between the 13th and 20th weeks of pregnancy.

Dinoprostone. Dinoprostone is administered intravaginally and is used to abort the fetus between the 12th and 20th weeks of pregnancy.

Sodium Chloride 20%. Sodium chloride is administered transabdominally into the amniotic fluid. This procedure is performed by the physician. It is used to abort the fetus during the second trimester of pregnancy, preferably between the 16th and 22nd weeks of pregnancy.

ADVERSE REACTIONS ASSOCIATED WITH ADMINISTRATION OF THE ABORTIFACIENTS

Carboprost. Adverse drug reactions to carboprost are usually temporary and disappear when therapy is completed. Adverse reactions include vomiting, diarrhea, nausea, headache, paresthesia, flushing, chills, and sweating. Rupture of the uterus has been reported.

Dinoprostone. After administration of dinoprostone, the most frequent adverse reactions seen are nausea, vomiting, hypotension, diarrhea, chills, and headache. Fever, joint inflammation and pain, and tightness in the chest may also be seen.

Sodium Chloride 20%. Accidental injection of the sodium chloride solution into the vascular system may occur when this drug is given. Additional adverse reactions include fever, flushing, fluid overload, pulmonary embolus, and changes in the blood coagulating mechanism.

NURSING MANAGEMENT

When carboprost is to be used, the physician may order an antiemetic or an antidiarrheal agent before administration of carboprost. Use a tuberculin syringe to measure and administer this drug. Give carboprost deep IM and rotate injection sites if more than one injection is necessary.

Administer dinoprostone as a vaginal suppository. Remove the suppository from the freezer and allow to reach room temperature before insertion. Carefully remove the foil wrapper from the suppository; avoid contact with the fingers. Place the patient in a supine position. Wearing a glove, the physician inserts the suppository high into the vagina. Keep the patient in the supine position for about 10 minutes after insertion of the suppository. The physician may allow ambulation after that time.

Sodium chloride is administered by the physician. About 250 mL is instilled into the amniotic sac by means of a transabdominal incision. The nurse is responsible for obtaining the necessary equipment for the procedure.

After administration of an abortifacient, observe for the onset of uterine contractions every 30 minutes to 1 hour. The time of the onset of labor, the length and intensity of each contraction, and the time interval between contractions are recorded. Monitor the blood pressure, pulse, and respiratory rate every 1 to 4 hours or according to unit policy or the physician's orders.

Notify the physician if adverse drug reactions occur and keep the physician informed of the patient's response to the abortifacient. Save all tissue expelled for examination either by the physician or by a laboratory. A vaginal examination may be performed by the physician after the fetus is passed.

Nursing Process
The Patient Receiving an Abortifacient

■ *Assessment*

Before the administration of an abortifacient, take the patient's vital signs. Some hospitals or clinics performing this procedure may also have additional assessments that are required before the procedure is begun.

■ *Nursing Diagnoses*
● **Anxiety** related to procedure
● **Knowledge Deficit** of abortion procedure

■ *Planning and Implementation*

The major goals of the patient may include a reduction in anxiety and an understanding of the abortion procedure.

Anxiety. Thoroughly explain the procedure to be performed to the patient. The physician or the nurse should also explain some of the adverse reactions that may occur during and after the procedure.

Emotional support is needed before, during, and after the administration of an abortifacient. Reassurance and understanding is required: the amount depends on the individual.

Knowledge Deficit. The amount of time spent in a hospital or clinic after the administration of an abortifacient varies. In addition, the instructions given to the patient about the passage of the fetus and postabortion examination also vary. Some hospitals or clinics may allow the patient to leave the facility and return when uterine contractions begin. The postdischarge instructions given to the patient are usually established by the facility performing the procedure or by a physician. Advise the patient to follow the instructions given by the physician or facility carefully.

■ *Expected Outcomes for Evaluation*

- Anxiety is reduced
- Patient verbalizes understanding of the abortion procedure
- Patient verbalizes understanding of the postprocedure directions given by the physician

Chapter Summary

- The three principal types of drugs used for their effect on the uterus are the oxytocics, the uterine relaxants, and the abortifacients. Oxytocic drugs stimulate the uterus. Ergonovine (Ergotrate) and methylergonovine (Methergine) are oxytocic drugs that increase the strength, duration, and frequency of uterine contractions and decrease uterine bleeding. They are useful after the delivery of the placenta to prevent postpartum and postabortal hemorrhage due to uterine atony. The major adverse reactions associated with ergonovine and methylergonovine are nausea, vomiting, diarrhea, elevated blood pressure, and chest pain.
- Oxytocin (Pitocin) is administered for starting or improving labor contractions to obtain an early vaginal delivery of the fetus. Administration of oxytocin may result in fetal bradycardia, uterine rupture, neonatal jaundice, nausea, and vomiting. The drug is administered by the intravenous route

with an electronic infusion device to control the infusion rate. A fetal monitor is used to detect any fetal distress. The physician establishes guidelines for the administration of the oxytocin solution and for increasing or decreasing the flow rate or discontinuing administration of oxytocin.

- Uterine relaxants are useful in the management of preterm labor. These drugs will decrease uterine activity and prolong the pregnancy to allow the fetus to develop more fully, thereby increasing the chance of fetal survival. Ritodrine (Yutopar) and terbutaline (Brethine) are used as uterine relaxants. The patient is monitored closely during administration since alterations in fetal and maternal heart rate and maternal blood pressure frequently occur.
- The use of terbutaline to manage preterm labor is investigational. However, most patients respond well when the drug is administered within established protocols. When used for the management of preterm labor, most agencies have the patient sign an informed consent prior to initiating therapy.
- Abortifacients are drugs that are used to abort or terminate a pregnancy. Carboprost (Hemabate) and dinoprostone (Prostin E2) are abortifacients that stimulate the uterus to contract. By stimulating uterine contractions, the uterus is emptied of the products of pregnancy, that is, the fetus, the placenta, and the amniotic fluid.
- After administration of an abortifacient, the patient is observed for the onset of uterine contractions every 30 minutes to 1 hour. The physician is notified if adverse drug reactions occur and kept informed of the patient's response to the abortifacient. All tissue expelled is saved for examination either by the physician or by a laboratory. A vaginal examination may be performed by the physician after the fetus is passed.

Critical Thinking Exercises

1. Develop a nursing care plan for Ms. Morris, a 28-year-old female, who is admitted to the obstetrical unit with premature labor. This is her second child and she has had two miscarriages. What nursing diagnoses would have the highest priority? How would you explore and plan to meet Ms. Morris' emotional needs?
2. Judith Watson, aged 28, is admitted to the obstetric unit and is to receive oxytocin to induce labor. What information would be necessary for her to receive from the nurse prior to the administration of oxytocin?

Drugs That Affect Other Body Systems

IX

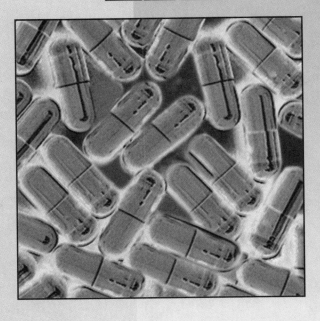

42

Drugs Used in the Management of Gastrointestinal Disorders

Chapter Objectives

On completion of this chapter the student will:

- *List the type of drugs prescribed or recommended for gastrointestinal disorders*
- *Discuss the actions and adverse reactions associated with gastrointestinal drugs*
- *Discuss the nursing implications to be considered when administering a gastrointestinal drug*
- *Use the nursing process when administering a gastrointestinal drug*

The gastrointestinal (GI) tract is subject to more diseases and disorders than any other system of the body. Some drugs used for GI disorders are available as nonprescription drugs, thereby creating potential problems of misuse and overuse, as well as disguising more serious medical problems.

Drugs Used in the Management of Gastrointestinal Disorders

The drugs presented in this chapter include the antacids, anticholinergics, GI stimulants, histamine H_2 antagonists, antidiarrheals, antiflatulents, digestive enzymes, emetics, gallstone-solubilizing agents, laxatives, and miscellaneous drugs. Some of the more common preparations and their individual uses are listed in Summary Drug Table 42-1.

ACTIONS OF THE DRUGS USED IN THE MANAGEMENT OF GASTROINTESTINAL DISORDERS

Antacids

Some of the cells of the stomach secrete *hydrochloric acid*, a substance that aids in the initial digestive process. *Antacids* (against acids) are drugs that neutralize or reduce the acidity of stomach and duodenal contents by combining with hydrochloric acid and producing salt and water. Examples of antacids include aluminum hydroxide gel (Amphojel), magnesia (magnesium hydroxide) and magaldrate (Riopan).

Anticholinergics

Anticholinergics (cholinergic blocking drugs) reduce gastric motility and decrease the amount of acid secreted by the stomach (see Chap. 20). Examples of anticholinergics used for GI disorders include propantheline (Pro-Banthine) and glycopyrrolate (Robinul).

Gastrointestinal Stimulants

Metoclopramide (Reglan) and dexpanthenol (Ilopan) increase the motility of the upper GI tract. The exact mode of action of these drugs is unclear. Cisapride (Propulsid) enhances the release of acetylcholine (a neurohormone necessary for normal intestinal function) thereby increasing GI motility.

Histamine H_2 Antagonists

These drugs inhibit the action of histamine at histamine H_2 receptor cells of the stomach, which then reduces the secretion of gastric acid. Examples of histamine H_2 antagonists include cimetidine (Tagamet), ranitidine (Zantac), famotidine (Pepcid), and nizatidine (Axid Pulvules).

Antidiarrheals

Antidiarrheals decrease intestinal peristalsis, which is usually increased when the patient has diarrhea. Examples of these drugs include difenoxin with atropine (Motofen), diphenoxylate with atropine (Lomotil), and loperamide (Imodium).

Antiflatulents

Simethicone (Mylicon) and charcoal are used as *antiflatulents* (against flatus or gas in the intestinal tract). Simethicone has a defoaming action that disperses and prevents the formation of mucus-surrounded gas pockets in the intestine. Charcoal is an absorbent that reduces the amount of intestinal gas.

Digestive Enzymes

The enzymes pancreatin and pancrelipase, which are manufactured and secreted by the pancreas, are responsible for the breakdown of fats, starches, and proteins. These enzymes are necessary for the breakdown and digestion of food. Both enzymes are available as oral supplements.

Emetics

The *emetic* (a drug that induces vomiting) apomorphine promotes vomiting by its direct action on the vomiting center (chemoreceptor trigger zone) of the medulla. Ipecac causes vomiting because of its local irritating effect on the stomach, as well as by stimulation of the vomiting center in the medulla. Examples of emetics include apomorphine and ipecac syrup.

Gallstone-Solubilizing Agents

Gallstone-solubilizing (gallstone-dissolving) agents, for example, ursodiol (Actigall) suppress the manufacture of cholesterol and cholic acid by the liver. The

Summary Drug Table 42-1. Drugs Used in the Management of Gastrointestinal Disorders

Generic Name	Trade Name*	Dose Ranges
ANTACIDS†		
aluminum carbonate gel, basic	Basaljel	2 capsules or tablets or 10 mL of suspension PO prn up to 12 times/d
aluminum hydroxide gel	Amphojel, *generic*	500–1500 mg tablets or capsules PO 3–6 times/d; 5–30 mL suspension PO prn between meals and hs
calcium carbonate	Dicarbosil, Tums, *generic*	0.5–1.5 g PO as needed
magaldrate	Riopan, *generic*	5–10 mL PO between meals and hs
magnesia (magnesium hydroxide)	Milk of Magnesia	5–15 mL PO up to 4 times/d; liquid concentrate: 2.5–7.5 PO up to 4 times/d; tablets: 622–1244 mg PO up to 4 times/d
sodium bicarbonate	Bell/ans, *generic*	0.3–2 g PO 1–4 times/d
ANTICHOLINERGICS		
glycopyrrolate	Robinul, Robinul Forte, *generic*	1–2 mg PO 2–3 times/d; 0.1–0.2 mg IM, IV 3–4 times/d
propantheline bromide	Pro-Banthine, *generic*	15 mg PO 30 min ac and hs
GASTROINTESTINAL STIMULANTS		
cisapride	Propulsid	10–20 mg PO qid 15 min ac and hs
dexpanthenol	Ilopan, *generic*	Postoperative ileus: 250–500 mg IM; treatment of paralytic ileus: 500 mg IM
metoclopramide	Reglan, *generic*	10–15 mg PO 30 min ac and hs; 10–20 mg IM, IV
HISTAMINE H₂ ANTAGONISTS		
cimetidine	Tagamet	300–2400 mg/d PO in divided doses; alternate dose schedules include: 400–800 mg PO hs; 300 mg PO qid; up to 2400 mg/d IM in divided doses; 300 mg intermittent IV infusion; 37.5 mg/h continuous IV infusion
famotidine	Pepcid, Pepcid IV	20–40 mg PO at hs or 20 mg PO bid or q6h; 20 mg IV q12h
nizatidine	Axid Pulvules	150 mg PO bid or 150–300 mg PO at hs
ranitidine	Zantac	150 mg PO bid or 300 mg PO hs; 50 mg q6–8h IM, IV
ANTIDIARRHEALS		
difenoxin hydrochloride with atropine sulfate	Motofen	Initial dose 2 tablets PO then 1 tablet after each loose stool
diphenoxylate hydrochloride with atropine sulfate	Lomotil, Lonox, *generic*	Initial dose 5 mg PO qid then as needed
loperamide hydrochloride	Imodium A-D, Maalox Anti-Diarrheal Caplets, *generic*	Initial dose 4 mg PO then 2 mg after each loose stool
ANTIFLATULENTS		
charcoal	CharcoCaps, *generic*	520 mg PO pc
simethicone	Gas-X, Mylicon, *generic*	125 mg capsules PO qid pc and hs, 40–125 mg tablets PO qid pc and hs
DIGESTIVE ENZYMES		
pancreatin	Entozyme Tablets, Dizymes Tablets	1–2 tablets PO with meals or snacks
pancrelipase	Cotazym Capsules, Viokase Powder, Ilozyme Tablets	4000–48,000 units lipase PO with meals and snacks

(continued)

Summary Drug Table 42-1 (Continued)

Generic Name	Trade Name*	Dose Ranges
EMETICS		
apomorphine hydrochloride	*generic*	2–10 mg SC; do not repeat
ipecac syrup	*generic*	15–30 mL PO followed by 3–4 glasses of water; children: dosage based on age: 5–15 mL PO followed by ½ to 2 glasses of water
GALLSTONE-SOLUBILIZING AGENTS		
ursodiol	Actigall	8–10 mg/kg/d PO in 2–3 divided doses
LAXATIVES‡		
Bulk-Producing Laxatives		
polycarbophil	FiberCon, Fiberall	1 g PO daily to qid or as needed
psyllium	Metamucil, Konsyl	1 rounded teaspoon stirred into 1 glass of liquid PO 1–3 times/d
Emollient Laxatives		
mineral oil	Agoral Plain, Kondremul Plain, *generic*	5–45 mL PO
Fecal Softeners		
docusate calcium	Surfak Liquigels, *generic*	240 mg PO daily
docusate sodium	Colace, Modane Soft, *generic*	50–500 mg PO
Hyperosmolar Agents		
glycerin	Sani-Supp, *generic*	1 rectal suppository
Irritant or Stimulant Laxatives		
bisacodyl	Dulcolax, *generic*	10–15 mg PO or one 10 mg rectal suppository; up to 30 mg PO as preparation for lower GI procedures
cascara sagrada	*generic*	5 mL or 1 tablet PO hs
phenolphthalein	Ex-Lax, Feen-a-mint	60–194 mg PO hs
senna	Senolax	2–8 tablets/d PO
Saline Laxatives		
magnesium hydroxide	Phillips' Milk of Magnesia, *generic*	15–30 mL PO
Miscellaneous Drugs		
mesalamine	Asacol, Pentasa, Rowasa	Tablets: 800 mg PO tid; capsules: 1 g PO qid; rectal suppository: one bid
misoprostol	Cytotec	100–200 mcg PO qid with food
olsalazine sodium	Dipentum	1 g/d PO in 2 divided doses
omeprazole	Prilosec	20–60 mg/d PO; doses up to 120 mg PO tid may be used
sucralfate	Carafate	1 g PO bid to qid
sulfasalazine	Azulfidine, *generic*	1–4 g/d PO in divided doses

*The term, *generic*, indicates the drug is available in a generic form.
†Some antacids offer a combination of drugs and may contain one or more of the agents listed.
‡Some laxatives offer a combination of drugs and may contain one or more of the agents listed.

suppression of the manufacture of cholesterol and cholic acid may ultimately result in a decrease in the size of radiolucent gallstones.

Laxatives

There are various types of laxatives (see Summary Drug Table 42-1). The action of each laxative is somewhat different, yet produces the same result—the relief of constipation.

- **Bulk-producing laxatives** are not digested by the body and therefore add bulk and water to the contents of the intestines. The added bulk in the intestines stimulates peristalsis, moves the products of digestion through the intestine, and encourages evacuation of the stool. Examples of

bulk-forming laxatives are psyllium (Metamucil) and polycarbophil (FiberCon).
- **Emollient laxatives** lubricate the intestinal walls and soften the stool, thereby enhancing passage of fecal material. Mineral oil is an emollient laxative.
- **Fecal softeners** promote water retention in the fecal mass and soften the stool. One difference between emollient laxatives and fecal softeners is that the emollient laxatives do not promote the retention of water in the stool. Examples of fecal softeners include docusate sodium (Colace) and docusate calcium (Surfak).
- **Hyperosmolar agents** dehydrate local tissues, which causes irritation and increased peristalsis with consequent evacuation of the fecal mass. Glycerin is a hyperosmolar agent.
- **Irritant or stimulant laxatives** increase peristalsis by direct action on the intestine. An example of an irritant laxative is cascara sagrada and senna (Senokot).
- **Saline laxatives** attract or pull water into the intestine, thereby increasing pressure in the intestine followed by an increase in peristalsis. Magnesium hydroxide (Milk of Magnesia) is a saline laxative.

Miscellaneous Drugs

Misoprostol (Cytotec) inhibits gastric acid secretion and increases the protective property of the mucosal lining of the GI tract by increasing the production of mucus by the lining of the GI tract. Sucralfate (Carafate) exerts a local action on the lining of the stomach. The drug forms a complex with the exudate of the stomach lining. This complex forms a protective layer over a duodenal ulcer, thus aiding in healing of the ulcer. Omeprazole (Prilosec) suppresses gastric acid secretion by blocking the final step in the production of gastric acid by the gastric mucosa.

Mesalamine (Asacol), olsalazine (Dipentum), and sulfasalazine (Azulfidine) are three drugs that exert a topical antiinflammatory effect in the bowel. The exact mechanism of action of these drugs is unknown.

USES OF DRUGS USED IN THE MANAGEMENT OF GASTROINTESTINAL DISORDERS

Antacids

Antacids are used in the treatment of gastric distress, such as heartburn and acid indigestion, and in the medical treatment of peptic ulcer. Many antacid preparations contain more than one ingredient, for example, Maalox, which consists of aluminum hydroxide *and* magnesium hydroxide.

Anticholinergics

Specific anticholinergic drugs are occasionally used in the medical treatment of peptic ulcer. These drugs have been largely replaced by histamine H_2 antagonists, which appear to be more effective and have less adverse drug reactions.

Gastrointestinal Stimulants

Oral preparations of metoclopramide are used in the treatment of symptomatic *gastroesophageal reflux disease* (GERD; a reflux or backup of gastric contents into the esophagus), and *gastric stasis* (failure to normally move food out of the stomach) in diabetics. This drug is given parenterally to prevent nausea and vomiting associated with cancer chemotherapy, and to prevent nausea and vomiting during the immediate postoperative period. Dexpanthenol may be given parenterally immediately after major abdominal surgery to reduce the risk of *paralytic ileus* (lack of peristalsis or movement of the intestines). Cisapride is used in the treatment of heartburn associated with GERD.

Histamine H_2 Antagonists

These drugs are used for medical treatment of a gastric or duodenal ulcer, gastric *hypersecretory* (excessive gastric secretion of hydrochloric acid) conditions, and GERD.

Antidiarrheals

Antidiarrheals are used in the treatment of diarrhea.

Antiflatulents

Antiflatulents are used to reduce gas formation in the intestines. Simethicone may also be included in some antacid products, for example, Mylanta Liquid and Di-Gel Liquid.

Digestive Enzymes

These drugs are prescribed as replacement therapy for those with pancreatic enzyme insufficiency. Conditions or diseases that may cause a decrease in or absence of pancreatic digestive enzymes include cystic fibrosis, chronic pancreatitis, cancer of the pancreas, the malabsorption syndrome, surgical removal of all or part of the stomach, and surgical removal of all or part of the pancreas.

Emetics

Emetics are used to cause vomiting and thereby empty the stomach rapidly when an individual has accidentally or intentionally ingested a poison or drug overdose. Not all poison ingestions or drug overdoses are treated with emetics.

Gallstone-Solubilizing Agents

These drugs are used in the nonsurgical treatment of radiolucent gallstones. They are not effective for all types of gallstones and require many months of drug therapy to produce results. Because of potential toxic effects associated with long-term use, these drugs are only recommended for carefully selected and closely monitored patients.

Laxatives

A laxative may be ordered for the short-term relief or prevention of constipation; for prevention of straining at stool when this is contraindicated; before examination of the rectum; and in preparation for surgery and diagnostic tests, such as radiographic examination of the bowel.

Miscellaneous Drugs

Mesalamine is used in the treatment of chronic inflammatory bowel disease. Olsalazine is used in the treatment of ulcerative colitis in those allergic to sulfasalazine. Sulfasalazine is used in the treatment of Crohn's disease and ulcerative colitis.

Omeprazole is used in the treatment of duodenal ulcer and GERD. Sucralfate is used in the treatment of duodenal ulcer. Misoprostol is used to prevent gastric ulcers in those taking aspirin or nonsteroidal antiinflammatory drugs in high doses for a prolonged time.

ADVERSE REACTIONS ASSOCIATED WITH THE ADMINISTRATION OF DRUGS USED IN THE MANAGEMENT OF GASTROINTESTINAL DISORDERS

Antacids

The magnesium-containing antacids may have a laxative effect and produce diarrhea. Aluminum-containing and calcium-containing products tend to produce constipation.

Anticholinergics

Dry mouth, blurred vision, urinary hesitancy, urinary retention, nausea, vomiting, palpitations, and headache are some of the adverse reactions that may be seen with the use of anticholinergic drugs (see Chap. 20).

Gastrointestinal Stimulants

The adverse reactions associated with metoclopramide are usually mild. Higher doses or prolonged administration may produce central nervous system symptoms, such as drowsiness, dizziness, Parkinson-like symptoms (tremor, masklike facial expression, muscle rigidity), depression, facial grimacing, motor restlessness, and involuntary movements of the eyes, face, or limbs. Dexpanthenol administration may cause itching, difficulty breathing, and urticaria. The adverse reactions that may be seen with the administration of cisapride include diarrhea, abdominal pain, nausea, constipation, and headache.

Histamine H₂ Antagonists

There is a low incidence of adverse reactions seen with the administration of these drugs. Mild and transient diarrhea, dizziness, and fatigue have been reported with the use of cimetidine. Famotidine administration may result in headache and dizziness.

Antidiarrheals

Diphenoxylate use may result in anorexia, nausea, vomiting, constipation, rash, dizziness, drowsiness, sedation, euphoria, and headache. This drug is a narcotic-related drug that has no analgesic activity but has sedative and euphoric effects and drug dependence potential. To discourage abuse, it is combined with atropine (an anticholinergic or cholinergic blocking drug), which causes dry mouth and other mild adverse effects. Loperamide is not a narcotic-related drug; minimal adverse reactions are associated with its use. Occasionally, abdominal discomfort, pain, and distention have been seen, but these symptoms are also seen with severe diarrhea and are difficult to distinguish from an adverse drug reaction.

Antiflatulents

No adverse reactions have been reported with the use of antiflatulents.

Digestive Enzymes

No adverse reactions have been reported with the use of digestive enzymes; however, high doses may cause nausea and diarrhea.

Emetics

Therapeutic doses of apomorphine may cause central nervous system depression. There are no apparent adverse reactions to ipecac. Although not an adverse reaction, a danger associated with any emetic is the aspiration of vomitus.

Gallstone-Solubilizing Agents

Diarrhea, cramps, nausea, and vomiting are the more common adverse drug reactions. A reduction in the dose may reduce or eliminate these problems. Prolonged use of these agents may result in hepatotoxicity (toxic to the liver).

Laxatives

Laxative use, especially high doses or use over a long time, can cause diarrhea and a loss of water and electrolytes. For some patients, this may be a serious adverse effect. Laxatives may also cause abdominal pain or discomfort, nausea, vomiting, perianal irritation, and weakness. Prolonged use of a laxative can result in serious electrolyte imbalances, as well as the "laxative habit," that is, a dependency on a laxative to have a bowel movement.

Miscellaneous Drugs

Oral administration of mesalamine administration may cause abdominal pain, nausea, headache, dizziness, fever, and weakness. The adverse reactions associated with rectal administration are less than those seen with oral administration but headache, abdominal discomfort, flulike syndrome, and weakness may still occur. Olsalazine administration may result in diarrhea, abdominal discomfort, and nausea. Sulfasalazine is a sulfonamide with adverse reactions the same as for the sulfonamide drugs (see Chap. 11 and Summary Drug Table 11-1).

The more common adverse reactions seen with omeprazole include headache, abdominal pain, and nausea. The adverse reactions seen with the administration of sucralfate are usually mild but constipation may be seen in a small number of patients. Misoprostol administration may result in diarrhea, abdominal pain, nausea, GI distress, and vomiting.

NURSING MANAGEMENT

Assess the patient receiving one of these drugs for relief of symptoms (diarrhea, pain, constipation, and so on). Notify the physician if the drug fails to relieve symptoms.

Monitor vital signs daily and more frequently if the patient has a bleeding peptic ulcer, severe diarrhea, or other condition that may warrant more frequent observation. Evaluate the effectiveness of drug therapy by a daily comparison of symptoms with those experienced before starting therapy. In some instances, frequent evaluation of the patient's response to therapy may be necessary.

Antacids

Antacids are not given within 2 hours before or after administration of other oral drugs. When antacids are given, keep a record of bowel movements because use of these drugs may cause constipation or diarrhea. If the patient expresses a dislike for the taste of the antacid or has difficulty chewing the tablet form, inform the physician. A flavored antacid may be ordered if the taste is a problem, or a liquid form if there is a problem chewing a tablet.

Anticholinergics

Urinary retention or hesitancy may be seen during therapy with these drugs. This can be avoided by instructing the patient to void before taking the drug. If urinary retention is suspected, monitor the intake and output. These drugs also may cause drowsiness, dizziness, and blurred vision, which may interfere with activities such as reading or watching television. If dizziness occurs, the patient will require assistance with ambulatory activities. If *photophobia* (aversion to bright light) occurs, the room may be kept semidark.

Gastrointestinal Stimulants

If drowsiness or dizziness occurs with the administration of metoclopramide, the patient will require assistance with ambulatory activities. Observe patients receiving high or prolonged doses of this drug for adverse reactions related to the central nervous system.

Dexpanthenol is administered to prevent paralytic ileus during the immediate postoperative period. The patient is therefore observed for signs of this complication, namely, abdominal pain and distention. The drug also may be given if a paralytic ileus has occurred, in which case bowel sounds will be diminished or absent. Auscultate the abdomen frequently for the presence or absence of bowel sounds and inform the physician of the results of these assessments.

Histamine H₂ Antagonists

When one of these drugs is given by the parenteral route, monitor the rate of infusion at frequent intervals. Too rapid an infusion has been reported to occasionally result in cardiac arrhythmias.

Antidiarrheals

Notify the physician if an elevation in temperature occurs or if severe abdominal pain or abdominal rigidity or distention occurs, because this may indicate a complication of the disorder, such as infection or intestinal perforation. If diarrhea is severe, addi-

tional treatment measures, such as IV fluids and electrolyte replacement, may be necessary.

Drowsiness or dizziness may occur with these drugs. The patient may require assistance with ambulatory activities. If diarrhea is chronic, encourage the patient to drink extra fluids. In some instances, the physician may prescribe an oral electrolyte supplement to replace electrolytes lost by frequent loose stools.

Digestive Enzymes

Observe the patient for nausea and diarrhea. If these occur, notify the physician before the next dose is due because dosage may need to be reduced. Check the patient's tray after each meal. If the diet is taken poorly or if certain foods are not eaten, bring this to the attention of the physician. Weigh the patient is weighed weekly (or as ordered) and bring any significant or steady weight loss to the attention of the physician.

Note and record the appearance of each stool. Periodic stool examinations, as well as ongoing descriptions of the appearance of the stools, help the physician determine the effectiveness of therapy.

Emetics

After the administration of an emetic, observe the patient closely for signs of shock, respiratory depression, or other signs and symptoms that may be part of the clinical picture of the specific poison or drug that was accidentally or purposely taken.

Laxatives

Record the results of administration on the patient's chart. If excessive bowel movements or severe prolonged diarrhea occurs or if the laxative is ineffective, notify the physician. If a laxative is ordered for constipation, encourage a liberal fluid intake to prevent a repeat of this problem.

Nursing Process
The Patient Receiving a Drug for a Gastrointestinal Disorder

■ *Assessment*

Review the patient's chart for the medical diagnosis and reason for administration of the prescribed drug. Question the patient regarding the type and intensity of symptoms (pain, discomfort, diarrhea, constipation, and so on) to provide a baseline for evaluation of the effectiveness of drug therapy.

■ *Nursing Diagnoses*

Depending on the patient's symptoms and reason for administration, one or more of the following nursing diagnoses may apply to a person receiving a GI drug:

- **Anxiety** related to diagnosis, symptoms, adverse drug reactions, other factors
- **Noncompliance** related to lack of knowledge, other factors
- **Risk for Ineffective Management of Therapeutic Regimen** related to lack of knowledge of medication regimen

■ *Planning and Implementation*

The major goals of the patient may include a reduction in anxiety and an understanding of and compliance to the prescribed therapeutic regimen. To make these goals measurable, more specific criteria must be added.

■ *Administration*

Special considerations for the administration of certain GI preparations are listed in the following sections.

Antacids. Shake liquid antacid preparations thoroughly immediately before administration. If tablets are given, instruct the patient to chew the tablets thoroughly before swallowing and then drink a full glass of water or milk. Liquid antacids are followed by a small amount of water or milk. Antacids may be ordered to be left at the patient's bedside for self-administration. Be sure an adequate supply of water and cups for measuring the dose are available.

Gastrointestinal Stimulants. Carefully time the administration of oral cisapride and metoclopramide. Cisapride must be given 15 minutes before each meal and oral metoclopramide 30 minutes before each meal.

Histamine H₂ Antagonists. Give ranitidine without regard to meals, but give oral cimetidine immediately before or with meals. Nizatidine and famotidine are given at bedtime. In certain situations or disorders, cimetidine and ranitidine may also be given by intermittent intravenous infusion or direct intravenous injection.

Antidiarrheals. These drugs may be ordered to be given after each loose bowel movement. Inspect each bowel movement before making a decision to administer the drug.

Digestive Enzymes. When digestive enzymes are given in capsule or enteric-coated tablet form, instruct the patient not to bite or chew the capsule or tablet. If the patient experiences difficulty swallowing the capsule form, open the capsule and sprinkle the contents on a small amount of soft food that is not hot, such as applesauce or flavored gelatin.

Emetics. Because treatment of poison ingestion is of an emergency nature, immediately obtain equipment for treatment. Along with the drug, obtain an emesis basin, towels, specimen containers (for sending contents of the stomach to the laboratory for analysis), and a suction machine and place them near the patient. Obtain the blood pressure, pulse, and respiratory rate and perform a brief physical examination to determine what other damages or injuries, if any, may have occurred.

Nursing Alert

Before an emetic is given, it is extremely important to know the chemicals or substance that have been ingested, the time they were ingested, and what symptoms were noted before seeking medical treatment. This information will probably be obtained from a family member or friend, but the adult patient may also contribute to the history. The physician or nurse may also contact the local poison center to obtain information regarding treatment.

An emetic must *not* be given when a corrosive substance (such as lye) or a petroleum distillate (paint thinner, kerosene, and so on) has been ingested. In many cases of poisoning, it is preferable to insert a nasogastric tube to empty stomach contents. These drugs are used with great caution, if at all, when the substance ingested is unknown or in question. An emetic is never given to a patient who is unconscious or semiconscious because aspiration of vomitus may occur.

Activated charcoal may be given before or after administration of apomorphine. Apomorphine is given by the subcutaneous route. Give oral fluids immediately after administration of apomorphine to dilute the poison and encourage vomiting. Position the patient on his or her side before or immediately after the drug is given. When emesis occurs, suction the patient as needed and observe closely for the possible aspiration of vomitus. Monitor vital signs every 5 to 10 minutes until stable.

Laxatives. Give bulk-producing or fecal-softening laxatives with a *full* glass of water or juice. Follow the administration of a bulk-producing laxative by an additional full glass of water. Mineral oil is preferably given on an empty stomach in the evening. Immediately before administration, thoroughly mix and stir laxatives that are in powder, flake, or granule form. If the laxative has an unpleasant or salty taste, explain this to the patient. Taste of some of these preparations may be disguised by chilling, adding to juice, or pouring over cracked ice.

Adverse Drug Reactions. Observe the patient for adverse drug reactions associated with the specific GI drug being administered and report any adverse reactions to the physician before the next dose is due.

Anxiety. Some patients may experience anxiety over circumstances, such as their diagnosis, the symptoms of their disorder, or the adverse drug reactions that may be seen with the administration of some of these drugs. Allow patients time to discuss their problems or to ask questions. Once problems that may be causing anxiety are identified, anxiety may be relieved by simple explanations. For example, a patient may be concerned over certain adverse reactions, such as a dry mouth (anticholinergics) or constipation (some antacids). Explain that these may need to be tolerated and that these adverse reactions may lessen over time. In addition, suggestions can be made to help relieve some adverse drug reactions, such as frequent sips of water to relieve a dry mouth or an increase in fluid intake to correct constipation.

Noncompliance. When a GI drug must be taken for a long time, there is a possibility that the patient may begin to skip doses or stop the drug. Encourage patients to take the prescribed drug as directed by the physician and emphasize the importance of not omitting doses or stopping the drug unless advised to do so by the physician.

■ *Patient and Family Teaching*
Include the following information in a patient and family teaching plan:

Antacids
- Do not use indiscriminately. Check with a physician before using an antacid if you have other medical problems, such as a cardiac condition (some laxatives contain sodium).
- Chew tablets thoroughly before swallowing and then drink a full glass of water.
- Adhere to the dosage schedule recommended by the physician. Do not increase the frequency of use or the dose if symptoms become worse. Instead, see the physician as soon as possible.
- Antacids impair the absorption of some drugs. Do not take other drugs within 2 hours before or after taking the antacid unless use of an antacid with a drug is recommended by the physician.
- If pain or discomfort remains the same or becomes worse, if the stools turn black, or if other symptoms occur, contact the physician as soon as possible.
- Antacids may change the color of the stool (white, white streaks); this is normal.

Anticholinergics
- If an aversion to light occurs, wear sunglasses when outside, keep rooms dimly lit, and schedule outdoor activities (when necessary) before the first dose of the drug is taken, such as early in the morning.
- If a dry mouth occurs, take frequent sips of cool water during the day. Take several sips of water before taking oral medications and sip water frequently during meals.
- Constipation may be avoided by drinking plenty of fluids during the day.
- Drowsiness may occur with these drugs. Schedule tasks requiring alertness during times when drowsiness does not occur, such as early in the morning before the first dose of the drug is taken.

Gastrointestinal Stimulants
- Take the drug as directed before each meal.
- Metoclopramide—if drowsiness or dizziness occurs observe caution while driving or performing hazardous tasks.
- Cisapride—avoid the use of alcohol while taking this drug as the sedative effects of alcohol may be increased.

Histamine H_2 Antagonists
- Keep the physician informed of the results of therapy, that is, relief of pain or discomfort.
- Take as directed (eg, with meals, at bedtime) on the prescription container.
- Follow physician's recommendations regarding additional treatment, such as eliminating certain foods, avoiding the use of alcohol, using additional drugs, such as an antacid, and so on.
- Cimetidine—If drowsiness occurs, avoid driving or performing other hazardous tasks.

Antidiarrheals
- Do not exceed the recommended dosage.
- The drug may cause drowsiness. Observe caution when driving or performing other hazardous tasks.

- Avoid the use of alcohol or other central nervous system depressants (tranquilizers, sleeping pills) and other nonprescription drugs unless use has been approved by the physician.
- Notify the physician if diarrhea persists or becomes more severe.

Digestive Enzymes
- Take as directed by the physician. Do not exceed the recommended dose.
- Do not chew tablets or capsules. Powder form may be sprinkled over small quantities of food. All the food sprinkled with the powder must be eaten.
- If capsules are difficult to swallow, open the capsule and sprinkle the contents on a small amount of soft food that is not hot.

Emetics (Ipecac Syrup)
- Ipecac is available without a prescription for use in the home. The instructions for use and the recommended dose are printed on the label.
- Read the directions on the label after the drug is purchased and be familiar with these instructions before an emergency occurs.
- In case of accidental or intentional poisoning, contact the nearest poison center *before* using or giving this drug. *Not all poisoning can be treated with this drug.*
- *Do not give this drug to semiconscious, unconscious, or convulsing individuals.*
- Vomiting should occur in 20 to 30 minutes. Seek medical attention immediately after contacting the poison center and giving this drug.

Gallstone-Solubilizing Agents
- Periodic laboratory tests (liver function studies) and ultrasound or radiologic examinations of the gallbladder may be scheduled by the physician.
- If diarrhea occurs, contact the physician. If symptoms of gallbladder disease (pain, nausea, vomiting) occur, contact the physician immediately.

Laxatives
- Avoid long-term use of these products unless use of the product has been recommended by the physician. Long-term use may result in the "laxative habit," which is a dependence on a laxative to have a bowel movement. Constipation may also occur with overuse of these drugs. Read and follow the directions on the label.
- Avoid long-term use of mineral oil. Daily use of this product may interfere with the absorption of some vitamins (vitamins A, D, E, K). Take on an empty stomach, preferably at bedtime.
- Do not use these products in the presence of abdominal pain, nausea, or vomiting.

- Notify the physician if constipation is not relieved or if rectal bleeding or other symptoms occur.
- Bulk-producing or fecal-softening laxatives—Drink a full glass of water or juice, followed by more glasses of fluid in the next few hours.
- Bisacodyl (Dulcolax)—Do not chew the tablets and do not take within 1 hour of taking antacids or milk.
- To avoid constipation, drink plenty of fluids, exercise, and eat foods high in bulk or roughage.

Miscellaneous Drugs
- Olsalazine—if diarrhea develops, contact the physician as soon as possible.
- Mesalamine—Swallow tablets whole; do not chew the tablets. Suppository: remove foil wrapper and immediately insert the pointed end into the rectum. Do not use force when inserting the suppository. Suspension: instructions are included with the product. Shake well. Remove the protective sheath from the applicator tip and gently insert the tip into the rectum.
- Omeprazole—Swallow tablets whole; do not chew the tablets.

■ Expected Outcomes for Evaluation
- Anxiety is reduced
- Adverse reactions are identified and reported to the physician
- Patient and family demonstrate understanding of drug regimen
- Patient verbalizes importance of complying with the prescribed treatment regimen
- Patient verbalizes an understanding of treatment modalities and importance of continued follow-up care

Chapter Summary

- The gastrointestinal (GI) tract is subject to more diseases and disorders than any other system of the body. Some drugs used for GI disorders are available as nonprescription drugs, thereby creating potential problems of misuse and overuse, as well as disguising more serious medical problems. The drugs presented in this chapter include the antacids, anticholinergics, GI stimulants, histamine H_2 antagonists, antidiarrheals, antiflatulents, digestive enzymes, emetics, gallstone-solubilizing agents, laxatives, and miscellaneous drugs.
- Antacids neutralize or reduce the acidity of stomach and duodenal contents and are used for treat-

ment of gastric distress and in the medical treatment of peptic ulcer. Anticholinergics reduce gastric motility and decrease the amount of acid secreted by the stomach and are used for treatment of peptic ulcer.

- The GI stimulants metoclopramide and dexpanthenol increase the motility of the upper GI tract. Cisapride enhances the release of acetylcholine. Metoclopramide is used in the treatment of symptomatic GERD and gastric stasis. Dexpanthenol may be given parenterally immediately after major abdominal surgery to reduce the risk of paralytic ileus. Cisapride is used in the treatment of heartburn associated with GERD.
- Histamine H$_2$ antagonists inhibit the action of histamine at histamine H$_2$ receptor cells of the stomach, which then reduces the secretion of gastric acid. These drugs are used for treatment of a gastric or duodenal ulcer, gastric hypersecretory conditions, and GERD.
- Antidiarrheals decrease intestinal peristalsis, which is usually increased when the patient has diarrhea, and are used for short-term treatment of diarrhea. Antiflatulents reduce the amount of gas present in the GI tract.
- Pancreatin and pancrelipase, which are manufactured and secreted by the pancreas, are responsible for the breakdown of fats, starches, and proteins and are necessary for the breakdown and digestion of food. Both enzymes are available as oral supplements for conditions causing a lack of these enzymes.
- The emetic apomorphine promotes vomiting by its direct action on the vomiting center of the medulla. Ipecac causes vomiting because of its local irritating effect on the stomach, as well as by stimulation of the vomiting center in the medulla. These drugs are used to empty stomach contents following ingestion of some poisons or accidental or intentional drug overdose.
- Gallstone-solubilizing agents suppress the manufacture of cholesterol and cholic acid by the liver. The suppression of the manufacture of cholesterol and cholic acid may ultimately result in a decrease in the size of radiolucent gallstones.
- Bulk-producing laxatives are not digested by the body and therefore add bulk and water to the contents of the intestines. Emollient laxatives lubricate the intestinal walls and soften the stool, thereby enhancing passage of fecal material. Fecal softeners promote water retention in the fecal mass and soften the stool. Hyperosmolar agents dehydrate local tissues, which causes irritation and increased peristalsis with consequent evacuation of the fecal mass. Irritant or stimulant laxatives increase peristalsis by direct action on the intestine. Saline laxatives attract or pull water into the intestine, thereby increasing pressure in the intestine followed by an increase in peristalsis.
- Misoprostol inhibits gastric acid secretion and increases the protective property of the mucosal lining of the GI tract by increasing the production of mucus by the lining of the GI tract. This drug is used to prevent gastric ulcers in those taking aspirin or nonsteroidal antiinflammatory drugs. Sucralfate exerts a local action on the lining of the stomach by forming a complex with the exudate of the stomach lining and is used in the treatment of duodenal ulcer. Omeprazole suppresses gastric acid secretion by blocking the final step in the production of gastric acid by the gastric mucosa and is used in the treatment of duodenal ulcer and GERD.
- Mesalamine, olsalazine, and sulfasalazine are three drugs that exert a topical antiinflammatory effect in the bowel and are used for inflammatory bowel disorders.

Critical Thinking Exercises

1. Ms. Harris, aged 76, tells you that she has been using various laxatives for constipation. She states that a laxative did help but now she is more constipated than she was before she began taking a laxative. What advice or suggestions would you give this patient?
2. Mr. Miller, aged 69, tells you that he is frequently constipated and asks you for the name of a good laxative. What patient teaching might be appropriate at this time?
3. Mr. Gates, your neighbor, has been given a prescription for diphenoxylate with atropine (Lomotil) to be taken if he should develop diarrhea while he is traveling in a foreign country. What warnings regarding this drug would you give to your neighbor?

43

Drugs Used in the Treatment of Musculoskeletal Disorders

Key Terms

Analgesic
Antiinflammatory
Antipyretic
Musculoskeletal
Prostaglandins

Chapter Outline

Chapter Objectives

On completion of this chapter the student will:

- *Discuss the actions and uses of drugs used in the treatment of musculoskeletal disorders*
- *List and discuss the adverse reactions of drugs used in the treatment of musculoskeletal disorders*
- *Discuss the nursing implications to be considered when administering drugs used in the treatment of musculoskeletal disorders*
- *Use the nursing process when administering drugs used in the treatment of musculoskeletal disorders*

A variety of drugs are used in the treatment of *musculoskeletal* (bone and muscle) disorders. The drug selected is based on the musculoskeletal disorder being treated, the severity of the disorder, and possibly other factors. For example, early cases of rheumatoid arthritis may respond well to the salicylates, whereas advanced rheumatoid arthritis not responding to other drug therapies may require the use of one of the gold compounds. The physician also may base the selection of a drug for treatment of a chronic musculoskeletal disorder on the patient's positive or negative response to past therapy.

Drugs Used in the Treatment of Musculoskeletal Disorders

ACTIONS OF THE DRUGS USED IN THE TREATMENT OF MUSCULOSKELETAL DISORDERS

The Salicylates

The *antiinflammatory* (against inflammation) action of aspirin is thought to be due to its ability to inhibit the synthesis of *prostaglandins*, a substance found in almost all body tissues and thought to increase the sensitivity of peripheral pain receptors to painful stimuli. When inflammation is reduced, pain is also relieved. In addition to an antiinflammatory action, the salicylates also have *analgesic* (relief of pain) and *antipyretic* (reduction of fever) activity.

Gold Compounds

The exact mechanism of action of the gold compounds, for example, gold sodium thiomalate (Myochrysine) and auranofin (Ridaura), in the suppression or prevention of inflammation is unknown.

Nonsteroidal Antiinflammatory Drugs

The nonsteroidal antiinflammatory drugs (NSAIDS) are so called because they do not belong to the steroid group of drugs; do not possess the adverse reactions associated with the steroids (corticosteroids); and, yet, have antiinflammatory activity. Their exact mechanism of action is unknown. In addition to their antiinflammatory action, they also possess analgesic (pain relieving) and antipyretic activity. Examples of these drugs include fenoprofen (Nalfon) and ibuprofen (Advil).

Drugs Used for Gout

The deposit or collection of urate crystals in the joints causes the symptoms (pain, redness, swelling, joint deformity) of gout. Allopurinol (Zyloprim) reduces the production of uric acid, thus decreasing serum uric acid levels and the deposit of urate crystals in joints. The exact mechanism of action of colchicine is unknown, but it does reduce the inflammation associated with the deposit of urate crystals in the joints. This probably accounts for its ability to relieve the severe pain of acute gout. Colchicine has no effect on uric acid metabolism.

In those with gout, the serum uric acid level is usually elevated. Sulfinpyrazone (Anturane) increases the excretion of uric acid by the kidneys, which lowers serum uric acid levels and consequently retards the deposit of urate crystals in the joints. Probenecid (Benemid) works in the same manner and may be given alone or with colchicine as combination therapy when there are frequent, recurrent attacks of gout. Probenecid also has been used to prolong the plasma levels of the penicillins and cephalosporins.

Skeletal Muscle Relaxants

The mode of action of many skeletal muscle relaxants, for example carisoprodol (Soma), baclofen (Lioresal), and chlorzoxazone (Paraflex), is not clearly understood. Many of these drugs do not directly relax skeletal muscles but their ability to relieve acute painful musculoskeletal conditions may be due to their sedative action. Cyclobenzaprine (Flexeril) appears to have an effect on muscle tone, thus reducing muscle spasm.

The exact mode of action of diazepam (Valium), a tranquilizer (see Chap. 25), in the relief of painful musculoskeletal conditions is unknown. The drug does have a sedative action, which may account for some of its ability to relieve muscle spasm and pain.

The Corticosteroids

The potent antiinflammatory action of the corticosteroids make these drugs useful in the treatment of many types of musculoskeletal disorders. The corticosteroids are discussed in Chapter 38.

Miscellaneous Drugs

Phenylbutazone (Butazolidin) and oxyphenbutazone are chemically related. These drugs have antiinflammatory, as well as antipyretic and analgesic, activity. The exact mode of their antiinflammatory action is not well understood. These drugs may inhibit prostaglandin synthesis, which may partially account for their antiinflammatory activity. The mechanism of action of penicillamine (Cuprimine), methotrexate, and hydroxychloroquine (Plaquenil) in the treatment of rheumatoid arthritis is unknown.

USES OF THE DRUGS USED IN THE TREATMENT OF MUSCULOSKELETAL DISORDERS

Although the drugs covered in this chapter are used in the treatment of musculoskeletal disorders, some of the drugs in each group have specific uses; these are listed in Summary Drug Table 43-1.

The **salicylates** are used in the treatment of rheumatoid arthritis and osteoarthritis, as well as relief of pain or discomfort resulting from musculoskeletal injuries such as sprains. The salicylates are also of value in relieving mild to moderate muscle or joint pain or tenderness. Aspirin (acetylsalicylic acid) has greater antiinflammatory activity than the other salicylates, and therefore is the preferred salicylate for the treatment of arthritic disorders. **Gold compounds** are used to treat active juvenile and adult rheumatoid arthritis not controlled by other antiinflammatory drugs. **Nonsteroidal antiinflammatory drugs** are used in the treatment of rheumatoid arthritis, osteoarthritis, and ankylosing spondylitis.

Drugs indicated for treatment of gout may be used to manage acute attacks of gout or in preventing acute attacks of gout (prophylaxis). **Skeletal muscle relaxants** are used in various acute, painful musculoskeletal conditions, such as muscle strains and back pain. The **corticosteroids** may be used to treat rheumatic disorders such as ankylosing spondylitis, rheumatoid arthritis, gout, bursitis, and osteoarthritis. **Phenylbutazone** and **oxyphenbutazone** are used in the management of gouty arthritis, rheumatoid arthritis, ankylosing spondylitis, and degenerative joint disease of the hips and knees when other drugs have not proven effective. **Penicillamine**, **methotrexate**, and **hydroxychloroquine** are used in the treatment of rheumatoid arthritis. The administration of **methotrexate** is reserved for severe, active rheumatoid arthritis.

ADVERSE REACTIONS ASSOCIATED WITH THE ADMINISTRATION OF DRUGS USED IN THE TREATMENT OF MUSCULOSKELETAL DISORDERS

The Salicylates

The adverse reactions associated with the administration of the salicylates are discussed in Chapter 15 and in Summary Drug Table 15-1. Because relatively high doses of these drugs may be required for some arthritic disorders, such as rheumatoid arthritis, adverse reactions that may be seen with high doses are tinnitus (ringing in the ears) and gastrointestinal (GI) distress. Easy bruising and prolonged bleeding or oozing from injuries also may be seen. At times, adverse reactions are severe and the dosage may need to be decreased or the drug discontinued.

Gold Compounds

Adverse reactions to the gold compounds may occur any time during therapy, as well as many months after therapy has been discontinued. Dermatitis and stomatitis are the most common adverse reactions seen. Pruritus often occurs before the skin eruption becomes apparent. Photosensitivity reactions (exaggerated sunburn reaction when the skin is exposed to sunlight or ultraviolet light) may also occur.

Nonsteroidal Antiinflammatory Drugs

GI symptoms are the most common adverse reactions seen with the nonsteroidal antiinflammatory drugs. These reactions may include nausea, vomiting, abdominal discomfort, diarrhea, constipation, gastric or

Summary Drug Table 43-1. Drugs Used in the Treatment of Musculoskeletal Disorders

Generic Name	Trade Name*	Uses	Adverse Reactions	Dose Ranges
THE SALICYLATES				
aspirin (acetyl-salicylic acid)	Bayer, Ecotrin, *generic*	Rheumatoid arthritis, osteoarthritis, pain and discomfort of musculoskeletal injuries; see also Summary Drug Table 15-1	Tinnitus, GI distress, easy bruising, prolonged bleeding from injuries; see also Chapter 15 and Summary Drug Table 15-1 and text of Chap. 43 for signs of salicylism	Arthritis and other rheumatic conditions: 3.2–6 g/d PO in divided doses
GOLD COMPOUNDS				
auranofin	Ridaura	Rheumatoid arthritis	Dermatitis, stomatitis, photosensitivity reactions, pruritus, hematologic changes, nausea, vomiting, anorexia, rash, urticaria, metallic taste	6 mg/d PO in single or divided doses
aurothioglucose	Solganal	Same as auranofin	Same as auranofin	Initial dose: 10 mg IM; dosage increased weekly until 0.8–1 g is given; dose may be continued at 50 mg IM every 3–4 wk
gold sodium thiomalate	Myochrysine	Same as auranofin	Same as auranofin	Initial dose: 10 mg IM; dosage increased weekly until 1 g has been given; dose may be continued at 25–50 mg IM every 3–4 wk
NONSTEROIDAL ANTIINFLAMMATORY DRUGS (NSAIDS)				
diclofenac	Cataflam, Voltaren	Osteoarthritis, rheumatoid arthritis, ankylosing spondylitis	Nausea, vomiting, abdominal discomfort, diarrhea, constipation, gastric or duodenal ulcer, GI bleeding	Osteoarthritis: 100–150 mg/d PO in divided doses; rheumatoid arthritis: 150–200 mg/d PO in divided doses; ankylosing spondylitis: 100–125 mg/d PO in divided doses
etodolac	Lodine	Osteoarthritis	Same as diclofenac	800–1200 mg/d PO in divided doses
fenoprofen calcium	Nalfon, *generic*	Rheumatoid arthritis, osteoarthritis	Same as diclofenac	Up to 3.2 g/d PO
flurbiprofen	Ansaid	Rheumatoid arthritis, osteoarthritis	Same as diclofenac	Up to 300 mg/d PO in divided doses
ibuprofen	Advil, Motrin, Rufen, *generic*	Rheumatoid arthritis, osteoarthritis	Same as diclofenac	Up to 3.2 g/d PO in divided doses
indomethacin	Indocin, *generic*	Rheumatoid arthritis, ankylosing spondylitis, osteoarthritis, bursitis, tendinitis, acute gouty arthritis	Same as diclofenac	Up to 150 mg/d PO in divided doses
ketoprofen	Orudis, *generic*	Rheumatoid arthritis, osteoarthritis	Same as diclofenac	Up to 300 mg/d PO in divided doses
meclofenamate sodium	Meclomen, *generic*	Rhematoid arthritis, osteoarthritis	Same as diclofenac	200–400 mg/d PO in 3–4 equal doses
nabumetone	Relafen	Rheumatoid arthritis, osteoarthritis	Same as diclofenac	1000–2000 mg/d PO as a single or divided dose

(continued)

Summary Drug Table 43-1 (Continued)

Generic Name	Trade Name*	Uses	Adverse Reactions	Dose Ranges†
naproxen	Naprosyn, Aleve, Anaprox, *generic*	Rheumatoid arthritis, osteoarthritis, ankylosing spondylitis, acute gout	Same as diclofenac	Arthritic disorders: up to 1.25 g/d PO in divided doses; acute gout: initial dose 750 mg PO then 250 mg q8h until attack subsides
oxaprozin	Daypro	Rheumatoid arthritis, osteoarthritis	Same as diclofenac	600–1200 mg/d PO as a single dose or up to 1800 mg/d PO in divided doses
piroxicam	Feldene, *generic*	Rheumatoid arthritis, osteoarthritis	Same as diclofenac	20 mg/d PO as a single or divided dose
sulindac	Clinoril, *generic*	Rheumatoid arthritis, osteoarthritis, ankylosing spondylitis, bursitis, tendinitis, acute gouty arthritis	Same as diclofenac	Arthritic disorders: 150 mg PO bid; bursitis, tendenitis, gouty arthritis: 200 mg PO bid
tolmetin sodium	Tolectin	Rheumatoid arthritis, osteoarthritis	Same as diclofenac	Up to 1800 mg/d PO in divided doses
DRUGS USED FOR GOUT				
allopurinol	Zyloprim, *generic*	Management of symptoms of gout	Rash, exfoliative dermatitis, Stevens-Johnson syndrome, nausea, vomiting, diarrhea, abdominal pain, hematologic changes	100–800 mg/d PO
colchicine	*generic*	Relief of acute attacks of gout, prevention of gout attacks	Nausea, vomiting, diarrhea, abdominal pain, bone marrow depression	Acute attack: Initial dose 1.2 mg PO or 2 mg IV then 0.5–1.2 mg PO q1–2h or 0.5 mg IV q6h until attack aborted or adverse effects occur; prophylaxis: 0.5–0.6 mg/d PO
probenecid	Benemid	Treatment of hyperuricemia of gout and gouty arthritis	Headache, anorexia, nausea, vomiting, urinary frequency, flushing, dizziness	0.25 mg PO bid for 1 wk then 0.5 mg PO bid
sulfinpyrazone	Anturane	Treatment of gouty arthritis	Upper GI disturbances	200–800 mg/d PO in 2 divided doses
SKELETAL MUSCLE RELAXANTS				
baclofen	Lioresal	Spasticity due to multiple sclerosis, spinal cord injuries	Dry mouth, euphoria, excitement, dyspnea, anorexia, rash	15–80 mg/d PO in divided doses
carisoprodol	Soma, *generic*	Relief of discomfort due to acute, painful musculoskeletal conditions	Dizziness, drowsiness, tachycardia, nausea, vomiting	350 mg PO tid, qid
chlorzoxazone	Paraflex, *generic*	Same as carisoprodol	GI disturbances, drowsiness, dizziness, rash	250–500 mg PO tid, qid
cyclobenzaprine hydrochloride	Flexeril	Same as carisoprodol	Tachycardia, drowsiness, dizziness, dry mouth, nausea, constipation	20–40 mg/d PO in divided doses

(continued)

Summary Drug Table 43-1   (Continued)

Generic Name	Trade Name*	Uses	Adverse Reactions	Dose Ranges†
dantrolene sodium	Dantrium	Spasticity due to spinal cord injury, stroke, cerebral palsy, multiple sclerosis	Drowsiness, dizziness, weakness, constipation, tachycardia, malaise	Initial dose: 25 mg/d PO then 50–400 mg/d PO in divided doses
diazepam	Valium	Relief of skeletal muscle spasm, spasticity due to cerebral palsy, paraplegia	Drowsiness, sedation, sleepiness, lethargy, constipation, diarrhea, bradycardia, tachycardia, rash	2–10 mg PO tid, qid; 2–10 mg IM, IV
CORTICOSTEROIDS†				
prednisolone	Delta-Cortef, *generic*	Ankylosing spondylitis, bursitis, acute gouty arthritis, rheumatoid arthritis	See Chap. 38	5–60 mg/d PO
prednisone	Deltasone, Ora-sone, *generic*	Same as prednisolone	See Chap. 38	5–60 mg/d PO
MISCELLANEOUS DRUGS				
hydroxychloro-quine sulfate	Plaquenil	Rheumatoid arthritis	Irritability, nervousness, alopecia, anorexia, nausea, vomiting, ophthalmic effects, hematological effects	200–600 mg/d PO
methotrexate	Rheumatrex Dose Pack, *generic*	Rheumatoid arthritis	Nausea, vomiting, decreased platelet count, leukopenia, stomatitis, diarrhea, alopecia	7.5 mg PO once a wk or 2.5 mg at 12-hr intervals for 3 doses once a week
oxyphenbutazone	*generic*	Rheumatoid arthritis, gouty arthritis, ankylosing spondylitis, de-degenerative joint disease of the hips and knees, painful shoulder	Abdominal discomfort, edema, nausea, rash, indigestion, heartburn, vomiting, constipation, diarrhea, epigastric pain, aplastic anemia, agranulocytosis	Arthritis disorders: 300–600 mg/d PO in divided doses; acute gouty arthritis: initial dose 400 mg PO then 100 mg PO q4h
penicillamine	Cuprimine, Depen	Rheumatoid arthritis	Pruritis, rash, anorexia, nausea, vomiting, epigastric pain, bone marrow depression, proteinuria, hematuria, increased skin friability, tinnitus	Initial dose: 125–250 mg/d PO and increased to obtain remission. Maximum daily dose is 1.5 g/d PO
phenylbutazone	Butazolidin, Azolid, *generic*	Same as oxyphenbutazone	Same as oxyphenbutazone	Same as oxyphenbutazone

*The term, *generic*, indicates that the drug is available in a *generic* form.
†See Chap. 38 for additional corticosteroid preparations and adverse reactions.

duodenal ulcer formation, and GI bleeding, which can be potentially serious. Hematologic changes can occur, and in some instances are serious. Other adverse reactions include jaundice, toxic hepatitis, visual disturbances, rash, dermatitis, and hypersensitivity reactions. Many of these adverse reactions are only seen with high doses or prolonged therapy.

Drugs Used for Gout

One adverse reaction associated with allopurinol is skin rash, which, in some cases, has been followed by serious hypersensitivity reactions such as exfoliative dermatitis and the Stevens-Johnson syndrome (see Chap. 11 for a description of this syndrome). Other adverse reactions include nausea, vomiting, diarrhea, abdominal pain, and hematologic changes.

Colchicine administration may result in nausea, vomiting, diarrhea, abdominal pain, and bone marrow depression. When this drug is given to patients with an acute attack of gout, the physician may order the drug given at frequent intervals until GI symptoms occur. Probenecid administration may cause headache, GI symptoms, urinary frequency, and hypersensitivity reactions. Upper GI disturbances may be seen with the administration of sulfinpyrazone. Even when the drug is given with food, milk, or antacids, GI distress may persist and the drug may need to be discontinued. The adverse reactions seen with other agents used in the treatment of gout are listed in Summary Drug Table 43-1.

Skeletal Muscle Relaxants

Drowsiness is the most common reaction seen with the use of skeletal muscle relaxants. Additional adverse reactions are given in Summary Drug Table 43-1. Some of the adverse reactions that may be seen with the administration of diazepam include drowsiness, sedation, sleepiness, lethargy, constipation or diarrhea, bradycardia or tachycardia, and rash.

The Corticosteroids

Corticosteroids may be given in high doses for some arthritic disorders. There are many adverse reactions associated with high dose and long-term corticosteroid therapy. Chapter 38 discusses some of the adverse reactions associated with corticosteroid therapy. A comprehensive list of adverse reactions may be found in Table 38-2.

Miscellaneous Drugs

Phenylbutazone and oxyphenbutazone have the same adverse reactions, which include abdominal discomfort, edema, nausea, rash, indigestion, and heartburn. Less common adverse reactions include vomiting, constipation, diarrhea, and epigastric pain. The adverse reactions seen with penicillamine include pruritus, rash, anorexia, nausea, vomiting, epigastric pain, bone marrow depression, proteinuria, hematuria, increased skin friability, and tinnitus. Penicillamine is capable of causing severe toxic reactions.

Methotrexate is a potentially toxic drug that is also used in the treatment of malignancies and psoriasis. Nausea, vomiting, a decreased platelet count, leukopenia (decreased white blood cell count), stomatitis (inflammation of the oral cavity), rash, pruritus, dermatitis, diarrhea, alopecia (loss of hair), and diarrhea may be seen with the administration of this drug.

Hydroxychloroquine administration may result in irritability, nervousness, alopecia, anorexia, nausea, vomiting, and diarrhea. This drug also may have adverse effects on the eye, for example, blurred vision, corneal edema, halos around lights, and photophobia. Hematologic effects, such as aplastic anemia and leukopenia, may also be seen.

NURSING MANAGEMENT

Periodic evaluation is an important part of therapy for musculoskeletal disorders. With some disorders such as acute gout, the patient can be expected to respond to therapy in hours. Therefore, it is important to inspect the joints involved every 1 to 2 hours to identify immediately a response or nonresponse to therapy. At this time, question the patient regarding the relief of pain, as well as adverse drug reactions. In other disorders, response is gradual and may take days, weeks, and even months of treatment. Depending on the drug administered and the disorder being treated, evaluation of therapy may be daily or weekly. These recorded evaluations help the physician plan present and future therapy including dosage changes, changes in the drug administered, institution of physical therapy, and so on.

Patients on complete bed rest require position changes and good skin care every 2 hours. The patient with an arthritic disorder may experience much pain or discomfort and require assistance with activities, such as ambulating, eating, and grooming.

The following discussion focuses on nursing assessments and management for specific drugs or drug groups.

The Salicylates

These drugs may be given with food or milk or a full glass of water. The physician may prescribe an antacid to be given with the drug to minimize GI distress.

When high doses are given, observe the patient closely for signs of salicylate toxicity. Periodic monitoring of plasma salicylate acid levels may be ordered. Therapeutic levels are between 100 and 300 mcg/mL. Levels greater than 150 mcg/mL may result in symptoms of mild salicylism, namely tinnitus, difficulty in hearing, dizziness, nausea, vomiting, diarrhea, mental confusion, central nervous system depression, headache, sweating, and hyperventilation (rapid, deep breathing). Levels over 250 mcg/mL may result in symptoms of mild salicylism plus headache, diarrhea, thirst, and flushing. Levels over 400 mcg/mL may result in respiratory alkalosis, hemorrhage, excitement, confusion, asterixis (involuntary jerking movements especially of the hands) pulmonary edema, convulsions, tetany (muscle spasms), fever, coma, shock, and renal and respiratory failure. Any one or more of these symptoms should be considered a sign of salicylate toxicity. Notify the physician before the next dose is due.

Check the color of the stools. Black or dark stools or bright red blood in the stool may indicate GI bleeding. Report any change in the color of the stool to the physician.

Gold Compounds

Aurothioglucose (Solganal) and gold sodium thiomalate are given intramuscularly, preferably in the upper outer quadrant of the gluteus muscle. Auranofin is given orally.

Observe the patient closely for evidence of dermatitis. Itching may occur before a skin reaction and should be reported to the physician immediately.

Inspect the mouth of the patient daily for evidence of ulceration of the mucous membranes. A metallic taste may be noted before stomatitis becomes evident. Advise the patient to inform the physician or nurse if a metallic taste occurs.

Good oral care is necessary. The teeth should be brushed after each meal and the mouth rinsed with plain water to remove food particles. Mouthwash may also be used but excessive use may result in oral infections due to the destruction of the normal bacteria present in the mouth.

Nonsteroidal Antiinflammatory Drugs

Indomethacin (Indocin) is given with an antacid (when prescribed by the physician), food, or milk. Sulindac (Clinoril) is given with food. The other nonsteroidal antiinflammatory agents may be given with food or milk if GI upset occurs.

GI reactions may occur with the use of these drugs and can be severe and even fatal, especially in patients with a history of upper GI disease, such as stomach ulcers. Withhold the next dose and notify the physician if diarrhea, nausea, vomiting, tarry stools, or abdominal pain occurs.

Advise the patient that the drug may take several days to relieve pain and tenderness.

For the diabetic patient, the insulin dosage may require adjustment when these drugs are given. Test the blood glucose (using a glucometer) as ordered and inform the physician of any marked change in blood glucose levels. If urine testing is ordered, test the urine four times per day and keep the physician informed of test results.

Drugs Used for Gout

Allopurinol, probenemid, and sulfinpyrazone are given with or immediately after meals to minimize GI distress. Colchicine usually can be given with food or milk. When this drug is used for the treatment of an acute gout attack, it may be given every 1 to 2 hours until the pain is relieved or the patient develops vomiting or diarrhea. The physician writes specific orders for administration of the drug and when the drug is to be stopped. Evaluate the patient carefully for relief of pain or the occurrence of nausea, vomiting, or diarrhea. After this evaluation, decide whether to administer or withhold the drug. Colchicine may be given with food or milk when it is given as a prophylaxis for gout. Check with the physician regarding administration with food when the drug is given at 1- to 2-hour intervals. Colchicine may be given intravenously for severe gout.

Encourage a liberal fluid intake and measure the intake and output. The daily urine output should be at least 2 L. An increase in urinary output is necessary to excrete the urates (uric acid) and prevent urate acid stone formation in the genitourinary tract.

Provide adequate fluids and remind the patient frequently of the importance of increasing fluid intake. If the patient fails to increase the oral intake, inform the physician. In some instances, it may be necessary to administer intravenous fluids to supplement the oral intake when the patient fails to drink about 3000 mL of fluid per day.

Skeletal Muscle Relaxants

These drugs may be given with food to minimize GI distress. In addition to drug therapy, rest, physical therapy, and other measures may be part of treatment.

These drugs may cause drowsiness. The patient should be evaluated carefully before being allowed to ambulate alone. If drowsiness does occur, assistance with ambulatory activities is necessary. If drowsiness is severe, notify the physician before the next dose is due.

Corticosteroids

When the patient is receiving one of these drugs on alternate days (alternate-day therapy), the drug *must be given before* 9 AM. It is extremely important that these drugs not be omitted or suddenly discontinued. These drugs are also discussed in Chapter 38.

Nursing Alert

When a corticosteroid is discontinued, the dosage must be tapered gradually over several days. If high dosages have been given, it may take a week or more to taper the dosage.

Phenylbutazone and Oxyphenbutazone

These drugs *must* be given with food or milk to minimize GI distress. If drowsiness occurs, the patient requires assistance with ambulatory activities. Once a therapeutic response is obtained, the dosage may be reduced or the drug discontinued.

Nursing Alert

Phenylbutazone and oxyphenbutazone may depress the bone marrow. Withhold the next dose and notify the physician if any of the following occur: sore throat, fever, soreness of the mouth, stomatitis, unusual bleeding or bruising, or tarry stools.

Penicillamine

This drug *must* be given on an empty stomach, 1 hour before or 2 hours after a meal.

Nursing Alert

Administration of penicillamine has been associated with many adverse reactions, some of which are potentially serious and even fatal. Carefully evaluate any complaint or comment made by the patient and report it to the physician.

Increased skin friability may occur, which may result in easy breakdown of the skin at pressure sites, such as the hips, elbows, and shoulders. The patient who is unable to ambulate must have his or her position changed and pressure sites inspected for skin breakdown every 2 hours.

Methotrexate

Nursing Alert

Methotrexate is potentially toxic and patients must be closely observed for development of adverse reactions. All adverse reactions or suspected adverse reactions must be immediately brought to the attention of the physician.

Observe the patient for signs of easy bruising and infection, which may indicate bone marrow depression, an adverse reaction related to the platelets and white blood cells. Inspect the oral cavity daily for signs of inflammation or ulceration. Inspect each stool for diarrhea or signs of GI bleeding.

Hydroxychloroquine

Give the drug with food or milk. Observe the patient closely for adverse reactions. Be alert to skin rash, fever, cough, easy bruising, or unusual bleeding, or the patient's complaints of sore throat, visual changes, mood changes, loss of hair, tinnitus, or hearing loss. Adverse reactions are reported immediately.

Nursing Process
The Patient Receiving a Drug for a Musculoskeletal Disorder

■ *Assessment*

The patient with a musculoskeletal disorder may be in acute pain or have longstanding mild to moderate pain, which can be just as difficult to tolerate as severe pain. Along with pain, there may be skeletal deformities, for example, the joint deformities seen with advanced rheumatoid arthritis. For many musculoskeletal conditions, drug therapy is a major treatment modality. Therapy with these drugs may keep the disorder under control (eg, therapy for gout), improve the patient's ability to carry out the activities of daily living, or make the pain and discomfort tolerable.

Obtain the patient's history, that is, a summary of the disorder including onset, symptoms, and current treatment or therapy. In some instances, it may be necessary to question patients regarding their ability to carry out activities of daily living, including employment when applicable.

For the physical assessment, generally appraise the patient's physical condition and limitations. If the patient has arthritis (any type), examine the affected joints in the extremities for appearance of the skin over the joint, evidence of joint deformity, and mobility of the affected joint. Take the vital signs and weight to provide a baseline for comparison during therapy. If the patient has gout, examine the affected joints and note the appearance of the skin over the joints and any joint enlargement.

■ *Nursing Diagnoses*

Depending on the drug, dose, and reason for administration, one or more of the following nursing diagnoses may apply to a person receiving a drug for a musculoskeletal disorder:

- **Anxiety** related to symptoms of disorder, other factors
- **Noncompliance** related to indifference, lack of knowledge, other factors
- **Risk for Ineffective Management of Therapeutic Regimen** related to lack of knowledge of medication regimen, adverse drug effects, treatment modalities

■ *Planning and Implementation*

The major goals of the patient may include a reduction in anxiety and an understanding of and compliance to the prescribed therapeutic regimen. To make these goals measurable, more specific criteria must be added.

Adverse Drug Reactions. Some of these drugs are toxic. Closely observe the patient for the development of adverse reactions. Should any one or more adverse reactions occur, notify the physician before the next dose is due. Notify the physician immediately of serious adverse reactions.

Anxiety. Patients with a musculoskeletal disorder often have anxiety related to the symptoms and the chronicity of their disorder. In addition to physical care, these patients often require emotional support, especially when a disorder is disabling and chronic. Explain to the patient that therapy may take weeks or longer before any benefit is noted. When this is explained before therapy is started, the patient is less likely to become discouraged over the slow results of drug therapy.

Noncompliance. To ensure compliance to the treatment regimen, the patient must understand the importance of complying with the prescribed treatment regimen and taking the drug exactly as directed to obtain the best results from therapy. To meet this goal develop an effective plan of patient and family teaching.

■ *Patient and Family Teaching*

The points included in a patient and family teaching plan depend on the type and severity of the musculoskeletal disorder being treated. Carefully explain that treatment for the disorder includes drug therapy, as well as other medical management, such as diet, exercise, limitations or nonlimitations of activity, periodic physical therapy treatments, and so on. Emphasize the importance of not taking any nonprescription drugs unless their use has been approved by the physician.

Include the following points for specific drugs in the teaching plan. Information included for the patient taking a corticosteroid is explained in Chapter 38.

Salicylates

- Take with food or milk to minimize GI distress.
- Notify the physician if nausea, vomiting, abdominal pain, easy bruising or bleeding, tinnitus, impaired hearing, sweating, thirst, diarrhea, or black tarry stools occur.

Gold Compounds

- The possibility of toxic reactions must be explained before therapy is started on an outpatient basis. This is usually the responsibility of the physician. Give the patient a list of the adverse reactions that require notifying the physician of their occurrence as soon as possible. Emphasize the importance of contacting the physician if a metallic taste is noted.
- Inform the patient that arthralgia (pain in the joints) may be noted for 1 or 2 days after the parenteral form is given.
- Avoid exposure to sunlight because a photosensitivity reaction may occur.

Nonsteroidal Antiinflammatory Drugs

- Do not take aspirin during therapy with this drug; aspirin may interfere with the drug's action.
- Take this drug with food or milk to prevent GI upset. Take indomethacin with food or milk; take sulindac with food.
- Notify the physician if skin rash, itching, visual disturbances, weight gain, diarrhea, black stools, nausea, vomiting, or persistent headache occurs.
- Diabetic patient—Closely monitor blood glucose (with a glucometer) as recommended by the physician. Notify the physician if the blood glucose is elevated despite adherence to the prescribed diet because an adjustment in insulin dosage may be needed.

Drugs Used for Gout

- Drink at least 10 glasses of water a day until the acute attack has subsided.
- Take this drug with food to minimize GI upset.
- If drowsiness occurs, avoid driving or performing other hazardous tasks.
- Acute gout—Notify the physician if pain is not relieved in a few days.
- Colchicine for acute gout—take at the intervals prescribed by the physician. Stop taking the medication when the pain is relieved or when diarrhea or vomiting occurs. If the pain is not relieved in about 12 hours, notify the physician.
- Allopurinol—Notify the physician if a skin rash occurs.
- Colchicine—Notify the physician if skin rash, sore throat, fever, unusual bleeding or bruising, unusual fatigue, or weakness occurs.

Skeletal Muscle Relaxants

- This drug may cause drowsiness. Do not drive or perform other hazardous tasks if drowsiness occurs.

Penicillamine

- The toxic effects associated with this drug must be explained before therapy is started. This is usually done by the physician. The patient must know which toxic reactions require contacting the physician immediately.
- Take this drug on an empty stomach 1 hour before or 2 hours after a meal.
- If other drugs are prescribed, penicillamine is taken 1 hour apart from any other drug.
- Observe skin areas over the elbows, shoulders, and buttocks for evidence of bruising, bleeding, or break in the skin. If these occur, do not self-treat the problem but notify the physician immediately.

Phenylbutazone and Oxyphenbutazone

- Take this drug with food or milk to prevent GI upset.
- Notify the physician immediately if any of the following occur: sore throat, sores in the mouth, unusual bleeding or bruising, fever, blurred vision, black tarry stools, or skin rash.

Methotrexate

- Take the drug *exactly* as directed. If a weekly dose is prescribed, use a calendar or some other method to take the drug on the same day each week. *Never* increase the prescribed dose of this drug.
- Notify the physician immediately if any of the following occur: sore mouth, sores in the mouth, diarrhea, fever, sore throat, easy bruising, rash, itching, or nausea and vomiting.

Hydroxychloroquine

- Take the drug with food or milk.
- Contact the physician immediately if any of the following are noted: hearing or visual changes, skin rash or severe itching, hair loss, change in the color of the hair (bleaching), changes in the color of the skin, easy bruising or bleeding, fever, sore throat, muscle weakness, or mood changes.
- It may be several weeks before symptoms are relieved.

■ Expected Outcomes for Evaluation

- Anxiety is reduced
- Adverse reactions are identified and reported to the physician
- Patient verbalizes importance of complying with the prescribed therapeutic regimen
- Patient and family demonstrate understanding of drug regimen

Chapter Summary

- A variety of drugs are used in the treatment of musculoskeletal (bone and muscle) disorders. The drug selected is based on the musculoskeletal disorder being treated, the severity of the disorder, and possibly other factors.

- The antiinflammatory action of aspirin is thought to be due to its ability to inhibit the synthesis of prostaglandins, a substance found in almost all body tissues and thought to increase the sensitivity of peripheral pain receptors to painful stimuli. The exact mechanism of action of the gold compounds, for example, gold sodium thiomalate and auranofin, in the suppression or prevention of inflammation is unknown.

- The nonsteroidal antiinflammatory drugs (NSAIDS) are so called because they do not belong to the steroid group of drugs, do not possess the adverse reactions associated with the steroids (corticosteroids) and yet have antiinflammatory activity. Their exact mechanism of action is unknown.

- Allopurinol reduces the production of uric acid, thus decreasing serum uric acid levels and the deposit of urate crystals in joints. The exact mechanism of action of colchicine is unknown, but it does reduce the inflammation associated with the deposit of urate crystals in the joints. This probably accounts for its ability to relieve the severe pain of acute gout. Sulfinpyrazone increases the excretion of uric acid by the kidneys, which lowers serum uric acid levels and consequently retards the deposit of urate crystals in the joints. Probenecid works in the same manner and may be given alone or with colchicine as combination therapy when there are frequent, recurrent attacks of gout.

- The mode of action of many skeletal muscle relaxants is not clearly understood. Many of these drugs do not directly relax skeletal muscles but their ability to relieve acute painful musculoskeletal conditions may be due to their sedative action. The potent antiinflammatory action of the corticosteroids make these drugs useful in the treatment of many types of musculoskeletal disorders.

- Phenylbutazone and oxyphenbutazone have antiinflammatory, as well as antipyretic and analgesic, activity. The exact mode of their antiinflammatory action is not well understood. These drugs may inhibit prostaglandin synthesis, which may partially account for their antiinflammatory activity. The mechanism of action of penicillamine, methotrexate, and hydroxychloroquine in the treatment of rheumatoid arthritis is unknown.

- Musculoskeletal disorders include diseases such as osteoarthritis, rheumatoid arthritis, ankylosing spondylitis, bursitis, muscular injuries such as sprains, and gout. Some of the drugs in this chapter are used for more than one type of musculoskeletal disorder whereas others are used for a specific disorder. With a few exceptions, response to therapy may take weeks or months.

- Some of the drugs used for the treatment of musculoskeletal disorders have the potential for causing serious and sometimes fatal adverse reactions.

Critical Thinking Exercises

1. Mary is a nurse who has returned to nursing after 15 years absence to raise a family. Mary asks you what should be included in a teaching plan for a patient with rheumatoid arthritis now taking high doses of salicylates. What information would you suggest Mary emphasize in a teaching plan?

2. Ms. Leeds is prescribed methotrexate for rheumatoid arthritis not responding to other therapies. She is nervous about starting the drug after she was told that the drug can cause many serious adverse reactions. What could you say to Ms. Leeds to relieve her anxiety? What specific instructions would you give her before she begins therapy with this drug?

44

Topical Drugs Used in the Treatment of Skin Disorders

Key Terms

Chapter Outline

Chapter Objectives

On completion of this chapter the student will:

* *Discuss the actions and uses of drugs used in the treatment of skin disorders*
* *List and discuss the adverse reactions of drugs used in the treatment of skin disorders*
* *Discuss the nursing implications to be considered when administering drugs used in the treatment of skin disorders*
* *Use the nursing process when administering drugs used in the treatment of skin disorders*

The skin forms a barrier between the outside environment and the structures located beneath the skin. The *epidermis* is the outermost layer of the skin. Immediately below the epidermis is the *dermis*. The dermis contains small capillaries, which supply nourishment to the dermis and epidermis, sebaceous (oil-secreting) glands, sweat glands, nerve fibers, and hair follicles. The epidermis and dermis are closely attached to one another.

Because of the skin's proximity to the outside environment, it is subject to various types of injury and trauma, as well as changes in the skin itself.

Topical Antiseptics and Germicides

An *antiseptic* is an agent that stops, slows, or prevents the growth of microorganisms. A *germicide* is an agent that kills bacteria.

ACTIONS OF TOPICAL ANTISEPTICS AND GERMICIDES

The exact mechanism of action of topical antiseptics and germicides is not well understood. These agents affect a variety of microorganisms. Some of these drugs have a short duration of action, whereas others have a long duration of action. The action of these agents may depend on the strength used and the time the drug is in contact with the skin or mucous membrane.

Benzalkonium. Benzalkonium (Zephiran) is a rapid-acting preparation with a moderately long duration of action. It is active against bacteria and some viruses, fungi, and protozoa. Benzalkonium solutions are *bacteriostatic* (slows or retards the multiplication of bacteria) or *bactericidal* (destroys bacteria), depending on their concentration.

Chlorhexidine. Chlorhexidine gluconate (Hibiclens) affects a wide range of microorganisms, including gram-positive and gram-negative bacteria.

Hexachlorophene. Hexachlorophene (pHisoHex) is a bacteriostatic cleansing agent. It has activity against staphylococci and other gram-positive bacteria. Cumulative action occurs with repeated use. The antibacterial residue left by this agent is resistant to

removal by many soaps, solvents, and detergents. Its activity may last for many days.

Iodine. Iodine has antiinfective action against many bacteria, fungi, viruses, yeasts, and protozoa. Povidone-iodine (Betadine) is a combination of iodine and povidone, which liberates free iodine. Povidone-iodine is often preferred over iodine solution or tincture because it is less irritating to the skin. Unlike iodine, treated areas may be bandaged or taped.

Nitrofurazone. Nitrofurazone (Furacin) has a broad spectrum of activity and is bactericidal against most bacteria commonly causing skin infections, including many that have become resistant to antibiotics.

Merbromin and Thimerosal. Merbromin (Mercurochrome) contains 25% mercury. It has only fair antiseptic activity. Thimerosal (Merthiolate) contains 49% mercury and has sustained bacteriostatic and fungistatic activity.

USES OF TOPICAL ANTISEPTICS AND GERMICIDES

Topical antiseptics and germicides are primarily used to reduce the number of bacteria on skin surfaces. Some of these agents, for example, chlorhexidine gluconate and hexachlorophene, may be used as a surgical scrub, as a preoperative skin cleanser, in washing the hands prior to and after caring for patients, and in the home to clean the skin. Others, such as iodine, merbromin, and thimerosal may be applied to minor cuts and abrasions to prevent infection. Some of these agents may also be used on mucous membranes. Nitrofurazone is frequently used in the prevention of infections in burns.

ADVERSE REACTIONS ASSOCIATED WITH THE USE OF TOPICAL ANTISEPTICS AND GERMICIDES

Topical antiseptics and germicides have few adverse reactions. Occasionally, an individual may be allergic to the drug and a skin rash or itching may occur. If an allergic reaction is noted, use of the topical agent is discontinued.

NURSING MANAGEMENT

Topical antiseptics and germicides are used, instilled, or applied as directed by the physician or the label of the product. Topical antiseptics and germicides are *not* a substitute for clean or aseptic techniques. They must be used as directed to obtain maximum effectiveness. Occlusive dressings (see Nursing Management under Topical Corticosteroids) are not to be used after application of these products unless a dressing is specifically ordered by the physician.

An occlusive dressing is not recommended following the use of benzalkonium. Iodine permanently stains clothing and temporarily stains the skin. Remove or protect the patient's personal clothing when iodine solution or tincture is applied.

Antiseptic and germicidal agents kept at the patient's bedside must be *clearly* labeled with the name of the product, the strength, and, when applicable, the date of preparation of the solution. Replace hard-to-read or soiled, stained labels as needed. Do *not* keep these solutions at the bedside of any patient who is confused or disoriented because the solution may be mistaken for water or another beverage and ingested.

Topical Antiinfectives

Localized skin infections may require the use of a topical antiinfective. The topical antiinfectives include antibiotic, antiviral, and antifungal drugs.

ACTIONS AND USES OF TOPICAL ANTIINFECTIVES

Topical Antibiotic Drugs

Topical antibiotics exert a direct local effect on specific microorganisms. Tetracycline (Achromycin), chlortetracycline (Aureomycin), chloramphenicol (Chloromycetin), erythromycin, and neomycin are examples of topical antibiotics. These drugs are used to prevent superficial infections in minor cuts, wounds, skin abrasions, and minor burns. Erythromycin is also indicated for treatment of acne vulgaris.

Topical Antiviral Drugs

Acyclovir (Zovirax) is the only topical antiviral agent currently available. This drug inhibits viral replication and is used in the treatment of initial episodes of genital herpes, as well as herpes simplex virus infections in *immunocompromised* patients, for example, patients with an immune system incapable of fighting infection.

Topical Antifungal Drugs

Antifungal drugs exert a local effect by inhibiting growth of the fungi. Examples of antifungal agents and their uses are:

- Miconazole (Micatin), ciclopirox (Loprox), and econazole (Spectazole)—used for treatment of tinea pedis (athlete's foot), tinea cruris (jock itch), tinea corporis (ringworm), and superficial candidiasis.
- Clioquinol (Vioform)—used for eczema, athlete's foot, and other fungal infections
- Triacetin (Fungoid)—used for nail fungus, athlete's foot, jock itch, ringworm, and monilial impetigo and dermatitis.

ADVERSE REACTIONS ASSOCIATED WITH TOPICAL ANTIINFECTIVES

Adverse reactions to topical antiinfectives are usually mild. Occasionally, the patient may develop a skin rash, itching, urticaria (hives), dermatitis, irritation, or redness, which may indicate a *hypersensitivity* (allergic) reaction to the drug. Prolonged use of topical antibiotic preparations may result in a superficial *superinfection* (an overgrowth of bacterial or fungal microorganisms not affected by the antibiotic being administered).

NURSING MANAGEMENT

Before each application, cleanse the skin with soap and warm water unless the physician orders a different method. Apply the antiinfective as prescribed (eg, thin layer, applied liberally) and either cover the area or leave it exposed, as directed.

Nursing Alert

Exercise care when applying antiinfectives or any topical drug near or around the eyes.

At the time of each application, inspect the affected area for changes (eg, signs of improvement or worsening of the infection) and for adverse reactions, such as redness or rash. Contact the physician and do not apply the drug if these or other changes are noted or if the patient complains of new problems, such as itching, pain, or soreness at the site.

Topical Corticosteroids

Topical corticosteroids vary in potency, with potency depending on factors such as the concentration of the drug (percentage); the vehicle in which the drug is suspended (lotion, cream, aerosol spray, and so on), and the area to which the drug is applied (open or denuded skin, nonbroken skin, thickness of the skin over the treated area).

Examples of topical corticosteroids include amcinonide (Cyclocort), betamethasone dipropionate (Diprosone), desonide (DesOwen), fluocinolone acetonide (Flurosyn), hydrocortisone (Cort-Dome), and triamcinolone acetate (Aristocort).

ACTIONS AND USES OF TOPICAL CORTICOSTEROIDS

Topical corticosteroids exert localized antiinflammatory activity. When applied to inflamed skin, they reduce itching, redness, and swelling. These drugs are useful in treating skin disorders, such as psoriasis, dermatitis, rashes, eczema, insect bite reactions, and first and second degree burns, including sunburns.

ADVERSE REACTIONS ASSOCIATED WITH TOPICAL CORTICOSTEROIDS

Localized reactions may include burning, itching, irritation, redness, dryness of the skin, and secondary infection.

NURSING MANAGEMENT

Prior to application, wash the area with soap and warm water unless the physician directs otherwise. Topical corticosteroids are usually ordered to be applied sparingly. The physician also may order the area of application to be covered or left exposed to the air. Some corticosteroids are applied as an occlusive dressing. The drug is applied while the skin is still moist following washing with soap and water; the area is then covered with a plastic wrap and sealed with tape or bandage and left in place for the prescribed period of time.

Topical Local Anesthetics

A topical anesthetic may be applied to the skin or mucous membranes.

ACTIONS AND USES OF TOPICAL ANESTHETICS

Topical anesthetics temporarily inhibit the conduction of impulses from sensory nerve fibers. These drugs may be used to relieve itching and pain due to skin conditions, such as minor burns, fungus infections, insect bites, rashes, sunburn, and plant poisoning, such as poison ivy. Some are applied to mucous membranes as local anesthetics. Examples of local anesthetics include benzocaine (Lanacane), dibucaine (Nupercainal), lidocaine (Xylocaine), and tetracaine (Pontocaine).

ADVERSE REACTIONS ASSOCIATED WITH TOPICAL ANESTHETICS

Occasionally, local irritation, dermatitis, rash, burning, stinging, and tenderness may be noted.

NURSING MANAGEMENT

Apply the anesthetic as directed by the physician. Prior to the first application, clean and dry the skin. For subsequent applications, remove all previous residue, if any, from the skin.

When a topical gel, such as lidocaine viscous, is used for oral anesthesia for the control of pain, instruct the patient not to eat food for 1 hour after use since local anesthesia of the mouth or throat may impair swallowing and increase the possibility of aspiration.

Topical Enzymes

ACTIONS AND USES OF TOPICAL ENZYMES

A topical enzyme aids in the removal of dead soft tissues by hastening the reduction of proteins into simpler substances. This is called *proteolysis* or a *proteolytic* action. The components of certain types of wounds, namely *necrotic* (dead) tissues and *purulent exudates* (pus-containing fluid) prevent proper wound healing. Removal of this type of debris by application of a topical enzyme aids in healing. Examples of conditions that may respond to application of a topical enzyme include second- and third-degree burns, pressure ulcers, and ulcers due to peripheral vascular disease.

Examples of topical enzymes include sutilains (Travase), collagenase (Santyl), and fibrinolysin and desoxyribonuclease (Elase).

ADVERSE REACTIONS ASSOCIATED WITH TOPICAL ENZYMES

The application of sutilains may cause mild, transient pain. Numbness and dermatitis also may be seen. Collagenase and fibrinolysin and desoxyribonuclease have a low incidence of adverse reactions.

NURSING MANAGEMENT

Certain types of wounds may require special preparations before applying the topical enzyme. Clean or prepare the area and apply the topical enzyme as directed by the physician. If bleeding occurs with the use of sutilains, discontinue applying the ointment and contact the physician.

Emollients

An *emollient* is a product that will soften or soothe the skin. Emollients are useful in treating dry skin and the discomfort associated with this problem. Most emollients are available as nonprescription products and often contain one or more ingredients. Examples of the ingredients found in emollients include mineral oil, aloe, glycerin, petrolatum, lanolin

oil, and vitamins A, D, and E. Adverse reactions to these preparations are rare.

Keratolytics and Cauterizing Agents

A *keratolytic* is a drug that removes excess growth of the epidermis (top layer of skin) in disorders, such as various types of warts. A *cauterizing* agent is one that uses a substance that destroys tissues and is used to remove warts, calluses, corns, seborrheic keratoses (benign variously colored skin growths arising from oil glands of the skin), and warts. Examples of keratolytics include salicylic acid, cantharidin, and podofilox. Monochloroacetic acid, dichloroacetic acid, trichloroacetic acid, and silver nitrate are cauterizing agents. Cauterizing agents and some keratolytics are only applied by a physician. Some strengths of salicylic acid are available as nonprescription products for the removal of warts on the hands and feet. Podofilox may be prescribed to be applied by the patient.

NURSING MANAGEMENT

The nurse may be responsible for checking the treatment sites 1 or more days after application. Alert the physician to any signs of extreme redness or infection at the application site.

Topical Antipsoriatics

Topical *antipsoriatics* are drugs used in the treatment of psoriasis. These agents help in the removal of the plaques associated with this disorder. Examples of antipsoriatics include anthralin (Anthra-Derm) and calcipotriene (Dovonex). Application of calcipotriene may cause burning, itching, and skin irritation. Anthralin may cause skin irritation, as well as temporary discoloration of the hair and fingernails.

NURSING MANAGEMENT

The nurse may be responsible for applying the product and inspecting the areas of application. Exercise care so that the product is only applied to the psoriatic lesions and not to surrounding skin. Signs of excessive irritation should be brought to the attention of the physician.

Nursing Process
The Patient Receiving a Topical Drug for a Skin Disorder

■ *Assessment*

Visually inspect the involved area. Describe the area including the size, color, and general appearance and record on the patient's chart.

■ *Nursing Diagnoses*
- **Anxiety** related to discomfort related to the skin disorder, appearance of the skin disorder
- **Risk for Ineffective Management of Therapeutic Regimen** related to knowledge deficit of use of topical drug

■ *Planning and Implementation*

The major goals of the patient may include a relief of anxiety and an understanding of the application or the reason for use of a topical drug. To make these goals measurable, more specific criteria must be added.

Anxiety. Some patients may exhibit anxiety over the symptoms or appearance of certain skin disorders. Allow time for the patient to verbalize concerns or ask questions about the application or use of a specific product. The application of some topical drugs may cause a brief stinging or burning sensation. Reassure the patient that the discomfort is brief. If the patient complains of severe discomfort or pain, discuss the problem with the physician.

■ *Patient and Family Teaching*

If the physician has prescribed or recommended the use of a topical drug, include the following in a teaching plan:
- Wash the hands thoroughly before and after applying the product.
- If the enclosed directions state that the product will stain clothing, be sure clothing is moved away from the treated area. If the product stains the skin, wear disposable gloves when applying the drug to prevent staining the fingers.
- Follow the directions on the label or use as directed by the physician. Read any enclosed directions for use of the product carefully.

- Prepare the area to be treated as recommended by the physician or described in the directions supplied with the product.
- Do not apply to areas other than those specified by the physician. Apply the drug as directed (eg, thin layer, apply liberally, and so on).
- Follow the directions of the physician regarding covering the treated area or leaving it exposed to air. The effectiveness of certain drugs are dependent on keeping the area covered or leaving it open.
- Keep this product away from the eyes (unless use in or around the eye has been recommended or prescribed). Do not rub or put the fingers near the eyes unless the hands have been thoroughly washed and all remnants of the drug removed from the fingers. If the product is accidentally spilled, sprayed, or splashed in the eye, wash the eye immediately with copious amounts of running water. Contact the physician *immediately* if burning, pain, redness, discomfort, or blurred vision persists for more than a few minutes.
- The drug may cause momentary stinging or burning when applied (when applicable).
- Discontinue use of the drug and contact the physician if rash, burning, itching, redness, pain, or other skin problems occur.

■ *Expected Outcomes for Evaluation*
- Anxiety is reduced
- Patient or family member demonstrates understanding of use and application of the prescribed or recommended drug

Chapter Summary

- The skin forms a barrier between the outside environment and the structures located beneath the skin. The epidermis is the outermost layer of the skin. Immediately below the epidermis is the dermis. The dermis contains small capillaries that supply nourishment to the dermis and epidermis, sebaceous (oil-secreting) glands, sweat glands, nerve fibers, and hair follicles. The epidermis and dermis are closely attached to one another. Because of the skin's proximity to the outside environment, it is subject to various types of injury and trauma, as well as changes in the skin itself.
- An antiseptic is an agent that stops, slows, or prevents the growth of microorganisms. A germicide is an agent that kills bacteria. The exact mechanism of action of topical antiseptics and germicides is not well understood. Topical antiseptics

and germicides are primarily used to reduce the number of bacteria on skin surfaces. Some of these agents may also be used on mucous membranes.

- Localized skin infections may require the use of a topical antiinfective. The topical antiinfectives include antibiotic, antiviral, and antifungal drugs.
- Topical antibiotics exert a direct local effect on specific microorganisms. Acyclovir is the only topical antiviral agent currently available. This drug inhibits viral replication. Topical antifungal drugs exert a local effect by inhibiting growth of the fungi.
- Topical corticosteroids exert localized antiinflammatory activity. When applied to inflamed skin, they reduce itching, redness, and swelling.
- Topical anesthetics temporarily inhibit the conduction of impulses from sensory nerve fibers.
- A topical enzyme aids in the removal of dead soft tissues by hastening the reduction of proteins into simpler substances.
- An emollient is a product that will soften or soothe the skin; it is useful in treating dry skin and the discomfort associated with it.

- A keratolytic is a drug that removes excess growth of the epidermis (top layer of skin) in disorders, such as various types of warts. A cauterizing agent is one that uses a substance that destroys tissues.
- Topical antipsoriatics are drugs used in the treatment of psoriasis.

Critical Thinking Exercises

1. A nurse tells you that she is upset because she was reprimanded over the labeling of a topical antiseptic used for cleaning a pressure ulcer, as well as over leaving the solution at the patient's bedside. She feels that her supervisor is unfair and that the entire situation is not as serious as the supervisor contends it to be. What would you say to this nurse?

2. What would you include in the daily assessment of a patient prescribed a topical drug?

45

Otic and Ophthalmic Preparations

Key Terms

Cycloplegia
Intraocular pressure
Miosis
Miotic
Mydriasis
Mydriatic
Myopia
Ophthalmic
Otic
Superinfection

Chapter Outline

Chapter Objectives

On completion of this chapter the student will:

- *Discuss the actions and uses of otic and ophthalmic preparations*
- *List and discuss the adverse reactions of otic and ophthalmic preparations*
- *Discuss the nursing management of a patient receiving an otic or ophthalmic preparation*
- *Use the nursing process when administering an otic or ophthalmic preparation*

Scherer JC, Roach S: INTRODUCTORY CLINICAL PHARMACOLOGY,
FIFTH EDITION © 1996 Lippincott-Raven Publishers

The eyes and ears are subject to various disorders, some of which are mild and others potentially or actually serious. Since the eyes and ears provide an interpretation of our outside environment, any disease or injury that has the potential for partial or total loss of function of these organs must be treated.

Otic Preparations

Various types of preparations are used for the treatment of *otic* (ear) disorders. Otic preparations can be divided into three categories: (1) antibiotics; (2) antibiotic and steroid combinations; and (3) miscellaneous preparations. The miscellaneous preparations usually contain one or more of the following ingredients:

- Benzocaine—a local anesthetic
- Phenylephrine—a vasoconstrictor decongestant
- Hydrocortisone, desonide—corticosteroids for anti-inflammatory and antipruritic effects
- Glycerin—an emollient and a solvent
- Antipyrine—an analgesic
- Acetic acid, boric acid, benzylkonium chloride, aluminum acetate, benzethonium chloride—provide antifungal or antibacterial action
- Carbamide peroxide, triethanolamine—aid in removing ear wax by softening and breaking up the wax

Examples of otic preparations are given in Summary Drug Table 45-1.

USES OF OTIC PREPARATIONS

Otic preparations are instilled in the external auditory canal and may be used to relieve pain, treat infection and inflammation, and aid in the removal of ear wax.

ADVERSE REACTIONS ASSOCIATED WITH THE ADMINISTRATION OF OTIC PREPARATIONS

Prolonged use of otic preparations containing an antibiotic may result in a *superinfection* (an overgrowth of bacterial or fungal microorganisms not affected by the antibiotic being administered).

NURSING MANAGEMENT

Nursing Alert

Only preparations labeled as *otic* are instilled in the ear. Check the label of the preparation *carefully* for the name of the drug and a statement indicating that the preparation is for otic use.

Prior to instillation of otic preparations, the container may be held in the hand for a few minutes to warm to body temperature. Cold and warm (above

Summary Drug Table 45-1. Otic Preparations

Generic Name	Trade Name*	Uses	Dose Ranges
chloramphenicol	Chloromycetin Otic	Superficial infections of the external auditory canal	2–3 drops into ear tid
hydrocortisone, neomycin sulfate, polymixin B	AntibiOtic, Otosporin, Oticair, *generic*	Same as chloramphenicol	4 drops into ear tid, qid
hydrocortisone, acetic acid propylene glycol diacetate sodium acetate, benzethonium chloride	Acetasol HC, VoSol HC Otic	Treatment of inflammatory conditions of external auditory canal	Insert saturated wick, leave in and keep moist for 24 h then remove wick and instill 5 drops tid, qid
benzocaine, antipyrine, glycerin	Allergan Ear Drops, Auralgan Otic, *generic*	Treatment of ear pain	Instill 2–4 drops, then insert saturated cotton pledget. Repeat 3–4/d
carbamide peroxide, anhydrous glycerin	Mollifene Ear Wax Removal System, Auro Ear Drops	Removal of ear wax	Instill 5–10 drops bid for 4 days

*The term, *generic,* indicates that the drug is available in generic form.

body temperature) preparations may cause dizziness or other sensations following instillation into the ear.

When instilling ear drops, have the patient lie on his or her side with the ear toward the ceiling. If the patient wishes to remain in an upright position, tilt the head toward the untreated side with the ear toward the ceiling. In the adult, the earlobe is pulled up and back. In children, the earlobe is pulled down and back. If the physician has not ordered a soft cotton plug to be placed in the opening of the external ear canal, keep the patient lying on the untreated side for 2 to 3 minutes. Once the patient is upright, the solution running out of the ear may be gently removed with gauze.

Nursing Process
The Patient Receiving an Otic Preparation

■ *Assessment*
The physician examines the ear and external structures surrounding the ear and prescribes the drug indicated to treat the disorder. The nurse may be responsible for examining the outer structures of the ear, namely the ear lobe and the skin around the ear.

■ *Nursing Diagnoses*
Depending on the physician's diagnosis and the patient's symptoms, one or more of the following may apply to the patient receiving an otic preparation:
- **Anxiety** related to ear pain or discomfort, changes in hearing, diagnosis, other factors
- **Risk for Ineffective Management of Therapeutic Regimen** related to lack of knowledge of correct technique for instilling ear medication, therapeutic regimen

■ *Planning and Implementation*
The major goals of the patient may include a reduction in anxiety and an understanding of the application and use of an otic preparation. To make these goals measurable, more specific criteria must be added.

Anxiety. Ear disorders may result in symptoms such as pain, a feeling of fullness in the ear, tinnitus, dizziness, or a change in hearing. Patients with

an ear disorder or injury usually have great concern over the effect the problem will have on their hearing. Reassure the patient that every effort is being made to treat the disorder and relieve the symptoms. Prior to instilling an otic solution, inform the patient that a feeling of fullness may be felt in the ear and that hearing in the treated ear may be impaired while the solution remains in the ear canal.

■ *Patient and Family Teaching*
Give the patient or a family member instructions or a demonstration in the instillation technique of an otic preparation. The following information may be given to the patient when an ear ointment or solution is prescribed:
- Wash the hands thoroughly before cleansing the area around the ear (when necessary) and instilling ear drops or ointment.
- Instill the prescribed number of drops or amount of ointment in the ear. Do not put the applicator or dropper tip in the ear.
- Immediately after use replace the cap or dropper. Refrigerate the solution if so stated on the label.
- Keep the head tilted or lie on the untreated side for 2 to 3 minutes to allow the solution to remain in contact with the ear. Excess solution and solution running out of the ear is wiped off with a tissue.
- Do not insert anything into the ear canal before or after applying the prescribed medication unless advised to do so by the physician.
- Complete a full course of treatment with the prescribed drug to achieve satisfactory results.
- Do not use nonprescription ear products during or after treatment unless use has been approved by the physician.
- Temporary changes in hearing or a feeling of fullness in the ear may occur for a short time after the medication has been instilled.
- Notify the physician if symptoms do not improve or become worse.

■ *Expected Outcomes for Evaluation*
- Anxiety is reduced
- Patient demonstrates ability to instill otic preparation in ear
- Patient verbalizes knowledge and importance of therapeutic regimen
- Patient and family demonstrate understanding of drug regimen

Ophthalmic Preparations

ACTIONS AND USES OF OPHTHALMIC PREPARATIONS

Various types of preparations are used for the treatment of *ophthalmic* (eye) disorders:

Sympathomimetic agents—have alpha- and beta-adrenergic activity (see Chap. 17 for a detailed discussion of adrenergic drugs). These drugs lower the *intraocular pressure* (IOP) (the pressure within the eye) by increasing the outflow of aqueous humor in the eye; they may be used to treat glaucoma. Some sympathomimetics, for example, tetrahydrozoline (Visine), are also used for their vasoconstrictor action to relieve minor eye irritation. The instillation of a sympathomimetic drug also results in *mydriasis* (dilatation of the pupil).

Beta-adrenergic blocking agents—decrease the rate of production of aqueous humor and thereby lower intraocular pressure. These drugs are used to treat glaucoma.

Miotics—contract the pupil of the eye (*miosis*), resulting in an increase in the space through which the aqueous humor flows. This increased space and improved flow results in a decrease in the intraocular pressure. Miotics may be used in the treatment of glaucoma.

Vasoconstrictors / mydriatics—dilate the pupil (mydriasis), constrict superficial blood vessels of the sclera, and decrease the formation of aqueous humor. Depending on the specific drug and strength, these agents may be used prior to eye surgery; in the treatment of glaucoma; for relief of minor eye irritation; and to dilate the pupil for examination of the eye.

Cycloplegic mydriatics—cause mydriasis and *cycloplegia* (paralysis of the ciliary muscle, resulting in an inability to focus the eye). These drugs are used in the treatment of inflammatory conditions of the iris and uveal tract of the eye and for examination of the eye.

Nonsteroidal antiinflammatory drugs—inhibit prostaglandin synthesis (see Chap. 15 for a discussion of the nonsteroidal antiinflammatory drugs), thereby exerting antiinflammatory action. These drugs are used to treat postoperative inflammation following cataract surgery (diclofenac); for the relief of itching of the eyes due to seasonal allergies (ketorolac); and during eye surgery to prevent miosis (flurbiprofen, suprofen).

Corticosteroids—possess antiinflammatory activity and are used for inflammatory conditions, such as allergic conjunctivitis, keratitis, herpes zoster keratitis, and inflammatory of the iris. Corticosteroids also may be used following injury to the cornea or after corneal transplants to prevent rejection.

Antibiotics—possess antibacterial activity and are used in the treatment of eye infections.

Sulfonamides—possess a bacteriostatic effect against a wide range of gram-positive and gram-negative microorganisms; they are used in the treatment of conjunctivitis, corneal ulcer, and other superficial infections of the eye.

Antiviral agents—interfere with viral reproduction by altering DNA synthesis. These drugs are used in the treatment of herpes simplex infections of the eye.

Antifungal agents—possess antifungal activity against a variety of yeast and fungi.

Silver—possesses antibacterial activity against gram-positive and gram-negative microorganisms. Silver protein, mild, is occasionally used in the treatment of eye infections. Silver nitrate is occasionally used to prevent gonorrheal ophthalmia neonatorum (gonorrhea infection of the newborn's eyes). Ophthalmic tetracycline and erythromycin have largely replaced the use of silver nitrate in newborns.

Artificial tear solutions and inserts—lubricate the eyes and are used for conditions such as dry eyes and eye irritation due to inadequate tear production.

Inactive ingredients may be found in some preparations. Examples of these agents include preservatives, antioxidants, which prevent deterioration of the product, and agents that slow drainage of the drug from the eye into the tear duct. Examples of the types of eye preparations are found in Summary Drug Table 45-2.

ADVERSE REACTIONS ASSOCIATED WITH THE ADMINISTRATION OF OPHTHALMIC PREPARATIONS

The incidence of adverse reactions is usually small. Since some ophthalmic preparations may be absorbed systemically, some of the adverse effects associated with systemic administration of the particular drug may be noted. When antibiotics are prescribed, a superinfection may be seen with prolonged or repeated use. Some ophthalmic preparations produce momentary stinging or burning on instillation.

Summary Drug Table 45–2. Ophthalmic Preparations

Generic Name	Trade Name*	Uses	Dose Ranges
SYMPATHOMIMETIC AGENTS			
dipivefrin hydrochloride	Propine	Treatment of glaucoma	1 drop q12h
epinephrine hydrochloride	Epifrin, *generic*	Same as dipivefrin hydrochloride	1–2 drops/d or bid
BETA-ADRENERGIC BLOCKING AGENTS			
betaxolol hydrochloride	Betoptic	Treatment of glaucoma	1 drop bid
carteolol hydrochloride	Ocupress	Same as betaxolol hydrochloride	1 drop bid
levobunolol hydrochloride	Betagen Liquifilm	Same as betaxolol hydrochloride	1 drop/d, bid
metipropranolol hydrochloride	OptiPranolol	Same as betaxolol hydrochloride	1 drop bid
timolol maleate	Timoptic	Same as betaxolol hydrochloride	1 drop/d, bid
MIOTICS			
carbachol, topical	Isopto Carbachol	Treatment of glaucoma	1–2 drops up to 3 times/d
isoflurophate	Floropryl	Treatment of glaucoma	0.25 inch strip of ointment into eye every 8–72 h
physostigmine (eserine)	Isopto Eserine, *generic*	Treatment of glaucoma	2 drops up to qid
pilocarpine hydrochloride	Isopto Carpine, *generic*	Treatment of glaucoma	1–2 drops up to 6 times/d
pilocarpine ocular therapeutic system	Ocusert Pilo-20, -40	Treatment of glaucoma	Insert new system every 7 d
VASOCONSTRICTORS/MYDRIATICS			
oxymetazoline hydrochloride	OcuClear, Visine	Relief of redness of eye due to minor irritation	1–2 drops 2–4 times/d
phenylephrine hydrochloride	Isopto Frin 0.12%, Ak-Dilate 2.5%, Neo-Synephrine 10%	0.12% for relief of redness of eye due to minor irritation; 2.5% and 10% treatment of uveitis, glaucoma; refraction procedures, prior to eye surgery	0.12% 1–2 drops up to 4 times/d; 2.5% and 10% 1 drop
tetrahydrozoline hydrochloride	Murine Plus, Visine, *generic*	Relief of redness due to minor eye irritation	1–2 drops up to 4 times/d
CYCLOPLEGIC/MYDRIATICS			
atropine sulfate	Isopto Atropine, *generic*	Eye refraction, treatment of acute inflammatory conditions of iris, uveal tract	1–2 drops up to 4 times/d
homatropine hydrobromide	Isopto Homatropine	Eye refraction, treatment of inflammatory conditions of uveal tract	1–2 drops q3–4h
NONSTEROIDAL ANTIINFLAMMATORY DRUGS			
diclofenac sodium	Voltaren	Postoperative inflammation following cataract surgery	1 drop qid
flurbiprofen sodium	Ocufen	Inhibition of intraoperative miosis	1 drop q1/2h beginning 2 hr before surgery
ketorolac tromethamine	Acular	Relief of ocular itching due to seasonal allergies	1 drop qid
suprofen	Profenal	Same as flurbiprofen	3 drops at 3, 2, and 1 h before surgery
CORTICOSTEROIDS			
dexamethasone phosphate	Ak-Dex, *generic*	Treatment of inflammatory conditions of the conjunctiva, lid, cornea, anterior segment of the eye	Solution: 1–2 drops qh during the day and q2h at night and reduced to 1 drop q4h when response noted; ointment: thin coating in lower conjunctival sac 3–4 times/d

(continued)

Summary Drug Table 45-2 (Continued)

Generic Name	Trade Name*	Uses	Dose Ranges
prednisolone sodium phosphate	AK-Pred, *generic*	Same as dexamethasone	1–2 drops qh during the day and q2h at night and reduced to 1 drop q4h when response noted
ANTIBIOTICS			
erythromycin	Ak-Mycin	Treatment of eye infections	See package insert
gentamicin	Garamycin, *generic*	Same as erythromycin	See package insert
tetracycline	Achromycin	Same as erythromycin	See package insert
SULFONAMIDES			
sodium sulfacetamide	Ak-Sulf, *generic*	Treatment of conjunctvitis, corneal ulcer, other superficial eye infections	1–2 drops q1–3h
ANTIVIRAL AGENTS			
idoxuridine	Herplex	Treatment of herpes simplex keratitis	1–2 drops qh during the day and q2h at night and reduced to 1 drop q2h during the day and q4h at night when response noted
vidarabine	Vira-A	Treatment of herpes simplex keratitis and conjunctivitis	0.5 inch of ointment into lower conjunctival sac 5 times/d at 3-hr intervals
ANTIFUNGAL AGENTS			
natamycin	Natacyn	Treatment of fungal infections of the eye	1 drop q1–2h
SILVER			
silver nitrate	*generic*	Prevention of ophthalmia neonatorum	2 drops of 1% solution in each eye
silver protein, mild	Argyrol S. S.	Treatment of eye infections	1–3 drops q3–4 h
ARTIFICIAL TEARS			
glycerin, sodium chloride	Dry Eye Therapy	Treatment of dry eyes	1–2 drops 3–4 times/d
benzalkonium chloride, polyvinyl alcohol, sodium chloride	Artificial Tears	Treatment of dry eyes	1–2 drops 3–4 times/d

*The term, *generic,* indicates that the drug is available in generic form.

NURSING MANAGEMENT

> **Nursing Alert**
>
> Only preparations labeled as *ophthalmic* are instilled in the eye. Check the label of the preparation *carefully* for the name of the drug, the percentage of the preparation, and a statement indicating that the preparation is for ophthalmic use.

Prior to instillation, ophthalmic solutions and ointments can be warmed in the hand for a few minutes. Ophthalmic ointments are applied to the eyelids or dropped into the lower conjunctival sac; ophthalmic solutions are dropped into the lower conjunctival sac. When eye solutions are instilled, apply gentle pressure on the inner canthus to delay drainage of the drug down the tear duct. Consult the physician regarding use of this technique *before* the first dose is instilled because this technique can be potentially dangerous in some eye conditions, such as recent eye surgery.

Some ophthalmic drugs produce blurring of vision, which can result in falls and other injuries. Warn the patient to exercise care when getting out of bed when the vision is impaired by these drugs. Patients admitted for treatment of acute glaucoma should be assessed every 2 hours for relief of pain.

Patients using the pilocarpine ocular therapeutic system must have the system replaced every 7 days. The system is inserted at bedtime since *myopia* (near-sightedness) occurs for several hours after insertion.

When a patient is scheduled for eye surgery, it is most important that the eye drops ordered by the physician are instilled at the correct time. This is especially important when the purpose of the drug is to change the size of the pupil.

Nursing Process
The Patient Receiving an Ophthalmic Preparation

■ *Assessment*
The physician examines the eye and external structures surrounding the eye and prescribes the drug indicated to treat the disorder.

■ *Nursing Diagnoses*
Depending on the physician's diagnosis and the patient's symptoms, one or more of the following may apply to the patient receiving an ophthalmic preparation:

- **Anxiety** related to eye pain or discomfort, diagnosis, other factors
- **Risk for Ineffective Management of Therapeutic Regimen** related to lack of knowledge of technique of instilling an eye medication, therapeutic regimen

■ *Planning and Implementation*
The major goals of the patient may include a reduction in anxiety and an understanding of the application and use of an ophthalmic preparation. To make these goals measurable, more specific criteria must be added.

Anxiety. Eye injuries and some eye infections are very painful. Other eye conditions may result in discomfort or a loss of or change in vision. The patient with an eye disorder or injury usually has great concern over the effect the problem will have on his or her vision. Reassure the patient that every effort is being made to treat the disorder.

■ *Patient and Family Teaching*
The patient or a family member will require instruction in the technique of instilling an ophthalmic preparation. The following information may be given to the patient and family member when an eye ointment or solution is prescribed:

- Hold the bottle (solution) or tube (ointment) in the hand for a few minutes before instilling.
- Wash the hands thoroughly before cleansing the eyelids, instilling eye drops, or applying an eye ointment.
- Instill the prescribed number of drops or amount of ointment. If more than one type of ophthalmic preparation is being instilled, wait the recommended time interval before instilling the second medication (usually 5 minutes for a solution and 10–15 minutes for an ointment).
- Close the eye gently; do not squeeze the eyes tightly shut after instilling the drug.
- The medication may cause a momentary stinging or burning sensation; this is normal.
- Complete a full course of treatment with the prescribed drug to achieve satisfactory results.
- Do not rub the eyes and keep hands away from the eyes.
- Do not use nonprescription eye products during or after treatment unless use has been approved by the physician.
- Replace the cap of the eye medication immediately after instilling the eye drops or ointment. Do not touch the tip of the container or tube.
- Temporary blurring of vision may occur. Avoid activities requiring visual acuity until vision returns to normal.
- Notify the physician if symptoms do not improve or worsen.

■ *Expected Outcomes for Evaluation*
- Anxiety is reduced
- Patient demonstrates ability to instill ophthalmic preparation in eye
- Patient and family demonstrate understanding of drug regimen
- Patient verbalizes knowledge and importance of treatment regimen

Chapter Summary

- The eyes and ears are subject to various disorders, some of which are mild and others potentially or actually serious. Since the eyes and ears provide an interpretation of our outside environment, any disease or injury has the potential for partial or total loss of function of these organs.
- Otic preparations can be divided into three categories: (1) antibiotics; (2) antibiotic and steroid combinations; and (3) miscellaneous preparations.

Otic preparations are instilled in the external auditory canal and may be used to relieve pain, treat infection and inflammation, and aid in the removal of ear wax. Prolonged use of otic preparations containing an antibiotic may result in a superinfection (an overgrowth of bacterial or fungal microorganisms not affected by the antibiotic being administered).

- Only preparations labeled as otic are instilled in the ear. The label of the preparation must be checked carefully for the name of the drug and a statement indicating the preparation is for otic use.
- Various types of preparations are used for the treatment of ophthalmic (eye) disorders and may include sympathomimetic agents, beta-adrenergic blocking agents, miotics, vasoconstrictors/mydriatics, cycloplegic mydriatics, nonsteroidal anti-inflammatory drugs, corticosteroids, antibiotics, sulfonamides, antiviral agents, antifungal agents, and artificial tear solutions and inserts. Inactive ingredients also may be found in some preparations.

- Only preparations labeled as ophthalmic are instilled in the eye. The label of the preparation must be checked carefully for the name of the drug, the percentage of the preparation, and a statement indicating that the preparation is for ophthalmic use.

Critical Thinking Exercises

1. Ms. Stone, aged 76, has glaucoma and is prescribed timolol (Timoptic) eye drops. Your initial assessment reveals that she has severe arthritis and appears to have difficulty following instructions. What further investigations would you make before developing a teaching plan for this patient?
2. Prepare a teaching plan for a patient prescribed an otic ointment for an infection in the outer ear canal.

46

Immunologic Agents

Key Terms

Chapter Outline

Chapter Objectives

On completion of this chapter the student will:

* *Discuss humoral immunity and cell-mediated immunity*
* *Define the terms used in immunology*
* *Distinguish between and define the three different types of immunity*
* *Discuss the positive and negative aspects of an immunization program*
* *Discuss nursing implications to be considered when administering an immunologic agent*

Scherer JC, Roach S: INTRODUCTORY CLINICAL PHARMACOLOGY,
FIFTH EDITION © 1996 Lippincott-Raven Publishers

Immunity refers to the ability of the body to identify and resist microorganisms that are potentially harmful. This ability enables the body to fight or prevent infectious disease and inhibit tissue and organ damage. The immune system has two distinct, but overlapping, mechanisms with which to fight invading organisms: the antibody-mediated defenses (*humoral* immunity) and cell-mediated defenses (cellular immunity).

HUMORAL IMMUNITY

In humoral immunity, special lymphocytes (white blood cells), called B-lymphocytes produce circulating antibodies to act against a foreign substance. This type of immunity is based on the antigen-antibody response. An *antigen* is a substance, usually a protein, that stimulates the body to produce antibodies. An *antibody* is a globulin (protein) produced by the B-lymphocytes as a defense against an antigen. Humoral immunity functions to protect the body against bacterial and viral infections.

Specific antibodies are formed for a specific antigen, that is, chickenpox antibodies are formed when the person is exposed to the chickenpox virus (the antigen). This is called an *antigen-antibody response.* Once manufactured, antibodies circulate in the bloodstream, sometimes for only a short time and at other times, for the life of the person. When an antigen enters the body, specific antibodies neutralize the specific invading antigen. This is called *immunity.* Thus, the individual with *specific* circulating antibodies is immune (or has immunity) to a *specific* antigen. *Immunity* then is the resistance that an individual has against disease.

CELL-MEDIATED IMMUNITY

Cell-mediated immunity is the result of the activity of the T-lymphocytes and macrophages (large cells that surround, engulf, and digest microorganisms and cellular debris). The macrophages and T-lymphocytes work together to destroy the antigen. T-lymphocytes are divided into three types: (1) circulating T-lymphocytes that function within the bloodstream identifying and destroying antigens; (2) noncirculating T-lymphocytes that produce lymphokines, a substance that causes macrophages to migrate to inflamed tissue; and (3) memory T-lymphocytes that recognize antigens and activate macrophages. These T-lymphocytes defend against

viral infections, fungal infections, and some bacterial infections. If cell-mediated immunity is lost, as in the case of acquired immunodeficiency syndrome, the body is unable to protect itself against many viral, bacterial, and fungal infections.

Cell-mediated and humoral immunity are interdependent, that is, cell-mediated immunity influences the function of the B-lymphocytes and humoral immunity influences the function of the T-lymphocytes.

Immunologic Agents

Some immunologic agents capitalize on the body's natural defenses by stimulating the immune response, thereby creating within the body protection to a specific disease. Other immunologic agents supply ready-made antibodies to provide passive immunity. Examples of immunologic agents include vaccines, toxoids, and immune globulins.

VACCINES, TOXOIDS, AND IMMUNE GLOBULINS

Antibody-producing tissues cannot distinguish between an antigen that is capable of causing disease (a live antigen) or an *attenuated* (weakened) antigen or a killed antigen. Because of this phenomenon, *vaccines,* which contain either an attenuated or killed antigen, have been developed to create immunity to certain diseases. The live antigens are either killed or weakened during the manufacturing process. Vaccines containing specific attenuated or killed antigens are used to create immunity to specific diseases.

A *toxin* is a poisonous substance produced by some bacteria, such as the *Clostridium tetani,* the bacteria that causes tetanus. A toxin is capable of stimulating the body to produce *antitoxins,* which are substances that act in the same manner as antibodies. Toxins are powerful substances and like other antigens, they can be attenuated. A toxin that is attenuated (or weakened), but still capable of stimulating the formation of antitoxins is called a *toxoid.*

Both vaccines and toxoids are administered to stimulate the immune response within the body to specific antigens or toxins. The initiation of the immune response, in turn, produces resistance to a specific infectious disease. The immunity produced in this manner is called *active immunity.*

Globulins are proteins present in blood serum or plasma; they contain antibodies. *Immune globulins* are solutions obtained from human blood containing antibodies that have been formed by the body to specific antigens. Because they contain ready-made antibodies, they are given for passive immunity against disease. Those receiving immune globulins receive antibodies only to those diseases to which the donor blood is immune.

ACTIVE IMMUNITY

When a person is exposed to certain infectious microorganisms (antigens), the body begins to form antibodies (or build an immunity) to the invading microorganism. This is called active immunity. There are two types of active immunity: naturally acquired active immunity and artificially acquired active immunity. Summary Drug Table 46-1 identifies agents that produce active immunity.

Naturally Acquired Active Immunity

Naturally acquired active immunity occurs when the person is exposed to a disease and develops the disease, and the body manufactures antibodies to provide future immunity to the disease. It is called *active* immunity because the antibodies were produced by the person who had the disease (Fig. 46-1).

An example is when the individual is exposed to chickenpox for the first time and has no immunity to the disease. The body immediately begins to manufacture antibodies against the chickenpox virus. However, the production of a sufficient quantity of antibodies takes time, and the individual gets the disease. At the time of exposure and while the individual still has chickenpox, the body continues to manufacture antibodies. These antibodies circulate in the individual's bloodstream for life. In the future, any exposure to the chickenpox virus results in the antibodies' mobilizing to destroy the invading antigen.

Artificially Acquired Active Immunity

Artificially acquired active immunity occurs when an individual is given a killed or weakened antigen, which stimulates the formation of antibodies against the antigen. The antigen does *not* cause the disease but the individual will still manufacture specific antibodies against the disease. When a vaccine con-

taining an attenuated antigen is given, the individual *may* develop a few minor symptoms of the disease or even a mild form of the disease but the symptoms are almost always milder and usually last for a short time.

The decision to use an attenuated or a killed virus for a vaccine is based on research that shows the results of such an administration. Some antigens, when killed, show a poor antibody response, whereas when the antigen is merely weakened, a good antibody response occurs.

An example is the administration of the measles vaccine to an individual who has not had measles. The measles (rubeola) vaccine contains the live, attenuated measles virus. The individual receiving the vaccine develops a *mild or modified* measles infection, which then produces immunity against the rubeola virus.

Artificially acquired immunity against some diseases may require periodic *booster* injections to keep an adequate antibody level (or antibody titer) circulating in the blood. A booster injection may be needed because the life of some antibodies is short. A booster injection is the administration of an additional dose of the vaccine to "boost" the production of antibodies to a level that will maintain the desired immunity. The booster is given months or years after the initial immunization. The immunization schedules for children are given in Table 46-1.

PASSIVE IMMUNITY

Passive immunity is obtained from the administration of immune globulins or antitoxins. This type of immunity provides the individual with ready-made antibodies from another human or by an animal (see Fig. 46-1). Passive immunity provides *immediate* immunity to the invading antigen, but lasts for only a short time. Summary Drug Table 46-2 identifies agents for passive immunizations.

An antitoxin is an solution obtained from the blood of animals that have been immunized with specific antigens, for example, the diphtheria antitoxin. Because diphtheria is extremely serious (sometimes fatal), it is necessary to provide the individual with *immediate* immunity by the administration of diphtheria antitoxin. The antitoxin that is given is produced by an animal (a horse) injected with the live diphtheria virus. The animal produces an antitoxin identical to the antitoxin that can be manufactured by a human. The individual exposed to diphtheria would also produce his or her own antitoxin, but this may take days or even weeks.

Summary Drug Table 46-1. Agents for Active Immunization

Generic Name	Trade Name*	Uses	Adverse Reactions	Dose Ranges
BACTERIAL VACCINES				
BCG vaccine	*generic*	Those with negative tuberculin skin tests exposed to sputum-positive cases of tuberculosis	Incidence is low	0.2–0.3 mL intradermally
cholera vaccine	*generic*	Travel to areas requiring cholera vaccination	Transitory local reactions, malaise, fever, headache	2 doses of 0.5 mL SC, IM 1 wk to 1 mo apart
hemophilus b conjugate vaccine	HibTITER, ProHIBIT, PedavaxHIB	Immunization for children 2 mo to 5 y against diseases caused by *Haemophilus influenzae b*	Redness at injection site, fever	0.5 mL IM, 3 doses, 2 mo apart, booster at 15 mo; ProHIBIT: 0.5 mL IM
meningococcal polysaccharide vaccine, groups A, C, Y, and W-135	Menomune-A/C/Y/W-135	Immunization for medical and laboratory personnel, travelers to endemic areas, household travelers to endemic areas, household contacts of meningococcal disease	Headache, malaise, fever, chills; tenderness, pain, and redness at injection site	0.5 mL SC
pneumococcal vaccine, polyvalent	Pneumovax 23, Pnu-Immune 23, *generic*	Immunization against pneumococcal pneumonia and bacterium	Erythema and soreness at injection site, fever, myalgia	0.5 mL SC, IM
poliovirus vaccine, inactivated (Salk, IPV)	*generic*	Immunization against poliomyelitis	Erythema, induration and pain at injection site	0.5 mL SC
typhoid vaccine	*generic*	Intimate exposure to known carrier, travel to area where typhoid is endemic	Local reactions, malaise, myalgia, fever	Primary immunization: 2 doses of 0.5 mL SC at intervals of ≥ 4 wk; children under 10: each dose is 0.25 mL; booster: 0.5 mL SC or 0.1 mL intradermal every 3 y
VIRAL VACCINES				
hepatitis B vaccine	Heptavax-B, Recombivax-HB, Engerix-B	Immunization against all known subtypes of hepatitis B virus	Local reactions, malaise, fatigue, headache, nausea, myalgia	See package insert of specific trade name for amount and dosage schedule
influenza virus vaccine	Fluogen, Fluzone, Fluvirin, *generic*	Annual vaccination of those at increased risk of consequences from infections of lower respiratory tract, older persons, those providing essential community services	Local reactions, fever, malaise, myalgia	See package insert for recommended dosage schedule; vaccine prepared for use during a specific year
measles (rubeola) virus vaccine, live, attenuated	Attenuvax	Given before or immediately after exposure to natural measles; immunization for children 15 mo or older	Fever, rash (between 5th and 12th days after administration)	1 ampule SC at 15 mo of age

(continued)

Summary Drug Table 46–1 (Continued)

Generic Name	Trade Name*	Uses	Adverse Reactions	Dose Ranges
measles (rubeola) and rubella virus vaccine	M-R-Vax II	Immunization for children 15 mo to puberty and adults	Fever, rash (between 5th and 12th days after administration)	0.5 mL SC
measles, mumps, and rubella virus vaccine	M-M-R II	Immunization for children 15 mo to puberty and adults	Fever, rash (between 5th and 12th days after administration)	0.5 mL SC
mumps virus vaccine, live	Mumpsvax	Immunization for children 15 mo or older and adults	Fever, parotitis, burning or stinging at site	0.5 mL SC
poliovirus vaccine live, oral, trivalent (Sabin, TOPV)	Orimune	Prevention of poliomyelitis in infants, children up to 18 y	Vaccine-associated paralysis (rare)	Primary series: 3 doses of 0.5 mL PO started at 6–12 wk of age; 2nd dose given 7 d after 1st dose; 3rd dose in 21 or 28 d after the 1st dose
rubella virus vaccine live	Meruvax II	Immunization for children aged 14 to puberty, adolescent and adult males, non-pregnant adolescent and adult females	Fever, joint pain, rash, malaise, sore throat, lymphadenopathy, headache	0.5 mL (preferably at 15 mo of age)
rubella and mumps virus vaccine, live	Biavax II	Immunization for children aged 1 mo to puberty	Fever, joint pain, rash, malaise, sore throat, lymphadenopathy, headache	0.5 mL (preferably at 15 mo of age)
TOXOIDS				
diphtheria and tetanus toxoids, combined (labeled for pediatric or adult use)	*generic*	Pediatric form used until age 6; adult form for children aged 7 or over and adults	Local reactions, fever, drowsiness, anorexia, vomiting, malaise, generalized aches and pains	Pediatric: 2–3 doses (depending on age) of 0.5 mL IM 4 wk apart, then 0.5 mL in 6–12 mo and a booster of 0.5 mL when starting school; adults: 2 doses of 0.5 mL IM 4–8 wk apart, reinforcing dose of 0.5 mL 6–12 mo later; booster dose of 0.5 mL every 10 y
diphtheria and tetanus toxoids and whole cell pertussis vaccine absorbed (DTP)	Tri-Immunol, *generic*	Immunization of infants and children through age 6	Local reactions, fever, chills, irritability	3 doses of 0.5 mL IM at 4–8 wk intervals; booster: 0.5 mL when child is 4–6 y old
diphtheria and tetanus toxoids and acellular pertussis vaccine (DTaP)	Acet-Immune, Tripedia	Immunization as the 4th or 5th dose in children (DTwP as 1–3 doses)	Local reactions, fever, chills, irritability	Fourth: 0.5 mL IM at approximately 18 mo of age (at least 6 mo after 3rd DTwP and Fifth: 0.5 mL at 4–6 y of age
diphtheria and tetanus toxoids and whole cell pertussis and Haemophilus influenzae type B conjugate vaccines (DTwP-HIB)	Tetramune	Immunization of infants and children through age 6	Local reactions, fever, chills, irritability	Beginning at 2 mo of age, 3 doses of 0.5 mL at 2 mo intervals; followed by a fourth dose of 0.5 mL at 15 mo of age

(continued)

Summary Drug Table 46-1 (Continued)

Generic Name	Trade Name*	Uses	Adverse Reactions	Dose Ranges
rabies vaccine, human diploid cell cultures (HDCV)	Imovax Rabies Vaccine	Preexposure and postexposure immunization	Local reactions, nausea, headache, muscle aches, abdominal pain	See package insert for dosage recommendation and suggested schedules
rabies vaccine, human diploid cell cultures (for intradermal use)	Imovax Rabies I.D. Vaccine	Preexposure immunization for those at risk	Same as for rabies vaccine, human diploid cell cultures	3 doses of 0.1 mL given intradermally; 2nd-dose given 7 d after 1st dose, 3rd dose in 21 or 28 d after the 1st dose
tetanus toxoid, fluid and tetanus toxoid, absorbed	generic	Immunization in adults and children	Local reactions, fever, chills, malaise, myalgia	Tetanus toxoid absorbed: 2 doses of 0.5 mL IM given 4–8 wk apart; booster every 10 y; tetanus toxoid, fluid: 3 doses of 0.5 mL IM, SC at 4–8 wk intervals and 4th dose 6–12 mo after 3rd dose: booster every 10 y

*The term, *generic,* indicates that the drug is available in generic form.

Because immediate immunity is required in this instance, passive immunity is the chosen method of providing temporary immunity to this disease.

Diphtheria antitoxin would be given if the individual: (1) has never had diphtheria (naturally acquired active immunity); (2) has never received the diphtheria vaccine (artificially acquired active immunity); or (3) was exposed to or began to develop the disease.

Another example of passive immunity is the administration of immune globulins (see Summary Drug Table 46-2), such as hepatitis B immune glob-

Active and passive immunity

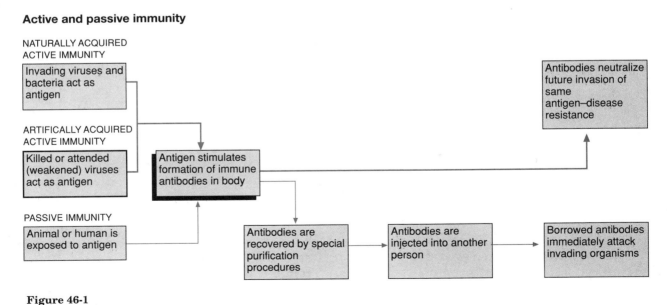

Figure 46-1

Active and passive immunity.

Table 46-1. Recommended Childhood Immunization Schedule (United States — January 1995)

Vaccine[1]	Birth	2 mos	4 mos	6 mos	12 mos[6]	15 mos	18 mos	4–6 yrs	11–12 yrs	14–16 yrs
Hepatitis B[2]	HB-1									
		HB-2		HB-3						
Diphtheria, tetanus, pertussis[3]		DTP	DTP	DTP	DTP or DTaP at 15 mos			DTP or DTaP	Td	
H. influenzae type b[4]		Hib	Hib	Hib	Hib					
Polio		OPV	OPV	OPV				OPV		
Measles, mumps, rubella[5]					MMR			MMR or MMR		

[1]Vaccines are listed under the routinely recommended ages. Shaded bars indicate range of acceptable ages for vaccination.

[2]Infants born to HB₁AG-negative mothers should receive the second dose of heptitis B vaccine between 1 and 4 months of age, provided at least 1 month has elapsed since receipt of the first dose. The third dose is recommended between 6 and 18 months of age. Infants born to HBsAG-positive mothers should receive immunoprophylaxis for hepatitis B with 0.5 ml Hepatitis B Immune Globulin (HBIG) within 12 h of birth, and 0.5 ml of either Merck, Sharpe & Dohme vaccine (Recombivax HB) or of SmithKline Beecham vaccine (Engerix-B) at a separate site. In these infants, the second dose of vaccine is recommended at 1 mo of age and the third dose at 6 months of age. All pregnant women should be screened for HBsAG in an early prenatal visit.

[3]The fourth dose of DTP may be administered as early as 12 months of age, provided at least 6 months have elapsed since DTP3. Combined DTP-Hib products may be used when these two vaccines are to be administered simultaneously. DTaP (diphtheria and tetanus toxoids and acellular pertussis vaccine) is licensed for use for the fourth and/or fifth dose of DTP vaccine in children 15 months of age or older and may be preferred for these doses in children in this age group. Td (diphtheria and tetanus toxoids for persons ≥ 7 years of age) is recommended at 11–12 years of age, provided at least 5 years have elapsed since the last dose of DTP or DT.

[4]Three H. influenzae type b conjugate vaccines are available for use in infants: HbOC [HibTITER] (Lederle Praxis); PRP-T [ActH1B; OmniH1B] (Pasteur Merieux, distributed by SmithKline Beecham; Connaught); and PRP-OMP [PedvaxH1B] (Merck, Sharp & Dohme). Children who have received PRP-OMP at 2 and 4 months of age do not require a dose at 6 months of age. After the primary infant Hib conjugate vaccine series is completed, any licensed Hib conjugate vaccine may be used as a booster dose at ages 12–15 months.

[5]The second dose of MMR vaccine should be administered EITHER at 4–6 years of age OR at 11–12 years of age, depending on state school requirements.

[6]Vaccines recommended in the second year of life (12–15 months of age) may be given at either one or two visits.

Approved by the Advisory Committee on Immunization Practices (ACIP), the American Academy of Pediatrics (AAP), and the American Academy of Family Physicians (AAFP).

ulin. Administration of this vaccine is an attempt to prevent hepatitis B *after* the individual has been exposed to the virus.

NURSING IMPLICATIONS

Immunization is an important method of controlling some of the infectious diseases that are capable of causing serious and sometimes fatal consequences. An example is the polio virus vaccine. Before the development of this vaccine, many children and adults were afflicted with this disease each year. Some years produced an epidemic of poliomyelitis (polio). Many persons were admitted to the hospital daily and often required weeks and even months of hospitalization. Many of these victims were permanently paralyzed. For some, the paralysis affected one or both arms or legs. Others developed a form of the disease that affected the respiratory center, resulting in

permanent respiratory paralysis requiring lifetime use of artificial ventilation because they would never be able to breathe on their own. Today, poliomyelitis is rare because administration of the poliovirus vaccine has provided immunity to a large number of the population.

History

Before the administration of any vaccine, an allergy history is obtained. If the individual is known or thought to have allergies of any kind, this is told to the physician before the vaccine is given. Some vaccines contain antibodies obtained from animals, such as the horse, whereas other vaccines may contain proteins or preservatives to which the individual may be allergic. A highly allergic person may have an allergic reaction (which could be serious and even fatal). If the patient has an allergy history, the

Summary Drug Table 46–2.   Agents for Passive Immunity

Generic Name	Trade Name*	Uses	Adverse Reactions	Dose Ranges
IMMUNE SERUMS				
hepatitis B immune globulin (HBIG)	H-BIG, HyperHep, Hep-B-Gammagee	Postexposure prophylaxis	Local reactions, fever, urticaria	0.06 mg/kg IM as soon as possible after exposure and repeated 28–30 d after exposure; see package insert for additional dosage and schedules
immune globulin intramuscular	Gamastan, Gammar	Hepatitis A (before or soon after exposure), rubeola (prevention and modification in those exposed < 6 d previously), immunoglobulin deficiency, passive immunization for varicella in immunosuppressed patients	Local reactions, fever, urticaria	0.02–1.3 mL/kg IM depending on reason for use
immune globulin, intravenous (IGIV)	Gamimune N, Sandoglobulin, Gammagard, Venoglobulin-I, Iveegam	Immunodeficiency syndrome, idiopathic thrombocytopenic purpura, B-cell lymphocytic leukemia	Hypersensitivity reactions, hypotension	See package insert of specific product (by trade name) for dosage
RHo(D) immune globulin	Gamulin Rh, RhoGAM	Prevention of sensitization to Rho(D) factor and of hemolytic disease in the newborn in a subsequent pregnancy; transfusion accidents (Rho-[D] negative patient transfused with Rho-[D] positive blood)	Local reactions, fever, urticaria	≥ 1 vial IM depending on reason for use
tetanus immune globulin	Hyper-Tet	Passive immunization	Tenderness, pain, muscle stiffness	Adults: 250 U IM; children: dose based on weight (4 U/kg)
varicella-zoster immune globulin (human)	*generic*	Passive immunization of immune deficient individuals in those meeting required criteria (see package insert)	Tenderness, pain at injection site	Dosage based on weight (125 U/10 kg; maximum dose: 625 U IM)
ANTITOXINS				
diphtheria antitoxin	*generic*	Prevention or treatment of diphtheria	Anaphylaxis, pain and redness at injection site	Therapeutic: 20,000–120,000 U IM, IV; prophylaxis: 10,000 U IM
tetanus antitoxin	*generic*	Tetanus: prevention of tetanus when tetanus immune globulin not available	Tenderness, pain at injection site	Prophylactic: 1500–5000 U IM, SC; treatment: 50,000–100,000 U IM and IV (part of dose given IV and remainder IM)

(continued)

Summary Drug Table 46–2 (Continued)

Generic Name	Trade Name*	Uses	Adverse Reactions	Dose Ranges
RABIES PROPHYLAXIS PRODUCTS				
antirabies serum, equine origin (ARS)	*generic*	Suspected exposure to rabies	Serum sickness, local pain, erythema, urticaria	1000 U/55 lbs (39.6 IU/g)
rabies immune globulin, human (RIG)	Imogam, Hyperab	Immunization for those suspected of exposure	Fever, soreness at injection site, low grade fever, anaphylaxis	20 IU/kg IM; ½ the dose may be used to infiltrate the wound
rabies vaccine human diploid cell cultures (HDCV)	Imovax Rabies Vaccine	Preexposure immunization for those in high risk group, post-exposure immunization	Hypersensitivity reactions, tenderness, pain at injection site	Preexposure: 3 IM injections of 1 mL each on d 0, 7, 21, or 28; Post-exposure: 5 IM injection or 1 mL on d 0, 3, 7, 14, and 28

*The term, *generic*, indicates that the drug is available in generic form.

physician may decide to skin test him or her for allergy to one or more of the components or proteins in the vaccine.

Administration

If a vaccine is not in liquid form and must be reconstituted, the nurse must read the directions enclosed with the vaccine. It is important to follow the enclosed directions carefully. Package inserts also contain information regarding dosage, adverse reactions, method of administration, administration sites (when appropriate), and, when needed, recommended booster schedules.

On occasion, it may be necessary to postpone the regular immunization schedule, particularly of children. This is of special concern to parents. The decision to delay immunization because of illness or for other reasons must be discussed with the physician. However, the decision to administer or delay vaccination because of febrile illness (illness causing an elevated temperature) depends on the severity of the symptoms and the specific disorder. In general, all vaccines can be administered to those with minor illness, such as a cold virus and those with low grade fever. However, moderate or severe febrile illness is a contraindication. In instances of moderate or severe febrile illness, vaccination is done as soon as the acute phase of the illness is over. Table 46-2 lists general contraindications for immunizations. Specific contraindications and precautions may be found in the package insert that comes with the drug.

Nursing Alert

Minor adverse reactions such as fever, rashes, and aching of the joints are possible with the administration of a vaccine. In most cases, these reactions subside within 48 hours. The physician may prescribe 10 to 15 mg/kg acetaminophen every 4 hours to control these reactions.

Patient and Family Teaching

Because of the effectiveness of various types of vaccines in the prevention of disease, nurses must inform the public about the advantages of immunization. Parents should be encouraged to have infants and young children receive the immunizations suggested by the physician.

Those traveling to a foreign country are advised to contact their physician or local health department well in advance of their departure date for information about the immunizations that will be needed. Immunizations should be given well in advance of departure because it may take several weeks to produce adequate immunity.

When an adult or child is receiving a vaccine for immunization, the patient or a family member is made aware of the possible reactions that may occur, for example, soreness at the injection site, fever, and so on.

There have been fatalities, as well as serious viral infections of the central nervous system, associated with the use of vaccines. Although the number of these incidents is small, a risk factor still remains when some vaccines are given. However, a risk is also associated with *not* receiving immunization against

Table 46-2. Contraindications for Immunization

1. Moderate or severe illness, with or without fever.
2. Anaphylactoid reactions (eg, hives, swelling of the mouth and throat, difficulty breathing (dyspnea), hypotension, and shock).
3. Known allergy to vaccine or vaccine constituents, particularly horse serum, eggs, or neomycin.
4. Individuals with an immunological deficiency should not receive the oral polio virus vaccine (virus is transmissible to the immunocompromised individual).
5. Immunizations are postponed during the administration of steroids, radiation therapy, and antineoplastic (anticancer) drug therapy.
6. Live virus vaccines against measles, rubella, and mumps should not be given to pregnant women.
7. Patients who experience encephalopathy (alterations in unconsciousness, unresponsiveness, or seizures) within 7 days of receiving the vaccine for diphtheria, tetanus, and pertussis should not be given any additional doses.

some infectious diseases. That risk may be higher and just as serious as the risk associated with the use of vaccines. It must also be remembered that when a large segment of the population is immunized, the small number of those not immunized are less likely to be exposed to and be infected with the disease-producing microorganism. But when large numbers of the population are *not* immunized, there is a great increase in the chances of exposure to the infectious disease and a significant increase in the probability that the individual will develop the disease.

Chapter Summary

- Immunity refers to the ability of the body to identify and resist organisms that are potentially harmful. The immune system has two distinct, but overlapping, mechanisms with which to fight invading organisms: the antibody-mediated defenses (humoral immunity) and cell-mediated defenses.
- In humoral immunity, special lymphocytes, B-lymphocytes, produce circulating antibodies to act against a foreign substance. Specific antibodies are formed for a specific antigen. This is called an antigen-antibody response. When an antigen enters the body, specific antibodies neutralize the specific invading antigen resulting in immunity.
- Cell-mediated immunity is the result of the activity of the T-lymphocytes and macrophages. The macrophages and T-lymphocytes work together to destroy the antigen.

- Vaccines that contain either an attenuated or killed antigen have been developed to create immunity to certain diseases.
- A toxin is a poisonous substance produced by some bacteria that is capable of stimulating the body to produce antitoxins, which act in the same manner as antibodies. A toxin that is attenuated, but still capable of stimulating the formation of antitoxins is called a toxoid. Both vaccines and toxoids are administered to stimulate the immune response within the body to specific antigens or toxins. The initiation of the immune response, in turn, produces resistance to a specific infectious disease.
- Immune globulins are obtained from human blood and contain antibodies to specific antigens. Because they contain ready-made antibodies, these immune globulins are given to provide immediate immunity to invading antigens.
- Naturally acquired active immunity occurs when the person is exposed to a disease and develops the disease, and the body manufactures antibodies to provide future immunity to the disease.
- Artificially acquired active immunity occurs when an individual is given a killed or weakened antigen, which stimulates the formation of antibodies against the antigen. The antigen does not cause the disease but the individual will still manufacture specific antibodies against the disease.
- Passive immunity provides the individual with antibodies made by another human or by an animal. Passive immunity provides immediate immunity to the invading antigen but this type of immunity lasts for only a short time.
- Immunization is an important method of controlling some of the infectious diseases that are capable of causing serious and sometimes fatal consequences. To properly administer the immunization, the enclosed directions must be followed carefully. Package inserts also contain information regarding dosage, adverse reactions, method of administration, administration sites (when appropriate) and, when needed, recommended booster schedules.

Critical Thinking Exercises

1. Ms. Wilson has brought her 6-month-old daughter, Michelle, to the clinic for the last of the series of three DPT and OPV immunizations. Ms. Wilson asks you to explain how a vaccination will keep her daughter from getting sick. How would you address this topic with Ms. Wilson?
2. Discuss the significance of all healthcare workers receiving the hepatitis b vaccine (Heptavax-B). Is this necessary for all health care personnel? Why or why not?

47

Antineoplastic Drugs

Chapter Outline

Chapter Objectives

On completion of this chapter the student will:

- *List the types of drugs used in the treatment of neoplastic diseases*
- *List the general adverse reactions associated with the administration of the antineoplastic drugs*
- *Discuss nursing management when administering an antineoplastic drug*
- *Use the nursing process when administering an antineoplastic drug*

Antineoplastic drugs are agents used in the treatment of malignant diseases (cancer). These agents can be used for cure, control, or palliative (relief of symptoms) therapy. Although these drugs may not always effect a complete cure of the malignancy, they often slow the rate of tumor growth and delay metastasis (spreading of the cancer to other sites). Use of these drugs is one of the tools in the treatment of cancer. The term *chemotherapy* is often used to refer to therapy with antineoplastic drugs.

Antineoplastic Drugs

The antineoplastic drugs covered in this chapter include the alkylating agents, antibiotics, antimetabolites, hormones, mitotic inhibitors, and miscellaneous drugs.

ACTIONS OF THE ANTINEOPLASTIC DRUGS

Generally, most antineoplastic drugs affect cells that rapidly proliferate (divide and reproduce). Malignant neoplasms or cancerous tumors usually consist of rapidly proliferating cells. The normal cells that line the oral cavity and gastrointestinal tract, and cells of the gonads, bone marrow, hair follicles, and lymph tissue are also rapidly dividing cells and are usually affected by these drugs. Thus, antineoplastic drugs may affect normal, as well as malignant (cancerous) cells.

Chemotherapy is administered in a series of cycles to allow for recovery of the normal cells and to destroy more of the malignant cells. Every malignant cell must be destroyed for the cancer to be cured. Each cycle of treatment with the antineoplastic drugs kills some, but by no means all, of the malignant cells. Therefore, repeated courses of chemotherapy are used to kill more and more of the malignant cells, until theoretically none are left.

Alkylating Agents

Alkylating agents interfere with the process of cell division of malignant and normal cells. The malignant cells appear to be more susceptible to the effects of the alkylating agents. Examples of alkylating agents include mechlorethamine (Mustargen) and chlorambucil (Leukeran).

Antibiotics

The antibiotics, unlike their antibiotic relatives, do not have antiinfective (against infection) ability. They appear to interfere with DNA and RNA synthesis, and therefore delay or inhibit cell division, including the reproducing ability of malignant cells. Examples of antineoplastic antibiotics include bleomycin (Blenoxane) and doxorubicin (Adriamycin).

Antimetabolites

The antimetabolites interfere with various metabolic functions of cells, thereby disrupting normal cell functions. These drugs are most effective in the treatment of rapidly dividing neoplastic cells. Examples of the antimetabolites include methotrexate (Folex) and fluorouracil (Adrucil).

Hormones

The exact method of antineoplastic action of hormones is unclear. These drugs also appear to counteract the effect of male or female hormones in hormone-dependent tumors (see Chap. 40). Examples of hormones used as neoplastic agents include testolactone (Teslac), an androgen; polyestradiol (Estradurin), an estrogen; and megestrol (Megace), a progestin.

Gonadotropin-releasing hormone analogues, for example, leuprolide (Lupron), appear to act by inhibiting the anterior pituitary secretion of gonadotropins, thus, suppressing the release of pituitary gonadotropins. These drugs primarily decrease serum testosterone levels and therefore are used in the treatment of advanced prostatic carcinomas.

Mitotic Inhibitors

Mitotic inhibitors interfere with or stop cell division. Examples of mitotic inhibitors include etoposide (VePesid) and vincristine (Oncovin).

Miscellaneous Antineoplastic Drugs

The mechanism of action of this unrelated group of drugs is not entirely clear. Examples of miscellaneous antineoplastics include interferon Alpha-2a (Roferon-A) and hydroxyurea (Hydrea).

USES OF THE ANTINEOPLASTIC DRUGS

Antineoplastic drugs may be given alone or in combination with other antineoplastic drugs. In many instances, a combination of these drugs produces better results than the use of a single antineoplastic agent.

Although many antineoplastic drugs share a similar activity (ie, they interfere in some way with cell division), their uses are not necessarily similar. The more common uses of specific antineoplastic drugs are given in Summary Drug Table 47-1.

ADVERSE REACTIONS ASSOCIATED WITH THE ADMINISTRATION OF ANTINEOPLASTIC DRUGS

Antineoplastic drugs often produce a wide variety of adverse reactions. Some of these reactions are dose dependent, that is, their occurrence is more common or their intensity is more severe when higher doses are used. Other adverse reactions occur primarily because of the effect the drug has on many cells of the body.

Some adverse reactions are desirable, for example, the depressing effect of certain antineoplastic drugs on the bone marrow because this adverse drug reaction is essential in the treatment of the leukemias. Other adverse reactions are not desirable, for example, severe vomiting or diarrhea.

Antineoplastic drugs are potentially toxic and their administration is often associated with many serious adverse reactions. At times, some of these adverse effects are allowed because the only alternative is to stop treatment of the malignancy. A treatment plan is developed that will prevent, lessen, or treat most or all of the symptoms of a specific adverse reaction. An example of prevention is giving an antiemetic before administering an antineoplastic drug known to cause severe nausea and vomiting. An example of treatment of the symptoms of an adverse reaction is the administration of an antiemetic, as well as intravenous (IV) fluids and electrolytes when severe vomiting occurs.

Adverse reactions seen with the administration of these drugs may range from very mild to life-threatening. Some of these reactions, such as the loss of hair (*alopecia*), may have little effect on the physical status of the patient but may definitely have a serious effect on the patient's mental health. Because nursing is concerned with the whole patient, some of these physically altering reactions can have a profound effect on the patient and must be considered when planning nursing management.

Some of the adverse reactions seen with antineoplastic agents are listed in Summary Drug Table 47-1. Appropriate references should be consulted when administering these drugs because there are a variety of uses, dose ranges, and, in some instances, many adverse reactions.

NURSING MANAGEMENT

Most hospitals and clinics require that nurses receive specialized training and standardized educational preparation prior to administering the antineoplastic drugs. The Oncology Nursing Society has developed guidelines and educational tools for credentialing nurses for certification in administering chemotherapy.

Management of the patient receiving an antineoplastic drug depends on factors such as the drug or combination of drugs given; the dosage of the drugs; the patient's physical response to therapy; the response of the tumor to chemotherapy; and the type and severity of adverse reactions.

In some hospitals, policies are established to provide nursing personnel with specific guidelines for the assessment and management of patients receiving a single or combination chemotherapeutic drug regimen. If guidelines are not provided, review the drugs being given prior to administration. Consult appropriate references to obtain information regarding the preparation and administration of a particular drug, the average dose ranges, all the known adverse reactions, and the warnings and precautions given by the manufacturer.

Preparing an Antineoplastic Drug for Administration

Although some of these drugs are given orally, others are given by the parenteral route. It is *most important* to follow the manufacturer's or physi-

Summary Drug Table 47-1. Antineoplastic Drugs

Generic Name	Trade Name*	Uses	Adverse Reactions	Dose Ranges
ALKYLATING AGENTS				
busulfan	Myleran	Chronic myelogenous leukemia	Leukopenia, anemia, cataracts, hyperpigmentation of skin, thrombocytopenia	1–8 mg/d PO
carboplatin	Paraplatin	Ovarian carcinoma	Bone marrow supression, pain, nausea, vomiting, diarrhea, electrolyte changes	360 mg/m² IV; smaller doses may be used when there is renal insufficiency or hematologic changes
carmustine	BiCNU	Brain tumors, multiple myeloma, Hodgkin's disease	Thrombocytopenia, burning at injection site, nausea, vomiting, azotemia, leukopenia	100–200 mg/m² IV
chlorambucil	Leukeran	Chronic lymphocytic leukemia, malignant lymphomas, Hodgkin's disease	Bone marrow depression, hyperuricemia, nausea, vomiting, diarrhea, hepatotoxicity	0.03–0.2 mg/kg/d PO
cisplatin (CDDP)	Platinol	Metastatic testicular and ovarian tumors, advanced bladder cancer	Nephrotoxicity, ototoxicity, marked nausea and vomiting, leukopenia, thrombocytopenia, hyperuricemia	Testicular tumors: 20 mg/m² IV; ovarian 50 mg/m² IV; bladder cancer: 50–70 mg/m² IV
cyclophosphamide	Cytoxan, Neosar	Malignant lymphomas, Hodgkin's disease, multiple myeloma, leukemia, carcinoma of the ovary and breast, neuroblastoma, retinoblastoma	Leukopenia, thrombocyto-, penia, anemia, anorexia, nausea, vomiting, diarrhea, cystitis, alopecia	Initial dose: 40–50 mg/kg IV; maintenance doses: 1–5 mg/kg/d PO; 3–15 mg/kg IV
ifosfamide	Ifex	Testicular cancer	Hemorrhagic cystitis, mental confusion, coma, alopecia, nausea, vomiting	1.2 g/m²/d IV
lomustine	CeeNu	Brain tumors, Hodgkin's disease	Nausea, vomiting, thrombocytopenia, leukopenia, alopecia, anemia	100–300 mg/m² PO
mechlorethamine hydrochloride	Mustargen	Hodgkin's disease, lymphosarcoma, bronchogenic carcinoma, leukemia	Nausea, vomiting, jaundice, alopecia, lymphocytopenia, granulocytopenia, thrombocytopenia, skin rash, diarrhea	0.4 mg/kg IV as a total dose for a course of therapy which may be given as a single or divided dose
melphalan	Alkeran	Multiple myeloma, carcinoma of the ovary	Nausea, vomiting, bone marrow depression, skin rash, alopecia	6–10 mg/d PO; dosage may also be based on weight, 16 mg/m² IV
pipobroman	Vercyte	Polycythemia vera, chronic granulocytic leukemia	Nausea, vomiting, abdominal cramping, diarrhea, rash	1–3 mg/kg/d PO
streptozocin	Zanosar	Carcinoma of the pancreas	Renal toxicity, severe nausea and vomiting, diarrhea	500–1000 mg/m² IV-depending on dosage intervals
thiotepa (triethylene thiophosphoramide)	*generic*	Carcinoma of the breast, ovary, Hodgkin's, lymphosarcomas, intracavity effusions due to localized metastatic disease	Nausea, vomiting, pain at injection site, bone marrow depression	0.3–0.4 mg/kg IV; dosage is higher for intracavity or intratumor administration

(continued)

Summary Drug Table 47-1 (Continued)

Generic Name	Trade Name*	Uses	Adverse Reactions	Dose Ranges
uracil mustard	*generic*	Chronic lymphocytic or myelogenous leukemia, non-Hodgkin's lymphomas	Bone marrow depression, nausea, vomiting, diarrhea	Adults: 0.15 mg/kg PO as a single weekly dose
ANTIBIOTICS				
bleomycin sulfate	Blenoxane	Carcinoma of the head and neck, lymphomas, testicular carcinoma	Pneumonitis, pulmonary fibrosis, erythema, rash, fever, chills, vomiting	0.25–0.5 U/kg IV, IM, SC
dactinomycin	Cosmegen	Wilms's tumor, choriocarcinoma, Ewing's sarcoma, testicular carcinoma	Anorexia, alopecia, bone marrow depression, nausea, vomiting	Up to 15 mcg/kg/d IV; may also be given by isolation perfusion at 0.035–0.05 mg/kg
daunorubicin hydrochloride	Cerubidine	Leukemia	Bone marrow depression, alopecia, acute nausea and vomiting, fever, chills	25–45 mg/m^2/d IV
doxorubicin hydrochloride	Adriamycin, Rubex	Acute leukemias, neuroblastoma, soft tissue and bone sarcomas, carcinomas of the breast, ovary, bladder, lymphomas, Wilms's tumor	Alopecia, acute nausea and vomiting, mucositis, chills, bone marrow depression, fever	30–75 mg/m^2 IV
idarubicin hydrochloride	Idamycin	Leukemia	Congestive heart failure, arrhythmias, chest pain, myocardial infarction, nausea, vomiting, alopecia	12 mg/m^2 daily X 3d IV
mitomycin	Mutamycin	Adenocarcinoma of the stomach, pancreas	Bone marrow depression, anorexia, nausea, vomiting, headache, blurred vision, fever	20 mg/m^2 IV
mitoxantrone hydrochloride	Novantrone	Leukemia	CHF, GI bleeding, jaundice, nausea, vomiting, diarrhea, infections, dyspnea, headache, conjunctivitis, stomatitis	12 mg/m^2 IV
pentostatin (2^1-deoxycoformycin)	Nipent	Alpha-interferon-refractory hairy cell leukemia	Leukopenia, anemia, thrombocytopenia, nausea, vomiting, rash, fever	4 mg/m^2 every other week IV
plicamycin (mithramycin)	Mithracin	Malignant tumors of the testes, hypercalcemia and hypercalcuria associated with neoplasms	Hemorrhagic syndrome (epistaxis, hematemesis, widespread hemorrhage in the GI tract, generalized advanced bleeding), vomiting, diarrhea, anorexia, nausea, stomatitis	Testicular tumors: 25–30 mcg/kg/d IV; hypercalcemia, hypercalcuria: 25 mcg/kg/d IV for 3–4 d
ANTIMETABOLITES				
cytarabine	Cystosar-U	Acute myelocytic or lymphocytic leukemia	Bone marrow depression, nausea, vomiting, diarrhea, anorexia	100–200 mg/m^2/d IV, SC
floxuridine	FUDR, *generic*	GI adenocarcinoma metastatic to the liver	Diarrhea, anorexia, nausea, vomiting, alopecia, bone marrow depression	0.1–0.6 mg/kg/d by arterial infusion
fludarabine	Fludara	Chronic lymphocytic leukemia	Bone marrow depression, fever, chills, infection, nausea, vomiting	25 mg/m^2 IV
fluorouracil (5-FU)	Adrucil, *generic*	Carcinoma of the breast, stomach, pancreas, colon	Diarrhea, anorexia, nausea, vomiting, alopecia, bone marrow depression	3–12 mg/kg/d IV

(continued)

Summary Drug Table 47-1 (Continued)

Generic Name	Trade Name*	Uses	Adverse Reactions	Dose Ranges
mercaptopurine (6-mercaptopurine, 6–MP)	Purinethol	Acute lymphatic leukemia, acute or chronic myelogenous leukemia	Bone marrow depression, hyperuricemia, hepatotoxicity	1.5–2.5 mg/kg/d PO
methotrexate (MTX)	Folex, *generic*	Lymphosarcoma, severe psoriasis, cancer of the head, neck, breast, lung	Ulcerative stomatitis, nausea, rash, pruritus, renal failure, bone marrow depression, fatigue, fever, chills	Antineoplastic dosages vary widely depending on type of tumor; psoriasis: 10–50 mg/wk IV, IM, PO or up to 6.5 mg/d PO
thioguanine	*generic*	Acute leukemias, chronic myelogenous leukemia	Bone marrow depression, hepatic toxicity, nausea, vomiting, stomatitis, hyperuricemia	2–3 mg/kg/d PO
HORMONES				
fluoxymesterone	Halotestin, *generic*	Inoperable breast carcinoma	Virilization, amenorrhea, menstrual irregularities	10–40 mg/d PO in divided doses
methyltestosterone	Android-10, *generic*	Breast carcinoma	Virilization, amenorrhea, menstrual irregularities	50–200 mg/d PO (25–100 mg buccal)
testolactone	Teslac	Breast cancer in post-menopausal women or premenopausal women when ovarian function has been terminated	Glossitis, anorexia, paresthesia, hypertension, nausea, vomiting, rash	250 mg PO qid
testosterone (aqueous suspension)	Tesamone, Histerone, *generic*	Breast carcinoma	Virilization, amenorrhea, menstrual irregularities	50–100 mg IM 3 times/wk
testosterone cypionate	Depo-Testos-terone, *generic*	Breast carcinoma	Virilization, amenorrhea, menstrual irregularities	200–400 mg IM every 2–4 wk
ANTIANDROGEN				
flutamide	Eulexin	Metastatic prostate carcinoma	Hot flashes, loss of libido, diarrhea, nausea, vomiting, impotence	250 mg PO tid at 8 h intervals
ANABOLIC STEROIDS				
nandrolone phenpropionate	Androlone, *generic*	Control of metastatic breast carcinoma	Nausea, vomiting, diarrhea, fluid and electrolyte imbalance, virilization	50–100 mg/wk IM
ESTROGENS				
chlorotrianisene	TACE	Prostatic carcinoma	Headache, dizziness, intolerance to contact lens, edema, thromboembolism, hypertension, nausea, weight changes, dysmenorrhea, testicular atrophy, acne, breast tenderness, gynecomastia	12–25 mg/d PO
conjugate estrogens, oral	Premarin	Breast and prostatic carcinoma	Headache, dizziness, intolerance to contact lens, edema, thromboembolism, hypertension, nausea, weight changes, dysmenorrhea, testicular atrophy, acne, breast tenderness, gynecomastia	Breast carcinoma: 10 mg PO tid; prostatic carcinoma: 1.25–2.5 mg PO tid

(continued)

Summary Drug Table 47-1 (Continued)

Generic Name	Trade Name*	Uses	Adverse Reactions	Dose Ranges
diethylstilbestrol (DES)	*generic*	Breast and prostatic carcinoma	Headache, dizziness, intolerance to contact lens, edema, thromboembolism, hypertension, nausea, weight changes, dysmenorrhea, testicular atrophy, acne, breast tenderness, gynecomastia	Breast carcinoma: up to 15 mg/d PO; prostatic carcinoma: 1–3 mg/d PO
diethylstilbestrol diphosphate	Stilphostrol	Inoperable prostatic carcinoma	Headache, dizziness, intolerance to contact lens, edema, thromboembolism, hypertension, nausea, weight changes, dysmenorrhea, testicular atrophy, acne, breast tenderness, gynecomastia	50–200 mg or more PO tid; drug may also be given IV
estradiol	Estrace	Breast and prostatic carcinoma	Headache, dizziness, intolerance to contact lens, edema, thromboembolism, hypertension, nausea, weight changes, dysmenorrhea, testicular atrophy, acne, breast tenderness, gynecomastia	Breast carcinoma: 10 mg PO tid; prostatic carcinoma: 1–2 mg PO tid
estramustine phosphate sodium (estradiol and nonnitrogen mustard)	EMCYT	Metastatic or progressive prostatic carcinoma	Nausea, diarrhea, anorexia, fluid retention, increased risk of thrombosis, leukopenia, rash, thrombopenia	14 mg/kg/d PO in 3–4 divided doses
ethinyl estradiol	Estinyl	Breast and prostatic carcinoma	Headache, dizziness, intolerance to contact lens, edema, thromboembolism, hypertension, nausea, weight changes, dysmenorrhea, testicular atrophy, acne, breast tenderness, gynecomastia	Breast carcinoma: 1 mg PO tid; prostatic carcinoma: 0.15–2 mg/d PO
polyestradiol phosphate	Estradurin	Prostatic carcinoma	Nausea, vomiting, painful swelling of breast, thrombophlebitis, pulmonary embolism, erythema multiforme	40–80 mg IM
ANTIESTROGEN				
tamoxifen citrate	Nolvadex,	Breast carcinoma in menopausal women	Hypercalcemia, ophthalmic changes, hot flashes, nausea, vomiting, vaginal bleeding and discharge	10–20 mg PO bid
PROGESTINS				
medroxyprogesterone acetate	Depo-Provera	Endometrial or renal carcinoma	Breast tenderness, pruritus, thromboembolitic phenomena, amenorrhea	400–1000 mg/wk IM
megestrol acetate	Megace	Advanced carcinoma of the breast, endometrium	Carpal tunnel syndrome, alopecia, deep vein thrombosis, weight gain, nausea and vomiting	Breast carcinoma: 40 mg PO qid; endometrial carcinoma: 40–320 mg/d PO in divided doses
GONADOTROPHIN-RELEASING HORMONE ANALOGUE				
leuprolide acetate	Lupron	Advanced prostatic carcinoma	Edema, headache, dizziness, bone pain, nausea, vomiting, anorexia, ECG changes, hypertension	1 mg/d SC in divided doses

(continued)

Summary Drug Table 47-1 (Continued)

Generic Name	Trade Name*	Uses	Adverse Reactions	Dose Ranges
goserelin acetate	Zoladex	Advanced prostatic carcinoma	Hot flashes, sexual dysfunction, lethargy, edema, vaginitis, headache, depression	3.6 mg SC every 28 d
MITOTIC INHIBITORS				
etoposide	VePesid	Testicular tumors, small cell lung cancer	Nausea, vomiting, anorexia, granulocytopenia, alopecia	Testicular cancer: 50–100 mg/m² IV; lung cancer: 35 mg/m² IV, oral dose is twice the IV dose
teniposide (WM-26)	VuMON	Leukemia	Nausea, vomiting, mucositis, diarrhea, alopecia, leukopenia, rash, thrombocytopenia, anemia	165–250 mg/m² IV
vinblastine sulfate (VLB)	Velban, Velsar, *generic*	Hodgkin's disease, lymphoma, testicular carcinoma, Kaposi's sarcoma	Leukopenia, nausea, vomiting, paresthesias, malaise, weakness, mental depression, headache	3.7–18.5 mg/m²/wk IV
vincristine sulfate (VCR)	Oncovin, *generic*	Acute leukemia, lymphosarcoma, neuroblastoma, Wilms's tumor, Hodgkin's disease	Ataxia, headache, oral ulceration, vomiting, weight loss, fever, diarrhea	1.4 mg/m²/wk IV
MISCELLANEOUS ANTINEOPLASTIC DRUGS				
aldesleukin (Interleukin-2; IL-2)	Proleukin	Metastatic renal cell carcinoma	Anemia, thrombocytopenia, mental changes, thyroid dysfunction, fever, chills, pruritis, GI effects	0.037 mg/kg IV
altretamine	Hexalen	Ovarian cancer	Nausea, vomiting, leukopenia peripheral neuropathy	260 mg/m²/d PO
asparaginase	Elspar	Leukemia	Hypersensitivity reactions (rash, urticaria, arthralgia, respiratory distress, acute anaphylaxis), depression, somnolence, fatigue, coma, anorexia, nausea, vomiting	200–1000 IU/kg/d IV; 6000 IU/m²/d IM
BCG	TICE BCG, TheraCys	Carcinoma of the bladder	Dysuria, urinary frequency, cystitis, hematuria, urinary incontinence	Three vials intravesically
cladribine	Leustatin	Hairy cell leukemia	Neutropenia, fever, infection, fatigue, nausea, headache	0.09 mg/kg/d
dacarbazine	DTIC-Dome	Melanoma, Hodgkin's disease	Anorexia, nausea, vomiting	Melanoma: 2–4.5 mg/kg IV or 250 mg/m² IV; Hodgkin's: 150–375 mg/m² IV
hydroxyurea	Hydrea	Melanoma, leukemia, carcinoma of the ovary	Bone marrow depression, stomatitis, anorexia, nausea, vomiting, diarrhea, headache	20–80 mg/kg PO
interferon alpha-2a	Roferon-A	AIDS-related Kaposi's sarcoma, hairy-cell leukemia	Fever, fatigue, myalgia, headache, chills, anorexia, nausea, diarrhea, vomiting, dizziness, cough, dyspnea, abdominal pain	Leukemia: 3 million IU per dose SC, IM; Kaposi's sarcoma: 36 million IU SC, IM per dose

(continued)

Summary Drug Table 47-1 (Continued)

Generic Name	Trade Name*	Uses	Adverse Reactions	Dose Ranges
interferon alpha-2b	Intron A	AIDS-related Kaposi's sarcoma, hairy-cell leukemia	Fever, fatigue, myalgia, headache, chills, anorexia nausea, diarrhea, vomiting, dizziness, cough, dyspnea, abdominal pain	Leukemia: 2 million IU/m² per dose SC, IM; Kaposi's sarcoma: 30 million IU/m² per dose IM, SC
levamisole Hcl	Ergamisol	Adjunct treatment with Dukes' Stage C colon cancer	Agranulocytosis, nausea, vomiting, rash, fever, chills, malaise	50 mg q8h PO
mitotane	Lysodren	Adrenocortical carcinoma	Anorexia, nausea, vomiting, diarrhea, skin rash	2–16 g/d PO in divided doses
pacLitaxel	Taxol	Ovarian and breast carcinoma	Bone marrow suppression, infection, hypersensitivity reactions, bradycardia, hypotension, peripheral neuropathy, nausea, vomiting, alopecia	135–175 mg/m² IV
pegaspargase (PEG-L-asparaginase)	Oncaspar	Acute lymphoblastic leukemia	Nausea, vomiting, fever, malaise, dyspnea, hypotension, diarrhea	2500 IU/m² IM or IV
procarbazine hydrochloride	Matulane	Hodgkin's disease	Leukopenia, anemia, nausea, vomiting, thrombocytopenia, anorexia	1–6 mg/kg PO

*The term, *generic,* indicates that the drug is available in generic form.

cian's directions regarding the type of solution to be used for dilution or administration. For example, when carmustine (BiCNU) is prepared for administration, the manufacturer warns that only the diluent supplied with the drug is to be used for the first step in diluting the drug.

When preparing an antineoplastic drug for parenteral administration, wear disposable plastic gloves. Some of these drugs can be absorbed through the skin of the individual preparing these drugs. Because antineoplastic agents are highly toxic and can have an effect on many organs and systems of the body, use measures to prevent absorption of the drug through the skin. Take precautions to prevent accidental spilling or spraying of the drug into the eyes or onto unprotected areas of the skin. Thoroughly wash hands before and after preparing and administering an antineoplastic agent. This is especially important when the drug is given by the parenteral route.

Special directions for administration, stated by either the physician or manufacturer, are also important. For example, cisplatin cannot be prepared or administered with needles or IV administration sets containing aluminum because aluminum reacts with cisplatin, causing a precipitate formation and loss of potency.

Administering an Antineoplastic Drug

Some antineoplastic agents have specific recommended administration techniques. For example, an infusion pump is recommended for the administration of cisplatin; lomustine (CeeNu) is given orally on an empty stomach; and plicamycin (Mithracin) is administered by slow IV infusion over 4 to 6 hours. If administration guidelines are not provided by the physician or the hospital, check with the appropriate authorities (physician, pharmacist) regarding the administration of a specific antineoplastic agent.

Read the package insert supplied with the drug thoroughly before the drug is prepared and administered. The manufacturer's recommendations may include information, such as storage of the drug, reconstitution procedures, stability of the drug after reconstitution, the rate of administration, the technique of administration, and so on.

Postadministration Management

After the administration of an antineoplastic agent, plan nursing management based on the following:

• The patient's general condition

- The patient's individual response to the drug
- Adverse reactions that may occur
- Guidelines established by the physician or hospital
- Results of periodic laboratory tests

The Patient's General Condition

The patient who is acutely ill with many physical problems requires different nursing management than one who is ambulating and able to participate in the activities of daily living. Once the patient's general condition is assessed and his or her needs identified, develop a nursing care plan to meet those needs. Patients receiving chemotherapy can be at different stages of their disease; therefore, individualize nursing management of each patient based on the patients needs and not only on the type of drug administered.

The Patient's Individual Response to the Drug

Not all patients respond in the same manner to a specific antineoplastic drug. For example, an antineoplastic agent may cause vomiting but the amount of fluid and electrolytes lost through vomiting may vary from patient to patient. One patient may require additional sips of water once nausea and vomiting has subsided, whereas another may require IV fluid and electrolyte replacement. Nursing management is not only geared to what may or what did happen, but is also based on the effects produced by a particular adverse reaction. In the example of the patient who is vomiting, it is important to accurately measure all fluid intake and all output from the gastrointestinal and urinary tracts, as well as to observe the patient for signs of dehydration and electrolyte imbalances. These measurements and observations aid the physician in determining if fluid replacement is necessary.

Adverse Drug Reactions

Alopecia. _Alopecia_ (loss of hair) is a common adverse reaction associated with some of the antineoplastic drugs. This problem occurs 10 to 21 days after the treatment cycle is completed. If hair loss is associated with the antineoplastic drug being given, tell the patient that hair loss may occur. Hair loss is temporary and hair will grow again when the drug therapy is completed. Warn the patient that hair loss may occur suddenly and in large amounts.

Depending on the patient, plans may need to be made in advance for the purchase of a wig or cap to disguise the hair loss until the hair grows back. Although this may seem to be a minor problem when compared to the serious reactions that may be seen during chemotherapy, the loss of hair _is_ a personal problem for most patients and requires as much nursing consideration as a serious or life-threatening situation.

Anorexia. _Anorexia_ (loss of appetite resulting in the inability to eat) is a common occurrence with the antineoplastic drugs. Assess the nutritional status of the patient before and during treatment. Small, frequent meals (five to six meals daily) are usually better tolerated than three large meals. Breakfast is often the most tolerable meal of the day. Stress the importance of eating meals high in nutritive value, particularly protein (eg, eggs, milk products, tuna, beans, peas, and lentils). Monitor weight weekly and report any weight loss.

Bone Marrow Depression. _Bone marrow depression_ is a potentially dangerous adverse reaction resulting in decreased production of blood cells. Bone marrow depression is manifested by abnormal laboratory test results and clinical evidence of leukopenia, thrombocytopenia, or anemia. For example, there is a decrease in the white blood cells or leukocytes (_leukopenia_), a decrease in the thrombocytes (_thrombocytopenia_) and a decrease in the red blood cells resulting in _anemia_.

Patients with leukopenia have a decreased resistance to infection and must be monitored closely for _any_ signs of infection.

> **_Nursing Alert_**
>
> Report any of the following signs of infection to the physician immediately: fever of 100.4° F (38° C) or higher, cough, sore throat, chills, frequent urination or a white blood cell count less than 2000/mm³.

Thrombocytopenia is characterized by a decrease in the platelet count (below 100,000/mm³). Patients with thrombocytopenia are monitored for bleeding tendencies and precautions are taken to prevent bleeding. Injections are avoided but, if necessary, pressure is applied to the injection site for 3 to 5 minutes to prevent bleeding into the tissue and the formation of a hematoma. Have the patient avoid the use of electric razors, nail trimmers, dental floss, firm toothbrushes, or use of any sharp objects. Monitor closely for easy bruising, skin lesions, and bleeding from any orifice (opening) of the body.

Nursing Alert

Report any of the following to the physician immediately: bleeding gums, easy bruising, increased menstrual bleeding, tarry stools, or coffee ground emesis.

Anemia occurs as the result of a decreased production of red blood cells in the bone marrow and is characterized by fatigue, dizziness, shortness of breath, and palpitations. On occasion, the administration of blood transfusions may be necessary to correct the anemia.

Nausea and Vomiting. Nausea and vomiting are common adverse reactions with the antineoplastic drugs. The physician may order a premedication antiemetic about 30 minutes before treatment with the antineoplastic drug begins and continue the antiemetic for several days following administration. Provide small, frequent meals to coincide with patients tolerance for food. Avoid greasy or fatty foods and unpleasant sights, smells, and tastes. Cold foods, dry foods, and salty foods may be more tolerable. Provide diversional activities such as music, television, books, and so on.

Stomatitis. Because the cells in the mouth grow rapidly, they are particularly sensitive to the effects of the antineoplastic drugs. *Stomatitis* (inflammation of the mouth) may occur 5 to 7 days after chemotherapy and continue up to 10 days after therapy. This adverse reaction is particularly uncomfortable since irritation of the mucous membrane of the mouth affects the nutritional aspects of care. Any foods or products that are irritating to the mouth, such as alcoholic beverages, spices, strong mouthwashes, or toothpaste are avoided. Provide soft or liquid food high in nutritive value. Inspect the oral cavity for increased irritation. Report any white patches on the tongue, throat, or gums; any burning sensation; and bleeding from the mouth or gums. Provide good mouth care every 4 hours with normal saline or alcohol-free mouthwash. Avoid lemon/glycerin swabs since they tend to irritate the oral mucosa and further complicate stomatitis. The physician may order a topical viscous anesthetic, such as lidocaine viscous, before meals to decrease discomfort when eating.

General Considerations. Knowing what adverse reactions may occur allows the nurse to prepare for any event that will happen. For example, a hemorrhagic syndrome may be seen with the administration of plicamycin. Knowing this, assessments for hemorrhage are incorporated in the nursing care plan. Another example is the development of hyperuricemia (elevated blood uric acid levels), which may be seen with drugs, such as melphalan (Alkeran) or mercaptopurine (Purinethol). When this adverse reaction is known to occur, intake and output measurements, as well as encouragement to increase fluid intake to at least 2000 mL of oral fluid per day are included in the nursing care plan.

Guidelines Established by the Physician or Hospital

During chemotherapy, the physician may write orders for certain nursing procedures, such as measuring intake and output; monitoring the vital signs at specific intervals; increasing the fluid intake to a certain amount; and so on. Even when orders are written, increase the frequency of certain assessments, such as monitoring vital signs, if the patient's condition changes.

Some hospitals have written guidelines for nursing management when the patient is receiving a specific antineoplastic agent. Incorporate these guidelines into the nursing care plan with nursing observations and assessments geared to the individual. Add assessments to the nursing care plan when there has been a change in the patient's condition.

Results of Periodic Laboratory Tests

There are different types of laboratory tests that may be used to monitor the patient's response to therapy. Some of these tests, for example, a complete blood count, may be used to determine the response of the bone marrow to an antineoplastic agent. Other tests, for example, liver function tests, may be used to detect liver toxicity, which may be an adverse reaction that can be seen with the administration of some of these drugs. Review all recent laboratory tests at the time they are reported. Report all significant changes or abnormal results to the physician immediately because it may be necessary to treat the abnormal situation, temporarily stop chemotherapy, or change the dosage regimen.

Abnormal laboratory tests may also require a change in the nursing care plan. For example, a significant drop in the platelet count may result in bleeding episodes and require measures, such as prolonged pressure on injection sites, to prevent bleeding or bruising episodes.

Important Points to Remember

Antineoplastic drugs are potentially toxic agents that can cause a variety of effects during and after their administration. Consider the following general areas when an antineoplastic drug is administered:

- Great care and accuracy are important in preparing and administering these drugs.
- Wear disposable plastic gloves when preparing any of these drugs for parenteral administration.
- Closely observe the patient before, during, and after the administration of an antineoplastic drug.
- Closely observe the IV site to detect any signs of extravasation (leakage into the surrounding tissues). Tissue necrosis can be a serious complication. Discontinue the infusion and notify the physician if discomfort, redness along the pathway of the vein, or infiltration occurs.
- Continually update nursing assessments, nursing diagnoses, and nursing care plans to meet the changing needs of the patient.
- Notify the physician of all changes in the patient's general condition, the appearance of adverse reactions, and changes in laboratory test results.
- Provide the patient and his or her family with both physical *and* emotional support during treatment.

Nursing Process
The Patient Receiving an Antineoplastic Drug

■ Assessment

The extent of assessment depends on the type of malignancy and the patient's general physical condition.

The initial assessment of the patient scheduled for chemotherapy may include the following:

- The type and location of the neoplastic lesion (as stated on the patient's chart)
- The stage of the disease; for example, early, metastatic, terminal
- The patient's general physical condition

- The patient's emotional response to his or her disease
- The anxiety or fears the patient may have regarding chemotherapy treatments
- Previous or concurrent treatments (if any), such as surgery, radiation therapy, other antineoplastic drugs
- Other current nonmalignant disease or disorder, for example, congestive heart failure or peptic ulcer, that may or may not be related to the malignant disease
- The patient's knowledge or understanding of the proposed chemotherapy regimen
- Other factors, such as the patient's age, financial problems that may be associated with a long-term illness, family cooperation and interest in the patient, the adequacy of health insurance coverage (which may be of great concern to the patient), and so on

Immediately before administering the first dose of an antineoplastic drug, take the vital signs. Obtain a current weight because the dose of some antineoplastic drugs is based on the patient's weight in kilograms or pounds. The dosages of some antineoplastic drugs also may be based on body surface measurements and are stated as a specific amount of drug per square meter (m^2) of body surface. Additional physical assessments may be necessary for certain antineoplastic agents.

A few antineoplastic agents require treatment measures before administration of the antineoplastic drug. An example of preadministration treatment is hydration of the patient with 1 to 2 liters of IV fluid infused before administration of cisplatin (Platinol), or administration of an antiemetic before the administration of mechlorethamine. These measures are ordered by the physician and, in some instances, may vary slightly from the manufacturer's recommendations.

When an antineoplastic drug has a depressing effect on the bone marrow, laboratory tests, such as a complete blood count, are ordered to determine the effect of the previous drug dosage. Before administering the first dose of the drug, pretreatment laboratory tests provide baseline data for future reference. Record all laboratory tests on the patient's chart and notify the physician of the results before the administration of successive doses of an antineoplastic agent. If these tests indicate a severe depressant effect on the bone marrow or other test abnormalities, the physician may reduce the next drug dose or temporarily stop chemotherapy to allow the affected body systems to recover.

■ *Nursing Diagnoses*

The nursing diagnoses for the patient with a malignancy are usually extensive and should be based on many factors, such as the patient's physical and emotional condition; the adverse reactions resulting from antineoplastic drug therapy; and the stage of the disease. The two diagnoses listed below apply only to the drug or drugs being administered and do not cover other possible areas that also may be added, for example, a risk for a fluid volume deficit due to prolonged vomiting secondary to an adverse drug reaction; altered oral mucous membranes due to an adverse drug reaction; or anticipatory grieving.

- **Anxiety** related to diagnosis, necessary treatment measures, the occurrence of adverse reactions, other factors
- **Risk for Ineffective Management of Therapeutic Regimen** related to lack of knowledge, adverse reactions, other factors (specify)

■ *Planning and Implementation*

The major goals of the patient may include a reduction in anxiety and an understanding of the prescribed treatment modalities. To make these goal manageable, more specific criteria must be added.

Anxiety. Patients and family members are usually devastated by the diagnosis of a malignancy. The emotional impact of the disease may be forgotten or put aside by members of the medical team as they plan and institute therapy to control the disease. Patients undergoing chemotherapy require a great deal of emotional support from all members of the medical team. Kindness and gentleness in giving care and an understanding of the strain placed on the patient and the family may help reduce some of the fear and anxiety experienced during treatment.

■ *Patient and Family Teaching*

When the patient is hospitalized, explain all treatments and possible adverse effects to the patient before the initiation of therapy. The physician usually discusses the proposed treatment and possible adverse drug reactions with the patient and family members. Briefly review the physician's explanations immediately before parenteral administration of a drug.

Some of these drugs are taken orally at home. The areas included in a patient and family teaching plan for this type of treatment regimen is based on the drug prescribed; the physician's explanation of the chemotherapy regimen; the physician's instructions for taking the drug; and the needs of the individual.

Some hospitals or physicians give printed instructions to the patient. Review these instructions after they have been read by the patient and allow time for the patient or family member to ask questions. The patient has a right to know the dangers associated with these drugs and what adverse reactions may occur.

Some patients are given antineoplastic drugs in a physician's office or outpatient clinic. Before the institution of therapy, explain the treatment regimen thoroughly to the patient and family. In some instances, a medication to prevent nausea may be prescribed to be taken before administration of the drugs in the physician's office or clinic. To obtain the best possible effects, stress to the patient that the drug must be taken at the time specified by the physician.

Include the following points in a patient and family teaching plan when oral therapy is prescribed:

- Take the drug only as directed on the prescription container. Follow specific directions, such as "take on an empty stomach" or "take at the same time each day"; they are extremely important.
- *Never* increase, decrease, or omit a dose unless advised to do so by the physician.
- If *any* problems (adverse reactions) occur, no matter how minor, contact the physician immediately.
- *All* recommendations given by the physician, such as increasing the fluid intake, eating, or avoiding certain foods are important.
- The effectiveness or action of the drug could be altered if these directions are ignored. Other recommendations, such as checking the mouth for sores; rinsing the mouth thoroughly after eating or drinking; or drinking extra fluids are given to identify or minimize some of the effects these drugs have on the body. It is important that these recommendations be followed.
- Keep all appointments for chemotherapy. These drugs must be given at certain intervals to be effective.
- Do not take *any* nonprescription drug unless the use of a specific drug has been approved by the physician.
- Avoid drinking alcoholic beverages unless the physician approves of their use.
- Always inform other physicians, dentists, and other medical personnel of therapy with this drug.
- Keep all appointments for the laboratory tests ordered by the physician. If unable to keep a laboratory appointment, notify the physician immediately.

■ *Expected Outcomes for Evaluation*

- Anxiety is reduced
- Patient verbalizes understanding of dosage regimen

- Patient verbalizes an understanding of treatment modalities and importance of continued follow-up care
- Adverse reactions are identified and reported to the physician
- Patient verbalizes importance of complying with the prescribed therapeutic regimen

Chapter Summary

- Antineoplastic drugs are agents used in the treatment of malignant diseases. These drugs are used to cure, to control, or for palliative therapy. While these drugs may not always cure the malignancy, they often slow the rate of tumor growth and delay metastasis. Chemotherapy is the term used to refer to therapy with the antineoplastic drugs. The antineoplastic drugs include: alkylating agents, antibiotics, antimetabolites, hormones, mitotic inhibitors, and various miscellaneous drugs.
- Most antineoplastic drugs exert their most potent effect on cells that rapidly proliferate. Since malignant cells proliferate rapidly, they are highly sensitive to the antineoplastic agents. However, these drugs also affect normal cells that divide and reproduce rapidly, such as the cells of the oral cavity, the gastrointestinal tract, the bone marrow, and the hair follicles. The mechanism of action of these drugs is not well understood. Generally, they affect one or more stages of cell growth or reproduction.
- Antineoplastic drugs are potentially toxic and their administration is associated with many adverse effects varying from mild to life-threatening. Some of the more common adverse reactions include alopecia, anorexia, leukopenia, thrombo-

cytopenia, anemia, nausea and vomiting, and stomatitis. Nursing management focuses on monitoring for these and other adverse reactions and planning interventions to control or lessen their effects.
- During chemotherapy, the physician may write orders for certain nursing procedures, such as measuring intake and output; monitoring the vital signs at specific intervals; increasing the fluid intake to a certain amount; and so on. Some hospitals or clinics have written guidelines for nursing management when the patient is receiving a specific antineoplastic agent. These guidelines are incorporated into the nursing care plan with nursing observations and assessments geared to the individual patient. Specific precautions are necessary when preparing and administering chemotherapy. Most agencies require specialized training and certification for nurses who will administer the antineoplastic drugs.

Critical Thinking Exercise

Patients with a malignant disease need special consideration, understanding, and emotional support. On occasion, these needs are unrecognized by members of the medical profession. If you were recently diagnosed as having cancer, what would be some of the feelings you would experience at this time? What would you want the nurse to do for you at this time? What would be your thoughts about your future? What would you want to know or not know? As you think about this or discuss these questions, remember that any patient may have these same emotional responses and may need the same things you would expect from the nurse or other members of the medical profession.

48

Fluids and Electrolytes

Key Terms

Blood plasma
Extravasation
Fluid overload
Half-normal saline
Hypocalcemia
Hypokalemia
Hyponatremia
Infiltration
Normal saline
Plasma expanders
Plasma protein fractions
Protein substrates

Chapter Outline

Chapter Objectives

On completion of this chapter the student will:

- *List the types and uses of solutions used in the management of body fluids*
- *Discuss the nursing implications to be considered when administering a solution used in the management of body fluids*
- *Use the nursing process when administering solutions used in the management of body fluids*
- *List the types and uses of electrolytes and their salts used in the management of electrolyte imbalances*
- *Discuss the more common signs and symptoms of electrolyte imbalance*
- *Discuss the nursing implications to be considered when administering electrolytes and their salts*
- *Use the nursing process when administering electrolytes and their salts*

Scherer JC, Roach S: INTRODUCTORY CLINICAL PHARMACOLOGY,
FIFTH EDITION © 1996 Lippincott-Raven Publishers

The composition of body fluids remains relatively constant despite the many demands placed on the body each day. On occasion, these demands cannot be met and electrolytes or electrolyte salts and fluids must be given in an attempt to restore equilibrium.

Two major areas are covered in this chapter: (1) the solutions used in the management of body fluids and (2) the electrolytes and electrolyte salts that may be administered to replace the one or more electrolytes that may be lost by the body.

Solutions Used in the Management of Body Fluids

Blood plasma, plasma protein fractions, protein substrates, plasma expanders, and *parenteral nutrients* are used to correct nutritional or fluid deficiencies, as well as to treat certain diseases and conditions.

TYPES AND USES OF SOLUTIONS USED IN THE MANAGEMENT OF BODY FLUIDS

Blood Plasma

Plasma is the liquid part of blood, containing water, sugar, electrolytes, fats, gases, proteins, bile pigment, and clotting factors. Human plasma, also called human pooled plasma, is obtained from donated blood. Although whole blood must be typed and crossmatched because it contains red blood cells carrying blood type and Rh factors, human plasma does not require this procedure. Because of this, plasma can be given in acute emergencies. Plasma administered intravenously (IV) is used to increase blood volume when severe hemorrhage has occurred and it is necessary to partially restore blood volume while waiting for whole blood to be typed and crossmatched. Another use of plasma is in treating conditions when plasma alone has been lost, as may be seen in severe burns.

Plasma Protein Fractions

Plasma protein fractions include human plasma protein fraction 5% and normal serum albumin 5% and 25%. Plasma protein fraction 5% is an IV solution containing 5% human plasma proteins. Serum albumin is obtained from donated whole blood and is a protein found in plasma. Plasma protein fractions are used to treat hypoproteinemia (a deficiency of protein in the blood), as might be seen in patients with the nephrotic syndrome and hepatic cirrhosis, as well as other diseases or disorders. Plasma protein fractions are also used to treat hypovolemic (low blood volume) shock. As with human pooled plasma, blood type and crossmatch is not needed when plasma protein fractions are given.

Protein Substrates

Protein substrates are amino acids, which are essential to life. Amino acids promote the production of proteins, enhance tissue repair and wound healing, and reduce the rate of protein breakdown. Amino acids are used in certain disease states such as severe kidney and liver disease, as well as in total parenteral nutrition solutions. Total parenteral nutrition (TPN) may be used in conditions such as impairment of gastrointestinal absorption of protein and as increased requirement for protein as seen in those with extensive burns or infections, and when the oral route for nutritional intake cannot be used.

Plasma Expanders

IV solutions of plasma expanders include hetastarch (Hespan); low-molecular-weight dextran (Dextran 40); and high-molecular-weight dextran (Dextran 70, Dextran 75). Plasma expanders are used to expand plasma volume when shock is due to burns, hemorrhage, surgery, and other trauma. When used in the treatment of shock, plasma expanders are not a substitute for whole blood or plasma but are of value as emergency measures until the latter substances can be used.

Parenteral Nutrients

Solutions used to supply nutrients and fluid include dextrose (glucose) in water or sodium chloride, alcohol in dextrose, and IV fat emulsion. Dextrose is a carbohydrate that is used to provide a source of calories and fluid. Alcohol (as alcohol in dextrose) also provides calories. Dextrose is available in various strengths (or percent of the carbohydrate) in a fluid, which may be water or sodium chloride (saline). Dextrose and dextrose in alcohol are available in various strengths (or percent of the carbohydrate and percent of the alcohol) in water. Dextrose solutions also are available with electrolytes, for example, Plasma-Lyte 56 and 5% dextrose. Calories provided by dextrose and dextrose and alcohol solutions are listed in Table 48-1.

IV fat emulsion contains soybean or safflower oil and a mixture of natural triglycerides, predominately unsaturated fatty acids. It is used in the prevention and treatment of essential fatty acid deficiency. It also provides nonprotein calories for those receiving parenteral nutrition when calorie requirements cannot be met by glucose.

ADVERSE REACTIONS ASSOCIATED WITH THE ADMINISTRATION OF SOLUTIONS USED IN THE MANAGEMENT OF BODY FLUIDS

One adverse reaction common to all solutions administered by the parenteral route is fluid overload, that is, the administration of more fluid than the body is able to handle. The term *fluid overload* (circulatory overload) is not a specific amount of fluid that is given. It describes a condition when the body's fluid requirements are met and the administration of fluid occurs at a rate that is greater than the rate at which the body can use or eliminate the fluid. Thus, the amount of fluid and the rate of administration of fluid that will cause fluid overload depends on several factors, such as the cardiac status and the adequacy of renal function. The signs and symptoms of fluid overload are listed in Table 48-2.

Table 48-1. Calories Provided in Intravenous Carbohydrate Solutions

Carbohydrate	Percentage	Calories/1000 mL
Dextrose	2.5%	85
Dextrose	5%	170
Dextrose	10%	340
Dextrose	20%	680
Dextrose	50%	1700
Dextrose	70%	2380
Alcohol in dextrose	5% alcohol and 5% dextrose	450
	10% alcohol and 5% dextrose	720

Table 48-2. Signs and Symptoms of Fluid Overload

Headache	Rapid breathing
Weakness	Wheezing
Blurred vision	Coughing
Behavioral changes (confusion, disorientation, delirium, drowsiness)	Rise in blood pressure
	Distended neck veins
Weight gain	Elevated central venous pressure (CVP)
Isolated muscle twitching	Convulsions
Hyponatremia	

Adverse reactions are rare when plasma protein fractions are administered but nausea, chills, fever, urticaria, and hypotensive episodes may occasionally be seen. Administration of protein substrates (amino acids) may result in nausea, fever, flushing of the skin, metabolic acidosis or alkalosis, and decreased phosphorus and calcium blood levels.

Administration of hetastarch, a plasma expander, may be accompanied by vomiting, a mild temperature elevation, itching, and allergic reactions. Allergic reactions are evidenced by wheezing, edema around the eyes (periorbital edema), and urticaria. Low- or high-molecular-weight dextran administration may result in allergic reactions, which are evidenced by urticaria, hypotension, nasal congestion, and wheezing. Hyperglycemia and phlebitis may be seen with administration of glucose.

NURSING MANAGEMENT

An IV infusion pump may be ordered for the administration of these solutions. Set the alarm of the infusion pump and check the functioning of the unit at frequent intervals. Check the needle site every 15 to 30 minutes and more frequently if the patient is restless or confused. When one of these agents is given with a regular IV infusion set, check the infusion rate every 15 minutes.

Inspect the needle site every 30 minutes for signs of *extravasation* (escape of fluid from a blood vessel into surrounding tissues) or *infiltration* (the collection of fluid into tissues). More frequent inspection may be necessary if the patient is confused or restless. If signs of extravasation or infiltration are apparent, restart the infusion in another vein.

Patients receiving an IV fluid should be made as comfortable as possible, although under some circumstances this may be difficult. The extremity used for administration should be made comfortable and supported as needed by a small pillow or other device.

The average length of time for infusion of 1000 mL of an IV solution is 4 to 8 hours. The only exception is when there is a written or verbal order by the physician to give the solution at a rapid rate because of an emergency situation. In this instance, the order must specifically state the rate of administration (as drops per minute) or the period of time over which a specific amount of fluid is to be infused.

When these solutions are given, a central venous pressure line may be inserted to monitor the patient's response to therapy. Take and record central venous pressure readings as ordered. During administration, take the blood pressure, pulse, and respiratory rate as ordered or at intervals determined by the patient's clinical condition. For example, a patient in shock and receiving a plasma expander may require monitoring of the blood pressure and pulse rate every 5 to 15 minutes, whereas the patient receiving dextrose 3 days after surgery may require monitoring every 30 to 60 minutes.

The rate of IV infusion ordered by the physician may be stated as drops per minute, milliliters (mL) per minute, or a given volume administered over a specified period, for example, 125 mL/h or 1000 mL in 8 hours. Calculation of IV flow rates is discussed in Chapter 3.

Observe patients receiving IV solutions at frequent intervals for signs of fluid overload. If signs of fluid overload are observed, slow the IV infusion rate and notify the physician immediately.

Nursing Process
The Patient Receiving a Solution for Management of Body Fluids

▪ Assessment

Before administering an IV solution, include in assessments an evaluation of the patient's general status, a review of recent laboratory test results (when appropriate), the patient's weight (when appropriate), and vital signs. Take the blood pressure, pulse, and respiratory rate to provide a baseline, which is especially important when the patient is receiving blood plasma, plasma expanders, or plasma protein fractions for shock or other serious disorders.

▪ Nursing Diagnoses

Depending on the diagnosis, type of fluid, and reason for administration, one or more of the following nursing diagnoses may apply to a person receiving one of these preparations:

- **Fluid Volume Deficit** related to inability to take oral fluids, abnormal fluid loss, other factors (specify cause of fluid volume deficit)
- **Altered Nutrition: Less Than Body Requirements** related to inability to eat, recent surgery, other factors (specify cause of altered nutrition)
- **Anxiety** related to diagnosis, invasive procedure (venipuncture), other factors (specify)
- **Knowledge Deficit** of administration procedure

▪ Planning and Implementation

The major goals of the patient may include a reduction in anxiety, correction of the fluid volume deficit (where appropriate), improved oral nutrition (where appropriate), and an understanding of the administration procedure. To make these goals measurable, more specific criteria must be added.

Fluid Volume Deficit and Altered Nutrition. Many times the solutions used in the management of body fluids are given to correct a fluid volume deficit and to supply carbohydrates (nutrition). Review the patient's chart for a full understanding of the rationale for administration of the specific solution.

When appropriate, include in a plan of care nursing measures that may be instituted to correct a fluid volume and carbohydrate deficit. Examples of these measures include offering oral fluids at frequent intervals and encouraging the patient to take small amounts of nourishment between meals, as well as eat as much as possible at mealtime.

Anxiety. Some patients may exhibit anxiety related to their diagnosis or the need to administer IV fluids. Explain to the patient the procedure, as well as the need for medical personnel to frequently inspect the solution and needle site.

Knowledge Deficit. Give the patient or family a brief explanation of the reason for and the method of administration of an IV solution. Patients and families have been known to tamper with or adjust the rate of flow of IV administration sets. Emphasize the importance of not touching the IV administration set or the equipment used to administer IV fluids.

■ *Expected Outcomes for Evaluation*
• Fluid volume deficit is corrected
• Nutrition deficit is corrected
• Anxiety is reduced
• Patient and family demonstrate understanding of the procedure

Electrolytes and Electrolyte Salts

Along with a disturbance in fluid volume (eg, loss of plasma, blood, or water) or a need for providing parenteral nutrition with the previously discussed solutions, an electrolyte imbalance may exist. In some instances, an electrolyte imbalance may be present without an appreciable disturbance in fluid balance. For example, a patient taking a diuretic is able to maintain fluid balance by an adequate oral intake of water, which replaces the water lost through diuresis, but is unable to replace the potassium that is also lost during diuresis. Commonly used electrolytes are listed in Summary Drug Table 48-1.

TYPES AND USES OF ELECTROLYTES AND ELECTROLYTE SALTS

Bicarbonate (HCO$_3$⁻)

This electrolyte plays a vital role in the acid–base balance of the body. Bicarbonate may be given IV as sodium bicarbonate (NaHCO$_3$) in the treatment of metabolic acidosis, a state of imbalance that may be seen, for example, in diseases or situations such as cardiac arrest, severe shock, diabetic acidosis, and severe renal disease. Oral sodium bicarbonate is used as a gastric and urinary alkalinizer, and may be used as a single drug or may be found as one of the ingredients in some antacid preparations. It is also useful as part of the treatment for gout because it is capable of minimizing the formation of uric acid crystals in the urine.

Calcium (Ca^{2+})

Calcium is necessary for the functioning of nerves and muscles, the clotting of blood (see Chap. 32), the building of bones and teeth, and other physiologic processes. Examples of calcium salts are calcium gluconate and calcium carbonate. Calcium may be given for the treatment of *hypocalcemia* (low blood calcium), which may be seen in those with parathyroid disease or following accidental removal of the parathyroid glands during surgery of the thyroid gland. Calcium may also be recommended for those eating a diet low in calcium or as a dietary supplement when there is an increased need for calcium, such as during pregnancy. Calcium may also be given during cardiopulmonary resuscitation.

Magnesium (Mg^{2+})

Magnesium plays an important role in the transmission of nerve impulses. It is also important in the activity of many enzyme reactions, for example, carbohydrate metabolism. Magnesium sulfate (MgSO$_4$) is used in the prevention and control of seizures in obstetrical patients with preeclampsia or eclampsia. It may also be added to total parenteral nutrition mixtures.

Potassium (K⁺)

Potassium is necessary for the transmission of impulses, the contraction of smooth, cardiac, and skeletal muscles, and other important physiologic processes. Potassium as a drug is available as potassium chloride (KCl) and potassium gluconate, and is measured in milliequivalents (mEq), for example, 40 mEq in 20 mL or 8 mEq controlled release tablet. Potassium may be given for *hypokalemia* (low blood potassium). Examples of causes of hypokalemia are a marked loss of gastrointestinal fluids (severe vomiting, diarrhea, nasogastric suction, draining intestinal fistulas), diabetic acidosis, marked diuresis, and severe malnutrition.

Sodium (Na⁺)

Sodium is essential for the maintenance of normal heart action and in the regulation of osmotic pressure in body cells. Sodium, as sodium chloride (NaCl), may be given by IV. A solution containing 0.9% sodium chloride is called *normal saline* and a solution containing 0.45% sodium chloride is called *half-normal saline*. Sodium also is available combined with dextrose, for example, dextrose 5% and sodium chloride 0.9%.

Sodium is administered for *hyponatremia* (low blood sodium). Examples of causes of hyponatremia are excessive diaphoresis, severe vomiting or diarrhea, excessive diuresis, and draining intestinal fistulas.

Summary Drug Table 48–1. Electrolytes

Generic Name	Trade Name*	Uses	Adverse Reactions	Dose Ranges
calcium carbonate	Os-Cal 500, Calcitrate 600, *generic*	Hypoparathyroidism, postmenopausal and senile osteoporosis, rickets, osteomalacia, dietary supplement when calcium intake is inadequate	Symptoms of hypercalcemia	500 mg to 2 g PO 2–4 times/d
calcium gluconate	*generic*	Same as calcium carbonate	Symptoms of hypercalcemia	500 mg to 2 g PO 2–4 times/d; 2.3–9.3 mEq IV as required
electrolyte mixtures	Pedialyte, Rehydralyte Solution	Electrolyte and water deficiency	Rare	Dosage calculated on requirements, patient's age
magnesium (oral), magnesium sulfate (parenteral)	Mag-200, Megatrate, *generic*	Dietary supplement, magnesium deficiency, preeclampsia eclampsia	Symptoms of hypermagnesemia	Up to 483 mg/d PO in divided doses; up to 2 mEq/kg IM; up to 40 mEq IV
potassium chloride	Kay Ciel, Kaochlor, Kaon-Cl, *generic*	Hypokalemia	Symptoms of hyperkalemia	16–100 mEq/d PO; up to 80 mEq IV added to 1000 mL IV fluid
potassium gluconate	Kaon, Kaylixir, *generic*	Hypokalemia	Same as potassium chloride	16–100 mEq/d PO
sodium bicarbonate, parenteral	Neut, *generic*	Metabolic acidosis	Symptoms of alkalosis	Varies with degree of acidosis
sodium chloride, oral	Slo-Salt, *generic*	Deficiency of sodium and chloride	Symptoms of hypernatremia	Up to 1 g PO
sodium chloride, parenteral	*generic*	Deficiency of sodium and chloride	Symptoms of hypernatremia	Adjusted to patient's needs

*The term, *generic*, indicates that the drug is available in generic form.

Combined Electrolyte Solutions

Combined electrolyte solutions are available for oral and IV administration. The IV solutions contain various electrolytes and dextrose. The amount of electrolytes, given as mEq per liter, also varies. The IV solutions are used to replace fluid and electrolytes that have been lost and to provide calories by means of their carbohydrate content. Examples of IV electrolyte solutions are dextrose 5% with 0.9% sodium chloride, lactated Ringer's injection, Plasma-Lyte, and 10% Travert (invert sugar—a combination of equal parts of fructose and dextrose) and Electrolyte No. 2. The physician selects the type of combined electrolyte solution that will meet the patient's needs.

Oral electrolyte solutions contain a carbohydrate and various electrolytes. Examples of combined oral electrolyte solutions are Pedialyte and Rehydralyte Solution. Oral electrolyte solutions are most often used to replace lost electrolytes, carbohydrates, and fluid in conditions such as severe vomiting or diarrhea.

ADVERSE REACTIONS ASSOCIATED WITH THE ADMINISTRATION OF ELECTROLYTES AND ELECTROLYTE SALTS

Many adverse reactions associated with the administration of electrolytes and electrolyte salts are related to overdose, which results in, for example, signs and symptoms of *hyper*kalemia or *hyper*natremia (Table 48-3). Adverse reactions other than those related to overdose are discussed below.

Calcium

Irritation of the vein used for administration, tingling, a calcium taste, and "heat waves" may occur when calcium is given IV. Oral administration may result in gastrointestinal disturbances.

Table 48-3. Signs and Symptoms of Electrolyte Imbalances

CALCIUM

Normal laboratory values: 4.5–5.3 mEq/L or 9–11 mg/dL*

Hypocalcemia

Hyperactive reflexes, carpopedal spasm, perioral paresthesias, positive Trousseau's signs, positive Chvostek's sign, muscle twitching, muscle cramps, tetany, laryngospasm, cardiac arrhythmias, nausea, vomiting, anxiety, confusion, emotional liability, convulsions

Hypercalcemia

Anorexia, nausea, vomiting, lethargy, bone tenderness or pain, polyuria, polydipsia, constipation, dehydration, muscle weakness and atrophy, stupor, coma, cardiac arrest

MAGNESIUM

Normal laboratory values: 1.5–2.5 mEq/L or 1.8–3 mg/dL*

Hypomagnesemia

Leg and foot cramps, hypertension, tachycardia, neuromuscular irritability, tremor, hyperactive deep tendon reflexes, confusion, disorientation, visual or auditory hallucinations, painful paresthesias, positive Trousseau's sign, positive Chvostek's sign, convulsions

Hypermagnesemia

Lethargy, drowsiness, impaired respiration, flushing, sweating, hypotension, weak to absent deep tendon reflexes

POTASSIUM

Normal laboratory values: 3.5–5 mEq/L*

Hypokalemia

Anorexia, nausea, vomiting, mental depression, confusion, delayed or impaired thought processes, drowsiness, abdominal distention, decreased bowel sounds, paralytic ileus, muscle weakness or fatigue, flaccid paralysis, absent or diminished deep tendon reflexes, weak irregular pulse, paresthesias, leg cramps, ECG changes

Hyperkalemia

Irritability, anxiety, listlessness, mental confusion, nausea, diarrhea, abdominal distress, gastrointestinal hyperactivity, paresthesias, weakness and heaviness of the legs, flaccid paralysis, hypotension, cardiac arrhythmias, ECG changes

SODIUM

Normal laboratory values: 132–145 mEq/L*

Hyponatremia

Cold clammy skin, decreased skin turgor, apprehension, confusion, irritability, anxiety, hypotension, postural hypotension, tachycardia, headache, tremors, convulsions, abdominal cramps, nausea, vomiting, diarrhea

Hypernatremia

Fever, hot dry skin, dry sticky mucous membranes, rough dry tongue, edema, weight gain, intense thirst, excitement, restlessness, agitation, oliguria or anuria

---

*These laboratory values may not concur with the normal range of values in all hospitals and laboratories. The hospital policy manual or laboratory values sheet should be consulted for the normal ranges of all laboratory tests.

Magnesium

Adverse reactions seen with magnesium administration are rare. If they do occur, they are most likely related to overdose and may include flushing, sweating, hypotension, depressed reflexes, muscle weakness, and circulatory collapse.

Potassium

Nausea, vomiting, diarrhea, abdominal pain, and phlebitis have been seen with oral and IV administration of potassium. If extravasation of the IV solution should occur, local tissue necrosis (death of tissue) may be seen. If extravasation occurs, the physician is immediately contacted and the infusion slowed to a rate that keeps the vein open.

Sodium

Sodium as the salt (eg, sodium chloride) has no adverse reactions except those related to overdose. In some instances, excessive oral use may produce nausea and vomiting.

Sodium Bicarbonate

Some individuals may use sodium bicarbonate (baking soda) for the relief of gastric disturbances, such as pain, discomfort, symptoms of indigestion, and gas. Prolonged use of oral sodium bicarbonate or excessive doses of IV sodium bicarbonate may result in systemic alkalosis.

NURSING MANAGEMENT

When electrolytes are administered parenterally, the dosage is expressed in mEq, for example, calcium gluconate 7 mEq IV. When administered orally, sodium bicarbonate, calcium, and magnesium dosages are expressed in milligrams (mg). Potassium liquids and effervescent tablets dosages are expressed in mEq; capsules or tablets dosages may be expressed as mEq or milligrams.

Administration of Calcium

When calcium is administered IV, the solution is warmed to body temperature immediately before administration and the drug is administered *slowly*. In some clinical situations, the physician may order the patient to be placed on a cardiac monitor because additional drug administration may be determined by electrocardiographic changes.

Administration of Potassium

When given orally, potassium may cause gastrointestinal distress. Therefore, it is given immediately after meals or with food and a full glass of water. Tablets must *not* be crushed or chewed. If the patient has difficulty swallowing the tablets, consult the physician regarding the use of a solution or an effervescent tablet, which effervesces (fizzes) and dissolves on contact with water. Potassium in the form of an effervescent tablet, powder, or liquid must be thoroughly mixed with 4 to 8 ounces of cold water, juice, or another beverage. Effervescent tablets must stop fizzing before the solution is sipped slowly over 5 to 15 minutes. Oral liquids and soluble powders that have been mixed and dissolved in cold water or juice are also sipped slowly over 5 to 15 minutes. Advise patients that liquid potassium solutions have a salty taste. Some of these products have a flavoring added, which makes the solution more palatable.

Patients receiving oral potassium should have their blood pressure and pulse monitored every 4 hours, especially during early therapy. Also observe the patient for signs of hyperkalemia (see Table 48-3), which would indicate that the dose of potassium is too high. Signs of hypokalemia may also occur during therapy and may indicate that the dose of potassium is too low and must be increased. If signs of hypokalemia or hyperkalemia are apparent or suspected, notify the physician. In some instances, frequent laboratory monitoring of the serum potassium may be ordered.

The maximum recommended concentration of potassium is 80 mEq in 1000 mL of IV solution, although certain acute emergency situations may require a larger concentration of potassium. The physician orders the dose of the potassium salt (in mEq) and the amount and type of IV solution, as well as the time interval over which the solution is to be infused. After addition of the drug to the IV container, it is gently rotated to ensure mixture in the solution. Use a large vein for administration; the veins on the back of the hand should be avoided. An IV containing potassium should infuse in *no less than* 3 to 4 hours, thus requiring frequent monitoring of the IV infusion rate even when an IV infusion pump is used. Also inspect the IV needle site every 30 minutes for signs of extravasation. Potassium is irritating to the tissues. If extravasation does occur, discontinue the IV immediately and notify the physician. The acutely ill patient and the patient with severe hypokalemia will require monitoring of the blood pressure and pulse rate every 15 to 30 minutes during the time of the IV infusion. Measure intake and output every 8 hours. Slow the infusion rate to keep the vein open and notify the physician if an irregular pulse is noted.

Administration of Magnesium

Magnesium sulfate may be ordered intramuscularly, IV, or by IV infusion diluted in a specified type and amount of IV solution. When ordered to be given intramuscularly, this drug is given undiluted as a 50% solution for adults and a 20% solution for children.

When magnesium sulfate is ordered to treat convulsions or severe hypomagnesemia, the patient requires constant observation. Obtain the blood pressure, pulse, and respiratory rate immediately before the drug is administered, as well as every 5 to 10 minutes during the time of IV infusion or after the drug is given direct IV. Continue monitoring of these vital signs at frequent intervals until the patient's condition has stabilized. Closely observe the patient for early signs of hypermagnesemia (see Table 48-3) and contact the physician immediately if this imbalance is suspected. Frequent plasma magnesium levels are usually ordered. Laboratory request slips for this procedure are marked "emergency" because results must be obtained as soon as possible. Notify the physician if the magnesium level is higher or lower than the normal range.

Administration of Sodium

When sodium chloride is administered by IV infusion, observe the patient during and after administration for signs of hypernatremia (see Table 48-3). Check the rate of IV infusion as ordered by the physician every 15 to 30 minutes. More frequent monitoring of the infusion rate may be necessary when the patient is restless or confused. Patients receiving a 3% or 5% sodium chloride solution by IV infusion are observed closely for signs of pulmonary edema (dyspnea, cough, restlessness, bradycardia). If any one or more of these symptoms should occur, slow the IV infusion to keep the vein open (KVO) and contact the physician immediately. Patients receiving sodium chloride by the IV route have their intake and output measured every 8 hours. Observe the patient for signs of hypernatremia every 3 to 4 hours and contact the physician if this condition is suspected.

Administration of Bicarbonate

Oral sodium bicarbonate tablets are given with a full glass of water; the powdered form is dissolved in a full glass of water. If oral sodium bicarbonate is used to alkalinize the urine, check the urine pH two or three times a day or as ordered by the physician. If the urine remains acidic, notify the physician because an increase in the dose of the drug may be necessary.

IV sodium bicarbonate is given in emergency situations, such as cardiac arrest or certain types of drug overdose when alkalinization of the urine is necessary to hasten drug elimination. Obtain the blood pressure, pulse, and respiratory rate immediately before administration of the drug (an exception may be cardiac arrest or other emergency situations), and then monitor at frequent intervals thereafter. In cardiac arrest, the initial and subsequent doses are given by IV push. Repeat doses at intervals of about 5 minutes until the patient's condition has stabilized. Extravasation of the drug requires selection of another needle site because the drug is irritating to the tissues.

When given in the treatment of metabolic acidosis, the drug may be added to the IV fluid or given as a prepared IV sodium bicarbonate solution. Frequent laboratory monitoring of the blood pH and blood gases is usually ordered because dosage and length of therapy depend on test results. Observe the patient is observed for signs of clinical improvement and monitor the blood pressure, pulse, and respiratory rate every 15 to 30 minutes or as ordered by the physician.

Nursing Process
The Patient Receiving an Electrolyte or Electrolyte Salt

■ *Assessment*
Before the administering any electrolyte, electrolyte salt, or a combined electrolyte solution, assess the patient for signs of an electrolyte imbalance (see Table 48-3). Review all recent laboratory and diagnostic tests appropriate to the imbalance. Obtain vital signs to provide a data base.

In some situations, administer electrolytes when an electrolyte imbalance may *potentially* occur. For example, the patient with nasogastric suction is prescribed one or more electrolytes added to an IV solution, such as 5% dextrose or a combined electrolyte solution, to be given IV to make up for the electrolytes that are lost through nasogastric suction. In other instances, electrolytes are given to replace those already lost, such as the patient admitted to the hospital with severe vomiting and diarrhea of several days duration.

■ *Nursing Diagnoses*
Depending on the drug, dose, route of administration, and reason for administration, one or more of the following nursing diagnoses may apply to a person receiving an electrolyte or electrolyte salt:
- **Anxiety** related to diagnosis, method of administration (IV), other factors (specify)
- **Noncompliance** related to indifference, lack of knowledge, other factors
- **Risk for Ineffective Management of Therapeutic Regimen** related to knowledge deficit of medication regimen, adverse drug effects

■ *Planning and Implementation*
The major goals of the patient may include a reduction in anxiety, compliance to the prescribed therapeutic regimen, and an understanding of the medication regimen and adverse drug effects. To make these goals measurable, more specific criteria must be added.

Anxiety. Some patients may exhibit anxiety related to their diagnosis or the method of administration of the drug (IV). Explain the procedure, as well as the need for medical personnel to frequently inspect the solution and needle site, to the patient as well as allow time for the patient or family members to ask questions.

Noncompliance. To ensure accurate compliance to the prescribed medication regimen, carefully explain the dose and time intervals to the patient or a family member. Because overdose (which can be serious) may occur if the patient does not adhere to the prescribed dosage and schedule, it is most important that the patient completely understands how much and when to take the drug. Stress the importance of adhering to the prescribed dosage schedule during patient teaching.

The physician may order periodic laboratory and diagnostic tests for some patients receiving oral electrolytes. Encourage the patient to keep all appointments for these tests, as well as physician or clinic visits.

■ Patient and Family Teaching

Warn persons with a history of using sodium bicarbonate (baking soda) as an antacid that overuse can result in alkalosis and could disguise a more serious problem. Advise those with a history of using salt tablets (sodium chloride) not to do so during hot weather unless it is recommended by a physician. Excessive use of salt tablets can result in a serious electrolyte imbalance.

Additional teaching points for specific electrolytes are the following:

Calcium Salts
- Contact the physician if the following occur: nausea, vomiting, anorexia, constipation, abdominal pain, dry mouth, thirst, polyuria (symptoms of hypercalcemia).
- Do not exceed the dosage recommendations.

Potassium Salts
- Take the drug *exactly* as directed on the prescription container. Do *not* increase, decrease, or omit the drug unless advised to do so by the physician. Take the drug immediately after meals or with food and a full glass of water. Avoid the use of nonprescription drugs and salt substitutes (many contain potassium) unless use of a specific drug or product has been approved by the physician.
- Contact the physician if tingling of the hands or feet, a feeling of heaviness in the legs, vomiting,

nausea, abdominal pain, or black stools should occur.
- If the tablet has a coating (enteric-coated tablets), swallow it whole. Do not chew or crush the tablet.
- If effervescent tablets are prescribed, place the tablet in 4 to 8 ounces of cold water or juice. Wait until the fizzing stops before drinking. Sip the liquid over 5 to 10 minutes.
- If an oral liquid or a powder is prescribed, add the dose to 4 to 8 ounces of cold water or juice and sip slowly over a 5 to 10 minutes. Measure the dose accurately.

■ Expected Outcomes for Evaluation
- Anxiety is reduced
- Patient complies to the prescribed drug regimen
- Patient and family demonstrate understanding of drug regimen
- Patient verbalizes importance of complying with the prescribed therapeutic regimen

Chapter Summary

- The composition of body fluids remains relatively constant despite the many demands placed on the body each day. On occasion, these demands cannot be met and electrolytes or electrolyte salts and fluids must be given in an attempt to restore equilibrium.
- Blood plasma, plasma protein fractions, protein substrates, plasma expanders, and parenteral nutrients are used to correct nutritional or fluid deficiencies, as well as to treat certain diseases and conditions.
- Plasma is the liquid part of blood, containing in solution, water, sugar, electrolytes, fats, gases, proteins, bile pigment, and clotting factors. Human plasma, also called human pooled plasma, is obtained from donated blood. Plasma protein fractions include human plasma protein fraction 5% and normal serum albumin 5% and 25%. Protein substrates are amino acids, which are essential to life. Plasma expanders are used to expand plasma volume when shock is due to burns, hemorrhage, surgery, and other trauma. Parenteral nutrients solutions used to supply nutrients and fluid include dextrose (glucose) in water or sodium chloride, alcohol in dextrose, and IV fat emulsion.
- Along with a disturbance in fluid volume or a need for providing parenteral nutrition with the previously discussed solutions, an electrolyte imbalance may exist. In some instances, an electrolyte

imbalance may be present without an appreciable disturbance in fluid balance.

- Bicarbonate plays a vital role in the acid–base balance of the body. Bicarbonate may be given IV as sodium bicarbonate in the treatment of metabolic acidosis. Oral sodium bicarbonate is used as a gastric and urinary alkalinizer.
- Calcium is necessary for the functioning of nerves and muscles, the clotting of blood, the building of bones and teeth, and other physiologic processes and is used to treat hypocalcemic states.
- Magnesium plays an important role in the transmission of nerve impulses and is important in the activity of many enzyme reactions. Magnesium sulfate is used in the prevention and control of seizures in obstetrical patients with preeclampsia or eclampsia. It may also be added to total parenteral nutrition mixtures.
- Potassium is necessary for the transmission of impulses, the contraction of smooth, cardiac, and skeletal muscles, and other important physiologic processes. Potassium is used to prevent or treat hypokalemia.
- Sodium is essential for the maintenance of normal heart action and in the regulation of osmotic pressure in body cells. Sodium, as sodium chloride (NaCl), may be given by IV. A solution containing 0.9% sodium chloride is called normal saline and a solution containing 0.45% sodium chloride is called half-normal saline. Sodium also is available combined with dextrose, for example, dextrose 5% and sodium chloride 0.9%. Sodium is administered for hyponatremia.

Critical Thinking Exercises

1. Ms. Land is receiving 20 mEq of potassium chloride (KCl) added to 1000 mL of 5% dextrose and water. What assessments would you make while her IV is infusing?
2. Mr. Kendall is prescribed an oral potassium chloride liquid. What instructions regarding preparing and taking the medication would you give to Mr. Kendall?
3. Mr. Parker is to receive 1000 mL of 5% dextrose and water over 8 hours. How many mL should infuse each hour?

49

Vitamins; Drugs Used in the Treatment of Anemia

Key Terms

Anemia
Ascorbic acid
Blepharospasm
Cheilosis
Fat-soluble vitamin
Folinic acid rescue
Glossitis
Hypervitaminosis A
Intrinsic factor
Iron-deficiency anemia
Isomer
Megaloblastic anemia
Pernicious anemia
Photophobia
Vitamin
Water-soluble vitamin

Chapter Outline

Chapter Objectives

On completion of this chapter the student will:

- *Name the water-soluble and fat-soluble vitamins*
- *Discuss the actions, uses, and adverse reactions of the water-soluble and fat-soluble vitamins*
- *Discuss nursing management when administering a water-soluble or fat-soluble vitamin*
- *Use the nursing process when administering a water-soluble or fat-soluble vitamin*
- *List the drugs used in the treatment of anemia*
- *Discuss the actions, uses, and adverse reactions of the drugs used to treat anemia*
- *Discuss nursing management when administering a drug used for the treatment of anemia*
- *Use the nursing process when administering a drug used for the treatment of anemia*

Vitamins are organic substances needed by the body in small amounts for normal growth and nutrition. The exact role of some of the vitamins in human nutrition remains unclear. In general, vitamins act as regulators of body processes and as coenzymes in certain chemical reactions that occur within the body.

Most vitamins are obtained from outside sources, namely food, because they cannot be manufactured by the body. The vitamins manufactured by the body are vitamin D, which is produced on exposure of the skin to sunlight, and vitamin K, which is synthesized by bacteria normally residing in the intestine.

Vitamins are divided into two main groups according to their solubility: the *water-soluble vitamins* and the *fat-soluble vitamins*. The B-complex vitamins and vitamin C are the water-soluble vitamins. Vitamins A, D, E and K are the fat-soluble vitamins. Recommended dietary allowances of vitamins for adults are given in Table 49-1.

The Water-Soluble Vitamins

The *water-soluble vitamins* are vitamin C (ascorbic acid) and the B-complex vitamins: vitamins B_1 (thiamine), B_2 (riboflavin), B_5 (pantothenic acid), B_6

Table 49-1. Recommended Dietary Allowances of Vitamins for Adults*

WATER-SOLUBLE VITAMINS

Vitamin C (ascorbic acid): 60 mg
Vitamin B_1 (thiamine): men, 1.2–1.5 mg; women, 1.1 mg
Vitamin B_2 (riboflavin): men, 1.4–1.8 mg; women, 1.2–1.3 mg
Vitamin B_5 (pantothenic acid): approximately 4–7 mg
Vitamin B_6 (pyridoxine): men, 2 mg; women, 1.6 mg
Niacin (nicotine acid): men, 15–20 mg; women, 15 mg

FAT SOLUBLE VITAMINS

Vitamin A: men, 1000 mcg RE; women, 800 mcg RE†
Vitamin D: 400 IU or 10 mcg
Vitamin E: men, 15 IU; women, 12 IU
Vitamin K: men, 80 mcg; women, 65 mcg

DRUGS USED TO TREAT ANEMIAS

Iron: men, 10 mg; women, 15 mg (higher during pregnancy and lactation)
Folic acid: 180–200 mcg
Vitamin B_{12}: 2 mcg

---

*Other references may vary slightly from the RDAs given here.
†Retinal equivalents.

(pyridoxine), niacin (vitamin B_3, nicotinic acid), and vitamin B_{12} (cyanocobalamin). These vitamins are soluble in water and are not stored in the body but are excreted in the urine.

ACTIONS OF THE WATER-SOLUBLE VITAMINS

Vitamin C (Ascorbic Acid)

Vitamin C is necessary for the development of teeth, bone, blood vessels, and collagen (a special type of connective tissue) and is also involved with carbohydrate metabolism. This vitamin also appears to aid in wound healing in building strong tissue, such as cartilage, collagen, and capillary walls. Vitamin C produces a substance that acts to "cement" the cells together, which is why it may be given during the postoperative period.

Vitamin C or *ascorbic acid* is found in citrus fruits and some vegetables (tomatoes, cabbage, berries, and melons). A deficiency of this vitamin results in scurvy, a condition characterized by swollen, red, bleeding gums; a loosening of the teeth; fatigue; pallor; anemia; and hemorrhage of the skin, joints, and muscles due to capillary fragility. In most instances, a normal diet provides sufficient amounts of this vitamin. Examples of situations that may require additional vitamin C are a decreased or inadequate food intake, pregnancy, patients having major surgery, and infants and growing children.

Vitamin B₁ (Thiamine)

Vitamin B_1 plays an important role in carbohydrate metabolism. When the diet is high in carbohydrates, there is an increased need for vitamin B_1. Vitamin B_1 acts as a coenzyme in the production of energy from glucose to make energy available for normal growth. This vitamin is found in many foods. Large amounts of this vitamin are found in wheat germ, whole grains, pork, and enriched grain products. Smaller amounts of the vitamin may be found in milk and milk products.

A deficiency of vitamin B_1 results in beriberi, a disease characterized by neurological, gastrointestinal (GI), and cardiovascular symptoms. Symptoms that may be seen with beriberi are muscle weakness, anorexia, peripheral neuritis, cardiac arrhythmias, and edema of the lower extremities. In most instances, a normal diet provides the recommended daily requirement of this vitamin. Situations that may require administration of vitamin B_1 include a limited dietary intake of the foods containing this vitamin; the chronically ill patient; the postoperative patient; the chronic alcoholic; and the elderly. This vitamin may be given alone, but very often it is given in combination with other B vitamins under the name *vitamin B-complex.*

Vitamin B_2 (Riboflavin)

Vitamin B_2 plays a vital role in numerous tissue respiration systems, making it essential for tissue maintenance and growth. This vitamin is found in small amounts in almost all foods. Larger amounts of the vitamin are found in milk and milk products, organ meats, and green leafy vegetables.

A deficiency of vitamin B_2 is characterized by changes in the cornea of the eye; *cheilosis* (disorder of the lips with cracking and fissures); *glossitis* (inflammation of the tongue); seborrheic dermatitis (especially in the skin folds); roughness of the eyelids; *blepharospasm* (twitching of the eyelid); and *photophobia* (unusual intolerance to light). Inadequate riboflavin contributes to poor wound healing and inflammation. Riboflavin deficiency rarely occurs alone and is often seen with deficiency of other B vitamins and protein.

Vitamin B_5 (Pantothenic Acid)

Vitamin B_5 is an essential element in cellular metabolism. As a coenzyme, it plays a vital role in activating coenzyme A, which controls cell metabolism in many cells of the body. A true deficiency of this vitamin rarely occurs in those eating a normal diet because this vitamin is found in a wide variety of foods.

Vitamin B_6 (Pyridoxine)

Vitamin B_6 is involved with the metabolism of protein, carbohydrates, and fats. This vitamin is found in wheat germ, pork, organ and muscle meats, bananas, and whole grain cereals.

A deficiency of vitamin B_6 is rare and is most likely accompanied by other vitamin B deficiencies. When there is a deficiency of vitamin B_6, nausea, depression, anemia, and dermatitis may be seen.

Vitamin B_{12} (Cyanocobalamin)

Vitamin B_{12} is discussed in the section on drugs used to treat anemia.

Niacin (Vitamin B_3, Nicotinic Acid)

Niacin is converted by the body to nicotinamide, which is involved with the metabolism of fats, carbohydrates, and proteins. Niacin is found in meat, poultry, fish, enriched bread and bread products, and peanut butter.

A deficiency of niacin results in pellagra, a disease characterized by dermatitis, diarrhea, inflammation of the mouth, tongue, and intestinal lining, and mental changes.

USES OF THE WATER-SOLUBLE VITAMINS

The water-soluble vitamins are not stored in the body to any great extent. One or more of the water-soluble vitamins may be administered to prevent or treat a deficiency of one or more of these vitamins. Examples of situations or diseases that may result in a deficiency of one or more water-soluble vitamins include the following:

- Diseases or disorders of the GI tract, such as prolonged episodes of vomiting or diarrhea, or an inability of the body to absorb vitamins from the GI tract
- Emotional or psychotic disorders, such as bulimia, anorexia nervosa, and severe depression, when food intake is limited
- Fad diets, starvation diets
- Poor eating habits or the inability to purchase food for proper nutrition
- Prolonged periods without food, such as the time after surgery
- Use of niacin (nicotinic acid) to lower the blood cholesterol

The specific uses of each water-soluble vitamin are given in Summary Drug Table 49-1.

Summary Drug Table 49–1. Vitamins

Generic Name	Trade Name*	Uses	Adverse Reactions	Dose Ranges
VITAMIN A PREPARATIONS				
vitamin A	Aquasol A, *generic*	Vitamin deficiency	None unless overdosage occurs	PO 100,000–500,000 IU/d for 3d, then 50,000 IU/d for 2 wk, then 10,000–20,000 IU/d for 2 mo; IM 100,000 IU/d for 3d then 50,000 IU/d for 2 wks depending on degree of deficiency
isotretinoin	Accutane	Severe cystic acne	Cheilitis, conjunctivitis, eye irritation, dry skin, fetal abnormalities, pruritus, epistaxis, nausea, vomiting	0.5–2 mg/kg/d PO in 2 divided doses
tretinoin	Retin-A	Acne vulgaris	Redness, blistering, rash, stinging, peeling, contact dermatitis	Apply daily hs
VITAMIN B PREPARATIONS				
vitamin B_1 (thiamine hydrochloride)	Thiamilate, *generic*	Prevention and treatment of thiamine deficiency	Feeling of warmth, sweating, nausea, tightness in the chest, cyanosis, pulmonary edema, angioneurotic edema, urticaria, restlessness	5–10 mg/d PO, up to 30 mg IV, 10–20 mg IM
vitamin B_2 (riboflavin)	*generic*	Prevention and treatment of riboflavin deficiency	Yellow discoloration of the urine	5–50 mg/d PO
vitamin B_5 (calcium pantothenate, pantothenic acid)	*generic*	Supplement when diet is low in this vitamin	GI cramping, allergic reactions	5–100 mg PO
Vitamin B_6 (pyridoxine hydrochloride)	*generic*	Prevention and treatment of pyridoxine deficiency	Paresthesia, somnolence, unstable gait, numbness of the feet, awkwardness of the hands, ataxia	10–20 mg/d PO; higher doses may be used under certain conditions
niacin (nicotinic acid, vitamin B_3	Nicobid, Nicolar, *generic*	Prophylaxis and treatment of pellagra, hyperlipidemia, niacin deficiency	Nausea, vomiting, diarrhea, abdominal pain, severe generalized flushing of the skin with severe itching, or tingling and sensation of warmth	Pellagra: up to 500 mg/d PO; hyperlipidemia: 1–2 g PO tid; niacin deficiency: up to 100 mg/d PO; drug may also be given IM, IV, SC
VITAMIN C PREPARATIONS				
ascorbic acid	Cevalin, Cecon *generic*	Prevention and treatment of ascorbic acid deficiency	Large doses; diarrhea, burning on urination	70–150 mg/d PO; up to 1 g/d for scurvey IM, SC, IV
VITAMIN D PREPARATIONS				
calcifediol	Calderol	Metabolic bone disease, hypocalcemia in those on chronic renal dialysis, osteomalacia, hypocalcemia	Weakness, headache, vomiting, dry mouth, constipation, muscle and bone pain, metallic taste, nausea, tinnitus	300–350 mcg/wk PO in divided doses given qd or every other day
calcitriol	Rocaltrol, Calcimar	Hypocalcemia in those on chronic renal dialysis, hypoparathyroidism	Weakness, headache, vomit-, ing, dry mouth, constipation, muscle and bone pain, metallic taste, nausea, tinnitus	0.25–1 mcg PO

(continued)

Summary Drug Table 49–1 (Continued)

Generic Name	Trade Name*	Uses	Adverse Reactions	Dose Ranges
dihydrotachysterol (DHT)	Hytakerol, *generic*	Acute, chronic, and latent tetany (post-operative, idiopathic) and hypoparathyroidism	Drowsiness, headache, nausea, diarrhea, athralgia, decreased bone development	0.8–2.4 mg/d for 1 wk; maintenance: 0.2–2 mg/d regulated by serum calcium levels
cholecalciferol	Calciferol, *generic*	Rickets, familial hypophosphatemia, hypoparathyroidism, vitamin D deficiency	Drowsiness, headache, nausea, diarrhea, arthralgia, decreased bone development	Up to 500,000 IU/d PO (dose may be as low as 400 IU/d)
VITAMIN E PREPARATIONS				
Vitamin E	Aquasol E, *generic*	Treatment and prevention of vitamin E deficiency	None	60–75 IU/d PO IM not to exceed 300 IU/d; higher doses may be used
VITAMIN K PREPARATIONS				
menadiol sodium diphosphate (K4)	Synkayvite	Hypoprothrombinemia due to antibacterial or salicylate therapy, obstructive jaundice, biliary fistulas	Nausea, vomiting, pain at injection site, headache, rash	2–10 mg/d PO, 5–15 mg PO, IM, IV
phytonadione (K1)	Mephyton, Konakion, Aqua-MEPHYTON	Anticoagulant-induced prothrombin deficiency (oral anticoagulants), prophylaxis and treatment of hemorrhagic disease of the newborn	Headache, nausea, decreased hives, function rash, urticaria, shock, cardiac arrest (IV only)	1–25 mg IM, SC, PO; newborn: 0.5–1 mg IM (Restrict IV use to situations where other routes not possible)

*The term, *generic,* indicates that the drug is available in generic form.

ADVERSE REACTIONS ASSOCIATED WITH THE ADMINISTRATION OF WATER-SOLUBLE VITAMINS

Vitamin C

Large doses of vitamin C may result in diarrhea. Burning on urination may also occur. Soreness may be noted at the intramuscular (IM) injection site, and rapid intravenous (IV) administration may result in temporary faintness and dizziness.

Vitamin B₁

A feeling of warmth, pruritus, urticaria, sweating, nausea, restlessness, tightness in the chest, angioneurotic edema, cyanosis, and pulmonary edema may be seen with the administration of vitamin B_1. Serious sensitivity reactions can occur and death has been reported with IV use. When taken orally in a multivitamin preparation, adverse reactions are rare unless the recommended dose is exceeded.

Vitamins B₂ and B₅

No adverse reactions are seen with the administration of these vitamins.

Vitamin B₆

Paresthesia (numbness or tingling sensation), somnolence, and low serum folic acid levels may be seen with the administration of vitamin B_6.

Niacin

Administration of niacin (nicotinic acid, vitamin B_3) may result in nausea, vomiting, abdominal pain, diarrhea, severe generalized flushing of the skin, and a sensation of warmth. Flushing of the skin may also be accompanied by severe itching or tingling, especially when large doses are administered.

NURSING MANAGEMENT

Nurses are in a unique position to provide support and identify nutritional problems. Problems identified range from general malnutrition requiring supplementation to underlying disease requiring a special diet.

The nurse works closely with the registered dietitian to determine the nutritional needs of the patient and to plan ways to meet those needs in each individual. In those eating poorly or with a severe nutritional problem, an evaluation is made of the patient's nutritional intake. The physician is contacted if the patient fails to eat the prescribed diet.

Signs of vitamin deficiency may include any of the following: loss of appetite, gastric distress, fatigue, cracks at the corners of the mouth, swollen or red tongue, dermatitis, neuritis, loss of appetite, poor would healing or easy bruising. Report symptoms of vitamin deficiency to the physician.

B-Complex Vitamins

Riboflavin may cause a yellow/orange color to the urine. Niocin is rapidly absorbed from the GI tract and reaches its peak concentration 45 minutes after ingestion. Transient flushing may occur with oral therapy.

Nursing Alert

When niacin (nicotinic acid) is given for treatment of elevated blood cholesterol, tell the patient that a feeling of warmth, flushing, and itching may occur. Often, high doses are necessary for the treatment of an elevated blood cholesterol and these adverse reactions may be severe. Inform the physician immediately of a severe adverse reaction to this vitamin.

Pyridoxine overdosage has been seen in patients taking 50 mg to 2 g over long periods of time. Observe for symptoms of overdosage which include: unstable gait, numbness of the feet, awkwardness of the hands, decreased sensation to touch, and somnolence.

Diabetics, patients with a history of renal calculi, those on sodium restricted diets, or those on anticoagulant therapy should not take large doses of vitamin C.

Nursing Process
The Patient Receiving a Water-Soluble Vitamin

■ *Assessment*
The history and physical assessment depend on the reason for the administration of any one or a combination of water-soluble vitamins. When the individual has an actual vitamin deficiency due to any cause, the history and assessment include vital signs, looking for signs of the deficiency, a record of the patient's dietary intake, and looking for possible causes of an impaired nutritional state.

■ *Nursing Diagnosis*
- **Risk for Ineffective Management of Therapeutic Regimen** related to lack of knowledge, indifference, adverse reactions or other (specify)

■ *Planning and Implementation*
The major goal of the patient may be an understanding of the treatment regimen and reason for use. To make this goal measurable, more specific criteria must be added.

■ *Patient and Family Teaching*
When the patient has a vitamin deficiency, emphasize the importance of improving or correcting eating habits. The first step in developing a teaching plan is to determine the reason for the inadequate dietary intake. Next, determine what steps are necessary to improve the patient's nutritional intake. For example, an elderly patient with a history of poor nutrition may have a problem shopping for food or may not have the financial means to eat a well-balanced diet. For this problem, contacting the hospital's social service department may be beneficial. After an interview, the social service worker may refer the patient to those persons or private or government agencies that may provide the funds and means for obtaining the types of food required for a well-balanced diet.

Some nutritional problems are difficult to solve, such as the nutritional deficiencies of the chronic alcoholic refusing treatment for his or her alcoholism or the young woman with anorexia nervosa. Many times, the family may be able to help the patient improve his or her nutritional status, but there are other times when an attempt to improve nutrition fails.

The hospital dietitian is a resource person who can assist the *willing* patient with meal planning and selecting foods that are high in the vitamins required to correct the deficiency. When contacting the dietitian, give a full history of the patient's problems; the disease that may be causing a nutritional deficit (when applicable); the diet recommended by the physician; and a list of medications (including vitamin supplements) that the patient will be taking at home. Emphasize to the patient the importance of good nutrition and of following the diet prescribed by the physician and outlined by the dietitian.

Providing information to the general public about the adverse effects associated with high vitamin dosages, as well as giving correct information regarding the role of vitamin therapy is an important role for the nurse. For example, the public needs to understand that water-soluble vitamins cannot be stored in the body for any appreciable length of time and what the body doesn't need is excreted, sometimes in a few hours. And, unless prescribed by the physician, massive doses of these vitamins are of no value.

When applicable, explain the adverse reactions that may be seen with these drugs to the patient. Information such as advising patients taking niacin (nicotinic acid) to contact their physician if intense flushing and itching occur will provide important information concerning the adverse reactions of niacin.

■ *Expected Outcomes for Evaluation*
- Patient and family demonstrate understanding of drug regimen
- Patient verbalizes importance of complying with the prescribed therapeutic regimen

The Fat-Soluble Vitamins

The *fat-soluble vitamins* are A, D, E, and K. These vitamins are stored in the body and used as needed.

ACTIONS OF THE FAT-SOLUBLE VITAMINS

Vitamin A

Vitamin A is necessary for the eye to adapt to night vision. Vitamin A also prevents retardation of growth and preserves the integrity of epithelial cells.

Some of the foods containing vitamin A include kidney, liver, whole milk, eggs, butter, and leafy yellow and green vegetables. Some foods such as skim milk and margarine are fortified with this vitamin. Because vitamin A is a fat-soluble vitamin, absorption of this vitamin requires the presence of bile salts, pancreatic lipase (a pancreatic digestive enzyme), and dietary fat. Vitamin A is stored in the liver.

A deficiency of vitamin A results in night blindness or the inability to see in the dark. Drying of the skin, a lowered resistance to infection, changes in the cornea of the eye, growth retardation, and fetal malformations may occur when a vitamin A deficiency exists.

Vitamin D

Vitamin D is necessary for the metabolism of calcium. It also promotes the absorption of calcium and phosphorus in the intestine, and increases the rate of accretion (accumulation) and resorption of minerals from the bone. Absorption of vitamin D from the intestine depends on an adequate amount of bile. Vitamin D is stored in the liver but is also found in fat, muscle, the skin, brain, spleen, and bones.

Several vitamin D preparations are available for replacement therapy (see Summary Drug Table 49-1). The physician's choice of a vitamin D preparation is based on the problem being treated and the pharmacologic activity of the product selected. Sources of this vitamin are mainly foods fortified with vitamin D. Milk is the main fortified source of this vitamin. Sunlight is also a major source of vitamin D because the skin converts dehydrocholesterol in the skin to vitamin D_3.

A deficiency of vitamin D results in rickets, which is a malformation of the long bones (arms, legs) of the body in children. In adults, a deficiency leads to osteomalacia, which is a loss of calcium from the bones, resulting in a weakening of the bones and an increased tendency toward bone fractures.

Vitamin E

Vitamin E is considered an essential element in human nutrition. It acts as an antioxidant to interrupt the oxidation process and protect the cell membrane fatty acids from damage. A deficiency of this vitamin is rare because it is found in a great many foods and the daily requirement for the vitamin appears to be small. This vitamin requires the presence of bile salts for absorption, and is stored in the liver and muscle.

Vitamin K

Vitamin K is needed by the liver to manufacture prothrombin and the other factors involved in the blood-clotting mechanism. This vitamin is found in cabbage, liver, egg yolks, cauliflower, and other leafy vegetables. Intestinal bacteria also synthesize vitamin K. This is probably the greatest source of the vitamin.

A deficiency of vitamin K is rare when the individual eats a normal diet and there is an adequate number of vitamin K–producing bacteria in the intestine. A deficiency may exist when drugs, such as the antibiotics, decrease the number of intestinal bacteria responsible for the manufacture of this vitamin. When a deficiency does occur, it is seen as an inability of the blood to clot within a normal time period.

USES OF THE FAT-SOLUBLE VITAMINS

Vitamin A

Vitamin A is given when a deficiency exists. Conditions that may cause a vitamin A deficiency include biliary tract or pancreatic disease, sprue, colitis, hepatic cirrhosis, celiac disease, regional enteritis, and a poor nutritional intake of foods containing this vitamin.

Isotretinoin (Accutane) and tretinoin (Retin-A) are products chemically related to vitamin A and are used in the treatment of acne. Isotretinoin is an isomer of retinoic acid. (An *isomer* is a chemical substance that has the same chemical formula but different chemical properties as its related substance). Isotretinoin is taken orally, whereas tretinoin is applied topically.

Vitamin D

Vitamin D, along with the parathyroid hormone, regulates calcium metabolism. Therefore, it may be used in persons with a certain type of calcium deficiency, such as the calcium deficiency seen in those patients on prolonged renal dialysis. Vitamin D is also used in the treatment of rickets in children. Although this condition is relatively rare in the United

States, it may be seen in persons living in areas where exposure to sunlight is limited and whose diet is deficient in this vitamin.

Vitamin E

The only established use of vitamin E is in the prevention or treatment of a vitamin E deficiency, which is rare. An unlabeled use of this vitamin is the administration to premature infants receiving oxygen to reduce the incidence of eye damage (retrolental fibroplasia) and lung damage (bronchopulmonary dysplasia) due to oxygen administration. There are also other unlabeled conditions or disorders for which this vitamin has been used.

Vitamin K

Vitamin K is used to correct a vitamin K deficiency. Menadiol sodium diphosphate (Synkayvite) is used in the treatment of hypoprothrombinemia due to antibacterial or salicylate therapy, obstructive jaundice, and biliary fistulas. Phytonadione (Mephyton, AquaMEPHYTON) is an oral anticoagulant antagonist and may be given to patients receiving anticoagulant therapy when an elevated prothrombin time results in bleeding or hemorrhage (see Summary Drug Table 32-1).

ADVERSE REACTIONS ASSOCIATED WITH THE ADMINISTRATION OF FAT-SOLUBLE VITAMINS

Vitamin A

The adverse effects seen with vitamin A administration are related to overdosage (*hypervitaminosis A*). Signs of overdosage include fatigue, malaise, headache, abdominal discomfort, anorexia, vomiting, arthralgia, fissures of the lips, drying and cracking of the skin, alopecia, bone pain, and vertigo. Treatment of hypervitaminosis A is immediate withdrawal of the drug along with supportive treatment.

Adverse reactions associated with the administration of isotretinoin for acne include conjunctivitis, dry skin and mucous membranes, rash, brittle nails, and dry mouth. Women who are pregnant or may become pregnant must not use this drug because of a high risk of fetal deformities. Adverse reactions seen with the administration of tretinoin include redness, blistering, and swelling of the skin.

Vitamin D

Administration of vitamin D in normal doses may result in weakness, headache, somnolence, nausea, vomiting, dry mouth, constipation, muscle and bone pain, and a metallic taste. Overdosage of this vitamin may produce hypercalcemia (see Chap. 48) and the loss of calcium from bone in adults. Severe hypercalcemia can result in a loss of renal function and cardiovascular failure. Deaths have been reported with vitamin D overdosage.

Vitamin E

There appear to be no adverse reactions associated with the administration of this vitamin, nor have there been any adverse reactions seen with overdosage.

Vitamin K

Oral administration of vitamin K may result in nausea, vomiting, and headache. Parenteral administration may cause pain at the injection site. Anaphylactoid reactions have been reported with the IV administration of AquaMEPHYTON.

NURSING MANAGEMENT

When a vitamin deficiency exists, monitor the patient's food intake. Check each meal tray and inform the physician if the food intake is below normal. Ingestion of mineral oil may interfere with absorption of the fat-soluble vitamins.

When administering vitamin A, do not exceed the recommended dosage. Administer orally with food to increase absorption. Notify the physician if symptoms of overdosage occurs (eg, nausea, vomiting, anorexia, malaise, night sweats, drying or cracking of the lips). Therapeutic response is observed by weight gain, absence of dry skin and mucous membranes and decreased night blindness.

If isotretinoin is prescribed for acne, the physician discusses with the patient the dangers associated with pregnancy while on this drug. The nurse may be responsible for evaluating the patient's understanding of the precautions to be observed while taking isotretinoin.

If bleeding occurs during vitamin K therapy, closely observe the patient for continued bleeding. When parenteral phytonadione is given, the effect on the bleeding time is noted within 1 to 2 hours and hemorrhage, when present, is usually controlled within 3 to 6 hours.

Nursing Process
The Patient Receiving a Fat-Soluble Vitamin

■ *Assessment*
When a patient is receiving a fat-soluble vitamin for a vitamin deficiency, record the signs of the deficiency in the patient's chart. If a decreased nutritional intake is the cause of the deficiency, weight the patient and take the vital signs.

■ *Nursing Diagnosis*
- **Risk for Ineffective Management of Therapeutic Regimen** related to lack of knowledge, indifference, adverse reactions or other (specify)

■ *Planning and Implementation*
The major goal of the patient may be an understanding of the treatment regimen and reason for use. For this goal to be measurable, more specific criteria must be added.

■ *Patient and Family Teaching*
If the vitamin deficiency is due to a decreased dietary intake, the information included under the water-soluble vitamins is applicable. Include the following information in a teaching plan:

Vitamin Preparations
- Take this drug as prescribed. Do not increase or decrease the dose unless told to do so by the physician.
- Eat the foods recommended by the physician. If there is difficulty in purchasing these foods, discuss this with the physician or a social service worker.
- Avoid the use of mineral oil, which can prevent the absorption of these (fat-soluble) vitamins. If a lax-

ative is needed, ask the physician for the type of laxative that will not interfere with vitamin and food absorption.

- Do not use multivitamin preparations unless their use is approved by the physician.

Isotretinoin

- Take this drug with meals. Do not crush the capsules but swallow whole.
- Follow the physician's recommendations regarding contraceptive measures before, during, and after therapy. If pregnancy is suspected, stop taking the drug and immediately notify the physician.
- Avoid prolonged exposure to sunlight because a photosensitivity reaction may occur.

Tretinoin

- Avoid prolonged exposure to sunlight because a photosensitivity reaction may occur.
- Apply the drug as directed. Keep the drug away from the eyes, mouth, and mucous membranes.

■ Expected Outcomes for Evaluation

- Patient and family demonstrate understanding of drug regimen
- Patient verbalizes importance of complying with the prescribed treatment regimen
- Patient demonstrates understanding of the dangers associated with pregnancy (isotretinoin)

Drugs Used in the Treatment of Anemia

Anemia is a decrease in the number of red blood cells, a decrease in the amount of hemoglobin in red blood cells, or *both* a decrease in the number of red blood cells and hemoglobin. There are various types and causes of anemia. Once the type and cause have been identified, the physician selects a method of treatment. Drugs used in treatment of anemia are summarized in Summary Drug Table 49-2.

Summary Drug Table 49-2. Drugs Used in Treatment of Anemia

Generic Name	Trade Name*	Uses	Adverse Reactions	Dose Ranges
ferrous fumarate (33% elemental iron)	Feostat, *generic*	Prevention and treatment of iron-deficiency anemia	GI irritation, nausea, vomiting, constipation, diarrhea, allergic reactions	100–200 mg PO of elemental iron qd in divided doses
ferrous gluconate (11.6% elemental iron)	Fergon, *generic*	Prevention and treatment of iron-deficiency-anemia	GI irritation, nausea, vomiting, constipation, diarrhea, allergic reactions	100–200 mg PO of elemental iron qd in divided doses
ferrous sulfate (20% elemental iron)	Feosol, Fer-In-Sol, *generic*	Prevention and treatment of iron-deficiency anemia	GI irritation, nausea, vomiting, constipation, diarrhea, allergic reactions	100–200 mg PO of elemental iron qd in divided doses
folic acid	Folvite, *generic*	Megaloblastic anemias due to deficiency of folic acid	Allergic sensitization	Up to 1 mg/d PO, IM, IV SC
iron dextran	InFeD, *generic*	Iron deficiency anemia	Anaphylactoid reactions, soreness & and inflammation at injection site, hypersensitivity reactions	Dosage based on body weight and grams percent (g/dL) of hemoglobin
leucovorin calcium	Wellcovorin *generic*	Megaloblastic anemias, to counteract effect of overdosage of folic acid	Allergic sensitization urticaria, anaphylaxis	Megaloblastic anemias: initial 3–6 mg/d IM thru 1 mg/d PO for life; overdosage of folic acid antagonists: up to 1 mg IM, 200 mg/m² IV
vitamin B¹² (cyanocobalamin)	Rubramin PC, *generic*	B12 deficiencies as seen in pernicious anemia, GI pathology; also used when requirements for the vitamin are increased; Schilling's test	Mild diarrhea, itching, pulmonary edema, CHF, anaphylaxis	Schilling's test: 100–1000 μg/d X2 wk, then 100–1000 μg IM q mo

*The term, *generic*, indicates that the drug is available in generic form.

ACTIONS AND USES OF DRUGS USED IN THE TREATMENT OF ANEMIA

Iron

Iron is a component of hemoglobin, which is in red blood cells. It is the iron in the hemoglobin of red blood cells that picks up oxygen from the lungs and carries it to all body tissues. Iron is stored in the body and is found mainly in the reticuloendothelial cells of the liver, spleen, and bone marrow. Iron salts, for example, ferrous sulfate or ferrous gluconate, are used in the treatment of *iron-deficiency anemia,* which occurs when there is a loss of iron that is greater than the available iron stored in the body. Iron is found in foods such as meats, fruits, eggs, fish, poultry, grains, and dairy products. Iron dextran is a parenteral iron that is also used for the treatment of iron-deficiency anemia. It is primarily used when the patient cannot take oral drugs or when the patient experiences GI intolerance to oral iron administration.

Folic Acid

Folic acid is required for the manufacture of red blood cells in the bone marrow. Folic acid is found in leafy green vegetables, fish, meat, poultry, and whole grains. A deficiency of folic acid results in megaloblastic anemia. *Megaloblastic anemia* is characterized by the presence of large, abnormal, immature erythrocytes circulating in the blood. Folic acid is used in the treatment of megaloblastic anemias that are due to a deficiency of folic acid.

Although not related to anemia, studies indicate there is a decreased risk for neural tube defects if folic acid is taken prior to conception and during early pregnancy. Neural tube defects occur during early pregnancy when the embryonic folds forming the spinal cord and brain join together. Defects of this type include anencephaly (congenital absence of brain and spinal cord), spina bifida (defect of the spinal cord), and meningocele (a saclike protrusion of the meninges in the spinal cord or skull). The U.S. Public Health Service recommends the use of folic acid for women of childbearing age in order to decrease the incidence of neural tube defects. Dosage for nonpregnant women of childbearing age should be less than 1 mg per day, unless the physician or-

ders otherwise. Dosages during pregnancy are prescribed by the physician.

Leucovorin

Leucovorin is a derivative of, and an active reduced form of, folic acid. The oral and parenteral form of this drug is used in the treatment of megaloblastic anemia.

Leucovorin may also be used to diminish the hematologic effects of (intentional) massive doses of methotrexate, a drug used in the treatment of certain types of cancer (see Chap. 47). This technique of administering leucovorin after a large dose of methotrexate is called *folinic acid rescue* or *leucovorin rescue.* Occasionally, high doses of methotrexate are administered to select patients. Leucovorin is then used either at the time methotrexate is administered or a specific number of hours after the methotrexate has been given to decrease the toxic effects of the methotrexate. Leucovorin may be ordered to be given IV, IM, or by the oral route.

Vitamin B$_{12}$ (Cyanocobalamin)

Vitamin B$_{12}$ is essential to growth, cell reproduction, the manufacture of myelin (which surrounds some nerve fibers), and blood cell manufacture. The *intrinsic factor,* which is produced by cells in the stomach, is necessary for the absorption of vitamin B$_{12}$ in the intestine. A deficiency of the intrinsic factor results in abnormal formation of erythrocytes because of the body's failure to absorb vitamin B$_{12}$, a necessary component for blood cell formation. The resulting anemia is a type of megloblastic anemia called *pernicious anemia.*

A deficiency of this vitamin due to a low dietary intake of vitamin B$_{12}$ is rare because it is found in meats, milk, eggs, and cheese. The body is also able to store this vitamin; a deficiency, for any reason, will not occur for 5 to 6 years. A vitamin B$_{12}$ deficiency may be seen in persons who: (1) are strict vegetarians; (2) have had a total gastrectomy or subtotal gastric resection (when the cells producing the intrinsic factor are totally or partially removed); (3) have intestinal diseases such as ulcerative colitis or sprue; (4) have gastric carcinoma; or (5) have a congenital decrease in the number of gastric cells secreting intrinsic factor.

Vitamin B_{12} is also used to perform the Schilling's test, which is used to diagnose pernicious anemia.

ADVERSE REACTIONS ASSOCIATED WITH THE ADMINISTRATION OF DRUGS USED IN THE TREATMENT OF ANEMIA

Iron Salts

Iron salts occasionally cause GI irritation, nausea, vomiting, constipation, diarrhea, and allergic reactions. The stools usually appear darker in color.

Iron dextran is given by the parenteral route. Hypersensitivity reactions, including fatal anaphylactic reactions, have been reported with the use of this form of iron. Additional adverse reactions include soreness, inflammation, and sterile abscesses at the IM injection site. Intravenous administration may result in phlebitis at the injection site.

Folic Acid and Leucovorin

Administration of these drugs may result in allergic sensitization.

Vitamin B_{12}

Mild diarrhea and itching have been reported with the administration of vitamin B_{12}. Other adverse reactions that may be seen include a marked increase in red blood cell production, acne, peripheral vascular thrombosis, congestive heart failure, and pulmonary edema.

NURSING MANAGEMENT

Administration

Iron salts are preferably given between meals with water but can be given with food or meals if GI upset occurs. If the patient is receiving other medications, check with the hospital pharmacist regarding the simultaneous administration of iron salts with other drugs.

Oral iron solutions may cause temporary staining of the teeth. Dilute the solution with 2 to 4 ounces of water or juice and use a straw when administering. Stool may appear darker in color or black.

> **Nursing Alert**
>
> Parenteral iron has resulted in fatal anaphylactic-type reactions. Report any of the following adverse reactions: dyspnea, urticaria, rashes, itching, and fever.

Administer intramuscular iron preparations using the Z-track technique (see Chap. 2) to prevent staining of the tissues. Iron dextran is given IM or IV.

When leucovorin is administered after a large dose of methotrexate, the timing of the administration is outlined by the physician. It is essential that the leucovorin be given at the *exact* time ordered because the purpose of folinic acid rescue is to allow a high dose of a toxic drug to remain in the body for only a limited time.

Patients with pernicious anemia are treated with vitamin B_{12} by the parenteral route (IM) weekly until stabilized. The parenteral route is used because the vitamin is ineffective orally due to the absence of the intrinsic factor in the stomach, which is necessary for utilization of Vitamin B_{12}. After stabilization, maintainence (usually monthly) injections are necessary for life.

> **Nursing Alert**
>
> Pernicious anemia must be diagnosed and treated as soon as possible because vitamin B_{12} deficiency that is allowed to progress for more than 3 months may result in degenerative lesions of the spinal cord.

Observations

Include the following assessments, evaluations, and nursing tasks in the nursing care plan:

- Take the vital signs daily; more frequent monitoring may be needed if the patient is moderately to acutely ill.
- Observe the patient for adverse reactions. Report any occurrence of adverse reactions to the physician before the next dose is due. Report severe adverse reactions immediately.

- Iron salt therapy—Inform the patient that the color of the stool will change. If diarrhea or constipation occurs, inform the physician.
- Iron dextran—Inform the patient that soreness at the injection site may occur. Check injection sites daily for signs of inflammation, swelling, or abscess formation.
- A special diet (eg, foods high in iron or foods high in folic acid) may be prescribed. If the diet is taken poorly, note this on the patient's chart and discuss the problem with the physician.
- Observe the patient for relief of the symptoms of anemia. Some patients may note a relief of symptoms after a few days of therapy.
- Periodic laboratory tests are necessary to monitor the results of therapy.

Nursing Process
The Patient Receiving a Drug Used in the Treatment of Anemia

■ Assessment
Obtain a general health history and the symptoms of the anemia. The physician may order laboratory tests to determine the type, severity, and possible cause of the anemia. At times, it may be easy to identify the cause of the anemia, but there are also instances where the cause of the anemia is obscure.

If iron dextran is to be given, an allergy history is necessary because this drug is given with caution to those with significant allergies or asthma. The patient's weight may be required for calculating the dosage.

Take the vital signs to provide a baseline during therapy. Other physical assessments may include the patient's general appearance and, in the severely anemic patient, an evaluation of the patient's ability to carry out the activities of daily living.

■ Nursing Diagnoses
Depending on the drug, dose, and reason for administration, one or more of the following nursing diagnoses may apply to a person receiving a drug used in the treatment of anemia:

- **Anxiety** related to diagnosis, other factors
- **Risk for Ineffective Management of Therapeutic Regimen** related to indifference, lack of knowledge, adverse drug effects, other factors

■ Planning and Implementation
The major goals of the patient may include a reduction in anxiety and an understanding of and compliance to the prescribed treatment regimen. To make these goals measurable, more specific criteria must be added.

Anxiety. Some patients may have varying degrees of anxiety because of their diagnosis or the necessity of treatment. The nurse should explain the purpose of treatment and allow the patient time to ask questions.

■ Patient and Family Teaching
Explain the medical regimen thoroughly to the patient and family. Emphasize the importance of following the prescribed treatment regimen.

Include the following points in a patient and family teaching plan:

Iron Salt
- Take this drug on an empty stomach with water. If GI upset occurs, take the drug with food or meals.
- Do not take other drugs (prescription or nonprescription) at the same time or 2 hours before or after taking iron without first checking with the physician.
- This drug may cause a darkening of the stools, constipation, or diarrhea. If constipation or diarrhea becomes severe, contact the physician.
- Avoid the indiscriminate use of advertised iron products. If a true iron deficiency occurs, the cause must be determined and therapy should be under the care of a physician.

Folic Acid
- Avoid the use of multivitamin preparations unless use has been approved by the physician.
- Follow the diet recommended by the physician because diet and medication are necessary to correct a folic acid deficiency.

Leucovorin
- Megaloblastic anemia—Adhere to the diet prescribed by the physician. If the purchase of foods high in protein (which can be expensive) becomes a problem, discuss this with the physician.
- Folinic acid rescue—Take this drug at the exact prescribed intervals. If nausea and vomiting occur, contact the physician *immediately.*

Vitamin B12
- Nutritional deficiency of vitamin B_{12}—Eat a well-balanced diet including seafood, eggs, meats, and dairy products.

- Pernicious anemia—Lifetime therapy is necessary. Eat a well-balanced diet including seafood, eggs, meats, and dairy products. Avoid contact with infections and report any signs of infection to the physician immediately because an increase in dosage may be necessary.
- Therapy for pernicious anemia almost always requires parenteral administration of the drug at periodic intervals (usually monthly). Emphasize the importance of receiving the monthly injection. In some instances, the patient or a family member is allowed to give the drug, and instruction in administration is necessary.

■ Expected Outcomes for Evaluation
- Anxiety is reduced
- Patient and family demonstrate understanding of drug regimen
- Patient verbalizes importance of complying with the prescribed treatment regimen

Chapter Summary

- Vitamins are organic substances needed by the body in small amounts for normal growth and nutrition. The vitamins act as regulators of body processes and as coenzymes in certain chemical reactions that occur in the body. Vitamins are divided into two main groups according to their solubility: the water-soluble vitamins and the fat-soluble vitamins. The B-complex vitamins and vitamin C are classified as water-soluble vitamins. Vitamins A, D, E, and K are the fat-soluble vitamins.
- Although no one food contains all of the vitamins, vitamins can generally be obtained from the diet. Two exceptions are vitamin K and vitamin D. Besides its food sources, vitamin K is manufactured by the intestinal bacteria within the body. Vitamin D is produced in the body after exposure to sunlight. Vitamin deficiency diseases produce specific symptoms, which can usually be treated with the administration of the specific vitamin.
- The nurse works closely with the registered dietitian to determine the nutritional needs of the patient and to plan ways to meet those needs in each individual. In those eating poorly or with a severe nutritional problem, an evaluation is made of the patient's nutritional intake. The physician is contacted if the patient fails to eat the prescribed diet.
- Anemia is a decrease in the number of red blood cells, a decrease in the amount of hemoglobin in red blood cells, or both a decrease in the number of red blood cells and hemoglobin. Iron-deficiency anemia occurs when there is a loss of iron that is greater than the available iron stored in the body. Iron dextran is used to treat iron deficiency anemia and is administered deep IM using the Z-tract technique.
- Megaloblastic anemia results from a folic acid deficiency. This type of anemia is treated with leucovorin, an active reduced form of folic acid.
- Another use for leucovorin is in the treatment of methotrexate toxicity. The technique of administering leucovorin after a large dose of methotrexate is called folinic acid rescue or leucovorin rescue. Leucovorin is administered after methotrexate to decrease the hematologic effects.
- Pernicious anemia occurs as a result of the lack of the intrinsic factor in the stomach. For vitamin B_{12} absorption to take place, the intrinsic factor must be present. Without the intrinsic factor, vitamin B_{12} cannot be absorbed, and blood cell formation is inhibited. This results in pernicious anemia. Treatment is parenteral administration of vitamin B_{12}, usually for life.

Critical Thinking Exercises

1. Ms. Klepper, aged 32, has been diagnosed with pernicious anemia. Even though the physician has explained the diagnosis and the treatment she is confused and frightened. She questions you stating "I just don't understand what is happening in my body to cause me to feel so weak and tired?" and "How is the treatment going to work?" How would you handle this situation with Ms. Klepper? What would you tell her that would decrease her anxiety and increase her understanding?
2. Discuss the nursing diagnosis **Altered Nutrition: Less Than Body Requirements,** related to vitamin A deficiency. Identify outcome criteria and plan five nursing interventions appropriate for this diagnosis.
3. Mr. Alperin, aged 68, has been taking excessively large doses of vitamin A for the last 3 months. The vitamin was not prescribed by the physician, but Mr. Alperin "felt he needed extra vitamin A because he was having trouble with his eyesight." He has come to the clinic complaining of fatigue, abdominal discomfort, and dryness of the skin. What assessments would be most important for you to make? What would be the most significant component of the patient teaching for Mr. Alperin?

50

Heavy Metal Antagonists

Chapter Objectives

On completion of this chapter the student will:

* *List actions, uses, and more common adverse reactions of heavy metal antagonists*
* *Discuss the reasons for using a heavy metal antagonist*
* *Discuss the nursing implications to be considered when administering a heavy metal or heavy metal antagonist*
* *Use the nursing process when administering a heavy metal antagonist*

Scherer JC, Roach S: INTRODUCTORY CLINICAL PHARMACOLOGY,
FIFTH EDITION © 1996 Lippincott-Raven Publishers

Certain situations may expose persons to a *heavy metal* (a metal with a relatively high density). Air pollutants, especially those containing heavy metals such as lead and arsenic, pose a hazard to living organisms, including humans. Other sources of heavy metal poisoning include exposure to gasoline fumes and certain pesticides and weed killers, and the eating of seafood such as fish, clams, oysters, and shrimp caught in waters polluted with heavy metals.

Heavy Metal Antagonists

Poisoning by or excessive blood levels of the heavy metals lead, iron, gold, arsenic, mercury, and copper can be treated with drugs called heavy metal antagonists (Summary Drug Table 50-1).

ACTIONS AND USES OF HEAVY METAL ANTAGONISTS

Deferoxamine

Deferoxamine (Desferal) is an iron chelating drug. A *chelating agent* selectively and chemically binds the ion of a metal to itself, thus aiding in the elimination of the metallic ion from the body. Deferoxamine chelates and then removes excess iron from the body. Excessive iron (or iron overload) may be seen in those who have accidentally or purposely ingested excessive amounts of a drug containing iron, for example, ferrous sulfate. This type of iron overload may be acute or chronic, depending on the amount of drug ingested. Acute iron overload may be seen in persons ingesting large doses of an iron preparation in a short time. Chronic iron overload may be seen in persons taking excessive doses of an iron preparation over a time, as well as in persons receiving multiple blood transfusions.

Dimercaprol

Dimercaprol (BAL in Oil) promotes the excretion of arsenic, gold, and mercury by chelation. It may also be used with edetate calcium disodium to promote the excretion of lead in acute lead poisoning. Arsenic poisoning may occur in persons who have been exposed to certain insecticides and weed killers, as well as those who have been exposed to this chemical in industry. Gold poisoning may be seen in persons

receiving gold compounds for arthritis. Mercury poisoning can occur in those eating fish caught in water contaminated with industrial wastes containing mercury. Lead poisoning is discussed next.

Edetate Calcium Disodium (Calcium EDTA)

The calcium in edetate calcium disodium (Calcium Disodium Versenate) is displaced by heavy metals, such as lead, to form a stable chemical that is excreted in the urine. This drug is used in the treatment of acute and chronic lead poisoning. Poisoning with this heavy metal may be seen in persons working in industries where lead is used, such as the petroleum industry, as well as in small children ingesting paint fragments containing lead. Federal regulations require all paint to be lead-free, but lead-based paint may still be seen in older homes.

Penicillamine and Trientine

Penicillamine (Cuprimine) and trientine (Cuprid) are chelating drugs that remove excess copper in those with Wilson's disease (a degenerative disease of the liver). Trientine is used when patients experience adverse reactions to penicillamine. Penicillamine is also used in the treatment of rheumatoid arthritis (see Chap. 42) and *cystinuria* (the presence of cystine, an amino acid, in the urine). Cystinuria is an inherited metabolic disorder that can cause recurrent stones in the urinary tract.

Succimer

Succimer (Chemet) is a chelating agent used in treating lead poisoning in children with blood levels greater than 45 mcg/dL.

ADVERSE REACTIONS ASSOCIATED WITH THE ADMINISTRATION OF HEAVY METAL ANTAGONISTS

Deferoxamine. Occasionally, pain and induration at the injection site may occur. Other adverse reactions that may occur during therapy for acute

Summary Drug Table 50-1. Heavy Metal Antagonists

Generic Name	Trade Name*	Uses	Adverse Reactions	Dose Ranges
deferoxamine mesylate	Desferal Mesylate	Acute iron intoxication, chronic iron overload	Pain and induration at injection site, urticaria, hypotension, generalized erythema	Acute: 1 g IM, IV, then 0.5 g q4h for 2 doses then 0.5 g q4–12h based on response; chronic: 0.5–2 g/d IM, 1–2 g/d SC
dimercaprol	BAL in Oil	Treatment of arsenic, gold, and mercury poisoning; acute lead poisoning when used with edetate calcium disodium	Hypertension, tachycardia, nausea, vomiting, headache	Mild arsenic or gold: 2.5 mg/kg IM qid for 2 d, then bid on third day, then daily for 10 d; severe arsenic or gold: 3 mg/kg q4h for 2 d, then qid on third day, then bid for 10 d; mercury poisoning: 5 mg/kg IM then 2.5 mg/kg d or bid for 10 d; acute lead encephalopathy: 4 mg/kg IM then 3 mg/kg q4h for 2–7 d
edetate calcium disodium (EDTA)	Calcium Disodium, Versenate	Acute and chronic lead poisoning, lead encephalopathy	Renal tubular necrosis	Up to 35 mg/kg IM bid; 200 mg IV bid for up to 5 d, interrupt therapy for 2 d then follow with another 5 d of therapy
penicillamine	Cuprimine	Cystinuria, Wilson's disease, rheumatoid arthritis	Bone marrow depression, nephrotic syndrome, pruritus, skin rash, nausea, vomiting, tinnitus, epigastric pain, diarrhea	Up to 2 g/d PO
succimer	Chemet	Lead poisoning in children	Nausea, vomiting, diarrhea, anorexia, rash, sore throat, pain in stomach, back, and head	10 mg/kg PO q8h for 5 d then 10 mg/kg PO q12h for 2 wk
trientine	Syprine	Wilson's disease	Anemia, heartburn, epigastric pain and tenderness, thickening and flaking of skin	0.5–2 g/d PO in divided doses

*The term, *generic*, indicates that the drug is available in generic form.

iron intoxication are urticaria, generalized erythema, and hypotension.

Dimercaprol. One of the most common adverse reactions is a rise in blood pressure accompanied by a rise in pulse rate. Nausea, vomiting, and headache may occur when doses higher than recommended are given.

Edetate Calcium Disodium. The principal toxic effect of this drug is renal tubular necrosis.

Penicillamine. This drug has a high incidence of adverse reactions, some of which are potentially fatal, such as bone marrow depression and the nephrotic syndrome. Other adverse reactions include pruritus, skin rash, anorexia, nausea, vomiting, tinnitus, and epigastric pain.

Trientine. Heartburn, epigastric pain and tenderness, thickening and flaking of the skin, and anemia may be seen with the use of this drug.

Succimer. Adverse reactions seen with the administration of succimer may include nausea, vomiting, diarrhea, anorexia, rash, sore throat, and back, stomach, and head pain.

NURSING MANAGEMENT

- Depending on the patient's condition, monitor the vital signs every 1 to 4 hours.
- Measure and record intake and output. For the acutely ill patient, it may be necessary to measure the urinary output hourly. As iron is chelated, it is

excreted through the kidneys, and the urine becomes a reddish color. Alkalinization of the urine is recommended when dimercaprol or penicillamine are given. The physician may order monitoring of the urinary pH and administration of a urinary alkalizer, such as sodium bicarbonate or potassium and sodium citrate. Patients with cystinuria who are receiving penicillamine are encouraged to drink copious amounts of fluid, because an excess fluid intake lowers the required drug dosage.

Nursing Alert

Patients receiving a heavy metal antagonist are observed closely for adverse reactions, especially those that may be seen with the administration of penicillamine. Report all adverse reactions to the physician immediately.

- Therapy may be evaluated by means of laboratory tests, as well as daily assessments of the patient's general condition and a comparison of these symptoms with those recorded during the initial physical assessment. Noticeable improvement may be slow in some cases.
- When a heavy metal antagonist is administered IM, inspect the previous injection sites for signs of induration and inflammation. If these occur, notify the physician of the problem.
- If dimercaprol is given, a rise in blood pressure and pulse are common responses to therapy. Notify the physician if these vital signs show a significant rise at any time during therapy.
- Some patients may exhibit a marked rise in temperature during therapy with penicillamine. Notify the physician if this occurs because a temporary interruption in therapy may be necessary.
- When edetate calcium disodium is used to treat lead poisoning, the drug may be given IM or IV. When given IM, the drug is given for 3 to 5 days, followed by a rest period of 4 days after which time a second course is given. When given IV, the drug is diluted in 250 to 500 mL of normal saline or 5% dextrose and given twice daily for up to 5 days, followed by a rest period of 2 days after which time another 5 days of treatment is given.
- Dimercaprol is only given IM for 10 days.
- A course of therapy with succimer, an oral drug, lasts 19 days.
- The length of treatment with a heavy metal antagonist may vary somewhat from manufacturer's recommendations and be based on the severity of the heavy metal poisoning and the response of the patient to therapy.

Nursing Process
The Patient Receiving a Heavy Metal Antagonist

■ *Assessment*

When the patient is diagnosed as having excessive levels of a heavy metal (regardless of the cause), obtain a complete history with a background of the circumstances surrounding the heavy metal poisoning. In many instances, the nurse must question the patient extensively regarding exposure to a heavy metal.

Before starting therapy, take the vital signs, weigh the patient, and document the signs and symptoms of the poisoning.

■ *Nursing Diagnoses*

Depending on the patient's general physical condition and the reason for use, one or more of the following nursing diagnoses may apply to the patient receiving a heavy metal antagonist:

- **Anxiety** related to diagnosis, severity of symptoms, necessary preventive measures, other factors
- **Risk for Ineffective Management of Therapeutic Regimen** related to lack of knowledge of therapeutic regimen, methods of prevention, indifference, lack of knowledge of seriousness of heavy metal poisoning

■ *Planning and Implementation*

The major goals of the patient may include a reduction in anxiety, knowledge of preventive measures, and an understanding of and compliance to the prescribed therapeutic regimen. To make these goals measurable, more specific criteria must be added.

Anxiety. There can be temporary or permanent serious consequences attached to heavy metal poisoning. The patient or the family may be concerned over the heavy metal poisoning that has occurred; the success or possible failure of therapy; and the possible effects the poisoning may have. Allow the patient or family time to ask questions about the problems that have occurred because of the heavy metal poisoning, as well as to discuss possible ways to prevent this problem in the future.

Children suffering from chronic lead poisoning may develop mental retardation and other problems. Methods of preventing lead poisoning in children exposed to lead-based paint may require expensive household renovations. Repainting the furniture or walls may not be sufficient because the lead from the lead-based paint that is painted over may still leach through. Some families may be unable to afford the extensive work that may be required because all lead-based paint must first be removed from the surface before lead-free paint is applied. Spend time with these families and attempt to find measures that may help them remove the offending paint from walls and furniture. In some instances, a referral to a social agency for financial assistance may be necessary.

■ Patient and Family Teaching

Penicillamine, trientine and succimer, which are given orally, may be prescribed for outpatient use. Depending on the patient and the drug to be given, hospitalization may be required.

To ensure compliance, emphasize the importance of treatment with a heavy metal antagonist, elimination of those elements that caused the poisoning, and continued and uninterrupted treatment and follow-up care. Strongly encourage the patient or family to keep all physician or clinic appointments for immediate treatment and for long-term follow-up care (when applicable).

When the cause of poisoning is known, work with the patient or family to eliminate those factors (whenever possible) that caused the heavy metal poisoning.

Penicillamine and Trientine

- Take this drug on an empty stomach 1 hour before or 2 hours after a meal. If iron therapy is prescribed, 2 hours must elapse between taking the penicillamine and iron preparation.
- Swallow the capsule form whole; do not chew.
- Notify the physician immediately if fever, skin rash, or other unusual symptoms occur.
- Do not take any nonprescription drug unless use of a specific drug has been approved by the physician.
- Notify the physician if any of the following occurs: skin rash or other types of skin lesions, unusual bruising, sore throat, fever, sores in the mouth, persistent anorexia, nausea, vomiting, diarrhea, unusual fatigue, blood in the urine, or any other unusual symptoms that were not present before therapy was started.
- Patients with cystinuria receiving penicillamine—Drink 4000 mL or more of water or other fluids per day; this is about 16 to 17 large glasses of fluid.
- Follow the diet outlined by the physician; this is an important part of therapy.

Succimer

- If rash occurs, contact the physician.
- Drink extra fluids.

- Child: if the capsule is difficult to swallow, it may be opened and the contents (medicated beads) added to a small amount of soft food such as apple sauce. All the food must be eaten.

■ Expected Outcomes for Evaluation

- Anxiety is reduced
- Patient or family verbalizes an understanding of treatment modalities and importance of continued follow-up care
- Patient or family member demonstrates understanding of drug regimen
- Patient verbalizes importance of complying with the prescribed therapeutic regimen, recommended preventive measures
- Patient discusses preventive measures and actively seeks assistance with preventive measures

Chapter Summary

- Certain situations may expose persons to a *heavy metal* (a metal with a relatively high density). Air pollutants, especially those containing heavy metals, such as lead and arsenic, pose a hazard to living organisms, including humans. Other sources of heavy metal poisoning include exposure to gasoline fumes and certain pesticides and weed killers, and the eating of seafood such as fish, clams, oysters, and shrimp caught in waters polluted with heavy metals. Poisoning by or excessive blood levels of the heavy metals lead, iron, gold, arsenic, mercury, and copper can be treated with drugs called heavy metal antagonists.
- Some heavy metal poisonings are treated with a *chelating agent*, which selectively and chemically binds the ion of a metal to itself, thus aiding in the elimination of the metallic ion from the body. Deferoxamine, dimercaprol, penicillamine, trientine, and succimer are chelating agents.
- Administration of a heavy metal antagonist may cause a variety of adverse effects, some of which are serious. Deferoxamine may cause pain and induration at the injection site. One of the most common adverse reactions seen with dimercaprol is a rise in blood pressure, accompanied by a rise in pulse rate. The principal toxic effect of edetate calcium disodium is renal tubular necrosis. Penicillamine has a high incidence of adverse reactions, some of which are potentially fatal, such as bone marrow depression and the nephrotic syndrome. Trientine administration may result in heartburn, epigastric pain and tenderness, thickening

and flaking of the skin, and anemia. Adverse reactions seen with the administration of succimer may include nausea, vomiting, diarrhea, anorexia, rash, sore throat, and back, stomach, and head pain.
• Patients receiving a heavy metal antagonist are closely monitored for adverse reactions, as well as their response to the drug.

Critical Thinking Exercise

1. A friend of yours, who has a small baby, has moved into an older home which she plans to remodel. What danger to her child might be present in this house? What precautions or advice would you give your friend?

51

Substance Abuse

Key Terms

Abstinence syndrome

Anorexiants

Compulsive substance abuse

Delirium tremens

Drug addiction

Drug habituation

Drug tolerance

Drug withdrawal

Flashbacks

Hallucinogen

Physical dependency

Psychological dependency

Substance abuse

Chapter Outline

Chapter Objectives

On completion of this chapter the student will:

- *Differentiate between physical and psychological drug dependency*
- *Define drug addiction and drug habituation*
- *Discuss the dangers associated with substance abuse*
- *Describe the methods of treating drug addiction*

ubstance or drug abuse may be defined as the use of a natural or synthetic substance to alter mood or behavior in a manner that differs from its generally accepted use. Substance (drug) abuse is a leading problem in today's social environment. The social and economic impact of drug addiction and abuse directly or indirectly affects every member of society. The terms *drug* and *substance* are both used in the literature.

DEFINITION OF TERMS

- *Substance abuse* is the use of a drug or chemical to produce a change in mood or behavior in a way that departs from approved medical or social patterns.
- *Compulsive substance abuse* is the need to use any drug or chemical substance repeatedly to produce a desired effect. The need to use a drug compulsively may be psychological, physical, or both.
- *Physical dependency* is a compulsive need to use a substance repeatedly to avoid mild to severe withdrawal symptoms; it is the body's dependence on repeated administration of a drug.
- *Psychological dependency* is a compulsion to use a substance to obtain a pleasurable experience; it is the mind's dependence on the repeated administration of a drug.
- *Drug tolerance* is a need to increase the dose or the frequency of use to obtain the original or desired effect.

Physical or psychological drug dependency results in a physical or mental need to use the drug repeatedly. Symptoms of *drug withdrawal* (also called the *abstinence syndrome*) occur if use of the drug is suddenly discontinued. The symptoms of drug withdrawal may range from mild to severe. The severity of the abstinence syndrome depends on factors such as the individual, the drug and dose used, the frequency of use, and the length of time the drug has been used.

Drug addiction may be defined to include the following:

- A compulsive desire or craving to use a drug or chemical
- An involvement with the drug to the exclusion of all other activities
- A strong tendency to return to the drug after going through withdrawal
- A tendency to increase the dose or frequency of use
- Physical dependence on the drug

- Moderate to severe physical reactions when the abstinence syndrome occurs
- Detriments to society can exist in the drug and its use, as well as in the user

Drug habituation may be defined to include the following:

- A desire to continually use a drug or chemical for the effects produced
- Usually little or no tendency to increase the dose
- Psychological dependence but no physical dependence
- When the drug is withdrawn, there is no true abstinence syndrome
- The detrimental effect, if any exists, is on the individual rather than society

NARCOTICS

Heroin

Heroin (diacetylmorphine) is obtained from morphine (see Chap. 16). Heroin is the principal alkaloid of raw opium and is an illegal drug in the United States. It is the strongest and most addicting of all the opium derivatives. Physical addiction to heroin usually occurs rapidly, often within several weeks of frequent use, but this varies.

Addiction to heroin creates serious socioeconomic problems; individuals, families, and the community are affected by heroin abuse. The cost of a drug habit is high. Finances may be quickly depleted and the user finds it necessary to obtain money by other means, such as stealing or prostitution.

Malnutrition and physical neglect are two of the many problems associated with the continued use of heroin. Intravenous (IV) self-administration of the drug, which is the most common method of using heroin, may result in serious and sometimes fatal problems. Septicemia (pathogenic bacteria in the blood) can occur if the needle, syringe, or equipment used to prepare heroin for injection are contaminated. Two very serious infections, hepatitis B and the acquired immunodeficiency syndrome (AIDS), can be transmitted from one individual to another when needles and syringes are shared among users.

Heroin may be used by inhaling the powder (sniffing) but most users prefer injecting heroin. The heroin, which is a powder, is dissolved in water by using heat. Spoons are often used to hold the liquid over a flame. The liquid is then drawn up into a syringe and injected subcutaneously ("skin popping") or IV ("mainlining").

Following injection of heroin, the user experiences euphoria and drowsiness. Mentally, there is an escape from reality. Other effects of heroin use are the same as those seen with the opiates, namely, anorexia, fixed pinpoint pupils, constipation, and a decreased pulse and respiratory rate. Continued IV use results in scarred veins called tracks.

Signs of early withdrawal from heroin (abstinence syndrome) usually include yawning, perspiration, tearing of the eyes, and increased nasal discharge. These signs and symptoms are often followed by gooseflesh, abdominal cramps, bone and muscle pain, nausea, vomiting, diarrhea, dilatation of the pupils, restlessness, increase in body temperature, increase in pulse and respiratory rate, marked mental depression or despair, and an intense craving for the drug. The symptoms of withdrawal usually begin when the next dose of heroin would have been taken by the user, reach a peak in 36 to 72 hours, and gradually diminish in 4 or 5 days.

Unfortunately, persons may accidentally or intentionally take or be given an overdose of the drug. Symptoms of overdose include stupor to coma, pinpoint pupils, nausea, vomiting, decreased pulse and respiratory rate, and signs of shock. If overdose is recognized and treated as soon as possible, the narcotic antagonist naloxone (Narcan) may be given to reverse the respiratory depressant effects of heroin. In addition to administration of a narcotic antagonist, other medical treatment, such as correcting fluid or electrolyte imbalances, oxygen, and creating and maintaining a patent airway are instituted. Unfortunately, many cases of overdose are never treated and the individual dies.

Heroin crosses the placental barrier. A child born of a mother addicted to heroin is also addicted to the drug and needs immediate treatment. Even after receiving treatment, some infants die.

Other Narcotic Analgesics

Opiates, such as morphine and hydromorphone (Dilaudid), and other narcotics, such as meperidine (Demerol), are legal drugs used medically in the treatment of pain. These legal narcotics are usually not as accessible to the addict buying heroin on the streets from a pusher but may be used (when they can be obtained) as substitutes when heroin is not available.

Individuals addicted to opiates and other narcotics experience an abstinence syndrome similar to that experienced by the heroin user. They are also prone to the same dangers, such as hepatitis, septicemia, and AIDS if materials for preparation and administration are shared with others.

Addiction to legal narcotics may occur in those receiving the drug while under the care of a physician, as in the case of a terminally ill cancer patient. However, addiction has occurred because of a physician's carelessness in prescribing the drug in the treatment of a nonterminal illness.

The Terminally Ill

Terminally ill cancer patients who require a narcotic eventually become addicted to the drug after it has been given for several weeks. *Addiction in these patients is morally and legally acceptable.* Terminally ill patients in need of pain relief should never be denied a prescribed analgesic because of the potential for addiction. If addiction has occurred, these patients should be given the drug as ordered and on time. Making the patient wait for the drug may result in withdrawal symptoms, which will only add to the pain of his or her illness.

COCAINE

Cocaine, an alkaloid obtained from coca leaves, is highly addicting and, presently, is the number one substance abuse problem. Cocaine use has created serious and sometimes deadly consequences that affect the individuals, families, and the community. It is used in medicine on rare occasions as a local anesthetic but this use has been largely discontinued.

Cocaine stimulates the central nervous system (CNS), producing marked euphoria and excitement. The powder form of cocaine can be snorted (inhaled through the nose). It also may be dissolved in water and injected IV. Crack, a purified form of cocaine with a crystalline or rocklike appearance, is smoked either by placing it in a pipe or by sprinkling it on or mixing it with tobacco. Cocaine may be freebased, a process which reduces it to its purest form. It is then smoked by sprinkling it on a cigarette or inhaling it through a pipe. Freebasing produces a more immediate rush than when the substance is used by nasal inhalation. Those addicted to heroin usually do not use cocaine as a heroin substitute but may mix cocaine with heroin and inject it IV to obtain a greater drug effect. This combination is called a "speed-ball."

Cocaine use most often results in physical and psychological dependency. The cost of a cocaine habit can reach astounding figures with the person spending as much as several thousand dollars a month to support a drug habit.

Signs and symptoms of acute toxicity include agitation, psychotic behavior, violent or aggressive behavior, hyperthermia, seizures, cardiac arrhythmias, hypertension, respiratory failure, and dilated pupils. Acute toxicity can occur at any time and with any dose. Death has been known to occur with acute cocaine toxicity.

Signs and symptoms of chronic toxicity include cardiac arrhythmias; hypertension; memory impairment; personality and behavioral changes; ulceration of the nasal mucosa and perforation of the nasal septum (in those who inhale cocaine); needle marks along the pathways of veins (in those who use cocaine IV); anorexia; weight loss; psychosis and hallucinations.

Use of cocaine results in physical and psychological dependence. In some, dependence occurs rapidly, especially when crack cocaine is used. Some users have reported intense craving for the drug after one or two uses. How soon physical dependence occurs appears to vary with the individual, the purity of the cocaine, and pattern of use. Withdrawal from cocaine usually is characterized by depression, psychosis, lethargy, restlessness, an intense craving for the drug, inability to concentrate, and irritability.

MARIJUANA

Marijuana is classified as a *hallucinogen*. A hallucinogen is a drug capable of producing a state of delirium characterized by visual and sensory disturbances that are bizarre and distorted. Marijuana belongs to a family of plants called *Cannabis*. The substance that produces the hallucinogenic effect is a resin, tetrahydrocannabinol (THC) from the dried plant. The resin extracted from the plant's flowers is called *hashish,* which is 5 to 10 times more potent than the resin from the dried leaves.

Marijuana use may produce various effects, which appear to depend on the individual, as well as the amount of tetrahydrocannabinol in the marijuana. The user may experience euphoria, drowsiness, dizziness, lightheadedness, visual disturbances, sensory distortions, hunger (especially for sweets), giddiness, and hallucinations. On occasion, other effects such as panic, depression, nausea, vomiting, diarrhea, dryness of the mouth, inflammation and burning of the eyes, decrease in blood pressure, increase in pulse rate, and dilatation of the pupils may be seen. On occasion, an individual may not experience any effect from using marijuana but this may be because the product they used contained fillers and

little marijuana. The effects of the drug usually last 2 to 4 hours but this is highly variable.

Signs of chronic marijuana use include a lack of interest in school, work, and other people; carelessness in personal hygiene and clothes; a preoccupied appearance; lack of motivation; memory difficulty; and passiveness or apathy.

Marijuana is used medically on a limited basis to lower intraocular pressure in those with glaucoma and in selected terminally ill cancer patients. Specific guidelines in dispensing the drug are required and legal use of the drug is limited to research institutions or physicians who have applied for government approval of marijuana use in certain patients.

PSYCHOTOMIMETIC DRUGS

A psychotomimetic (hallucinogenic) drug produces an acute change in the perception of reality. Examples of drugs in this group are mescaline, lysergic acid diethylamide (LSD), 2,5-dimethoxy-4-methylamphetamine (also called STP), psilocybin, phencyclidine (PCP, angel dust) and dimethyltryptamine (DMT).

Use of these agents causes visual hallucinations and mood changes, which vary from person to person and even within the same person. These variances in drug effects may be attributed to the drug itself, the purity of the drug, and the circumstances under which the drug was used. Psychotic episodes, which appear to be more prevalent in those with underlying emotional problems, may occur during, as well as after, use. Another problem associated with use of a hallucinogen is the occurrence of *flashbacks* (brief episodes of the original sensations experienced during use of the substance). The frequency of flashbacks, which is more common with LSD use, is variable and may occur for many years after use of the hallucinogen has been discontinued. Some persons never experience flashbacks despite repeated use of a hallucinogen.

Although physical dependence on these drugs does not appear to occur, the user can develop a psychological dependence. No physical withdrawal symptoms occur if use of the substance is discontinued.

AMPHETAMINES

Amphetamine, dextroamphetamine, and methamphetamine are adrenergic drugs medically used as CNS stimulants and *anorexiants* (drugs that suppress the appetite). The use of these drugs in the treatment of obesity has declined because of their abuse potential but they still are of value in the treatment of narcolepsy (an uncontrollable desire to sleep during daytime hours) and attention deficit disorders with hyperactivity in children.

Amphetamines produce euphoria, alertness, and a sense of excitation or exhilaration. The user is talkative, restless, excitable, and perspires freely. The pupils also may be dilated. These drugs have addiction potential. The reasons for using amphetamines vary. Some may use the drug to stay awake for long periods of time, whereas others wish to experience the euphoria produced by the drug.

Amphetamines usually are taken orally. The drug is sometimes dissolved in water and injected by IV to produce an instant euphoric effect or "rush" that is greater in intensity than that produced by the oral route.

There are various ways that amphetamines are used. Some people will take the drug every few hours for several days. During this time, the user is in a constant state of euphoria, excitement, and sleeplessness. The drug is ultimately discontinued because of exhaustion, confusion, or disorientation, or the user may take a tranquilizer or barbiturate to come down off the high produced by repeated amphetamine use.

Those using amphetamines may be belligerent; repeated use may cause a severe psychosis. Depression and suicidal tendencies may occur when the drug is withdrawn.

METHCATHINONE

Methcathinone, also called "cat," is a chemical that has never been used in medicine. Although produced by a drug company many years ago, it was never marketed. The use of cat began about 1990, at which time it was made by a small number of people, one of whom had found the recipe for the drug while working for a drug company. Methcathinone produces effects similar to the amphetamines but it appears that the effects of this drug may be more intense than those produced by the amphetamines. It appears that the drug is physically addicting, however, more research and studies will be necessary to confirm facts, such as tolerance to the drug, addiction potential, type of addiction (physical, psychological, or both) and the type of symptoms experienced when the drug is withdrawn (abstinence syndrome).

Little is known about the drug and what long-term effects may occur with use. The drug is appar-

ently snorted, much like cocaine. It is easy and cheap for an individual to produce this drug with very minimal equipment. The raw materials can be obtained from hardware stores and chemical supply houses.

BARBITURATES AND NONBARBITURATES

Barbiturate and nonbarbiturate drugs have their proper use in medicine but are also subject to abuse. Drug tolerance can develop in the chronic barbiturate user and, in some instances, tolerance may develop within a week or two. These drugs have physical and psychological addiction potential when used for a period of time. The length of time required for physical and psychological dependence varies. While some of the nonbarbiturates have a low addiction potential, taking large doses for a long time can result in physical and psychological addiction.

Nursing Alert

When these drugs are subject to abuse or are used under a physician's supervision for a long time, they must *never* be suddenly discontinued. Instead, the dose must be slowly tapered over time.

When a barbiturate is suddenly discontinued, there is an abstinence syndrome characterized by abdominal cramps, nausea, vomiting, weakness, and tremors. *In some persons, withdrawal from barbiturates can be more harmful physically than withdrawal from heroin.*

An overdose of these drugs can result in convulsions, delirium, coma, and in some instances, death.

TRANQUILIZERS

Tranquilizers have been subject to widespread abuse by those involved in substance abuse, as well as by persons who do not consider themselves "drug users." When first used medically, tranquilizers were not believed to be physically addicting and were frequently prescribed by physicians for mild cases of anxiety and stress. Although tranquilizers still play an important role in the treatment of various types of psychiatric disorders, they were and occasionally still are overprescribed by some physicians. Unfortunately, the overuse of tranquilizers has resulted in many individuals being physically addicted to these drugs.

Addiction to tranquilizers appears to occur fairly rapidly, although the time required to produce addiction often depends on factors, such as the type of tranquilizer, the individual, and the tendency of the user to increase the dose to produce the desired effect.

Withdrawal, when it does occur, resembles barbiturate withdrawal, with the intensity of symptoms depending on the length of time the drug was used and the dose most frequently used. Withdrawal symptoms include extreme anxiety and nervousness and a strong desire to return to the drug.

> **Nursing Alert**
>
> Tranquilizer withdrawal symptoms can be severe. When an individual has been taking tranquilizers for a period of time they must *never* be suddenly discontinued. Instead, the dose must be slowly tapered.

ALCOHOL

Alcohol abuse and alcoholism is a major problem. Alcohol is subject to widespread abuse among all ages and socioeconomic levels. There are many and diverse problems associated with alcohol abuse, some of which are malnutrition, physical disease, broken marriages, loss of employment, and accidents resulting in injury or death. The chronic and even occasional alcohol user may also abuse other drugs, such as tranquilizers, amphetamines, barbiturates, and cocaine. Drinking alcohol and taking one or more of these drugs may have serious consequences because alcohol can increase the action of these and other drugs. For example, the use of alcohol *and* a CNS depressant such as a narcotic, tranquilizer, barbiturate, or nonbarbiturate can produce effects greater than that produced by the CNS depressant when used alone. Deaths have been reported with the use of alcohol along with a CNS depressant.

Every year many people are killed by drivers who are under the influence of alcohol, as well as other drugs. Television commercials, newspaper and magazine articles, and raising the drinking age in some states are being used to discourage alcohol abuse. Groups have formed to encourage stricter laws for those convicted of driving while impaired, and many businesses have programs available to help employees with a drinking problem.

Alcohol is a potentially physically addicting substance. The time or amount of alcohol consumption required to produce physical addiction is variable. Some will become physically addicted to alcohol in a relatively short time whereas others may drink for years before addiction occurs.

Signs of withdrawal from alcohol usually appear within 12 to 72 hours after the last drink.

> **Nursing Alert**
>
> Closely observe patients with a suspected or known alcohol problem for signs and symptoms of alcohol withdrawal from the time of admission and up to approximately 5 days. If alcohol withdrawal is suspected, contact the physician immediately.

Signs and symptoms of withdrawal, usually referred to as the DTs (*delirium tremens*), may range from mild to intense. These usually include tremors, weakness, anxiety, restlessness, excessive perspiration, nausea, and vomiting. The patient may be incoherent and pick at the bedclothes or nearby objects. Hallucinations, which are frequently terrifying, are often experienced. Seizures have occurred in some individuals during the first 24 hours of withdrawal. Recovery from withdrawal usually occurs within 5 to 7 days. During the period of alcohol withdrawal ("drying out"), the patient should be under medical supervision.

VOLATILE HYDROCARBONS

Benzene, acetone, carbon tetrachloride, gasoline, trichloroethylene, and toluene are examples of volatile hydrocarbons. Many of these chemicals are found in ordinary household products, such as cleaning solutions, nail polish removers, disposable lighters, and various types of glue. Some spray can products, such as hair spray, paint, and lacquers, use a volatile hydrocarbon as a propellant. Because they are relatively inexpensive and legal, the inhaling of a volatile hydrocarbon has become popular among the young, as well as those unable to afford other illegal substances. "Huffing" is a street term used to describe inhalation of a volatile hydrocarbon to produce lightheadedness, exhilaration, excitation, euphoria, and hallucinations.

To obtain the desired effect, the substance usually is sprayed into a handkerchief, plastic bag, or piece of clothing and then inhaled. It also may be directly inhaled from the container. The effects usually last 30 minutes or less.

Overdose can produce cardiac arrhythmias, hypotension, violent behavior, delirium, depression, and respiratory failure. Prolonged use results in damage to the heart, lungs, brain, kidneys, liver, and bone marrow. In some instances, the damage is so severe that death occurs.

Treatment may require respiratory support with mechanical ventilation and drug therapy for cardiac arrhythmias and hypotension. Rehabilitation must focus on the seriousness and consequences of this behavior. If permanent damage to one or more organs has occurred, treatment is aimed at preserving any remaining function.

METHODS OF TREATING SUBSTANCE ABUSE

There are different methods of treating substance abuse. There appears to be no one best way to treat the substance abuser. Some physicians and drug rehabilitation centers advocate a certain method of treatment and claim good results, whereas others, using a different method, claim equally good results. Emotional as well as physical support is necessary for the substance abuser *and* the immediate family since there often are many problems associated with substance abuse. Counseling and other types of support for the abuser, as well as immediate family members, are usually provided during and after the treatment period.

When one method of treatment fails, an effort must be made to determine if another method of treatment would produce better results. Thus, it may be necessary for some individuals to try more than one treatment method. Success in treating drug abuse usually depends on a person's desire to become and remain drug-free. When forced to enter a drug treatment program, a person is less likely to achieve and maintain a drug-free state.

Addiction to a narcotic can be treated in facilities, some of which are outpatient clinics, whereas others require the patient to be admitted for treatment. Most treatment facilities first attempt to reduce or eliminate withdrawal symptoms. Once the drug is eliminated from the body, treatment is aimed at helping the patient attain and maintain a drug-free state.

One method of treating narcotic addiction is by administration of methadone (Dolophine), a synthetic narcotic. Methadone administration prevents withdrawal symptoms and satisfies the craving for the narcotic. Although addiction to methadone does occur, the patient can be gradually withdrawn from methadone and ultimately become drug-free. Withdrawal from methadone appears to be less severe than withdrawal from heroin and other narcotics.

Another method of treating narcotic addiction is the administration of naltrexone (Trexan), which is a narcotic antagonist (see Chap. 16). The drug is used to maintain an opioid-free state in those who have been addicted to an opioid narcotic and are in a detoxified state. Treatment is not begun until the individual has been without a narcotic (opioid-free state) for 7 to 10 days. Individuals taking naltrexone on a regular basis will not obtain any effect from an opioid narcotic should there be an attempt to return to these drugs.

Addiction to other drugs such as cocaine, tranquilizers, or barbiturates may be treated by a physician, in individual clinics, or in public or private drug rehabilitation centers. Withdrawal from these drugs is necessary. Counseling and support therapy is an important part of treatment.

Chronic alcoholism, with or without a history of other substance abuse, may be treated by a physician or in public or private treatment centers. Alcoholics Anonymous is a support group that has done much to help the alcoholic attain and maintain an alcohol-free state. Recently, a small number of selected patients with a history of alcohol abuse have been treated with naltrexone (ReVia). Naltrexone, when used in those with a history of alcohol abuse, appears to eliminate the "high" associated with drinking and stops the craving for alcohol but does not eliminate the effects of alcohol, such as slowed reflexes, staggering gait, and slurred speech. At present, the recommended dose is one 50 mg tablet per day for 3 to 6 months.

Another drug used in the treatment of chronic alcoholism is disulfiram (Antabuse). When this drug is taken on a daily basis, ingestion of even small amounts of alcohol results in severe headache, respiratory difficulty, nausea, copious vomiting, sweating, thirst, chest pain, palpitations, dyspnea, hyperventilation, tachycardia, hypotension, syncope, blurred vision, and confusion.

The success of disulfiram and naltrexone in the treatment of chronic alcoholism usually depends on the individual's desire to remain in an alcohol-free state.

CONCLUSION

As members of the healthcare profession, nurses must be aware of the signs of substance abuse and overdose. It is not unusual to see a substance abuser being involved with more than one drug. Any patient entering a general hospital, clinic, retirement home, or nursing home may have a hidden history of substance abuse, including alcohol. This includes patients on a pediatric, as well as an adult, hospital unit. Closely observe any patient showing unusual behavior, asking for narcotics, or showing physical signs that do not appear related to the diagnosis or disease. Document all observations carefully in the patient's record and report them to the physician and supervisory personnel.

Members of the medical profession administer, prescribe, and dispense narcotics. A few may be tempted to experience the effects of a narcotic and subsequently may continue to use the drug. In some instances, addiction is kept well-hidden and may never be detected. At other times, a change in work performance or personality may give rise to suspicion among fellow workers. Nurses have taken narcotics meant for a patient, and the only clue to misappropriated narcotics is a patient's complaint about failure of the drug to relieve pain. Any suspicion of addiction is brought to the attention of the head nurse or supervisor.

Regardless of the drug used, substance abuse is dangerous. In addition to the danger of physical dependency with many of these agents, the social, legal, and economic implications may be devastating. Substance abuse can lead to various physical and mental disorders, such as malnutrition, weight loss, mental changes, and psychotic episodes. Instravenous drug users may develop hepatitis, septicemia, or acquired immunodeficiency syndrome, all of which can be fatal.

duce a desired effect. The need to use a drug compulsively may be psychological, physical, or both.

- Physical dependency is a compulsive need to use a substance repeatedly to avoid mild to severe withdrawal symptoms; it is the body's dependence on repeated administration of a drug.
- Psychological dependency is a compulsion to use a substance to obtain a pleasurable experience; it is the mind's dependence on the repeated administration of a drug.
- Drug tolerance is a need to increase the dose or the frequency of use to obtain the original or desired effect.
- Drug addiction may include the following: a compulsive desire or craving to use a drug or chemical; an involvement with the drug to the exclusion of all other activities; a strong tendency to return to the drug after going through withdrawal; and a tendency to increase the dose or frequency of use.
- Regarding physical dependence on the drug, when the abstinence syndrome occurs, there are moderate to severe physical reactions. Detriments to society can exist in the drug and its use, as well as in the user.
- Drug habituation may include the following: a desire to continually use a drug or chemical for the effects produced; usually little or no tendency to increase the dose; psychological dependence but no physical dependence; when the drug is withdrawn, there is no true abstinence syndrome; and the detrimental effect, if any exists, is on the individual rather than society.

Chapter Summary

- Substance (drug) abuse is a leading problem in today's social environment. The social and economic impact of drug addiction and abuse directly or indirectly affects every member of society.
- Substance abuse is the use of a drug or chemical to produce a change in mood or behavior in a way that departs from approved medical or social patterns.
- Compulsive substance abuse is the need to use any drug or chemical substance repeatedly to pro-

Critical Thinking Exercises

1. Ms. Ellis, aged 69, is admitted for surgical repair of a fractured hip. When taking her history, you suspect that she may have a drinking problem. What would you include in a nursing care plan for this patient? What specific assessments would you include in the plan?
2. There are some who feel that trying a drug or chemical substance "just once" is not harmful. What arguments can you give for not experimenting with or trying one or more substances that are subject to abuse?

Abbreviations

AC	before meals		**IM**	intramuscular
ADL	activities of daily living		**IOP**	intraocular pressure
AIDS	acquired immunodeficiency syndrome		**IU**	international units
ARC	AIDS-related complex		**IV**	intravenous
bid	twice a day		**KVO**	keep vein open
BPH	benign prostatic hypertrophy		**LOC**	level of consciousness
BUN	blood urea nitrogen		**mcg**	microgram
CBC	complete blood count		**MI**	myocardial infarction (heart attack)
CHF	congestive heart failure		**mL**	milliliter
CNS	central nervous system		**otc**	over-the-counter (non-prescription)
CTZ	chemoreceptor trigger zone		**PC**	after meals
d	daily		**PO**	by mouth
/d	per day		**qh**	every hour (q2h, q3h, q4h, q6h, etc—every 2, 3, 4, 6 hours and so on)
ECG	electrocardiograph			
g	gram		**qid**	4 times a day
GERD	gastroesophageal reflux disease		**REM**	rapid eye movements
GI	gastrointestinal		**SC**	subcutaneous
GU	genitourinary		**tid**	three times a day
hs	hour of sleep		**UTI**	urinary tract infection, pl. **UTIs**

Glossary

adrenergic drugs: drugs that act like or mimic the action of the sympathetic nervous system

afferent nerve fiber: a sensory nerve that carries an impulse toward the brain

agranulocytosis: a decrease or lack of granulocytes (a type of white blood cell)

alopecia: abnormal loss of hair; baldness

anabolism: tissue building process

analeptic: a drug that stimulates the respiratory rate and depth

analgesia: relief of pain

analgesic: a drug that relieves pain

anaphylactic reaction: a sudden, severe hypersensitivity reaction with symptoms that progress rapidly and may result in death if not treated

anemia: a decrease in the number of red blood cells and a below normal hemoglobin

androgens: testosterone and its derivatives

angioedema: localized wheals or swellings in subcutaneous tissues or mucous membranes which may be due to an allergic response. Also called angioneurotic edema

angioneurotic edema: see angioedema

anorexia: loss of appetite

anorexiant: a drug used to suppress the appetite

anthelmintic: a drug used to treat helminthiasis

antibacterial: active against bacteria

antiemetic: a drug used to treat or prevent nausea or vomiting

antiinfective: a drug used to treat infections

antipyretic: a drug that lowers an elevated body temperature

antiseptic: an agent that stops, slows, or prevents the growth of microorganisms

aplastic anemia: a blood disorder caused by damage to the bone marrow resulting in a marked reduction in the number of red blood cells and some white blood cells

arrhythmia: abnormal heart rate or rhythm; also called dysrhythmia

assessment: the collection of subjective and objective data

ataxia: unsteady gait; motor incoordination

atherosclerosis: a disease characterized by deposits of fatty plaques on the inner walls of arteries

atrial fibrillation: quivering of the atria

attenuate: weaken

aura: a sensation preceding a paroxysmal attack, as in the aura that occurs before a convulsion

auscultation: the process of listening for sounds within the body

bactericidal: a drug or agent that destroys (kills) bacteria

bacteriostatic: a drug or agent that slows or retards the multiplication of bacteria

bigeminy: an irregular pulse rate consiting of two beats followed by a pause before the next two paired beats

biliary colic: pain caused by the pressure of passing of gallstones

blepharospasm: a twitching or spasm of the eyelid

bradycardia: slow heart rate (below 60 beats per minute)

bronchospasm: spasm or constriction of the bronchi resulting in difficulty breathing

bursa: padlike sac found in connecting tissue usually located in the joint area

candidiasis: infection of the skin or mucous membrane with the species candida

cardiac output: amount of blood discharged from the left or right ventricle per minute

catabolism: tissue depleting process

catalyst: a substance that accelerates a chemical reaction without itself undergoing a change

cheilosis: cracking at the edges of the lips

chemotherapy: treatment with a drug, often used when referring to treatment with an antineoplastic drug

cinchonism: quinidine toxicity or poisoning

conjunctivitis: inflammation of the conjunctiva (mucous membrane lining the inner surfaces of the eye)

convulsion: paroxysm of involuntary muscular contractions and relaxations

cross-allergenicity: allergy to drugs in the same or related groups

cross-sensitivity: see cross-allergenicity

crystalluria: formation of crystals in the urine

cyanosis: bluish, grayish, or dark purple discoloration of the skin due to abnormal amounts of reduced hemoglobin in the blood

cycloplegia: paralysis of the ciliary muscle resulting in an inability to focus the eye

decaliter: 10 liters or 10,000 mL

dermis: a layer of skin immediately below the epidermis

diaphoresis: increased sweating or perspiration

diluent: a fluid that dilutes

diplopia: double vision

dyscrasia: disease or disorder

dyspnea: labored or difficult breathing

dystonia: prolonged muscle contractions that may cause twisting and repetitive movements or abnormal posture

dysuria: painful or difficult urination

efferent: carrying away from a central organ or section

endogenous: manufactured by the body

epidermis: outermost layer of the skin

epiphysis: a center of ossification (conversion of tissue to bone) at each extremity of long bones

epistaxis: nosebleed

Escherichia coli: a nonpathogenic colon bacillus; when found outside of the colon may cause infection

estrogens: female hormones

evaluation: a decision-making process determining the effectiveness of nursing action

exacerbation: increase in severity

exogenous: originating outside of the body

extravasation: escape of fluid from a blood vessel into surrounding tissues

febrile: related to fever (elevated body temperature)

germicide: an agent that kills bacteria

gingival hyperplasia: overgrowth of gum tissue

gingivitis: inflammation of gums

glossitis: inflammation of the tongue

glucagon: hormone secreted by the alpha cells of the pancreas that increases the concentration of glucose in the blood

granulocytopenia: a reduction or decrease in the number of granulocytes (a type of white blood cell)

helminthiasis: invasion by helminths (worms)

helminths: worms

hemolytic anemia: disorder characterized by chronic premature destruction of red blood cells

hirsutism: excessive body hair in a masculine distribution pattern

hyperglycemia: high blood glucose

hyperinsulinism: elevated levels of insulin in the body

hyperkalemia: increase in potassium in the blood

hyperlipidemia: an increase in the lipids in the blood

hypersensitivity reaction: allergic reaction to a drug or other substance

hypertension: high blood pressure

hypnotic: a drug that induces sleep

hypoglycemia: low blood glucose (sugar)

hypoinsulinism: low levels of insulin in the body

hypokalemia: low blood potassium

hyponatremia: low blood sodium

hypotension, orthostatic: a decrease in blood pressure occurring after standing in one place for an extended period

hypotension, postural: a decrease in blood pressure following a sudden change in body position

hypoxia: inadequate oxygen at the cellular level

immunocompromised: having an immune system incapable of fighting an infection

implementation: the carrying out of a plan of action

infiltration: the collection of fluid into tissues

intraocular pressure: the pressure within the eye

ketonuria: ketones in the urine

laryngospasm: spasm of the larynx resulting in dyspnea and noisy respirations

lethargic: sluggish, difficult to rouse

leukopenia: a decrease in the number of leukocytes (white blood cells)

lipids: a group of fats or fatlike substances

lipodystrophy: atrophy of subcutaneous fat

lumen: inside diameter, the space or opening within an artery

malaise: discomfort, uneasiness

melena: tarry stools

methemoglobinemia: clinical condition in which more than 1% of hemoglobin in the blood has been oxidized to the ferric form

miosis: constriction of the pupil

mydriasis: dilatation of the pupil

myopia: nearsightedness

narcolepsy: a chronic disorder that results in recurrent attacks of drowsiness and sleep during daytime

necrosis: death of tissue (adj. necrotic)

nephrotoxic: harmful to the kidney

nephrotoxicity: damage to the kidneys by a toxic substance

neuromuscular blockade: acute muscle paralysis and apnea

neurotoxicity: damage to the nervous system by a toxic substance

neutropenia: abnormally small number of neutrophil cells (type of white blood cell)

nonsteroidal: not a steroid

nursing diagnosis: a description of patient problems and their probable or related cause

nursing process: a framework for nursing action, consisting of problem-solving steps, that helps members of the healthcare team provide effective patient care

nystagmus: an involuntary and constant movement of the eyeball

objective data: information obtained by means of a physical assessment or physical examination

oliguria: a decrease in urinary output

ophthalmic: pertaining to the eye

opportunistic infection: infection resulting from microorganisms commonly found in the environment, which normally do not produce an infection unless there is an impaired immune system

orthostatic hypotension: see hypotension, orthostatic

osteomalacia: a softening of the bones

osteoporosis: a loss of calcium from the bones, resulting in a decrease in bone density

otic: pertaining to the ear

ototoxic: harmful to the ear

ototoxicity: damage to the organs of hearing by a toxic substance

overt: not hidden; clearly evident

palliative: therapy designed to treat symptoms, not to produce a cure

pancytopenia: a reduction in all cellular elements of the blood

parasite: an organism living in or on another organism (the host) without contributing to the survival or well-being of the host

parenteral: administration of a substance, such as a drug, by any route other than the oral route

paresthesia: an abnormal sensation such as numbness, tingling, prickling, or heightened sensitivity

pathogenic: disease-causing

petechiae: tiny purple or red spots that appear on the skin as a result of pinpoint hemorrhages within the outer layers of the skin

phlebitis: inflammation of a vein

photophobia: an aversion to or intolerance of light

photosensitivity: sensitivity to light

photosensitivity reaction: exaggerated sunburn reaction when the skin is exposed to sunlight or ultraviolet light

polydipsia: excessive thirst

polyphagia: eating large amounts of food

polyuria: excessive production and voiding or urine

postural hypotension: see hypotension, postural

prepubertal: before puberty

progesterones: female hormones

progestins: natural and synthetic progesterones

prophylaxis: prevention

prostaglandins: a fatty acid substance found in almost all tissues of the body and thought to increase the sensitivity of peripheral pain receptors to painful stimuli

pruritus: itching

pseudomembranous colitis: a severe, life-threatening form of diarrhea

rales: abnormal lung sounds often described as crackles

remission: periods of partial or complete disappearance of signs and symptoms

retinitis: inflammation of the retina of the eye

rhinitis; vasomotor rhinitis: inflammation of the nasal passages resulting in increased nasal secretions

sedative: a drug producing a relaxing, calming effect

somnolence: prolonged drowsiness; sleepiness

spru: a disease characterized by weakness, anemia, weight loss, and malabsorption of essential nutrients

Stevens-Johnson syndrome: fever, cough, muscular aches and pains, headache, and lesions of the skin, mucous membranes, and eyes. The lesions appear as red wheals or blisters, often starting on the face, in the mouth or on the lips, neck, and extremities

stomatitis: inflammation of the mouth

striae: lines or bands elevated above or depressed below surrounding tissue, or differing in color or texture

subjective data: information supplied by the patient or family

sublingual: under the tongue

superinfection: an overgrowth of bacterial or fungal microorganisms not affected by the antibiotic being administered

sympathomimetic: acting like the sympathetic nervous system

tachycardia: heart rate above 100 beats per minute

thrombocytopenia: low platelet count

thrombus: a blood clot (pl., thrombi)

tinnitus: ringing in the ears

toxicity: poisonous or harmful

trigeminy: an irregular pulse rate consisting of three beats followed by a pause before the next three beats

urticaria: hives

vasodilatation: an increase in the size of blood vessels, primarily small arteries and arterioles

vasopressor: a constriction of the blood vessels, which when widespread results in a rise in blood pressure

venous: pertaining to the veins

vertigo: a feeling of a spinning or rotation-type motion

Metric—Apothecary Equivalents and Conversions

Liquid Measurements

Metric	Approximate Apothecary Equivalents	Approximate Household Equivalents
1000 mL	32 fluid ounces (1 quart)	1 quart
500 mL	16 fluid ounces (1 pint)	1 pint
250 mL	8 fluid ounces	1 measuring cup
30 mL	1 fluid ounce	2 tablespoonfuls
15 mL	4 fluid drams	1 tablespoonful
4 or 5 mL	1 fluid dram	1 teaspoonful
1 mL*	15 or 16 minims	
0.06 mL	1 minim	1 drop

*1 milliliter (mL) is the approximate equivalent of 1 cubic centimeter (cc).

Weights

Metric	Approximate Apothecary Equivalents
30 g	1 ounce
15 g	4 drams
4 g	60 grams (1 dram)
1 g	15 or 16 grains
300 mg	5 grains
60 mg	1 grain
30 mg	$\frac{1}{2}$ grain
10 mg	$\frac{1}{6}$ grain
6 mg	$\frac{1}{10}$ grain
1 mg	$\frac{1}{60}$ grain
0.6 mg	$\frac{1}{100}$ grain
0.5 mg	$\frac{1}{120}$ grain
0.4 mg	$\frac{1}{150}$ grain
0.3 mg	$\frac{1}{200}$ grain
0.2 mg	$\frac{1}{300}$ grain
0.1 mg	$\frac{1}{600}$ grain

Other Equivalents and Conversions

Metric

1 kg = 1000 g
1 g = 1000 mg
1 mg = 0.001 g
1 g = 0.001 mg
1 liter = 1000 mL

Weight

1 kg = 2.2 pounds (lb)
1 lb = 453.6 g (0.454 kg)

Length

1 cm = 0.39 in
1 inch = 2.54 cm

Celsius (Centigrade) and Fahrenheit Temperatures

Celsius (Centigrade) 0	Fahrenheit 32
36.0	96.8
36.5	97.7
37.0	98.6
37.5	99.5
38.0	100.4
38.5	101.3
39.0	102.2
39.5	103.1
40.0	104.0
40.5	104.9
41.0	105.8
41.5	106.7
42.0	107.6

FAHRENHEIT

98.6°

NORMAL

CELSIUS

37°

To convert degrees F. to degrees C
    Subtract 32, then multiply by 5/9
To convert degrees C. to degrees F
    Multiply by 9/5, then add 32

Comparative Scales of Measures, Weights, and Temperatures

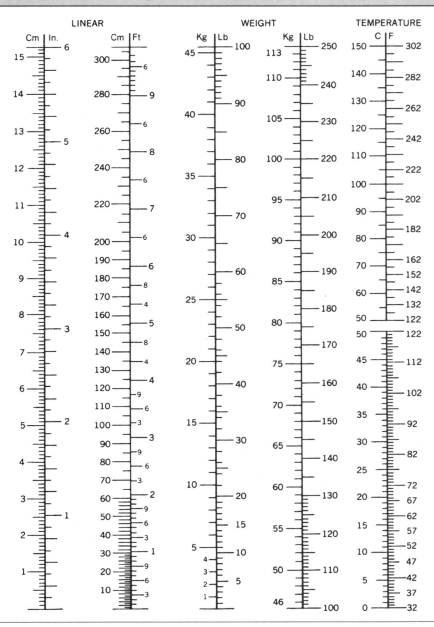

LINEAR   WEIGHT   TEMPERATURE

*2.5 cm = 1 inch   1 kg = 2.2 lb

Body Surface Area Nomograms

Nomogram for Estimating Body Surface Area of Infants and Young Children

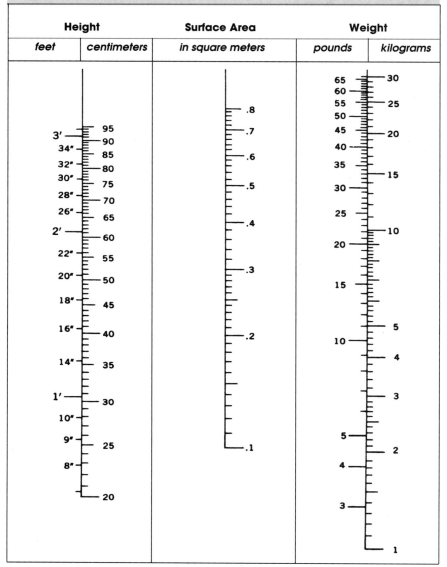

Height		Surface Area	Weight	
feet	*centimeters*	*in square meters*	*pounds*	*kilograms*

To determine the surface area of the patient, draw a straight line between the point representing his height on the left vertical scale to the point representing his weight on the right vertical scale. The point at which this line intersects the middle vertical scale represents the patient's surface area in square meters. (Courtesy of Abbott Laboratories)

Nomogram for Estimating Body Surface Area of Older Children and Adults

Height		Surface Area	Weight	
feet	*centimeters*	*in square meters*	*pounds*	*kilograms*

Height (feet / centimeters):
7′ — 220, 215
10″ — 210
8″ — 205
6″ — 200
4″ — 195
2″ — 190
6′ — 185, 180
10″ — 175
8″ — 170
6″ —
4″ — 165
2″ — 160
5′ — 155, 150
10″ — 145
8″ — 140
6″ — 135
4″ — 130
2″ — 125
4′ — 120
10″ — 115
8″ — 110
6″ — 105
4″ — 100
2″ — 95
3′ — 90
10″ — 85
8″ — 80
6′ — 75

Surface Area (in square meters):
3.00, 2.90, 2.80, 2.70, 2.60, 2.50, 2.40, 2.30, 2.20, 2.10, 2.00, 1.95, 1.90, 1.85, 1.80, 1.75, 1.70, 1.65, 1.60, 1.55, 1.50, 1.45, 1.40, 1.35, 1.30, 1.25, 1.20, 1.15, 1.10, 1.05, 1.00, .95, .90, .85, .80, .75, .70, .65, .60

Weight (pounds / kilograms):
440 — 200
420 — 190
400 — 180
380 — 170
360 — 160
340 — 150
320 — 140
300, 290 — 130
280, 270 — 120
260, 250, 240 — 110
230, 220 — 100
210 — 95
200 — 90
190 — 85
180 — 80
170 — 75
160 — 70
150 —
140 — 65
130 — 60
120 — 55
110 — 50
100 — 45
90 — 40
80 — 35
70 — 30
60 — 25
50 —
20

(Courtesy of Abbott Laboratories)

Index

Drugs are indexed under their generic names. Page numbers followed by f indicate illustrations; t following a page number indicates tabular material.

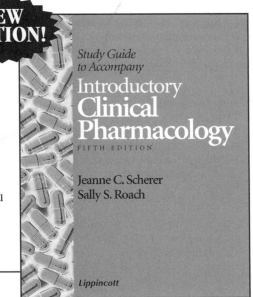
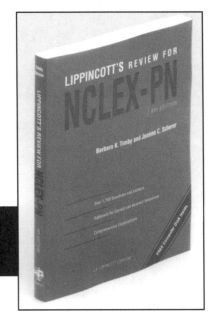
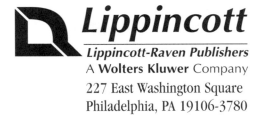

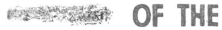
DATE DUE	
OCT 2 8 2001	
DEC 1 3 2002	
APR 2 3 2006	